PSYCHOSOMATIC MEDICINE

The Clinical Application of Psychopathology
To General Medical Problems

EDWARD WEISS, M. D.

Professor of Clinical Medicine,
Temple University Medical School, Philadelphia

O. SPURGEON ENGLISH, M. D.

Professor of Psychiatry,
Temple University Medical School, Philadelphia

SECOND EDITION

PHILADELPHIA AND LONDON

W. B. SAUNDERS COMPANY

Spanish edition: Medicina Psicosomatica
Lopez and Etchegoyan, S.R.L., 1949

Portuguese edition: Medicina Psicossomatica
Editora Guanabara, 1946

MADE IN U. S. A.

PRESS OF

W. B. SAUNDERS COMPANY

PHILADELPHIA

"For this is the great error of our day. . .
that physicians separate the soul from the body."

PLATO

PREFACE TO SECOND EDITION

Since the publication of the first edition of this book the psychosomatic concept has been widely accepted. The experience of military medicine was largely responsible. Physicians who served in the military forces returned to civilian practice with a healthy respect for the psyche as a factor in producing illness and a genuine desire to learn more about the subject. Our book has been revised with these points in mind. We have tried to introduce the lessons learned from military medicine and have also included many new studies on the relationship between the emotions and physiological disturbances.

The chapters have been rearranged so that the material of a general nature makes up Part I while the applications to special problems occur in Part II. Much has been rewritten and considerable new clinical material has been added. In particular there is a new chapter on psychosomatic diagnosis which includes advances in psychological testing that have been applied in psychosomatic diagnosis and prognosis. Material on social work in relation to psychosomatic medicine; on orthopedic and physical medicine; and, where necessary, new illustrative case material, has been added. New charts and tables summarizing diagnostic points and treatment suggestions are included.

Even more strongly than before, we believe that the psychosomatic concept has an important contribution to make, especially in relation to chronic illness and disease which remain the greatest challenge to medical science.

We continue to be indebted to our colleagues for their assistance. Dr. Morris Kleinbart and Dr. H. Keith Fischer have been unfailingly helpful. Dr. William H. Perloff advised us regarding the chapters on endocrinology. Dr. Leon Saul very generously made his material available to us. Dr. W. C. Menninger, director of the neuropsychiatric consultants division of the Surgeon General's office during World War II, was very kind in obtaining statistical material regarding psychosomatic problems in the army. Mr. George L. Cantzlaar gave us valuable editorial assistance.

EDWARD WEISS
O. SPURGEON ENGLISH

PREFACE TO THE FIRST EDITION

Understanding illness and treating sick people consists of something more than a knowledge of disease. This the senior author learned quite forcibly some twenty years ago shortly after he had entered clinical medicine through the doors of pathology. At that time he was consulted by a young woman whose headaches were of obscure origin. With pathological knowledge and scientific zeal, he vigorously proceeded to investigate, by means of physical examination and laboratory studies, her various organs and tissues. In the course of the "complete investigation" lumbar puncture was done. Following this she became worse than ever; she developed even more severe headaches, pain in her back, and various intestinal disturbances. She remained bedridden for nine months. During this period still more physical investigations were made. While the diagnosis, despite all these efforts, puzzled him at that time, the fact that the family continued to employ him remains a mystery to this day. At long last, however, the family's patience was exhausted and they decided to dispense with such services. They then asked an old physician, who had looked after the patient during her childhood, to take care of her. He knew what the young "scientist" had not attempted to discover: that the patient's only brother, to whom she was closely attached and who acted in the capacity of head of the family, was interested in a young woman whom he would probably marry. The patient's illness was her infantile way of expressing disapproval of her brother's marriage and, when the meaning of the illness was made clear to her, she promptly recovered.

It was a valuable lesson for the young doctor. It brought the realization that his training in medical school and hospital, supplemented by a study of diseased organs and tissues, had not fitted him for the practice of medicine. He has been trying to remedy that deficiency since, and in the course of that re-education he has been fortunate enough to associate himself with the psychiatrist-author of this book.

He has discovered that cases similar to the above are by no means the exception in the practice of medicine. On the contrary, many authorities agree that they constitute about a third of all cases, and that still another third of all patients have emotional factors which complicate and add to the burden of their physical disease. These are the problems dealt with in this book.

For many years the authors have been working together on clinical problems and teaching at the Temple University Medical School. A particular part of that teaching has been known as a "psychosomatic conference," a teaching exercise for senior medical students. It consists of the presentation of patients from the general medical wards, who have been studied psychologically as well as medically. The idea and the case material for this book grew out of those conferences. We are indebted to Dr. C. L. Brown, Professor of Medicine, for his encouragement and support of that teaching and for his kind permission to use the clinical material.

In January, 1939, a new periodical appeared under the title of Psychosomatic Medicine. Commenting upon this publication, an editorial in the "Journal of the American Medical Association" paid tribute to the dynamic psychology of Sigmund Freud in its fundamental application to this new synthesis in medicine. No work on psychosomatic medicine could have been attempted without the biologically oriented psychology of Freud. Following his discoveries, Ferenczi, Abraham, Jones, Jelliffe, and more recently, Felix Deutsch, Wittkower, Menninger, Alexander and his associates at the Chicago Institute of Psychoanalysis, and Flanders Dunbar and her associates at the Presbyterian Hospital in New York, by their important researches, have added materially to our knowledge of this subject. In 1935 Dunbar, in addition to her valuable studies, collected the widely scattered literature in this field in what must have been a tremendous task, and published it under the title "Emotions and Bodily Changes."

The epochal discoveries of Freud, the researches mentioned and the compilation of literature by Dunbar, made the present work possible. Accordingly we have borrowed freely from these sources, as well as from numerous other contributors, to whom references will be made.

With this latest development in research, all medicine tends to become psychosomatic medicine. We believe, therefore, that future textbooks of medicine will have to embody this approach.

Few illustrations such as are found in the usual medical book could be used in the present work. In dealing with the emotional life the only picture which can be reproduced is a verbal one in the form of an illustrative case. This requires more time from the reader than it takes to glance at a photograph, but we feel sure that he will be rewarded for his effort by a better understanding of the psychic forces that produce illness.

The book is constructed so that the busy practitioner can read the first seven chapters and get a general idea of the subject. If he is encouraged to read more we will consider our work well done. For the specialist we recommend that he do the same basic reading and, in addition, the section devoted to his subject. For the reader whose interest runs deeper, we suggest the liberal use of the index, which has been fashioned so that the material on a given subject is indicated from the standpoint of general discussion and as it applies to specific cases.

We are indebted to many of our colleagues for their support in this undertaking and wish especially to express our gratitude to Dr. Paul Sloane, Dr. Morris Brody and Dr. Hugo Roesler for their studies and notes on special cases, and to the many other consultants whose advice had to be sought in the psychosomatic approach to medical problems.

EDWARD WEISS
O. SPURGEON ENGLISH

CONTENTS

PART I

GENERAL ASPECTS OF PSYCHOSOMATIC MEDICINE

CHAPTER I

PSYCHOSOMATIC MEDICINE

CHAPTER II

PERSONALITY DEVELOPMENT AND PSYCHOPATHOLOGY

Chapter III

Psychosomatic Diagnosis

CHAPTER IV

TREATMENT—GENERAL PRINCIPLES OF PSYCHOTHERAPY

CHAPTER V

TREATMENT—"NORMAL" PROBLEMS IN PSYCHOTHERAPY

CHAPTER VI

TREATMENT—SPECIAL PSYCHOTHERAPEUTIC PROCEDURES

Chapter VII

Training in Psychosomatic Medicine

PART II. SPECIAL APPLICATIONS TO GENERAL MEDICINE AND THE SPECIALTIES

Chapter VIII

The Cardiovascular System

CHAPTER IX

THE CARDIOVASCULAR SYSTEM—EMOTIONAL FACTORS IN ORGANIC
HEART DISEASE

CHAPTER X

THE CARDIOVASCULAR SYSTEM—ESSENTIAL HYPERTENSION

CHAPTER XI

THE GASTROINTESTINAL SYSTEM

CHAPTER XII

THE GASTROINTESTINAL SYSTEM (*Continued*)

CHAPTER XIII

THE GASTROINTESTINAL SYSTEM (*Concluded*)

Chapter XIV

Endocrine System and Metabolism

Chapter XV

Endocrine System and Metabolism (Continued)

Chapter XVII

The Genito-Urinary System and the Sexual Function

CHAPTER XVIII

THE GENITO-URINARY SYSTEM AND THE SEXUAL FUNCTION (*Concluded*)

Chapter XIX

The Respiratory System

Chapter XX

The Respiratory System (*Concluded*)

Chapter XXI

The Central Nervous System

Chapter XXIV

Dentistry, Arthritis and Orthopedic Problems

Part One

GENERAL ASPECTS OF PSYCHOSOMATIC MEDICINE

Chapter I

PSYCHOSOMATIC MEDICINE

Psychosomatic is a relatively new term but it describes an approach to medicine as old as the art of healing itself. It is not a specialty but rather a point of view which applies to all aspects of medicine and surgery. It does not mean to study the soma less; it only means to study the psyche more. It is reaffirmation of the ancient principle that the mind and the body are one, that they function as interactive and interdependent organs—a principle which has always guided the intelligent general practitioner. As a science psychosomatic medicine aims at discovering the precise nature of the relationship of the emotions and bodily function. Research in the subject is founded on the confluence of modern physiological investigation, as developed by laboratory science and animal experimentation and by the discoveries of psychoanalysis, both representing dynamic outgrowths of medicine. These modern streams of thought and investigation are in the process of integration and the combination gives promise of establishing real progress in medicine. The whole subject has been given a great impetus as a result of World War II. Indeed it may be said that psychiatry was established on a firm scientific basis in World War I and has seen a substantial integration into general medicine in World War II. This, then, is psychosomatic medicine. When the integration is complete we may not have to use the term, for good medicine will be psychosomatic.

Physicians have always known that the *emotional life* had something to do with illness, but the structural concepts introduced by Virchow led to the separation of illness from the psyche of man and a consideration of disease as only a disorder of organs and cells. With this separation of diseases into many different ailments came the development of specialists to attend to all of these distinct diseases. With the specialists came the introduction of instruments of precision and the mechanization of medicine began. Medicine now contented itself with the study of the organism as a physiological mechanism, impressed by blood chemistry, electrocardiography, and other methods of investigation, but unimpressed by and, indeed, often holding in contempt the psychological background of the patient, which was not considered so scientific as the results of laboratory studies. This period may, in truth, be referred to as the "machine age in medicine." It is not to be denied that remarkable developments have occurred during this period of laboratory ascendancy,

3

but it also must be admitted that the emotional side of illness has been almost entirely neglected.

PSYCHOSOMATIC PROBLEMS IN THE PRACTICE OF MEDICINE

Between the small number of obviously psychotic persons whom a physician sees and the larger number of patients who are sick solely because of physical disease are a vast number of sick people who are not "out of their minds" and yet who do not have any definite bodily disease to account for their illness. Psychosomatic medicine is chiefly concerned with them (Group I). It is reliably estimated that about a third of the patients who consult a physician fall into this group. These are the so-called purely "functional" problems of medical practice.

Approximately another third of the patients who consult a physician have symptoms that are in part dependent upon emotional factors, even though organic findings are present (Group II). This second group is even more important than the first from the standpoint of diagnosis and treatment. These psychosomatic problems are often very complicated and, because serious organic disease may be present, the psychic factor is capable of doing more damage than in the first group. This phase of the subject will be referred to especially in the discussion of organic heart disease.

Group III comprises a group of disorders generally considered wholly within the realm of "physical disease," which have to do with the vegetative nervous system, such as migraine, asthma, and essential hypertension. Psychosomatic medicine is much interested in these disorders because it believes that the psychic factor may be of great importance in their etiology and, even more importantly, in their management.

Here we touch upon a fourth problem, in which studies are just beginning to be made, that is, the possible relationship of psychological disturbances to structural alteration. The viewpoint of disease bequeathed to us from the nineteenth century could be indicated in the following formula:

Cellular disease→Structural alteration→Physiological (or functional) disturbance.

In the twentieth century this formula underwent alteration in some situations. For example, in essential hypertension and vascular disease the formula was altered to read:

Functional disturbance→Cellular disease→Structural alteration.

We are still in the dark as to what may precede the functional disturbance, as in the example just cited of essential hypertension and the resulting vascular disease. It seems probable that future investigations will permit us to say that it is possible for a psychological disturbance to antedate the functional alteration. Then the formula would read:

Psychological disturbance—▶Functional impairment—▶Cellular disease—▶Structural alteration.

With the last problem, however, this book is not greatly concerned. We restrict ourselves, for the most part, to known psychosomatic relationships; in other words, we discuss *clinical problems* for which there are immediate, practical applications.

THE PRESENT MANAGEMENT OF PSYCHOSOMATIC PROBLEMS

The Illness Is "Functional"

How does modern medicine handle the above groups of patients? When we review our present management we find that the patients in Group I are commonly told that no organic disease is present and that the whole thing is "functional." They are often dismissed without further care, only to land eventually in the hands of some irregular practitioner or quack healer. Certainly in dealing with many of these patients it is necessary to do more than assure the patient of the absence of physical disease. Nor does it do to dismiss a patient with the statement that his illness is functional.

To the physician this term usually means "psychogenic," although he does not always admit it, even to himself. To the patient the term may mean anything from obscure illness of physical origin to "imagination" depending on the attitude and manner of the physician. Certainly if the physician is not clear in his own mind as to the nature of these problems he cannot give a satisfactory explanation to his patient. Slapping the patient on the back, with the statement, "It's all in your mind; forget it" is surely to be resented. The patient either says or thinks "You mean I'm going crazy?"—a thought which already may be disturbing him greatly—or he suspects that the doctor is suggesting that the trouble is "imaginary," which is resented more than anything else, and justifiably so. We will discuss the problem again but here it may be stated that once we are straight as to the nature of the problem and know that the emotions are involved, we must tell the patient so in terms which he can understand. There will be more respect for the psyche as a force producing illness when we deal honestly with it. Physicians take all kinds of twists and turns to avoid the use of the hated term, psychogenic. Often "neurogenic" replaces it and thus the physician is permitted to hold on to the notion that somehow there is a physical answer to the problem. We shall discuss this point shortly.

Hamman has written with a great deal of understanding on this subject: "When I was a student, the course in psychiatry consisted of lectures upon insanity and the demonstration of patients with gross disorders of thought and conduct. I had no interest in the topics and the patients distressed and disturbed me. I was greatly relieved when the course was over and never dreamed that I should find any occasion upon which to apply what I had heard and seen. I fully determined to have nothing further to do with psychiatry and unfortunately I held very obstinately to this determination. As a matter of fact, I still hold to it as regards what I then considered to be the province of psychiatry. I say that this determination was unfortunate because it prevented me from understanding what is the true domain of psychiatry, and so blinded me that it was many years before I could see the fruitful application of psychiatry to the daily problems of practice.

"In a word, the practicing physician is not at all interested in what he scornfully regards as the medicine of the madhouse and the asylum; but he is vitally interested in what we may call everyday psychiatry. At least he becomes interested in it when his interest is properly aroused by the demonstration of the importance and value of the application of psychiatry to his daily work. He must know a little about gross disorders of the mind, but only enough to see clearly that these extreme alterations are merely exaggerations of trends and reactions that he may observe in himself, in his friends, in his patients. If a physician is once persuaded to look within himself and to learn to identify unaccountable variations in mood and energy as the analogue of a manic-depressive cycle, the habit of ascribing failure and disappointment to ill luck or persecution as the promptings of paranoia, daydreams (in which satisfaction is secured for the rubs and indignities of life and retributive disaster showered upon enemies) as the harmless whisperings of schizophrenia, certain exaggerated reactions as the masks for defects and inadequacies, various somatic symptoms as excuses for retreat from difficult or unpleasant situations, he will forever after have an enduring interest in psychiatry."

Suspicion of Physical Disease

Sometimes the patient is told that the physician does not think that anything is the matter, but suspicion is cast upon some organ or system which needs watching and care. For example, the patient with symptoms referred to the heart region is told that his heart is all right. Nevertheless he is cautioned to rest, medicine is given, and each time that he visits the physician his heart is examined again, or his blood pressure is taken. It is impossible to eradicate the suspicion of organic disease under such circumstances. We will consider this point later, but here it may be emphasized that in dealing with the majority of functional problems we must examine thoroughly, satisfy ourselves as to the *absence of organic disease* and then stop examining with the firm statement, "You have no organic disease."

Pathologic Curiosities

Very frequently, following "thorough study" by means of the usual medical history, physical examination and laboratory investigation, some "pathologic curiosity"* is discovered which really has nothing to do with the illness, and the patient is then treated as though organically diseased, and is subjected to unnecessary medical or surgical treatment, which in many instances intensifies the neurotic condition.

In other words the attitude of modern medicine is not so very different toward these patients from that described in 1884 by Clifford Allbutt, the great English clinician, who said in speaking of the visceral neuroses: "A neuralgic woman seems thus to be peculiarly unfortunate. However bitter and repeated may be her visceral neuralgias, she is told either that she is hysterical or that it is all uterus. In the first place she is comparatively fortunate, for she is only slighted; in the second case she is entangled in the net of the gynecologist, who finds her uterus, like her nose, is a little on one side, or again, like that organ, is running a little, or it is as flabby as her biceps, so that the unhappy viscus is impaled upon a stem, or perched upon a prop, or is painted with carbolic acid every week in the year except during the long vacation when the gynecologist is grouse-shooting, or salmon-catching, or leading the fashion in the Upper Engadine. Her mind thus fastened to a more or less nasty mystery becomes newly apprehensive and physically introspective and the morbid chains are riveted more strongly than ever. Arraign the uterus, and you fix in the woman the arrow of hypochondria, it may be for life."

THE ORGANIC TRADITION IN MEDICINE

As a consequence of this structural and physiologic tradition in medicine a large number of physicians pride themselves upon their unwillingness to concede the absence of physical disease when dealing with an obscure illness. In discussing such a patient they are apt to say "but there must be something the matter," meaning that there must be a physical basis for the illness. And they furthermore believe that future researches along the lines of physical medicine will eventually uncover the hidden causes—infectious, allergic, endocrine, or metabolic—responsible for such obscure illnesses.

Still another group of physicians are willing to believe that psychic factors have something to do with illness but they have only a vague

* By "pathologic curiosity" is meant some congenital or acquired lesion that has no significance from the standpoint of health. Slight deviations of the nasal septum and calcified primary tuberculous lesions in the lung are examples.

notion of the part that such factors play. These physicians recognize that there is a "neurogenic factor" or a "large nervous element" present, but they look upon this feature as a secondary one and probably a consequence of the physical disorder. While freely acknowledging the relation of psychic causes to such physiologic phenomena as blushing, weeping, gooseflesh, vomiting, and diarrhea, they nevertheless find it difficult to believe that more prolonged (chronic) disturbances of a physiologic nature can possibly be psychic in origin.

They are the physicians who often remark about a patient, "but he doesn't look neurotic," perhaps imagining that such a patient should by his general apprehension or by evidences of physical nervousness betray the fact that neurosis is present. Their approach to the emotional problem is apt to consist of the question, "Are you worried about anything?" Unfortunately most neurotics do not betray their neurosis in their appearance, nor is the approach to their emotional problem so simple that the direct question, "Are you worried about anything?" will produce material of importance.

DIAGNOSTIC PROBLEMS IN PSYCHOSOMATIC MEDICINE

More specifically then, what are some of the diagnostic and therapeutic problems of psychosomatic medicine and how are they to be approached?

For example, there is the *failure to recognize neurosis* and treatment of the patient as organically diseased. This happens most frequently as already suggested, because modern clinical medicine attempts to establish the diagnosis of "functional" disease by ruling out organic disease through medical history, physical examinations and laboratory investigation. The point that we particularly wish to make is that *the diagnosis of "functional" illness must be established not simply by exclusion of organic disease, but on its own characteristics as well.* In other words neurosis has its own distinctive features to be discovered by psychosomatic study, for only in this way can serious errors in diagnosis and treatment be avoided. If the above statements are admitted, it must naturally follow that personality study is just as important in the problems of illness as laboratory investigation.

This kind of approach will do a great deal to relieve the fear of the physician that he is missing something organic because it will supply him with additional information to confirm his diagnosis of functional disease. It is perfectly true, of course, that organic disease can be overlooked and the patient treated as a neurotic, which is the reverse of the situation above mentioned. Later on we shall cite such cases. Physicians are constantly harassed by this fear of overlooking organic disease. They are of the opinion when dealing with this class of patients that the structural disease is hidden and will come to light with the passage of time. Again this may be true but in the majority of instances it is not.

A recent study from the Mayo Clinic is illuminating in this regard: Macy and Allen studied the records of 235 patients approximately six years after the diagnosis of chronic nervous exhaustion had been made, with the idea that if the clinical picture at the first examination was due to unrecognized organic disease, such organic disease should be detected by subsequent examinations over a period of years. The accuracy of the diagnosis proved to be 94 per cent, which seems to indicate that this kind of functional illness, at any rate, is not due to organic disease. It is interesting to note in passing that 289 separate operations had been performed on 200 patients of the group that they studied.

In an excellent study of psychoneurotic patients encountered in the general medical clinic of the New York Hospital, who were examined at the end of five years, Friess and Nelson found that of 269 consecutive patients only 8 per cent had been incorrectly diagnosed as psychoneurotic. They, too, called attention to the errors which can be avoided if the physician is aware that positive evidence of neurotic personality traits and neurotic behavior is essential for a diagnosis of psychoneurosis. The diagnosis should never be established, they say, solely on the basis of exclusion of organic disease, for this common practice frequently results in postponement of the correct diagnosis until such time as therapy may be of no avail. They suggest that it is far more prudent to confess ignorance of the diagnosis rather than to make a diagnosis of psychoneurosis in a patient with unexplained complaints but no evidence of neurotic personality traits. Bennett undertook a detailed analysis of 150 patients from the psychiatric department of a general hospital, who had been treated previously for "organic disease." Two hundred forty-four surgical operations had been performed upon these 150 patients, to say nothing of the many expensive laboratory investigations and unnecessary medical treatments. When the patients finally were treated by psychotherapy full recovery occurred in eighty and improvement in twenty-eight. The study once more demonstrates how an illness basically psychic is not recognized as such until it develops into a frank psychiatric syndrome.

The "Either-Or" Concept

When emotional factors are associated with actual organic disease too little attention is paid to the emotional factors. The feeling exists and the statement is made that "the physical findings are sufficient to account for the illness." In this connection let us again emphasize that just as we cannot limit ourselves simply to the exclusion of organic disease in dealing with the purely functional group, so even more importantly in the second group is there the necessity for not resting content with the finding of an organic lesion. As Barr stated in an excellent essay devoted to the responsibilities of the internist, "Recognizable organic diseases . . . do not remove the patient from the category of those who suffer adversely from emotional reactions. Indeed organic disease may exaggerate anxieties, fears and obsessions. On the other hand, freedom from disease and excellent nutrition will not necessarily bring happiness, contentment, or freedom from psychological deterioration or emotional disaster." *The day is near at hand for the final outmoding of the "either-or" concept (either functional or organic) in diagnosis and to place in its stead the idea of how much of one and how much of the other, that is, how much of the problem is emotional and how much is physical* and what is the relationship between them. This is truly the psychosomatic concept in medicine.

In a very clear consideration of the "cause" of illness, Halliday indicates the approach to this complicated problem with a simple illustration.

"Let us take," says Halliday, "a fragment of conversation which may be overheard when a toddler begins to howl in the street:

"Onlooker to mother—'Why is he crying?'

"Mother—'Oh, he cries at anything; he is just a baby.'

"Small brother—'He saw a cat and it frightened him.'

"Onlooker—'Well, he has got a fine pair of lungs anyway.'

"These remarks provide an explanation of the child's mode of behaviour in terms of the three fields of etiological discourse. In the field of the *individual* the cause is announced to be the characteristic of 'being a baby'; in the field of *environment*, the encounter with a cat; in the field of *mechanism*, the lungs in their instrumental perfection. It will be noted that if any mode of behavior is to take place, 'cause' must operate in all three fields at a particular point in time. In the example quoted, we may assume that the behaviour called 'crying' would not have appeared in the absence of (*a*) the characteristic of being a baby, or (*b*) the environmental factor of the cat, or (*c*) the mechanismic integrity of the respiratory organs."

Halliday then explains that when the findings as to cause in each of the three fields of "etiological discourse" can be related to one another, we may say that the illness is explained. Thus in diphtheria "the cause in the first field is the characteristic summarized by the phrase 'being Schick-positive'; cause in the second field is an encounter with the diphtheria bacillus; cause in the third field is the toxin produced on the fauces . . . "

When we think in terms of the psychosomatic point of view we must employ the same approach. In peptic ulcer, for example, we must think of (1) the individual: What kind of person is he? (predisposition, physical and psychological); (2) the environment: What has he met? (tobacco, food, social and psychological problems); and (3) mechanism: What happened? (vascular supply, hyperacidity, hypermotility, et cetera).

Here the psychic element is an integral part of the study, one of many and diverse etiological factors emerging at various levels of the personality development.

Functional and Organic

At this point it may not be amiss to quote further from Halliday in regard to that long-confused subject "Functional versus Organic Disease":

"Another source of obscurity is to confuse the technique of approach with the object of study. A common example is the mysterious phrase 'mind and body.' This seems to indicate that an individual is composed of two distinct and contrasted entities, a mind entity and a body entity. If the phrase has any meaning, it is this: The individual may be studied by a psychological approach and the individual may be studied by a structural or physical approach. It is our techniques or methods of investigation which are diverse and multiple, not the individual, who is a unity."

He goes on, "The words 'functional' and 'organic' suggest that illness may be divided into two distinct kinds, and much has been written on this faulty premise. For example, it has been stated that if an unorthodox healer cures a patient the illness must have been functional and, presumably, not the concern of the scientific medical man, who deals only in true or organic illness. Again, it has been stated that the word 'functional' is applicable to a morbid process which is 'reversible.'

"But what of lobar pneumonia, warts and, on occasion, even lipoma? A little consideration shows that the words organic and functional are merely examples of technical slang, which express in convenient form the following: In certain illnesses or in certain stages of these illnesses a structural technique or approach (e. g., anatomical, histological) provides a positive finding; in slang terms this illness is organic. In other illnesses the application of the structural approach yields a negative finding, whereas the application of other techniques of approach provides a positive finding; in slang terms, this illness is functional. Many writers, failing to appreciate the only meaning which can be given to these terms, seem to have imagined that by using them a fundamental etiological basis for the division of illness has been achieved."

THE NATURE OF EMOTIONAL PROBLEMS

These patients are suffering from disturbances in their emotional. lives; that is, the illness is wholly or in part of *psychological* origin and can be satisfactorily studied and treated only if this factor is adequately dealt with. It is true that the ill health may arise in a predisposed individual from long standing dissatisfactions in business, social or home life. (Why he is predisposed will be discussed in the next chapter, which deals with personality development.) Here we may state that the experiences of military psychiatry have demonstrated that everyone has his "breaking point" and that illness is determined by the impact of an upsetting event on a sensitized individual. If the environmental factor is powerful enough the staunchest personality may break down; conversely if the personality is sensitive enough, because of neurotic predisposition, a comparatively minor episode may be the precipitating factor for a psychotic, psychoneurotic, or psychosomatic illness. Failure of adjustment to environment is manifested by a disturbance in some part of the personality, either as bodily symptoms of various kinds or as affections of the spirit resulting in attacks of anxiety, obsessions, phobias, depression, and other disturbances of mood.

What is not so generally realized is that the mere discovery of the so-called dissatisfactions or unpleasant occurrences in the life situation of the individual is not a sufficient explanation nor even an adequate indication of the psychic background of the illness. In other words, besides excluding physical disease in the one case and correctly evaluating the part it plays in another, it is of the greatest importance to know *the patient's ability to adjust to certain life situations, his pattern of reacting to them, the degree of anxiety in his make-up and the nature and seriousness of his conflicts.* Psychosomatic study is necessary if we are to establish a specific relationship of the psychic situation to the personality of the individual. Just as the typhoid bacillus, specific for typhoid fever, depends upon the susceptibility of the individual, so does specificity of the psychic event depend upon personality structure of the person. To make such studies one must have some training in psychopathology. When psychopathology is given an equal place with tissue pathology in our medical curriculum and is as well taught, we will finally realize that psychotherapy is an integral part of our medical discipline.

PSYCHOSOMATIC STUDY IN ILLNESS

Can any advice be given as to how to proceed with this kind of study? Although this will be developed in a subsequent chapter, in a general way it may be stated now that, in addition to the physical study, it consists simply in getting to know the patient as a *human being* rather than as a mere medical case. Too often, as already stated, the patient is looked upon as a physiological mechanism and is studied by means of medical history and physical examination aided by "instruments of precision" and chemical tests. Tape measure and test tubes carry the erroneous notion of exactness and thoroughness—erroneous because the emotional life of the individual, which may hold the key to the solution of the problem, is not investigated or, at best, inadequately so.

While the subject will be discussed in connection with many of the cases that are to be presented, and in detail in the chapters on treatment, we state here briefly what is probably the best procedure in dealing with these patients: First, to satisfy ourselves and establish their confidence, a thorough *medical history* would be taken; this must contain more information regarding the family and social background of the patient than our present histories do. Then we should make a complete *physical examination* and such *laboratory tests* as are necessary to exclude physical disease or to establish the precise nature of the organic problem and the amount of disability which it in itself is capable of causing.

Having assured the patient that no physical disease is present in the first instance, or that it is present to a certain extent in the second group, but that *the disability is out of proportion to the disease*, it is usually easy by examples of psychic causes for such physiologic disturbances as blushing, gooseflesh, palpitation, and diarrhea to make the patient understand that *a disturbance in his emotional life may be responsible for the symptoms*. Then, important clues for this disturbance can usually be found by encouraging a discussion of problems centering around vocational, religious, marital, and parent-child relationships. This is usually best accomplished *indirectly* rather than by direct questions. Often it will help to mention a similar problem, describing a case which illustrates the emotional background. The more one can persuade such a patient to talk about "his other troubles" the sooner do we come to an understanding of "the present trouble." *The greater our success in switching the conversation from symptoms to personal affairs, the sooner do we come into possession of the real problem disturbing the patient.* We are all familiar with the patient who is preoccupied with his bowel function and wants to talk about nothing else, whose whole life really seems to surround his daily bowel movement. It is the physician's duty tactfully to switch him from a discussion of his symptoms to a discussion of his personal life. Encourage him to talk about himself as a person rather than as a medical case. In adults, domestic problems and professional and business relationships play a large part in functional illness. In young, unmarried people, family relationships, choice of a career, and often religious and sexual problems are important topics for discussion.

ORGAN LANGUAGE

A method of helping patients to understand their symptoms which we find useful is based upon the *symbolism of symptoms*. Patients are told that if they cannot find an outlet for tension of emotional origin by word or action, the body will find a means of expressing this tension through a kind of "organ language." While this is by no means a complete explanation of the mechanism responsible for disorders of emotional origin, as we shall discuss in the next chapter, it will suffice for illustrative purposes. Many clinical instances can be cited:

For example, if a patient cannot *swallow* satisfactorily and no organic cause can be found, it may mean there is something in the life situation of the patient that he "cannot swallow." *Nausea*, in the absence of organic disease, sometimes means that the patient "cannot stomach" this or that environmental factor. Frequently, a *feeling of oppression* in the chest accompanied by sighing respirations, again in the absence of organic findings, indicates that the patient has a "load on his chest" that he would like to get rid of by talking about his problems. The patient who has *lost his appetite* and as a consequence has become severely undernourished (so-called "anorexia nervosa," which in its minor manifestations is such a common problem) is very often emotionally starved just as he is physically starved. The common symptom *fatigue* is frequently due to emotional conflict which uses up so much energy that little is left for other purposes. Again emotional tension of unconscious origin frequently expresses itself as *muscle tension* giving rise to aches and pains and sometimes these are represented by sharp pains such as *atypical neuralgia*. Thus, we suggest that atypical neuralgia of the arm or face may be due to *focal conflict* as well as "focal infection." An *ache in the arm*, instead of representing the response to a focus of infection, may mean that the patient would like to strike someone but is prevented from doing so by the affection or respect that is mingled with his hostility. *Itching* for which no physical cause is found very often represents dissatisfaction with the environment which the individual takes out upon himself; martyr-like, he scratches himself instead of someone else. "All-gone" feelings in the epigastrium, "shaky legs," and even vertigo are common physical expressions of anxiety, and the *anxiety attack*, so frequently called a "heart attack," a gallbladder disturbance, hyperthyroidism, neurocirculatory asthenia and hyperinsulinism, is still far from being understood in general clinical medicine in spite of the fact that Freud described it more than forty years ago.

Many more examples could be given, but they are unnecessary because these and other similar problems will be discussed in detail among the case reports that follow. Only one more point remains before concluding this part of the discussion and that is that *the gastrointestinal tract is, above all other systems, the pathway through which emotions are often expressed in behavior.* Why this is so will become apparent in the chapter dealing with psychopathology.

This whole approach can be summed up in the following fashion: *If symptoms exist without a physical basis or, if physical disease fails to explain the symptoms completely, look for their meaning from the standpoint of behavior.* Such an approach can be applied to a wide variety of symptoms and can be utilized very generally in talking with patients. Nor does it require a very high degree of intelligence on the part of the patient to follow this simple explanation. Patients in the clinic as well as those in private care can be dealt with in this fashion and, as the material in this book will abundantly illustrate, they are just as susceptible to these psychosomatic disorders.

SEXUAL FACTORS

This again is a subject that will be treated in more detail later, but one point of importance does deserve consideration at this juncture, and that is the relation of sexuality to neuroses.

Ever since the introduction of the epoch-making studies of Freud to the problems of neurosis, medicine has misunderstood his conception of sexuality. He has often been quoted to the effect that disturbances in genital activity are the sole cause of the neuroses. This is very far from the truth. It is rather that difficulty in the sexual sphere appears as a revealing index to a neurotic personality and can be looked upon in that light. In other words, in much the same manner that urea retention serves as an index to an impending uremia, so do disturbances in the sexual life of the individual, such as varying degrees of frigidity in the female and varying degrees of impotence in the male, serve as a reliable index to the kind of personality that is very apt to develop a neurosis. Sexual difficulties are rarely in themselves the cause of the kind of the illness under consideration; when they are important and the patient has a satisfactory relationship to the physician, sufficient confidence will eventually be gained to permit discussion of these intimate matters. In women questions regarding menstruation and childbearing will often lead naturally to such a discussion.

In this connection let us suggest a cautious attitude in regard to *marital maladjustments,* which are often in the background of obscure illness. The better these problems are understood from the standpoint of personality study the clearer it becomes that serious emotional maladjustment is behind the marital problem. Consequently, casually to give advice regarding marriage and childbearing, divorce and extramarital relationships as short cuts to involved emotional problems is to assume knowledge beyond present human understanding.

PSYCHOTHERAPY

And now to come to one of the questions frequently raised by physicians regarding these matters, "Suppose you *do* find something of importance in the emotional life of a patient, some conflict that is causing illness—What good does it do the patient to know? What can you do about it?"

First of all, it is often a great help to the patient to know that the ailment is not organic in origin but is due to a disturbance in his emotional life. *When a neurotic symptom is divorced from a fear of organic disease—cancer, for example—it loses its force, whereupon the slogan, "carry on in spite of symptoms," often helps the patient a great deal.* This is especially true if the psychological approach which we have discussed is combined with the study and the emotional background of the illness is made clear to the patient.

What Is Psychotherapy?

"What, indeed, *is* psychotherapy?" Too often it is assumed to b" something vaguely referred to as "the application of the art of medicine.e This defies analysis but seems to represent a combination of the experience and common sense of the seasoned practitioner, an intuitive knowledge of people, the cultivation of a charming bedside manner, such trifles as serving food in attractive dishes, and the generous use of reassurance. The psychological approach in medicine, essential for psychotherapy, consists of something more. It is a *medical discipline* to an equal degree with internal medicine itself. It is an effort to understand the personality structure of patients, the mental mechanisms which are at work, and the specific relationships of psychological situations in the precipitation of the illness. We try to utilize this knowledge to promote the patient's emotional development so that no longer does he have to find the answer to his problems through illness. Thus, instead of treating symptoms we try to improve the patient's emotional adjustment in order that his symptoms will no longer be necessary to him. What the physician, nurse, and social worker may mean to the patient in terms of emotional significance is an integral part of this procedure to which we shall later devote some attention.

Reassurance, in the majority of instances, unless combined with an analysis of the illness from the standpoint of the behavior, gives only temporary help and, depending upon the degree of anxiety, has to be constantly repeated, like a dose of digitalis in a failing heart. Closely allied to reassurance is another superficial treatment which rarely results in more than temporary help, *i. e., environmental manipulation* without any attempt to give the patient insight into his conflicts.

Real psychotherapy, which is directly the opposite of simple reassurance, tries to make the patient understand the meaning of his symptoms and the nature of his conflicts. It is a re-educational process and when properly done leads to sufficient emotional development so that the necessity for symptom-formation is abolished. It may be defined as a process which utilizes psychodynamic principles to bring about emotional growth, thus permitting greater development of the individual's capacities and better social adjustment.

The best example of psychotherapy is psychoanalysis, but for various reasons this method cannot be applied directly to the majority of patients. Nevertheless, psychoanalytic insight and guidance in management combined with re-education and reassurance prove adequate to handle the emotional factor in the majority of psychosomatic disturbances. Between simple reassurance at one end of the scale and adequate psychoanalysis at the other, there are all degrees of psychotherapy which can be applied depending upon the degree of illness and the circumstances of the patient.

It is our hope that every physician will be trained in psychological medicine so that he may be able to understand and manage the many emotional problems that are presented to him daily. Possibly some internists will wish to perfect themselves in psychosomatic medicine in the same way that others interest themselves chiefly in cardiology, gastroenterology, and other fields. Certainly better training facilities in psychiatry should be developed for interns and residents in medicine to provide them with a psychosomatic approach to medical problems. At the same time an opportunity for residents in psychiatry to have more medical training would do a great deal to break down the hitherto false alignment between psychiatry and medicine. It would provide us with capable teachers who could cooperate in giving medical students the psychosomatic point of view. Therein lies our hope for an important development in medicine. As a part of this process and essential for its development, general hospitals must establish departments of psychiatry for the observation and treatment of psychoneurotic and psychosomatic problems. The time has passed for psychiatry to lead an isolated existence; until it is brought into physical proximity with general medicine it cannot achieve final integration into the general body of medical knowledge.

Major and Minor Psychotherapy

A considerable number of patients whom we have been seeing cannot be sent to psychiatrists, nor is it even necessary. Not that there is anything reprehensible about consulting a psychiatrist—this too is a problem of education—but there are not enough psychiatrists to take care of the thousands of such patients; moreover, as we have tried to show, a great part of this work lies in the field of general medicine.

Now, many general practitioners feel themselves capable of doing minor surgery but only a few have the skill to attempt major operations. They would not permit themselves to attempt something for which they are not prepared. This is just as true of psychotherapy. The general physician must be able to treat minor ailments but he must also be able to recognize when the problem is beyond him, and in such cases refer the patient elsewhere for major psychotherapy. Such knowledge and such an approach frequently will save the patient from unnecessary, troublesome, and expensive medical or surgical treatment with a resulting further degree of invalidism. So much for some of the more obvious benefits to be obtained through the psychosomatic approach. An inescapable part of any practical introduction to psychosomatic medicine, however, is the cost of psychotherapy.

Cost of Psychotherapy

What of the question of the time, effort, and expense of psychotherapy? True it is, that all of this takes time and effort, and it must be paid for, yet when we look into the time, effort, and expense consumed by many patients or by institutions taking care of these patients in the traditional medical approach, we realize that an hour or two well spent in a discussion of the life situation of such patients might have obviated a great deal of this expenditure. It is really amazing what the total expense of a great many of these needless studies amounts to, so far as the institution is concerned, and of course the same thing is true in the case of private patients. The day is close at hand when we shall regard some of these thick-chart patients, this *polyphysical approach* with the same amusement and disdain with which we now regard the polypharmacy of a bygone age in medicine.

Emotional Illness and Public Health

From the standpoint of the neglect of the psychosomatic approach, hospitals are beginning to understand that it is not only intelligent but economical to command the services of a psychiatrist in the general medical division, and the same question has applied in the past to the pensioning and disability ratings of veterans. Besides, we are aware of the great cost in terms of money and wastage of human resources in the problems of insurance and total disability. Taken together, these three problems—the unnecessary cost of private and public medical care, pension payments to veterans, and total disability benefits paid by insurance companies—constitute a staggering burden to the economy of

America. And there is one important, common denominator that applies to all of them: the unrecognized or inadequately dealt with *emotional component of illness.*

In addition to what has been said, in view of the proposals for health insurance and socialized medicine that are confronting us nowadays, the public health program faces a real need for attention to the psychic component in illness. The major weakness of all such systems has been the lack of knowledge concerning the emotional factor in illness. It is chronic illness in which the psychic component is of the greatest importance from the standpoint of diagnosis and treatment.

Admittedly the evaluation of the emotional component is a very difficult problem. It enters in such subtle ways and makes for such complications that it challenges evaluation under even the best of circumstances; when there is added, as it sometimes must be, the conscious effort to deceive, the problem is multiplied. How disabled is the patient with hypertensive vascular disease, how disabled the patient who has suffered a coronary occlusion? One personality refuses to give in to his illness, fights hard, and makes an excellent recovery; another with the seeds of passivity and dependency within him succumbs to chronic invalidism, and his unconscious desire to remain sick is nurtured by disability payments.

Understanding such problems really depends on a knowledge of psychopathology and the personality structure of the patient. Perhaps personality tests will be helpful, especially the Rorschach (described and evaluated in chapter III), an objective test which is often useful in the evaluation of the personality. Nothing, however, will take the place of a skiltull inverview for which the examining physician has been firmly grounded in both disciplines, tissue pathology and psychopathology, so that he may use both approaches simultaneously in his study of the patient. Psychotherapy can help patients, who would otherwise be anxious to obtain total disability, to understand that it would be better for them from the standpoint of their health and their character to continue to work, even part time, accepting income for which they themselves are responsible. The insurance examiner, identified with the company, is in a difficult position to make this evaluation, but the outside physician trained in the psychosomatic approach should not find it difficult to determine just what part the somatic aspect plays in the disability and how much of the condition can be attributed to emotional factors, and deal with his patient accordingly.

SUMMARY

The main point of this discussion can be stated briefly: The study and treatment of illness constitutes much more than the investigation and eradication of disease.   Yet there is nothing new or startling in this viewpoint.   We have heard a great deal in recent years about the study of the organism-as-a-whole, but for the greater part we have only been paying lip service to the concept.   We have been led to believe that the art of the physician, having to do with his common sense or intuition, as opposed to his "science," is sufficient to grasp the problems which we have been considering here.   It is not enough.   A real understanding of psychodynamics is necessary in order properly to study the emotional life in relation to ill health.   In other words, the physician must be able to define the specific mental factors producing an illness, rather than be satisfied with vague generalizations about "neurogenic background." Just as we would criticize the physician of today who would call all fevers malaria, so must we criticize the physician who hints obscurely at "nervous" factors in the background of an illness and makes no real effort to understand the psychic situation.

In his *History of Medicine* Garrison stated that the fundamental error of medieval medical science, as originally pointed out by Guy de Chauliac and later elucidated by Allbutt, was in the divorce of medicine from surgery.   He might have added that the fundamental error of modern medical science has been in the divorce of both from psychiatry.

Chapter II

PERSONALITY DEVELOPMENT AND PSYCHOPATHOLOGY*

PERSONALITY DEVELOPMENT

To understand the problems of psychosomatic medicine it is necessary to have a knowledge of psychopathology as well as of tissue pathology. Pathology of the psyche, or as some would prefer to say, pathology of the personality, develops early in life but may go unnoticed for many years. The onset is insidious and detection is not easy because our methods of measurement are still not precise and the public has not been educated to recognize the early manifestations of personality disturbance. Just as we have had campaigns to focus public attention upon the early evidences of tuberculosis, cancer, and appendicitis, so do we need further education regarding the early manifestations of psychopathology.

If one is to deal with the whole field of psychiatry he must command a very extensive knowledge of psychopathology. In this chapter, however, we shall try to limit ourselves to the psychopathology most pertinent to the problems of general medicine.

The psyche or personality is an organ which has many parts and many functions. It acts as a coordinating center to achieve such immediate physical and emotional satisfactions as are socially permissible and at the same time makes plans for those which are best reserved for the future. The parts of the personality have to work together harmoniously in order to gain the emotional rewards which maintain adequate self-esteem. A marked and prolonged fall in self-esteem may be as devastating to the functioning of the organism as a marked and prolonged reduction in the blood count. The personality must have an optimum number of sound, logical ideas well related to all environmental activities, for a *poverty of ideas* may be as disastrous as a poverty of red or white blood cells. The personality must have a sufficient quantity of good will in relation to other human beings (society) to serve as an energy reservoir in the carrying out of good ideas. A serious defect in the quantity of good will is as unfortunate as

* Although few direct references are made in this chapter, the material is derived from the fundamental contributions of Freud, his associates and students. References for the chapter and further references to the subject of psychosomatic medicine as a whole will be found at the end of the book.

a serious defect in a vital organ. During its development the personality must avoid the acquisition of too much *hate* because this pathological emotion may be as obstructive to good functioning of the person socially and economically as an accumulation of scar tissue in a heart valve would be obstructive to the normal circulation of the blood.

Psychopathology Established Early in Life

There is a greater tendency for psychopathology to begin early in personality growth than for tissue pathology to begin early in physical growth. It is not difficult to see why this should be so. At birth, with few exceptions, the structure of the body organs and organ systems is complete. Expansion in size of the structure follows but the structure is complete when extra-uterine life begins. Such is not the case with personality structure and growth. At birth the child has only the faintest rudiments of personality structure. The brain, which serves as the area of the body in which the personality gradually takes shape, is like a clean slate ready to be written upon by experience, or, viewed in a three-dimensional way, a bare plot of ground upon which an edifice will be constructed.

We must recognize that there are varying degrees of capacity in the nervous system, as well as in other systems of the body, to deal with stimuli both from within and without the organism. However, there are two points to be kept clearly in mind when trying to evaluate the importance of heredity versus environment in personality formation. First, the *constitution* is a relatively fixed and unchanging factor and therefore can usually be regarded as only of theoretical importance in the individual case. Second, constitution is in most cases a small component in personality formation when compared with the importance of the impact of *experiences* on the individual.

The system of scientific observation which has told us most about the growth of personality is psychoanalysis. The psychology of Freud is unusually well suited to be a medical psychology because it relates mental processes to biological processes. This will be discussed in greater detail later.

Anxiety

As we study the relation of these processes one to the other, the first and most important psychopathological phenomenon to be considered is anxiety. *Anxiety is a specific unpleasurable state of tension which indicates the presence of some danger to the organism.* When danger is real we speak of fear; when it is fancied, we call it anxiety (conscious or unconscious ideas of a frightening nature). One cannot be well oriented in the field of psychiatry or psychosomatic medicine without considerable knowledge of the role of anxiety in the development of illness of emotional origin. It lies at the root of all psychopathology and for that matter plays an important part in normal behavior.

There are two basic causes of anxiety: *fear of harm* and *fear of loss of love*. Later in life secondary causes of anxiety are situations which threaten to bring about either of these conditions, such as battle experience or loss of money or loss of social prestige.

The human being from birth onward has a need for optimum conditions of comfort as the growth processes advance. During the first months of life the body needs food and warmth not only because of their importance for physical growth but also for the tactile pleasure derived therefrom. The world of the infant is small and events which would seem to be of little consequence to the adult may have the greatest significance for the infant, in regard to both his immediate and his later responses. W. C. Menninger summarized the problem as follows:

"A child is born—as any quadruped—primitive, cannibalistic, asocial and uninhibited. The personality at birth is endowed with the two recognized fundamental drives of aggressiveness and erotism, perhaps more broadly described as destructive and constructive urges, as hostility and love. With growth and training the personality develops its individuality, with a conscious regulating portion which becomes the ego. The child learns to curb his instinctive infantile behavior through the training and supervision of his parents. Initially all restraint is exercised by these external powers. The child learns to control his aggression and is rewarded with love. Beginning in his early childhood, he unconsciously incorporates this control function within himself and psychologically includes this function of his parents within his own personality as his conscience.

"When the personality is mature, failure on the part of the ego to control the aggressive impulse is always accompanied by anxiety. Consequently anxiety comes to be a signal of disturbance within the personality. The impulse acts as a threat to the security of the ego, which has from experience the foreknowledge of the disapproval from the conscience. The picture becomes complicated when there is, in addition to the internal threat, an external threat in the form of danger. Psychiatrically it may or may not be rather simple to differentiate anxiety which arises because of a disturbance within the personality from the apprehension or fear which is precipitated by the external situation, for the compulsive individual may manifest anxiety without any external danger or threat. In some instances we see great apprehension or fear due entirely to external danger which superficially may resemble anxiety. Or they may be combined, as in the case of the combat soldier.

"Thus in a very oversimplified condensation of the dynamics of anxiety, we see that its origin is the unconscious aggressive impulses which threaten the ego."

The Feeding Process. The sensual pleasure derived from the feeding process is an example. The total nutritional process will leave a pleasant memory impression upon the mind if the good will and esteem of those who take care of the child are added to the feeding process. A sufficiency of food of the right kind, given at regular intervals and administered by one who loves the child, does much to lay the groundwork for a relaxed personality which regards the world as a friendly place. Thus the nutritional process, a feeling of security, and the capacity to love, are harmoniously combined.

If, on the other hand, there is insufficient food or a sudden change in the type of food or method of feeding, or if there is impatience or hostility on the part of the one who feeds the child, then the distress of hunger or of cold, or the lack of emotional warmth, permits anxiety to appear. There seems to be a blind sense (which we may be permitted to call instinct) that if such conditions continue long enough death will ensue. In the beginning, this apprehension that something threatens the integrity of the self is a reflex pattern and, as a matter of fact, much of it remains reflex throughout life. An important part of the therapeutic educational process is the effort to help the individual to understand the *source* of his anxiety and to teach him *what he must do to relieve it.* It is fundamental to our understanding of personality development to realize how much basic insecurity and resulting anxiety may occur through deprivation of food, warmth or love, or through misunderstanding of the physiological rhythms, during the early weeks and months of life, and that such difficult situations in the life of a child will produce anxiety through a definite physiological mechanism.

The Components of Anxiety. Anxiety has two elements: a *psychic* and a *somatic* (or physiological) component. The psychic component of anxiety is the sensory cortical registration of displeasure and apprehension, the instinctual awareness that something is wrong; and the somatic component is the motor response of rapid heart action, rapid or embarrassed respiration, flushing and perspiration, and even a disturbance in the function of the gastrointestinal tract. Anxiety can make its effects felt in every tissue of the body although in many cases it seems to limit its expression predominantly to those organs and tissues supplied by the autonomic nervous system.

The Unconscious. Parents unaware of the serious effects which trauma and deprivation have upon the personality of the child may permit much psychopathology in the form of anxiety to develop during the first year of life. Children are often neglected and fed carelessly as to rhythm or improperly as to the type of food; or they are weaned forcibly and without regard for the limited adaptive powers of the infant to a new experience. Depending upon the constitution of the infant such treatment is very apt to cause anxiety. Memory impressions are made and psychological reflexes are built up. These patterns are "forgotten" with the passing of time, but if numerous or highly charged with anxiety they may form the nucleus of illness later on. Very little of what happens to us is truly forgotten. Each event is registered on the brain as a memory with varying degrees of intensity and what cannot be recalled is referred to as unconscious. That part of the mental mechanism which holds these memories and their accompanying charges of emotion is called *the unconscious* (commonly referred to as the *unconscious mind*). The more pain, shame, disgust, or other painful effect that occurs during development, the more likely that *repression* will occur, and the more difficult it will be to recall the traumatic event in later life. The emotions combined with the memories and ideas accumulated during growth make the unconscious a dynamic center of psychic energy rather than a static storehouse of innocuous impressions.

Anxiety and the Gastrointestinal Tract. The digestive processes form the most important phase of the child's life during the first year. If this function has been exposed to and associated with too much strife, deprivation, or ill will, they become associated in the mind of the infant. One is "conditioned" to the other. The memories of unpleasant experiences associated with the gastrointestinal function exist in that part of the mind we call the unconscious. As the child grows older life conditions often improve but a revival of the same situation of deprivation at the hands of fate or ill will from classmates, business associates, or spouse may reactivate anxiety. Now if this anxiety and its cause are recognized and can be dealt with through escape, compromise, or through sharing the experiences and their effects with some stronger person, thus gaining reassurance and new strength, a solution is found. If the anxiety is not recognized and is not adequately discharged it finds no release and must exert its force upon the body itself. Then some organ or organ system is very apt to bear the brunt of this potent force and will function badly as a result. If during the years when the swallowing and digestive processes are of paramount importance in the life of the child there were anxiety-producing experiences, then similar experiences, later in life, are likely to reproduce symptoms of the upper gastrointestinal tract.

Efforts to Prevent Anxiety Formation. Already one thing is clear which we must emphasize in respect to preventive medicine and that is, that mothers must make an effort to prevent the formation of anxiety in the early months of life by an intelligent management of the nursing and feeding habits and this includes warmth and affection. So many modern mothers refuse to nurse their children, feeling that they have done their duty if they provide sufficient calories by means of bottle and formula. Little do they realize that the emotional satisfaction of nursing is an important safeguard against the development of emotional difficulties. Not, of course, that nursing guarantees that such difficulties will not arise, but they are less likely to occur if the infant can begin his career with adequate emotional satisfactions. Judging by the frequency of gastrointestinal symptoms of "functional" nature it can readily be understood that there must be a great deal of psychopathology taking place during this period of development.

Accumulation of Anxiety. Up to this time in our discussion we have talked of the child as being most dependent upon, indeed at the mercy of his caretakers. He is the *receiver* of good will or neglect indiscriminately, depending upon how much of each of these attitudes those around him have to offer. He can cry but his cries may be misunderstood or go unheeded. Should the latter happen and the child be left for long periods of time to cry alone, a marked sense of insecurity with correspondingly *large stores of anxiety* may be amassed, without the opportunity for relief that comes from contact with someone he trusts. Later these stored quantities of anxiety may be released by a stimulus similar to the one of childhood. Thus arises the "anxiety attack." We shall have more to say about this.

Pressure of Social Demands. As already stated, the early weeks and months of the life of the child are those in which he receives food, warmth, love, and affection. There comes a time, however, toward the end of the first year when the pressure of certain social demands is made upon our young human being. He is asked to change his pattern of voiding his excretions at will and to accept the pattern of depositing them in a specified place at a specified time. In the beginning this is by no means easy but with a repetition of the request in a friendly manner over a period of time the aim is accomplished, and no conflict is engendered. Some children have the good fortune to receive their training in these important tasks in such an environment. Let no one believe that this is not a very important time in the education of the child and the development of the personality. We glibly speak of the friendly manner necessary in carrying out this educational process. But in the weeks and months necessary for toilet training there is opportunity for many unfortunate incidents to occur. There are many mothers, nursemaids, and others who come in contact with the child, who themselves have great anxiety regarding the idea that the human being must rid himself of the waste products of metabolism. They dislike the odor, the "uncleanliness" of the untrained child, and show anxiety, anger, and disgust when the child does not learn the appointed task quickly enough. They make such an issue of rapid conformity to an established toilet routine that the child can be made most tense and apprehensive lest he displease. The mother or nurse may be so insistent upon the importance of rapid learning of sphincter control that she forgets the influence of relaxed play in a friendly environment; thus, many other aspects of the child's life also become entirely secondary to his mastery of toilet training.

The Compulsive Personality

To the unreasonable demands mentioned above there are two broad general lines of reaction—*conformity* and *rebellion*. If either departs from a reasonable norm it is difficult to say which is the more disastrous. In the child who is forced to be too compliant out of fear of punishment, temporary disapproval, or permanent loss of love, there are many possibilities for the development of psychopathology. He may become excessively docile and obedient with an inordinate urge for order and punctuality in every activity with which he is connected. He becomes anxious and tends to live too much for the approval of others or the approval of his own overstrict conscience. He may develop symptoms, such as a fear of going out socially—parties, sports events, and the like—lest he have the need to go to the toilet and either none would be available or he would be ashamed to release the stool when the opportunity came. We speak here of the bowel being "too well-trained" when, of course, we mean a personality that during childhood was made too anxious over a mishap in bowel control. This "fear of the upbringer" gradually becomes one of those memory impressions lodged in that great reservoir for registering past events—the unconscious. In later life it may manifest itself as a fear of society.

Rebellion. The other pathological direction, taken by emotions and ideas stirred up during this period of toilet training, is toward rebellion. Some children are able to resent and fight back at the parent or nurse whose demands are too great or made too unsympathetically. They react with soiling or later with enuresis, and may even insist on being incontinent during the day. They ignore requests to use the toilet or demands to keep their clothing clean. They may even smear the walls with excreta partly because children are attracted to their own excretions but partly because they resent the manner of training or the lack of love interest in the trainer and act as if to say: "I ignore your wishes. I'll have my own way. Since you treat me unkindly I'll make it unpleasant for you." It is not always easy to see why one child conforms too well while another takes the other extreme. Undoubtedly the more rebellious has been made to feel a little more secure during his early months of life so that he can better endure the displeasure of those around him over his failure to conform. Moreover, it is not to be assumed that the first reaction of apparent docility does not have its element of resentment also. But by swallowing his fear and resentment at being treated so strictly he often does more harm to his personality development than that which occurs in the more rebellious child.

Obedience. The overobedient child often turns out to be overserious, lacking in buoyancy and ease of manner, overmeticulous and disapproving of others who are not so fastidious. Having been given little love or tolerance such people are apt to be stingy both with love and material things. They tend to worship duty and do not learn to participate fully in life's pleasures. Their attention has been focused unduly upon the relatively unimportant problem of early and complete mastery of their excretions and they remain slaves to the correct management of the material details of life. They may be unable to understand or decide bigger and more human issues. Such characters are called the compulsive type of personality as opposed to the hysterical type which we shall discuss later.

We are indebted to Abraham for many valuable additions to Freud's original observations on the emotional accompaniments to feeding and excretion in the life of the young child.

Organ Language

The nonconformist or rebellious child shows his hostility to his overstrict and unfriendly upbringer by a series of "dirty tricks." He uses the bowel and bladder to express something he wants to say because he has neither the words nor the courage to do so directly. After a period of struggle with his superiors he usually ends by giving in and accepting the wishes of those who would have him control himself. But during this time an attitude and a pattern of organ function have been associated and remain stored in the unconscious mind. Later in life it may happen that when hostility is felt toward someone, or in regard to some situation, and the emotion cannot adequately express itself, it may seek expression by resorting to this old childish pattern, that is, with a return of urinary urgency or bowel frequency.

Role of Environment. If the reader up to this point has been able to project himself into the life of the young child he has had further evidence of the value of Freud's insistence on the role of the environment in the development of control of the physiological functions. Control of the physiological functions in a socially acceptable manner makes a lasting imprint upon the mind and becomes part of the mental processes. As we learn to control our bodies and their functions we build up our psychic structure. The mind is not created independently of the body but is very definitely linked with it. The function of the mind is to promote the control of ourselves and our relations to other people. When feelings and thoughts exist which cannot be expressed by word or action, they may find expression through some organ or organ system. The result is a "language of the organs" which may express itself in illness if the personality is not sufficiently developed to solve its problems through other channels. The organ which "speaks" is most likely to be the organ whose function was in the ascendancy when environmental conditions were bad and produced pain (anxiety) in the mind. But constitutional predisposition, identification with a parent, or other factors, may also determine the "choice of organ."

Much work remains to be done in respect to the choice of organ for the expression of neurosis. Very often an organ or system which is diseased quite naturally continues to engage the neurotic interest of the individual. It is obvious why this should be so. But the site of selection in the organ or system which is apparently free of disease is not so obvious. Why should it become the focal point for an organ neurosis? It has been proposed, for example, that bronchial asthma occurs in the person predisposed by heredity plus frequent or prolonged respiratory illness, such as whooping cough in early childhood, but definite proof is lacking. Explanations are offered elsewhere (Alexander) regarding the role of vector influences in certain organ systems. The gastrointestinal tract, for example, a system adapted to the physiological functions of intaking, retaining, and eliminating, may lend itself readily to the expression of similar psychological trends within the individual.

Sexuality

Having solved the problem of bowel and bladder control, the child is nearing the age of three. By this time his interest in himself and the outside world has increased. He wants to know the why and wherefore of things with an ever-expanding curiosity. Most of his questions are answered except in one sphere, that of sexuality. Grown-ups often regard this as something about which the child must not have information. When these same grown-ups are questioned as to why the child should not be enlightened they are rather vague. They say it is "dangerous" or that it "just isn't done" but when pressed for a good reason as to why it is dangerous they have difficulty finding an answer, showing that they have been blindly following tradition and not thinking about the real cause for their stand. Now it is true that young children are bewildered, excited, and often made anxious by witnessing the sexual act itself before having any facts about its meaning or before they have reached an age to appreciate its significance. And of course it repeatedly happens, especially with large families occupying small quarters, that a young child does witness the sexual act. However, there is a great difference between a sudden unwarranted exposure to the sexual act and the gradual education of the child by giving factual information about love and reproduction as the child asks for such information. No child of any age can assimilate all the information about sex at once. When such information is given gradually the knowledge is incorporated into the rest of the personality in a healthy way. Thus children learn to control that aspect of their personality just as they control other privileges.

Masturbation. Some adults feel that there are certain aspects of life against which the impressionable minds of children must always be guarded, for example, birth, sexuality, bodily injury, and death. But it must be remembered that these are all events which have to be met some day and there is a proper time to begin acquaintance with them. About as good a guide as any as to the best time for imparting this information is when the child asks to have it. If circumstances force him prematurely into contact with these events the child is likely to start his questioning at that time and if he does not we should wonder why and help him to understand the meaning of the event. Some recent experiments have shown how wise animals and children can be in choosing a correct diet for themselves. Giving them a chance to choose their own ideational diet we believe is equally safe. When their curiosity in these matters is satisfied and any necessary reassurance given, no psychopathology should arise. However, there are many homes where any interest on the part of the children in sexual matters is met with disapproval followed by threats, punishment, or misinformation. Such an attitude results only in anxiety due to fear of loss of love or to fear of physical harm. Karl Menninger states, "All psychiatric experience confirms the view that the boy who refrains from masturbation out of fear and guilt is more unstable, more subject to physical and 'nervous' breakdown, more likely to develop character disturbances than is the boy who is able to masturbate without feelings of guilt or to control such guilt feelings as masturbation arouses in him."

Threats of Injury. As the child learns about the world he wants to know where he comes from. As he inquires about the use of things in general he naturally questions the use of his genital organ. As he touches himself and finds this part of the body unusually sensitive to pleasure he has a desire to handle it more; this we call masturbation. This "playing with the self" is regarded as reprehensible by many adults and the child is told of the dire consequences supposed to follow in its wake. It is said to make one feebleminded, it "dries up the brain and causes it to run out through the spinal cord," it "weakens the lungs, the heart," it "makes one anemic, causes cancer, tuberculosis, syphilis; it causes pimples on the face and produces an effect on the posture *that anyone can detect,*" and so on!

This misinformation may remain a fairly fixed belief in the minds of some adults. It may produce or influence many symptoms because these persons feel that they have been guilty of doing a bad thing and *deserve* to be punished by heart disease, cancer, syphilis, etc. The fears instilled, or the threats of injury to the genitals or other punishment, may so impede the development of the sexual impulse as to cause impotence, frigidity, or sexual perversion. Some parents so discourage social activity in the growing child, because of its sexual implications, as to curtail seriously the sources of love, good will, prestige, and pleasure which are essential for a happy and efficient life. A strict, lonely or selfish, unhappy parent may so usurp the life activity and emotions of a child of the opposite sex as to interfere seriously with its emotional development. Because of this attachment such individuals later may have difficulty in marrying or if they do marry they cannot be happy. We shall deal with this subject more extensively among the case reports.

Masturbation a Normal Phenomenon. Masturbation is regarded by most psychiatrists, psychologists, and educators as a normal phenomenon for all ages from birth until marriage. It may occur in children less than a year old and then be present off and on until in adult life a better sexual adjustment is established. At about the age of five years there may be some increase in the tendency to masturbate. This coincides with an increase in the feeling of rivalry with the parent of the same sex. Growing out of this conflict there is an increase in the need for love in order to quell the consequent tension. If this fear of loss of love is met with added attentions and the play life is normal, no serious conflict need be engendered; nor is there any prolonging of the urge to self-gratification through masturbation which the child in his loneliness uses as a substitute gratification for love. There is also an increased tendency to masturbation at the time of puberty due to the increased activity of the sex glands and to the closer contact with the opposite sex which occurs at this age.

Anxiety Attacks Due to Sexual Influences. Because of these life situations anxiety attacks are a little more prone to occur at these times than at other periods of life. The attacks may occur either during the day in their characteristic form or at night as frightening dreams or nightmares. The dream picture often takes the form of pursuing men or animals or of falling from heights or of being in some other dangerous situation. Thus the dream usually represents in disguise some sexual or aggressive act or a punishment for the same. The accompanying sexual tension or the hallucinated threat of punishment calls forth larger quantities of anxiety than can be coped with by the psychic apparatus and there is an overflow through the autonomic nervous system to involve organs under its control. Palpitation of the heart, sweating, respiratory embarrassment, and even gastrointestinal and urinary symptoms may be present. If the anxiety attack occurs at night it is often followed by a period of weakness and insomnia. If it occurs during the day the same psychic stimuli, as seen in the dream, are at work although there is, of course, no conscious knowledge of the sequence of events.

Formation of a Phobia

Anxiety attacks are followed by weakness and fatigue and, if they occur frequently enough over a long period, they may result in an avoidance of the place or situation which activates the anxiety. The place or situation may be any group of people—a theater, a closed room, an open place, a subway—and the impulse to avoid these places is called a *phobia*.

Other Manifestations of Anxiety

Instead of occurring in attacks anxiety may show itself in other ways. Children may be jealous of a younger sibling; they may be unhappy at school, they may fear to take responsibility. They cannot gracefully accept an inferior position in a game even when it is their turn. They cannot "dare to lose or fail" because they have been allowed to believe that failure is shameful. They must always be in the center of attention to be happy, or go off by themselves and enjoy the fantasy of being superior. The more normal child joins readily in games with playmates, finds a place for himself in group activity and tends to imitate and identify himself with older people whose traits and personality qualities he admires.

The Hysterical Personality

Fantasy or daydreaming is to an extent a normal phenomenon in the life of everyone. However, the more the child has been prevented from living an active, well-rounded life the more he tends to seek gratification in daydreaming. If sexual information has been withheld by those upon whom the child depends for other information he will either obtain the facts from some outside and often undesirable source, or he will make up his own theories as to the physical relations between the sexes and live them out in his mind by means of fantasies. When living out the romantic and competitive ideas is not encouraged through social contacts and games, the pleasure in daydreams grows more satisfying with the years. As these people grow older they fear that they may fail or be laughed at for trying to express themselves through sports, music, public speaking, and like the sensitive child, they continue to excel only in their imaginations. In personality formation it is important that the growing child should identify himself with older persons whom he idealizes but it is also important that he should not be made to feel that he must always measure up to their standards of behavior.

This highly imaginative person, who is very emotional and yet whose emotions are not too well in control, who is quite romantic and erotic in his fantasy life, who tends to act frequently more by impulse than by reason, is regarded as the hysterical type of personality in contrast with the compulsive type alluded to earlier in this chapter. Such people love and hate in a more plastic and volatile way but for this very reason can be helped more quickly by psychotherapy. They can bring more feeling into personal contacts and if they have confidence in their physician they are able to adopt new ideas more rapidly and are more willing and better able to see a new point of view about living or about symptoms than the compulsive type of personality.

The Normal Personality

The abnormal personality is only a deviation from the normal or, perhaps better referred to as "the average personality." There are no set standards for personality. There are wide variations in the kind of personality which will make a successful social adaptation. However, for our purposes we should attempt some standard even though it is crude. Edward Glover of London has defined the normal personality as being (1) *free of symptoms*, (2) *unhampered by mental conflict*, (3) *having a satisfactory working capacity* and (4) *being able to love someone other than himself.*

As to the first criterion of the normal personality we have already referred to the way in which symptoms may register a complaint or act out an attitude by means of "body language." In the presence of anxiety the eye may refuse to see unpleasant sights or the ear to hear unpleasant words. The stomach may become "sick" because of an unsatisfactory life situation, or the same situation may cause a headache or a pain in the neck. Symptoms may be regarded as an evidence of physical disease by the family and the physician too, but when finally proved to be "functional" are looked upon, often with ill-concealed contempt, as the mark of an inadequate personality.

Regarding the second criterion, "unhampered by mental conflict," obviously much hangs upon the word *unhampered*. Everyone has a certain amount of mental conflict. There are always decisions to be made but the well-adjusted person makes his choices with a minimum of conflict, after weighing all factors. An example of hampering conflict is the girl who cannot make a choice of marriage between two suitors or who cannot make a choice of leaving her parents to marry some man whose work requires her residence in a distant city. She is miserably torn in her loyalties and either makes a choice and is not happy or postpones her decision until chances for marriage no longer exist. The girl unhampered by conflict makes her choice and once having made it is no longer tormented by regrets.

To have a *satisfactory working capacity* is most important in a well-adjusted personality. In the preceding paragraphs we have discussed its value to the individual as a means of livelihood, and as a source of pleasure, prestige, and a sense of usefulness.

NORMAL PERSONALITY	
EMOTIONAL FEATURES A minimum of mental conflict	BEHAVIOR Ability to reach a decision without too much stress or delay.
Satisfactory work capacity	Enjoys work. No undue fatigue. No need for frequent change. Maintains optimum efficiency.
Ability to love someone other than self	Takes pleasure in social relationships, marital relationships, parental relationships. Understands the emotional needs and point of view of others and makes appropriate response.
PHYSICAL STATUS Absence of symptoms (of neurotic origin)	

Capacity for Love

The capacity to love someone other than oneself is an important consideration not yet adequately discussed. The child in the beginning is entirely selfish. His needs are many and great and he is concerned only in having them satisfied. He learns that this involves interest in him and some sacrifice on the part of someone else. If the child gets a satisfactory amount of food, care, good will, and pleasure and is gradually taught that these things must be shared with others, he should learn how to love other people. In other words, he must learn by example more than by direct instruction that others' needs, as well as his own, have to be considered in order to have a happy home, and of course beyond the home, a contented community. He learns that selfishness to some degree must be relinquished for altruism and that this is not a stupid rule of life but that there are compensations for accepting it. The person who has the capacity to love is usually loved in return. The capacity to extend good will and consideration into every aspect of life, familial, social, marital, sexual, and parental, has a marked constructive effect upon the person who extends such feelings as well as upon the person who receives them, and thus brings pleasure to both.

Many children have had too little love given to them. They have tried to trust their parents but have been disappointed, and for this reason become afraid or unwilling to love. In adolescence they are fearful of expressing positive feelings lest they be repulsed or laughed at or regarded as sexually wicked. By the time they are young adults they have little or no desire to marry. They know or care very little for the things that must be shared in marriage or in any other relationship. They are interested only in *receiving* love and favors. They make poor members of a work organization and poor marital partners. They have no love or interest for children and if they become parents they nag, reproach, and quarrel with their children instead of enjoying them. The kind of personality that has little capacity for love does great harm to others even though there may be a fair degree of efficiency in that personality. Needless to say the person who cannot love has some disturbance in his ability either to give or to receive sexual pleasure.

Adolescence

As we have discussed the different phases of the development of the personality we have emphasized what has to be *given to* the child at various ages in the way of love, affection, patience, tolerance, warmth, information, and good ideas, which he gradually integrates according to the patterns he feels and sees around him. We must emphasize this statement. So many intelligent but neurotic parents bring their children up according to the directions outlined in manuals of psychology only to rear a child with a behavior problem which later becomes a neurotic illness. On the contrary many well-adjusted couples who love each other and love their children never see the inside of a book on child-raising and are rewarded with emotionally stable offspring. The point, of course, is that *the atmosphere of the home which the child absorbs is ever so much more important than any psychological precepts which his parents obtain from books.*

Preparation for Adult Life. Positive feelings and intelligent handling must, of course, continue during adolescence but here in most cases we reach the end of the state of dependency. Adolescence offers the last chance to play and at the same time the first chance to prepare seriously for the responsibilities of adult existence. In the years from fourteen to twenty much important work must be done in choosing and preparing for a vocation. At the same time much needs to be done in learning to play, to relax, and to adopt hobbies. Work alone is rarely the only goal which humans can follow exclusively and there are some good reasons why this should be so even though it may be possible for a few individuals to devote themselves entirely to work and remain emotionally healthy. First, work should not be regarded as a curse, a burden laid upon man without participation in which he should be ashamed to eat or have shelter. Work should be pictured to the growing child as something honorable and dignified, an important field for gaining a sense of usefulness and prestige, and therefore a source of pleasure as a means of livelihood.

Attitude toward Work. If the young child is praised and rewarded for the little duties of childhood, if interest is shown in his school and other work activities, and the necessity of productive activity is pointed out, he should never develop a work problem. There are, of course, pathological attitudes toward work. We are not trying to be amusing when we say that some people have no interest in work whatever. They have been given everything they wanted without any effort having been demanded of them in return, and consequently they do not feel that they need ever make any effort. Others have been given too little in the way of love and interest. They have been urged to work from an early age without reward, praise, or unselfish interest from their elders until they grow "sick of it." Possibly other younger people were at play while they toiled, and a sense of bitterness crept into their minds. In some cases early entry into the responsibility for support of the family is necessary but we are speaking of cases in which children have been forced to work because the parent felt that it would make for a sterling character. The result has been a bitter and resentful person who, hating authority and dull routine, either cannot work when he is on his own responsibility or becomes grossly inefficient. Where we find one person who is lazy because of youthful overindulgence (the common reason ascribed to laziness) we will find three or four who are lazy because of premature emphasis on work at the expense of the normal recreations of youth.

Sometimes, during adolescence, not enough attention is given to the *choice of vocation*. A boy is forced to follow in his father's footsteps whether he wants to or not. Latent talents are not exploited to their fullest possibilities. Often a young person is kept at work in uncongenial surroundings or with undesirable home conditions when work in another environment would be more successful.

Recreation. We have spoken of work first because of its importance in character development. But it must be emphasized that some attention to play, social relaxation, and the cultivation of hobbies is also important. How unfortunate is the overeducated and overtrained individual whose degrees, appointments, honorary societies, and medals form an imposing list but who is too shy to speak before a group or talk to colleagues or, if he can bring himself to do so, is too tactless or boring to make friends or hold the respect of fellow workers. Even the person who is friendly but is such a fiend for work that he has never had time to enjoy his family or develop other emotional resources, is in a sad plight when ill health, loss of job or retirement overtakes him. He then becomes a burden to his family and friends as well as poor company for himself.

Social Life. To prevent such unfortunate results there must be more attention given to the social processes during adolescence. If children have been well adjusted until puberty they usually continue so through adolescence. Many parents, however, believe that the added interest which the sexes take in each other will have terrible consequences, namely sexual promiscuity and the dangers of venereal disease and pregnancy. It is remarkable how many families, in which there has been a fair degree of harmony between parents and children until puberty, are troubled by distrust and suspicion afterward. The parent seems to expect the worst rather than the best of the adolescent—a dance or party is not regarded as a pleasant occasion for the young people to learn to play together and to share each other's lives, but instead is looked upon as a meeting where free sensual indulgence and the satisfaction of all curiosity will leave these young people satiated with life at twenty-one. It is true that in some cases things are done and said which would not be done or said in the presence of the parents but the results will, in most cases, be far less unfortunate than when the youngsters are sitting at home lonely and brooding, and hating the parent because they are missing those pleasures of companionship which make life worthwhile. The constant prohibitions from social opportunities force upon many young people so much loneliness, boredom, and frustration that they really tire of life and turn away from it into a neurosis or psychosis. Prevention, in part at least, consists in the recognition that there is an important place for social and personal recreation during adolescence. Dancing, games, and sports which can be indulged in alone or with a group; the cultivation of talents for music, art, and public speaking; the pursuit of a craft, handiwork, collecting, photography, etc., tend to divert the mind and give a wholesome completeness to living in the midst of which work is not just a drudgery or the be-all and end-all of existence. A great deal of responsibility can be taken and more accomplished when work is combined with the joy of living. An optimum intake in pleasant interpersonal relationships is a pretty safe guarantee for an efficient output in work.

PSYCHOPATHOLOGY

Neurasthenia

Deviations from the normal personality are often subtle and fade into one another, but when pronounced they are classifiable. One such group frequently referred to is neurasthenia. The neurasthenic individual is one who has been deprived of love during the early years of life. He has been neglected by busy or self-centered parents. He grows up fearful and lonely. He is unhappy, morose, irritable, and depressed, and he finds difficulty in concentrating and making decisions. He makes verbal complaints against fate, and his body and its various organs add their own complaints in the form of symptoms. The outstanding symptoms are fatigue, irritability, and gastrointestinal discomforts such as anorexia, nausea, belching, fullness in the stomach, distress after meals, constipation, etc. In some cases the distress is so prolonged and the concern with the functions of the body so intense, especially with regard to the function of the gastrointestinal tract and its appendages, that the syndrome is referred to as *hypochondria*.

NEURASTHENIA

EMOTIONAL FEATURES	PHYSICAL DISABILITY
Lack of initiative and ambition	Fatigue—lack of energy
Difficulty in concentration	Headache—dizziness
Feelings of inferiority	Muscular soreness
Pessimism	Fleeting back and chest pains
Suicidal ideas	Anorexia—indigestion—heart burn
Need to be dependent (unconscious)	Flatulence—constipation—pain in the abdomen

Some impairment in the sexual function

Hysteria

Conversion Hysteria. Another psychopathological phenomenon is hysteria. People who fall into this personality group have not received such severe rejection and deprivation during the earliest years of life as the neurasthenics. Their greatest emotional problems center around their relationships to people, especially the erotic component of such relationships. During the time when the sexual tendencies are predominant in personality development environmental influences have injected shame, guilt, fear, and taboos into intimate personal relationships, especially when they are accompanied by genital erotic tensions. Such feelings are not accepted directly in consciousness and the emotion and ideas connected with them are repressed into the unconscious mind. The result is an unintended yet necessary diversion of this erotic feeling into some other part of the body where the sexual tension, mixed with pain or discomfort, becomes satisfied in an often unnatural way. This is known as the phenomenon of *conversion* and is the most simple and the most obvious kind of psychogenic symptom formation. Because of this perverted satisfaction of erotic tension there has arisen the widespread belief that the neurotic consciously *enjoys* his symptoms. A great deal of mischief in the handling of patients with illness of emotional origin has come about through this misunderstanding.

Symptom Formation. The personality characteristics of the hysterical person have already been described and we have said that although he is emotionally unstable he is able, with the minimum of help, to "pull himself together" and control his behavior or symptoms. In other words, it is easier to help an hysterical person than one with a compulsive or neurasthenic personality. Nevertheless, there are different degrees of severity of hysterical illness, some being more resistant to psychotherapy than others. When the hysterical personality must resort to symptom formation in order to attempt a solution of a mental conflict he often uses one or at most two or three organs or sites of the body to convey the "organ language," whereas the neurasthenic may have aches and pains "all over." Although we have referred to the fact that the neurotic person satisfies certain emotional tensions by his symptoms we hope it has been made clear before now that there is no conscious enjoyment of symptom formation. Neither is there any conscious desire to escape from a difficult life situation.

When symptoms of illness are *consciously* simulated to escape from some unpleasant situation the phenomenon is known as *malingering*. This is a rare phenomenon in every-day civil life. It is more often seen in prisons and in the army or navy, particularly in war time. As regards the neurotic it is true that his symptoms sometimes result in escape from trying situations but this is not known consciously by the patient. Any escape from life which comes through neurosis is dearly paid for by the neurotic in anxiety, physical discomfort, inefficiency, and the loss of prestige which results from his inability to keep up in his work and his inability to enjoy life with his fellows.

CONVERSION HYSTERIA

EMOTIONAL FEATURES	PHYSICAL DISABILITY
Emotionally unstable and capricious—ambivalent feelings clearly shown	*Motor:* Tics—convulsions—paralysis—astasia—abasia
Emotionally immature	*Sensory:* Anesthesias — paresthesias —in body or in organs of special sense
Tendency to react emotionally rather than logically	
Vivid imagination and active fantasy life	*Visceral:* Esophageal spasm—cramps —vomiting—diarrhea
Amnesia. Dual or multiple personality	*Vasomotor:* Blushing

Some impairment in the sexual function

Anxiety Hysteria. A somewhat different hysterical disorder called anxiety hysteria is distinguishable from conversion hysteria. The onset is marked by the *anxiety attack*, and these attacks increase in frequency. The symptoms are at first limited to those organs most directly under the control of the autonomic nervous system. The attack is characterized by the sudden onset of anxiety with apprehension and dread. There is a feeling of weakness, sweating, and a sensation that something terrible is about to happen. There is dyspnea, palpitation, and sometime nausea. The attacks usually last only a few minutes and subside rather quickly but may last for an hour or more. Weakness and fatigue follow. The emotional as well as the physical distress is so marked as to cause the patient to conclude that some very serious physical disability is present. Almost never does he conclude that his difficulty is emotional.

Most people prefer to think that physical distress means physical disease, and unfortunately physicians have too frequently assisted them in this belief. When a patient with an acute anxiety attack is first examined the physician notes the rapid pulse and listens to the pounding heart and all too often permits the patient to believe that the heart is diseased, that hyperthyroidism is present, or covers his unwillingness to make a diagnosis of a psychological disorder by using some such term as neurocirculatory asthenia or autonomic imbalance.

As we have said the attacks tend to grow more frequent and as time goes on anxiety manifests itself in other ways. There is enough present so that there is a constant flow to the body causing such symptoms as weakness and fatigue, aches and pains in muscles and joints, vertigo and buzzing in the ears, and all sorts of bizarre symptoms just as occur in conversion hysteria. Eye disturbances are fairly frequent with the patient complaining of a halo appearing aroung electric lights or flashes of light or a sensation of seeing through a mist or seeing the world as unreal.

Severity of the Illness. Anxiety hysteria is more distressing and in-capacitating then conversion hysteria and harder to cure. Failure to understand its significance is the starting point for a great deal of con-fusion and mismanagement with regard to chronic illness. The patient with anxiety hysteria has had more reason as a child to distrust human beings and as an adult remains *skeptical.* Hence he distrusts the value of psychotherapy, and it is not easy to keep him in treatment routine. He may appear to have confidence when comfortable but when anxious he is more likely to draw his own conclusions as to the cause of his malady than to listen to his physician. He is intellectually willing to believe that his distress is due to emotion but when uncomfortable he can't "feel" that his physician knows what he is talking about. Moreover, as previously suggested, after having had drug treatment, operations, physiotherapy, glandular therapy, and other organic approaches to his illness, it is little wonder that he remains confused and skeptical.

ANXIETY HYSTERIA

EMOTIONAL FEATURES	PHYSICAL DISABILITY
Fear—apprehension—nameless dread	Anxiety attacks
Anxiety in attacks with cardiac palpitation—or general anxiety over social acceptance	Sudden weakness
	Cardiac palpitation
Nightmares—irritability	"All gone feeling"—tension—feeling of "going to pieces"
Moodiness—depression of spirits— tendency to seclusion. Fear of losing mind—fear of fainting or failing in street—fear of dying or being victim of some disease—fear of violence to self or others. Fear of jumping from heights	"Jittery"—dizziness—visual disturbance—feeling of "tightness" in body
	Nausea—belching—vomiting
	Urinary urgency—diarrhea
	Chest pain—back pain

Some impairment in the sexual function

Obsessional and Compulsion Neurosis

The last of the neuroses to be discussed here is compulsion (obsessional) neurosis. What part constitutional predisposition plays in determining this neurosis is impossible to estimate although it is held by many to be a significant factor. However, the environment is one in which children have led lives *deprived of emotional satisfaction*. There has been too little friendliness shown to the child and too much emphasis placed upon his gaining control of himself. He is submitted to harsh discipline, beginning with the period of toilet training. He is made to feel shame and humiliation if he does not quickly master bowel and bladder control. He is criticized if he does not achieve neatness, cleanliness, punctuality, memory for details—in short, he is forced to live up to adult standards in many things at an early age. One patient, for instance, could remember that in addition to strict training in early childhood, his father, being a tennis enthusiast, began to teach him tennis at the age of six. When the boy could not manage to do as well or progress as fast as the father expected, he would be scolded and shouted at until he was so hurt he would rebel, and then his father would call him a poor sport. All through life he was urged to master skills before he was able and was reproached instead of encouraged. This led him to be most critical of and unrelenting toward others. He was impatient and intolerant of punctuality, of awkwardness, of mistakes of any kind. He had "taken over," so to speak, and "incorporated" within himself the standards of his strict parents, and as he became an adult he made this the only code of behavior for both himself and others. He would have to cut his lawn on the same day each week and could not change his schedule for any pleasure which might present itself. He did his duty on schedule and he expected others to do the same.

Displacement. Even though such character traits as those just described are carried to the extreme they may not absorb all the anxiety instilled into the personality during childhood nor will they take care of the regressed hatred which such inconsiderate treatment produces. This anxiety and hostility can become *displaced* onto the symptomatic acts or ideas such as a compulsion to return home repeatedly to see if the door is locked, if the gas is turned off, or if the fire is under control. Such persons may be compelled to wash the hands repeatedly lest they infect or poison themselves or others. They may be compelled to hide all sharp instruments lest harm come to someone. They become obsessed with such thoughts as "Is there a God?" "Is life worth living?" "What if the sun and earth crashed together?" etc. In all their symptoms one does not have to look far to see a persistence of childish doubt, defiance, hostility, and a wish to retaliate against the overstrict parents. At the same time there is anxiety about these wishes, and defenses are erected against them, until much of the personality energy is utilized in fruitless thought and activity.

Ambivalence. The double attitude of conscious friendliness, with so much unconscious hostility that has to be kept concealed, is referred to as *ambivalence*. Compulsion neurosis can be a very crippling disorder and one not easy to treat. Little tolerance has been shown to such people as children and they in turn have little tolerance for the ideas of the one who tries to help them; in fact, there is so little desire to gratify the hopes of the therapist that they often defeat their own desire to get well. Here, as in all neuroses, the symptom itself has obtained a component of satisfaction which is not readily relinquished for pleasures which are more nearly normal.

COMPULSION NEUROSES
(*Obsessional Neuroses*)

EMOTIONAL FEATURES	PHYSICAL DISABILITY
Need to dwell upon an idea or carry out an act repetitiously, accompanied by inability to concentrate on the main issues of life	Theoretically there is none, but actually the amount of anxiety present is usually sufficient to cause fatigue and gastrointestinal tract symptoms and to interfere with adequate sex function
Serious personality, little sense of humor, intolerant of human foibles	
Difficulty in identifying with others	
Doubts about sincerity of others	
Limited capacity to enjoy life	
Temper outbursts. Efforts to control behavior of others	

Some impairment in the sexual function

Mental Elation and Depression (*Manic-Depressive Personality*)

No physician practices long without having contact with the pheno-menon of mental depression, *i. e.*, depression of spirits. All victims of neuroses suffer from feelings of inferiority, lowered self-esteem, fatigue, lack of energy, and difficulty in concentrating. However, in the neuroses these symptoms are mild or fleeting compared with the same phenomena in the manic-depressive psychoses. In the latter there is a more clear-cut and definite beginning to the period of depression and the degree of incapacity is more marked. Due to lack of interest and lack of will power the patient is nearly or completely paralyzed in carrying on his usual occupation. He may sleep poorly and lose appetite, lose weight, have an extremely pessimistic attitude toward the future, and be very derogatory toward himself and his abilities. He may falsely believe that he has sinned and harmed others in so doing. All this may lead to thoughts of or even attempts at suicide. If such a state is encountered after forty, the history may reveal similar attacks that have occurred within the previous twenty years. Persons subject to attacks of depression may also have cyclic phenomena of exalted spirits, a feeling of well-being, overconfidence, and overactivity, resulting in acts displaying bad judg-ment and even delusions of grandeur.

AFFECTIVE PSYCHOSES (*Manic-depressive Psychoses*)			
MANIC PHASE Overproductivity of $\begin{cases} \text{thought} \\ \text{speech} \\ \text{action} \end{cases}$		DEPRESSED PHASE Underproductivity of $\begin{cases} \text{thought} \\ \text{speech} \\ \text{action} \end{cases}$	
Mood Change	$\begin{cases} \text{Euphoria} \\ \text{Elation} \\ \text{Exaggerated sense of} \\ \quad \text{well being} \\ \text{Irritability} \\ \text{Truculence} \end{cases}$	Mood Change	$\begin{cases} \text{Depression} \\ \text{Pessimism} \\ \text{Hopelessness} \\ \text{Feeling of inferiority} \\ \text{Irritability} \end{cases}$
Impaired judgment. Disregard of everyday values Ambivalence, with hostility and aggression clearly evident Delusions of grandeur		Lack of initiative. Inability to love Inability to understand and use everyday values in work and social relationships Hate and aggression hidden under passivity Ideas of unworthiness or delusions of having sinned or harmed others	

Suicide. The lack of emotional and ideational control character-izes either phase of this state as a *psychosis* rather than a neurosis. How-ever, a depressed patient in the early stages of development may come to the general physician complaining primarily of physical symptoms and if the physician is thinking in terms of physical disease and has a blind spot for the emotional side of the illness he may find himself treating a severe emotional illness along physical lines. A sudden suicide may shock him into a realization that he has made a serious diagnostic error. As general medical men we must learn to recognize the early signs of suicidal tendencies just as we recognize the early evidences of pulmonary tuberculosis.

Schizophrenia

Finally we come to the most serious personality disturbance of all— schizophrenia. Since over 20,000 schizophrenics are entering our mental institutions yearly, *the practicing physician is seeing many such cases in his practice during the early course of their development*. Schizophrenia is a mental illness which does not break out suddenly but has a long incubation period. In the course of development these cases pass through a stage in which physical complaints are in the foreground. Many of them come to physicians with vague or bizarre complaints during what may be called the hypochondriacal stage. A careful history which touches on the personality will often elicit delusional beliefs about the body or about some outside influence which is affecting them such as electricity, poisoned food, etc.

Failure in Adaptation. The history of these people's lives shows that they attempt adaption somewhat as follows: They are sensitive in all human relations from infancy onward. They are lacking in those early life "feeling experiences" and ideas which would enable them to draw emotional sustenance from others, be they relatives or friends. This leaves them walled off emotionally from others. They are particularly unable to accept and utilize the sexual experience for its emotional value. They fit poorly into the social scene at all ages. They do not establish close and satisfying personal relationships. They have great emotional investment in fantasy. As they come in contact with other people they are hurt or ignored and at the same time frustrate themselves by their own inadequacies. There occurs disorganization in thinking so that they cease to be logical in both thought and action. There comes to be a splitting apart of ideas and feelings appropriate to the ideas. There is gradual social and economic failure. Anxiety and conflict are settled through false beliefs and false conclusions which lead to hallucinated punishment or gratification. Because of hypochondriacal pain they may conclude that cancer is present. Because of great loneliness the schizophrenic, for example, may believe that he can talk through the air to celebrated personages. From repressed sexual desire a woman may conclude that she is sought after by rich and important admirers who wish to marry her. A progressive lack of interest in the world's activities of the patient's environment both near and remote is the rule. The extension of the conflict *beyond* somatic distress to a relatively complete loss of emotional and ideational control shows the much greater seriousness of the psychosis over neurosis.

SCHIZOPHRENIA

1. Sensitive to impersonal stimuli and in personal relations from infancy onward.
2. Lacking in the early life "feeling experiences" and ideas which would enable them to draw emotional sustenance from others.
3. Particularly unable to accept and utilize sexual experiences for their emotional value.
4. Fit poorly into social scene at all ages.
5. As growth continues they do not establish close and satisfying personal relationships.
6. Great emotional investment in fantasy.
7. Frustrate themselves as well as being easily hurt by others.
8. Disorganization in thinking.
9. Splitting apart of idea and appropriate affect.
10. Gradual social and economic failure.
11. Gradual rejection of real world.
12. Regression to childish thinking and behavior.
13. Anxiety and conflicts settled through false conclusion and belief (delusion) and through hallucinated punishment or gratification.
14. Very little spontaneous tendency or conscious desire to leave this adaptation for normal world and its values.

Paranoia

There is a special type of psychotic personality reaction called paranoia. It is characterized by a slowly developing system of false beliefs without the sufferer having passed through the outward manifestations of personality disorganization seen in most schizophrenias and manic-depressive psychoses. Much anxiety has been present in these personalities and they have been deeply hurt. Their psychosexual development has encountered many frustrations and they are thought to have pronounced unconscious homosexual conflicts. While much is unknown about the development of the paranoid personality the end result is that the sensitive spots in the psyche are healed to some extent by false conclusions about themselves or the world about them. If they have failed economically they may acquire the belief that they are fabulously rich. If they have not succeeded socially they either compensate for this by believing that they are important and sought after or project the blame onto someone else and censure that person for their failure or unhappiness. Aside from sharply localized false beliefs the personality functions are intact. In some cases the amount of feeling accompanying the belief is quite intense and, in contrast to the situation in schizophrenia (where there is little cohesion between belief and appropriate feelings to the belief), there is considerable emotion corresponding with the idea. The result may be that the one believing himself an important religious personage must deliver impassioned sermons, and the one who believes his career has been interfered with by jealous persons seeks justice and in his zeal to see justice done may take the law into his own hands and be homicidal.

PARANOIA

1. Sensitive to psychic as well as more impersonal stimuli from childhood onward but limited in emotional and ideational capacities.
2. Limited capacity to identify with others and accept and correlate other points of view.
3. Psychosexually immature with tendency toward latent homosexuality.
4. Not pliable in adaptations and hence frustrate themselves and are hurt by others.
5. Social and economic adjustment is poor and relief from painful realization of this fact has to be false belief (delusion) through mechanism of overcompensation or projection. This occurs without passing through the personality disorganization of schizophrenia or manic-depressive psychoses.

Projection. Between the fixed delusions of the true paranoiac and the average individual there are many degrees of *compensatory and projection mechanisms*. The sensitive, frustrated wife who has paranoid tendencies may feel that her husband or husband's relatives have ruined her conjugal happiness whereas the fault has been her own inability to make a good adjustment in life. The busband may feel that his lack of business success has been due to favoritism shown to his colleagues by the boss. The belief in such cases is not absolute—it varies from day to day, and when challenged the holder will admit some doubt as to the truth of his assertions—but the delusions of true paranoia are constant and unchangeable. Nevertheless, these so-called "paranoid" personalities are not easy to live with or to work with. Their friendliness will not stretch to the point of permitting insight into their "nearly false" beliefs. They lack the flexibility which is necessary for a correction of personality inadequacies. They can bring neither a sense of humor nor a sense of fairness to bear upon their shortcomings when the latter are pointed out and this makes for difficulties in their personal relationships. Much anxiety in the neurosis of a husband or wife may be stimulated by a paranoid spouse. The sense of righteousness which the paranoid person shows, combined with his cold unwillingness to try to put himself in the other fellow's place—to try to sense his feelings or see his point of view—can be quite disturbing to the husband, wife, or child dependent upon such a person for affection and understanding.

DIFFERENTIAL DIAGNOSIS

The diagrams are an effort to put in concise form for ready reference the cardinal features of the personality study of each neurosis and of the psychogenic psychoses. We would like to repeat that we are not omitting the fact that constitution and physical factors such as nutrition, vitamin deficiencies, and childhood illness, all play a role in normal and and disturbed personality development. Nevertheless, we feel that the psychological and environmental factors are important to be understood and dealt with. To neglect them is to neglect the most modifiable part of the illness. We would also like to make clear that neuroses and often psychoses rarely follow a fixed and clearly defined pattern. They overlap so much in symptomatology that differential diagnosis is sometimes difficult. However, this attempt to give the essential features of each may be helpful. Additional diagnostic problems with respect to the various neuroses are summarized in an outline prepared by Dr. Maurice Levine and published with his kind permission (see Appendix).

PSYCHOPATHOLOGY OF PSYCHOSOMATIC DISORDERS

We have tried to indicate that the psychopathology of psychosomatic disorders does not differ essentially from that of the neuroses. Freud's theory of the libido and his concept of anxiety prove just as useful in this as in the latter field. The psychopathology of psychosomatic disorders is merely an extension or a fuller utilization of what we have learned about the neuroses. It is a further application of our knowledge that disturbed emotions may disturb bodily functions, not only temporarily but permanently, so that finally even structural changes may occur.

The study of the total reaction of the organism in contrast to the study of isolated functions has received a new impetus from animal psychology. Taking their departure from the school of Pavlov, which dealt mainly with circumscribed conditioned reflexes, a vigorous group of animal experimentors in this country have succeeded in producing neurotic symptoms in animals by increasing the difficulties of certain tasks with which the animals were confronted if they were to satisfy their hunger. In these studies the investigator's interest was directed toward the behavior of the whole animal.

Such observers as Masserman, Gantt, and Liddell by their important researches have thrown interesting light on this subject. It is difficult to predict what such observations will prove in regard to human behavior and human illness but it does offer a technic for studying psychological reactions in which the factors involved are few in number and therefore lend themselves to manipulation and exact observation.

Physiological Responses to Emotions

Alexander, who has made notable contributions to this subject, develops the concept somewhat after the following fashion:

It is well known from everyday experience that emotions such as fear, anger, resentment, guilt, or embarrassment have definite physiological effects, since the classic experiments of Cannon on the physiological effects of fear, hunger, pain, and rage laid the basis for many of the psychosomatic studies of today. We are well aware that weeping, laughing, blushing, and even disturbances in bowel and bladder control occur under the influence of strong emotions. These, however, are all transitory processes occurring in the everyday life of healthy persons. Systematic psychosomatic studies have shown not only that transitory physiological changes may be caused by the emotions but that sustained emotional strain may lead to chronic disturbances of physiological functions. These in turn may be responsible for certain bodily diseases.

Alexander continues by stating that these ideas introduced a cleavage in medical thinking because the emotions as a cause of illness and disease were not so tangible as germs or allergens. Moreover, the medical man took refuge in the fact that these physiological processes did after all have to originate in the body. For example, that such an emotion as embarrassment may cause *blushing* was answered by the medical scientist thus:

"Well, blushing can be explained physiologically. The dilatation of the blood vessels in the cheek is caused by nerve impulses conducted from higher brain centers via the autonomic nervous system. What the psychologist or psychoanalyst calls embarrassment, in the last analysis, is *nothing but some physiological process in the brain*. This physiological process in the brain which is conducted through the nervous system to the blood vessels of the cheek is the only thing which merits scientific consideration."

"This response," Alexander goes on, "is correct except for the statement 'embarrassment is nothing but a process in the brain.' Embarrassment certainly is a distinct process in the brain, but at the same time it is a subjective sensation which can be described in psychological terms and which also merits scientific consideration. In fact, at the present state of our knowledge it can be described only in psychological terms. We do not know much about the nature of that assumed physiological process which takes place in the brain when a person feels embarrassment. However, embarrassment as a psychological phenomenon can be most precisely described by the person who blushes. The person can tell us— of course, only if he wants to—whether he was embarrassed because he lied, or because he was praised, or because he suddenly heard the voice of his sweetheart.

"It is obvious, therefore, that at present if we want to study scientifically the phenomenon of blushing, we do better if we examine its causes in psychological terms. We may hope that some time in the future we shall also know the concomitant physiological processes, but even then it is an open question whether we shall dispense with our psychological understanding of embarrassment. For example: One person blushes when praised by the teacher in the presence of others because in childhood he had competed with his brother for parental approval and, remembering the illicit means by which he often obtained this approval, he now feels guilty and ashamed. Could the most minute physiological description explain as much as does this psychological one? Even so common a process as blushing from embarrassment can be understood fully only in the light of the life history of the individual. The same is true for weeping or laughter. Only when we know what makes Smith so sensitive to certain human events can we understand why his eyes fill with tears over a sentimental scene in the movies, whereas Jones in the same situation remains completely composed. Only the history of Mr. Smith and Mr. Jones will explain to us how and why the one became highly sensitized to seeing an old, helpless man peering through a window at a happy family on a Christmas Eve and why the other found the same scene trite and boring. Whether the most advanced brain physiology will ever be able to substitute for this type of knowledge is certainly an open question. It is difficult to imagine that it will."

Relation to Illness

"Certain it is, however, that at the present state of our knowledge the factors which cause weeping, laughing, or blushing cannot be properly described without using both psychological and physiological methods. The innervation of the tear gland in weeping or the dilatation of the blood vessels in blushing, the conduction of the nerve influences from the brain cortex to the eyes and the cheek can only be described in physiological terms, whereas the causative emotions are definable only in psychological terms. Similarly the local processes which immediately cause the ulceration of the stomach or an asthmatic attack must be described in strictly physiological terms; the causative emotional tensions, on the other hand, must be described and understood in psychological terms. Omitting this psychological part of the whole process does not increase the scientific nature of our description. On the contrary, understanding the local mechanisms involved in the development of an ulcer or asthma is only half of the story. Omitting the other half, the part which requires at our present state of knowledge psychological descriptions, would be to give up the most important aim of medicine, the understanding of causes. An appropriate use of psychological and physiological methods of description—each in its proper place—is the essence of the psychosomatic approach."

Alexander concludes that the interrelation of biochemical changes and emotions is today beyond question. Emotional tensions through the autonomic nervous system do influence the body chemistry and the changed body chemistry in turn reacts upon the emotional life. With the clear recognition of such mutual influences the cleavage between emotional and organic factors can be relegated to the past. Body chemistry and emotions do not represent two different sets of facts, one physical, the other mental. When we speak of emotions we refer always to definite physical processes in the brain which, however, can be studied psychologically because these brain processes are perceived subjectively as emotions and can be communicated to others by the use of language. The combined biochemical and psychological approach is now only in its beginnings but will undoubtedly become the main trend of future research and therapy.

THE ADAPTATION SYNDROME

Of importance in any consideration of the role of the emotions in physiologic integrations are the studies of Selye which culminated in his description of the "Adaptation Syndrome." Selye postulates that exposure of the organism to stress (any nonspecific noxious stimulus of sufficient intensity) will cause the liberation of toxic metabolites in the tissues and the production of the first stage of the syndrome, viz., the alarm reaction. This stage is divisible into two distinct phases. The first or shock phase is characterized by tachycardia, decrease in muscle tone and body temperature, formation of gastric and intestinal ulcers, hemo-concentration, anuria, edema, hypochlorhydria, leukopenia followed by leukocytosis, acidosis, a transitory hyperglycemia followed by a decrease in blood sugar, and a discharge of epinephrine from the adrenal medulla.

Mirsky, interested in the endocrine as well as emotional aspects of the *adaptation syndrome*, summarizes Selye's studies as follows:

"If the damage is not too severe and permits survival, the toxic metabolites stimulate the anterior lobe of the pituitary to discharge adrenocorticotropic hormone which, in turn, stimulates the secretion of adrenal cortical hormones, and thereby raises the resistance of the body. This results in the second phase of the alarm reaction, viz., the counter-shock phase. This phase is characterized by an enlarged and hyperactive adrenal cortex, rapid involution of the thymus and other lymphatic organs and a reversal of most of the signs characteristic of the shock phase.

"If the noxious stimulus is continued, the counter-shock phase gives way to the second stage of the general adaptation syndrome, the stage of resistance, at which time there is a regression of most of the morphological lesions observed in the first stage; and resistance to the continued stimulus reaches a minimum. This stage is attributed to the continued secretion of cortical hormones. The third and final stage of the syndrome appears after prolonged exposure to the noxious stimuli and is called the stage of exhaustion and is attributed to a failure in the adaptive mechanisms. When this occurs, the lesions characteristic of the alarm reaction re-appear, and death ensues.

"Under special experimental conditions, exposure to non-specific noxious agents may cause hypertension, nephrosclerosis, myocardial lesions and arthritides. These Selye attributed to the excessive amounts of pituitary and adrenal cortical hormones which are produced to increase the resistance to the action of the noxious stimuli. Selye calls these the 'diseases of adaptation.' The clinical studies of Albright, of Brown and of others lend support to Selye's concept and indicate that stress situations in man also may induce the adaptation syndrome."

ORGAN NEUROSIS

As we have already indicated, conversion symptoms are symbolic substitute expressions for an unbearable emotion which the individual represses and therefore cannot express through the normal channels of voluntary behavior. In addition to this conversion mechanism Alexander describes a different type of emotionally conditioned bodily disturbance which manifests itself in the viscera and is referred to as *vegetative neurosis*.

A simple example is the elevation of blood pressure under the influence of emotion such as rage and fear. Here the elevation of blood pressure has no direct psychological meaning. It is not a symbolic expression of rage or fear; rather it is a physiological concomitant of the emotional states of rage and fear. Whereas a conversion symptom is a symbolic expression of a well-defined psychological content (an attempt at relief), a vegetative neurosis is not an attempt to express an emotion but is the normal physiological accompaniment of constant or period-ically recurring emotional states. Chronic emotional tension causes chronic vegetative changes, and it is the chronicity of the condition which makes it morbid. Alexander suggests that the clarification of this issue has both theoretical and practical significance. It saves us from erroneous and futile therapeutic attempts to "interpret" such bodily expressions psychologically. Instead the physician who correctly understands the nature of these disturbances will try to help the patient to overcome certain chronic unrelieved emotional states which have a disturbing influence upon the vegetative functions of the organism.

Specificity

According to one assumption, any emotional tension may influence any vegetative function. The choice of symptom depends upon the history of the patient and his constitution: If he has a weak stomach, he might have a stomach upset when he gets angry; if he has a labile vasomotor system, he might develop high blood pressure under the influence of unrelieved aggressions. A quite different assumption, which may be called the theory of specificity, has guided the work of Alexander and his associates. According to their view, "physiological responses vary with the *quality* of the emotional state. Just as external behavior varies according to the nature of the emotion, so responses in the nervous control of the visceral organs vary. We know from experiments with animals that every emotional state has its specific vegetative tonus. The vegetative reactions to rage and fear are different, for example, from those due to relaxation during the process of digestion. It is to be expected therefore that the vegetative disturbance will vary in correspondence with the chronic unrelieved emotional state. The question is still undecided, however, to what extent constitutional factors or preexisting organic pathology or sensitivity influence different clinical pictures. Further careful clinical studies will have to decide this important issue."

Thus in the chapter on gastrointestinal problems we shall again quote from the studies of Alexander and his associates and show that in peptic ulcer the major problem surrounds a conflict between a conscious desire for independence and success, and strong unconscious cravings of passivity and dependence.

Personality Trends

In regard to this question Saul calls attention to the fact that it is the oral form of attachment to the mother, consisting of a mixture of impulses, desires, and feelings which become interwoven with sucking and later the eating mechanisms, that enters into psychosomatic gastrointestinal problems. Other biological mechanisms and forms of attachment to the mother seem to be important in the allergies. These are the dermal and respiratory. In other words, in many persons the form of attachment to the mother as seen in fantasies, dreams, and real life is not, as in many instances of gastrointestinal disorders, strongly "oral," but consists rather in a desire for shelter. The longings are represented not by wishes to be fed and all that this can imply emotionally, but by wishes to be sheltered and protected. Such individuals often gravitate to modes of life which gratify these tendencies. Perhaps it could be said that, given a choice, they would prefer snug housing to good food. Here, too, can be points of weakness and fixation, to form a physiological pathway for the attachment to the mother and become interwoven with powerful feelings and longings.

When the relationship to the mother, with all of its significance to the child (and in later life, unconsciously, to the adult) is threatened, or when a person is under stress, the longings for help or consolation are expressed in various combinations or forms in different persons—wanting to be fed, wanting to be carried or led, wanting to be snuggled and sheltered, and so on—reflecting the oral, ambulatory, dermal, respiratory, and other mechanisms and forms of attachment to the mother. The impulses may be gratified by personal relationships, sexual or sublimated, which reestablish in some degree the relationship to the mother. Examples of sublimated forms of gratification are: oral, eating and drinking; respiratory, talking and crying; dermal, baths and massage. The impulses may be repressed so that symptoms appear when the tension disturbs organ function. Of course, oral as well as dermal and respiratory trends can exist in the same individual.

Saul concludes, "The dermal and respiratory mechanisms, trends, and relations to the mother are analogous to the oral ones. They are fundamental to an understanding of psychobiological functioning. Preliminary observations strongly suggest that they play a role in the skin and respiratory allergies similar to that of the oral trends in the gastrointestinal disorders."

THE LESSONS OF MILITARY EXPERIENCE

In a notable discussion of the lessons to be learned from World War II Gregg points out that "psychiatry changed from a specialty to a generality—so to speak—and the psychiatric or psychological component of illnesses previously considered as exclusively medical or surgical began to be recognized as never before. Such discoveries also brought into sharp focus the inadequacies of the usual medical history-taking and the painful incompetence and even the contempt that a large number of our medical officers commonly showed for psychiatry. No experience could have revealed more effectively than the war the nonsense of isolating psychiatry from the rest of medicine."

Later he refers to the fact that "the promptness, the ease, the frequency, and the value of psychiatric consultations on medical and surgical wards in military hospitals suggest that psychiatric consultations in our civilian hospitals could bring equal advantage to patients and to the doctors responsible for bringing every helpful resource to bear upon the patients' problems." Moreover, Gregg recommends "a major revision of medical education, for only a radical change will provide the opportunity for adequate training in the psychiatric care of human beings for a full and happy life as well as a symptom-free existence." Next he asks, what are the causes for the percentage of men between 18 and 35 who were disqualified by reason of some kind of disorder of personality—14 per cent of all the men examined? "Does a social structure in peacetime which shows one in seven so definitely deviant not deserve profound reflection and study? From the war experience psychiatrists learned many of the factors of successful leadership: the value of the leader's example, his awareness of the emotional needs of his men, his constant and manifest solicitude, his knowledge of individual men under him and his personal interest in them. Are industrial relations and problems of civilian leadership likely to be solved in complete disregard of these factors of leadership proved in the war?"

Incidence of Psychosomatic Reactions

W. C. Menninger, chief of the division of psychiatry for the army during World War II, comments that the war gave added emphasis to the psychosomatic point of view. "Every army physician was confronted with a far greater number of patients having physical complaints in which no organic pathology could be found, than he saw in civilian life. . . . The stresses and strains of military life contributed to the high incidence of such functional complaints as were seen in patients on both medical and psychiatric wards." He quoted from a study by the internists of eleven army general hospitals in the United States who found that about one fourth of the patients on the cardiovascular wards and one fifth of the patients on the gastrointestinal wards were suffering from functional conditions. General Menninger added that a survey made by or with a psychiatrist, who would be more cognizant of psychological factors, would have disclosed an even greater number of such cases.

On the other hand, an investigation of the incidence of physical complaints in psychoneurotic patients was reported by Norman Brill as observed in six hundred unselected cases of psychoneuroses in six army general hospitals. In two thirds of the patients some organ dysfunction was a major symptom. Of the entire group, 29 per cent had gastrointestinal reactions, 14 per cent had cardiovascular reactions, and 9 per cent had rheumatic reactions.

One third of 1,800 consecutive cases referred to mental hygiene clinics in basic training camps presented psychosomatic complaints. These were classified as follows:

Complaints	Per Cent
Asthenic	24.9
Gastrointestinal	22.6
Rheumatic	19.9
Cardiovascular	13.7
Genito-urinary	10.7
Allergies and headache	8.2

(Menninger, W. C.: Somatization Reactions as Seen in Mental Hygiene Consultation Services, Bull. U. S. Army Med. Dept., 5:640-642, June 1946)

The chief significance of these figures, says Menninger, lies in their emphasis on the emotional factors in the illness of incapacitated, hospitalized men in the military service. As the statistics indicate, functional illness was frequently found on medical or surgical wards and somatic complaints were numerous in psychiatric patients. Medical personnel in every medical specialty were brought face to face with the need for greater understanding of the physiology, anatomy, and pathology of the psyche.

"In general," he declared, "there are four body systems used most frequently for emotional expressions which repeatedly and continuously come under the scrutiny of every physician: the cardiovascular, the gastrointestinal, the allergies, and the great group of aches and pains included in the cephalalgias, arthralgias and myalgias."

We are greatly indebted to W. C. Menninger for his kindness in obtaining the following chart comparing the incidence of certain disorders in World Wars I and II. References will be made to this material in succeeding chapters.

Selected Diagnoses, U. S. Army
Net Admissions and Annual Rates Per 1,000 Strength
World War I versus World War II

Diagnosis	WORLD WAR I (APR., 1917—DEC., 1919)		WORLD WAR II* (JAN., 1942—DEC., 1945)	
	Number of Admissions	Annual Rate Per 1,000	Number of Admissions	Annual Rate Per 1,000
Diabetes mellitus.........	718	0.17	6,267[a]	0.25[a]
Neurocirculatory asthenia.	4,377	1.06	35,763	1.40
Total peptic ulcers.......	2,919	0.71	69,955[b]	2.75[b]
Peptic ulcer: stomach...	1,755	0.43	6,259[b]	0.25[b]
Peptic ulcer: duodenum.	1,164	0.28	63,696[b]	2.50[b]

* Provisional data based on preliminary tabulations.

[a] Includes diabetic coma and diabetic gangrene.

[b] Includes estimated admission figures for the year 1943. Overseas admissions for that year are based on overseas experience for the first nine months of the year. Complete tabulations not yet available.

From the Medical Statistics Division, Surgeon General's Office, U. S. Army, November 1947, through the kindness of Dr. W. C. Menninger.

THE CONCEPT OF MATURITY

We began this chapter with a consideration of emotional immaturity as the background for psychoneurotic and psychosomatic disorders. We close with an excerpt from Saul's excellent discussion of the concept of maturity.

Speaking of the war neuroses Saul states: "Neurotic breakdown is caused in the reactive cases by external stress acting upon points of specific emotional vulnerability in the individual's personality. Thus combat, isolation, discipline, loss of buddies, all affected different men differently according to their makeups and emotional vulnerabilities. In the independent or 'internal' cases, this vulnerability is so great that little or no external stress is required as a precipitant. The vulnerability is caused by defects in the emotional development. Such defects cause not only susceptibility to classical neurosis, but also all sorts of neurotic manifestations in the broad sense of emotional disturbances and immaturity of behavior.

"Prevention of these defects and of their consequences requires thorough understanding of the course of emotional development to maturity. Causal psychotherapy reopens the emotional development and enables us to see what our patients would have been if traumatic childhood influences had not hindered and warped their growth. This leads to further understanding of maturity. Its fundamental characteristics reflect the ideal attitudes of parents toward children, in contrast with childish attitudes toward siblings and parents. These characteristics in proper balance involve:

1. predominance of independence and responsibility, with little need to regress,

2. predominance of giving and productivity, although with the capacity to receive normally,

3. lack of egotism and competitiveness,

4. a well-integrated conscience which furthers development,

5. sexuality free and integrated with mating and responsible, productive activity,

6. hostility toward self and others minimal but freely available for defense and constructive use,

7. grasp of reality unimpared by persisting childhood reactions, and

8. freedom from childhood patterns of reaction and hence full capacity for discrimination and adaptability.

"Of course," continues Saul, "this is an ideal. In reality childhood feelings will always persist to some degree, since these are important components of the unconscious. But a predominance of the mature attitudes, the overcoming of untoward reactions of childhood caused by traumatic upbringing and influences, and an integration of the normal persisting infantile impulses in adult loving, work, and play, is a proper realistic and justifiable goal.

"Clarification of the concept of maturity and of the development toward it is valuable for psychiatric theory and practice. Moreover, if the above description of maturity is correct, then the man-made evils and miseries of the world are for the most part the results of faulty up-bringing of children. Psychiatry, experienced in correcting these faults and in handling immature emotional reactions, therefore has valuable knowledge to contribute to the solution of present world problems. The difference between dealing with individuals and with groups, except for the greater support and sanctions to infantile impulses in groups, is essentially only practical. Hence psychiatric experience with therapy is applicable. Palliative measures for relieving external stresses and controlling aggressive reactions are the immediate functions of government, including world government. But in the long range, the only security for the world must rest upon a predominantly mature population. What this means and how to achieve it are questions for dynamic psychiatry to answer. They comprise mankind's central problem."

SUMMARY

As has been said, all illness is a problem of disturbance of psyche and soma, hence *all medicine is psychosomatic medicine*. In fact when this is thoroughly understood there will no longer be a necessity for the term psychosomatic medicine; both parts of the term will be implicit in the word medicine. However, disease has been regarded for many decades as being due to tissue pathology alone, and it is only in recent years that psychiatry, by gaining greater knowledge of the neuroses, has shown that the first cause of certain disease pictures is psychopathology rather than tissue pathology. Therefore, psychosomatic medicine at the present time embraces the neuroses plus an extension of our knowledge of neuroses to the psychopathology of other conditions previously thought to be in the realm of purely physical medicine. In succeeding chapters attempts will be made to demonstrate not so much that a medical problem is purely functional or purely physical but that psychological and physical factors are both present and that the question becomes: How much of the one and how much of the other is present and what is the relationship between them?

NORMAL PERSONALITY		NEUROSES	PSYCHOSES
EMOTIONAL FEATURES			
Unhampered by mental conflict	Ability to reach a decision without too much stress or delay.	Hampering mental conflicts Mild mood disturbances Capacity for decision impaired	Mental conflicts Severe mood disturbances Capacity for decision impaired
Satisfactory work capacity	Enjoys work No undue fatigue No need for frequent change Maintains optimum efficiency	Work not enjoyed Fatigue a frequent and pronounced symptom Impairment of work efficiency	Severe disturbances in efficiency; concentration upon or participation in work may be totally impossible
Ability to love someone other than self	Takes pleasure in social relationships, marital retionships, parental relationships. Can understand the emotional needs and point of view of others and make appropriate response	Disturbances in ability to enjoy social relations, i.e., inability to relate themselves to others in such a way as to gain security and emotional response. Limited capacity to give emotionally yet some conventional relation to others is maintained even though imperfect and at the cost of anxiety	Severe disturbances in ability to relate themselves to others, in fact, they tend to renounce their relations to others more or less completely
PHYSICAL STATUS Absence of symptoms (of neurotic origin)		Conversion of emotional stress (anxiety) into somatic symptoms in one or many parts of body	Somatic symptom formation during onset of illness but eventually symptoms are in sphere or control of emotion, thought, speech, action
			Varying amount of loss in control of well integrated thought, emotion and speech, and regressions to childish levels— and/or solution of anxiety through false beliefs or false sensory perception

Chapter III

PSYCHOSOMATIC DIAGNOSIS

Diagnosis depends much more upon the history than it does upon physical examination or laboratory studies. This is especially true in regard to psychosomatic affections.* In the first chapter we discussed the faulty concept of functional versus organic disease and the necessity for giving up the "either-or" diagnostic approach. In other words, personality study will show that psychosomatic disorders have their own distinctive features and that diagnosis must be established by the simultaneous application of physiological and psychological technics. In other words, the diagnosis of a "psychosomatic" affection can only be established by positive data from a psychological standpoint *in addition* to an evaluation of the part that physiological and "organic" factors play.

We frequently use the diagrams on page 60 in illustrating this topic. The upper diagram illustrates the usual approach in the study of illness which will presumably lead to a diagnosis. It consists of the bare facts of the medical history, the physical examination, and the various laboratory investigations. It is *diagnosis by exclusion* and fails in so many instances simply because the life situation of the patient—in other words, a study of the emotional life—which may provide the key to the solution of the problem, is completely neglected or at most inadequately investigated. One of the purposes of this book is to help repair this deficiency. The *proper psychosomatic approach* is shown in the *lower* diagram.

When a person gets sick he is sick all over; that is, the body and mind are one, and he gets sick for a variety of reasons, physical and psychic. In other words, it is usually not one thing that determines illness; it is many things, multiple factors, acting together. As we pointed out in the first chapter, in our approach to illness we must ask ourselves

---

* The term psychosomatic as used in this book indicates a method of approach to general medical problems, that is, the simultaneous application of physiological and psychological technics to the study of illness in an effort to make a definitive diagnosis and in preparation for comprehensive medical care. We also apply the term in a more limited sense to a specific affection, indicating that the disorder is one which can be understood only when psychological as well as physiological factors are taken into consideration (Halliday).

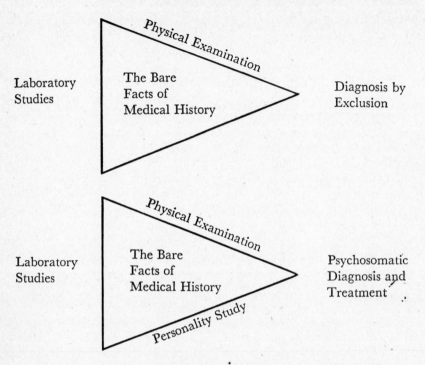

What kind of person are we dealing with? (inherited and acquired characteristics, physical and psychological)

What has he met? (germs, allergens, or emotionally disturbing events)

What has happened? (physiological mechanism or pathogenesis of the disorder)

For example, allergic responses occur when a prepared organism, possessing certain physical and psychological characteristics, meets certain elements, physiological and psychological. In some allergic disorders a single preponderant factor may be largely responsible, for example, in pollen hay fever; in others, such as asthma, frequently there are multiple interrelated factors, allergens and psychic disturbances, which act in a complementary fashion to produce the disorder.

THE PSYCHOSOMATIC POINT OF VIEW

This is the psychosomatic point of view: that the psyche enters, or better, emerges as one of the several factors, which acting together disturb the function of the organism. We will leave aside the great problem—how much of the illness depends upon constitutional factors and to what extent special life experiences are responsible. It is the old question of heredity and environment, nature and nurture, and we have no way of delimiting these factors with exact measurements.

Generally speaking, physicians look upon the problem of psychic factors in illness in several ways. There is a group which considers the physical factors as being all important and indeed wholly responsible for any personality change: "Why shouldn't he be nervous after having had such a serious disease so long?" In a smaller group one finds protagonists for *psychogenesis:* "The psychic factor is fundamental and all important in determining illness." A third group believes that physical and psychological factors are but different phases of the disordered constitution, perhaps parallel manifestations of the same basic fault, existing together and related to one another. To put it another way, psychological forces and somatic manifestations may have their roots in the same unconscious processes which discharge partly on the level of psychic representation through thoughts and feelings and partly on the physiological level through the autonomic nervous system (Kubie). This is the viewpoint which we favor, the psychosomatic viewpoint. We are not interested in proving psychogenesis, we are only interested in studying the psychic factor in illness, just as we study physical factors, and in relating them where possible. We would like the psyche to be treated with as much respect as germs or allergens.

Just as we insist on this unity regarding the nature of illness ("The body and the mind are one"), just so do we urge that the means of investigation are *two* (that is, physical and psychological) and that their simultaneous application represents psychosomatic diagnosis. And they are applied simultaneously although their application is often unconscious and unscientific. The physician in his usual approach to the patient, even when using the orthodox methods of medical history, physical examination, and laboratory studies, is at the same time making many intuitive observations about the unconscious mental processes of the patient as exhibited in his language and behavior. What we suggest is that order be brought into this intuitive process. We now have enough understanding so that we can begin to forge a scientific instrument in the exploration of unconscious processes. In other words, we are trying to establish rules of psychological exploration as exact as those of physical investigation.

Rather than be satisfied with loose terminology—"neurogenic factors," "emotional upsets," "physical and mental fatigue," "emotional stress and strain"—we must make an effort to define the specific emotional problem and relate it to the total personality make-up of the individual.

Postulates for Psychosomatic Diagnosis

Just as we try to establish a kind of "Koch's postulates" for an allergic problem, hay fever, for example:

1. heredity,
2. seasonal history,
3. skin tests,
4. antibodies,
5. induction of an attack with pollen,
6. hyposensitization or avoidance of the offending substance in controlling attacks,

so in the psychosomatic problem we try to establish:

1. a family history which suggests a background for psychological difficulties (heredity and pseudoheredity),
2. evidences for a childhood neurosis,
3. sensitivity to specific emotional factors (temporal relationship of present illness and emotionally disturbing event) especially at epochal or crucial life periods (puberty, marriage, childbirth, climacteric, etc.),
4. a specific personality structure (other evidences of neurosis or character disturbance),
5. demonstration of specific behavior on taking the history (artificial exposure to a conflict situation),
6. hyposensitization by psychotherapy or the avoidance of the provocative situation.

1. **A Family History Which Suggests a Background for Psychological Difficulties.** It is impossible to separate constitutional and hereditary factors in the development of psychosomatic disorders. What is often attributed to heredity is in fact pseudoheredity, that is, acquired as a result of environmental influences. Later in the chapter attention is paid to the various familial factors which suggest a background for psychological difficulties. How much of this is transmitted through the germ plasm and how much may be acquired by "social contagion" is difficult to say. Unconscious identification with a sick parent or parent figure is an important cause of psychoneurotic and psychosomatic disturbances.

2. **Evidences for a Childhood Neurosis.** Evidences for childhood neurosis will often be missing. Neither the individual nor his family can recall the indications of disturbed behavior or bodily dysfunction. Nevertheless, it is well known that almost invariably disturbed behavior or psychosomatic illness of adult life has been preceded by illness of emotional origin in childhood.

The fact that every child in his normal development shows some evidence of disturbed behavior or disorder of emotional origin makes this problem difficult to evaluate. It is a question of degree. Physicians so often say "The child will grow out of it." And so he may seem to do, but the nucleus of the disorder remains and may manifest itself later in life with a more severe illness. Apparently the adolescent period is the crucial one in which the emotional disorders of childhood may be submerged and adequately compensated or may undergo recrudescence and leave a mark which will be felt later in life.

3. **Sensitivity to Specific Emotional Factors.** When we ask ourselves why a psychosomatic disorder begins at a particular time we must attempt to sketch a cross-section of the individual's life situation at that time in order to discover emotionally disturbing events. We know that these are apt to occur at certain epochs in life, such as puberty, marriage, childbirth, climacteric, and during the senescent period. If the person is heavily predisposed, the incident that precipitates illness may be trivial; if he is comparatively well adjusted, it may require a major event to disturb him or precipitate a psychosomatic affection. In either event the incident is related to his personality structure.

4. **A Specific Personality Structure.** Almost never does a symptom of emotional origin exist alone. There are always other evidences of personality disturbance, either in the mental or the physical sphere. Both cross-section and longitudinal studies of the life situation, as well as the personality make-up, will show characteristic trends which indicate the predisposition to certain behavior manifestations or to a particular type of disorder.

5. **Demonstration of Specific Behavior.** When meaningful material is touched upon in taking the history the evidence in the patient's behavior is unmistakable. We must of course allow for the stress incident to the first contact between the patient and the physician but usually there is no difficulty in determining from the patient's behavior that a specific vulnerability exists when certain subjects are broached. It is like the dentist searching for crevices with his sharp-pointed instrument. We too must search for defects in the personality but it is the experienced interviewer who discovers the defect and yet avoids causing pain.

6. **Hyposensitization by Psychotherapy or by the Avoidance of Provocative Situations.** That a patient improves by means of psychotherapy may be much more obvious to the physician and to the family than to the patient. Indeed the patient will often deny that he is better even while members of his family attest to his improvement. One often obtains a better impression from what the patient does than from the way he says he feels. We do not ask people how they feel; we prefer to ask "What have you done?"

It is also true that manipulation of the environment can bring about improvement in a great many instances. This is the area in which the social worker can be so helpful. The failure to improve when the environment is improved is in itself an indication for psychotherapy.

A last word in regard to this topic: One must be very cautious about attributing improvement to psychotherapy. So often something in the environment has changed and the physician does not know it. The physician may take credit when it belongs elsewhere. Of course, it also may happen that the patient will give credit elsewhere when it belongs to the physician.

One special point that we would emphasize: Neurosis or psychosomatic ailment usually does not make its first appearance in middle life; one must always suspect organic disease.

In so far as allergy is concerned the fact that the removal of an allergen or a hyposensitization process "cures" the patient proves only that one factor has been removed and the morbid chain of events interrupted; and exactly the same reasoning can be applied to psychological factors.

Halliday's Six-Point Formula

Halliday develops his concept of a psychosomatic affection in a six-point formula. The following material is taken from his excellent discussion of the subject.

1. EMOTION AS PRECIPITATING FACTOR

"Examination of patients in series shows that in a high proportion of cases the bodily process emerged, or recurred, on meeting an emotionally upsetting event."

"When we investigate patients with psychosomatic affections, we find that the illness is often precipitated by an emotional disturbance which was an understandable response to a clearly recognizable disturbing event or events. Sometimes, however, the nature of the event seems petty in the objective sense and inadequate by itself to account for a profound emotional reaction in any "normal" person; but when consideration is given to the personality of the patient and to his previous life history, such minor events can often—and with good reason—be interpreted as acting as the last straw."

2. PERSONALITY TYPE

"A particular type of personality tends to be associated with each particular affection."

"When we meet an individual we receive certain impressions, and experience certain feelings, which provide us with a sense of the person-as-a-whole—his total characteristics—and to this we give the name of personality. Most medical men, especially perhaps those in general practice, come, as their clinical experience grows, to sense that certain kinds of disease tend to go with certain types of person. The impression of types depends on the general configuration of the patient: on his external expression (which is a matter not only of the facies but also of attitude, posture and manner of movement); on his 'internal expressions' (as revealed outwardly in pallor, flushings, throbbings, size of pupils); and also on impacts that are often indescribable but which arouse intuitions belonging to the order of 'hunches.' Psychological investigation of disposition does, however, allow some of these hunches to be described in a communicable way.

"The intuitive idea that different types of syndrome or disease may be expressions of different types of personality applies especially to psychosomatic affections. Studies of personality in relation to disease have made little progress partly because of the complicated statistical procedure involved and partly because of the difficulty of ascertaining which of the innumerable aspects of a person are most relevant. A psychological approach to personality takes account of traits relating to intelligence, dispositions and character. This approach is still being developed but it may be said that so far no adequate method of assessing types has yet been devised. Four broad types have, however, been described:

"*Hysterical or histrionic type.* This is associated with hysteria in its somatic manifestations whether sensori-motor disturbances (such as paralysis or spasms, anaesthesias or severe pains), or autonomic disturbances (such as vasomotor flushes or rashes).

"*Hypersensitive or allergic type.* Exemplified in asthma.

"*Self-assertive, self-sufficient, over-active, 'ulcer' type.* Exemplified in peptic ulcer and certain cases of fibrositis and hypertension.

"*Self-restricting, self-sacrificing, 'rheumatoid' type.* Exemplified in rheumatoid arthritis.

"Persons who develop psychosomatic affections commonly show notable obsessional trends—a term which refers to certain compulsive performances in daily routine such as always being punctual, always orderly and tidy, always very clean, always 'doing one's duty,'—in short, being generally fixed in one's way and set in one's ideas."

3. SEX RATIO

"*A marked disproportion in sex incidence is a finding in many, perhaps most, of these disorders.*"

"The excess is in males for some affections (*e. g.* childhood asthma, duodenal ulcer), and in females for others (*e. g.* chorea of childhood, exophthalmic goitre, gallbladder disease, rheumatoid arthritis). This suggests, among other things, the importance of the endocrine system as a mechanism in the mediation of these affections. It cannot, however, be related to physiological sex differences only, because with changes in the social environment of a community we find the phenomenon of alterations in the sex incidence and this sometimes brings about a complete reversal of the ratio over a period of years.

"For example, during the last century peptic ulcer preponderated in females, but during recent years came to preponderate definitely in males. Conversely, diabetes which during the last century was a disease of males, has now become a disease which preponderates in females. These facts suggest that the emotions must be taken into account in any adequate understanding of these affections. It is evident, however, that though disproportion in the sex incidence seems to be a finding for most psychosomatic organic affections, it cannot be postulated as a sine qua non of all psychosomatic disorders at all periods of time. Lastly, the sex disproportion in the incidence of psychosomatic affections is in striking contrast to the approximately equal sex incidence found in the infectious diseases."

4. ASSOCIATIONS WITH OTHER PSYCHOSOMATIC AFFECTIONS

"*Different psychosomatic affections may appear in the same individuals simultaneously, but the more usual phenomenon, as revealed in their natural history, is that of the alternation or of the sequence of different affections.*"

"Adequate records of associated, alternating and sequent affections are not yet available and except for the definite grouping of asthma, eczema, prurigo, migraine and enuresis, only occasional remarks on the subject are found in the literature.

"The sequence of peptic ulcer, fibrositis, and bronchitis is not uncommon in the medical history of middle-aged insured persons who have been for long periods on the sick list. It is possible that the changing endocrinological setting associated with particular phases of the life cycle may be one of the factors determining such sequences. The adult, like the child, may 'grow out' of one affection, but he may grow into another."

Mental Disorders as Associated Affections

"*Psychoneuroses.* A study of the natural history of psychosomatic affections shows that psychoneurotic illnesses may accompany psychosomatic organic diseases or may appear as preceding, alternating, or sequent disorders. During the course of psychoanalytical treatment this switching over is sometimes illustrated dramatically when, as a mental symptom becomes alleviated, a somatic manifestation takes its place. Such somatic manifestations are not necessarily one of the usual accepted bodily disturbances of anxiety state or hysteria, but may take the shape of organic expressions such as sore throat, hemorrhoids, bronchitis, skin eruptions or fibrositis."

"*Idiopathic psychoses* (*schizophrenia, manic-depressive psychosis, paranoia*). It has been suggested that the appearance of an idiopathic psychosis renders a psychosomatic expression unnecessary—a statement which is only partially true, since patients with these disorders often show functional disorders of the skin, as well as abnormalities in posture. There is, however, some rather loose evidence suggesting that among sufferers from the psychoses certain common psychosomatic affections such as peptic ulcer, rheumatoid arthritis and fibrositis are relatively rare. Psychosis and psychosomatic organic disease may alternate."

"*Mental illness and the psychosomatic formula*. A study of relevant data provided by textbooks of psychiatry shows that the separate mental disorders classed under the headings of the psychoneuroses and the idiopathic psychoses comply with the psychosomatic formula in respect of precipitating emotions, personality type, disproportion in sex incidence, positive family history and phasic manifestations—a finding which points to some kind of correspondence, connexion, equivalence, or relationship between psychosomatic affections and mental disorders."

5. FAMILY HISTORY

"A significantly high proportion of cases give a history of the same or of an associated disorder in parents, relatives and siblings."

"The method of familial transmission is still undecided. Only a proportion of a family becomes affected. In certain cases no positive family history is obtainable. Genetic (or mendelian) inheritance has not been established in respect of individual psychosomatic affections but there does seem to be inherited a kind of weakness, sensitiveness or inadequacy. There may perhaps also be inherited a predisposition to special patterns of bodily reaction, but this cannot be stated with certainty because of the difficulty of disentangling inherited predisposition from predispositions acquired early through 'psychological infection' from the parents giving rise to habits of faulty reaction which become fixed. A psychologist described a similar idea in these words: 'Parent-child resemblances in function and dysfunction need not be inherited but may arise through psychological tensions which recur in succeeding generations through unrecognized imitation and identification' (Wilson, 1939). But whether biologically inherited or very early acquired, the *predisposition* seems to be woven into the structure of the personality.

"Finally it may be noted how common speech assumes that there are family repertories of disease: One family is 'highly-strung', another, 'queer', another has weak stomachs, another is 'not strong', another 'chesty' ."

6. PHASIC MANIFESTATION

"*The course of the illness tends to be phasic with periods of crudescence, intermission and recurrence.*"

"Rhythmic manifestations are a feature of all life whether viewed somatically or psychologically, but in the case of psychosomatic affections the rhythm is an irregular one, as may be noted from studying over a period of time patients with peptic ulcer, asthma, rheumatoid arthritis, fibrositis and gall-bladder disease. Each major phase of recrudescence varies in severity and has no standard duration. In different people and in the same people on different occasions, the duration may vary from hours or days to months. Each stage is followed naturally by an interval of absence or subsidence, but this is of no constant length. The study of the behaviour of these affections indicates that this negative phase does not necessarily represent—as is sometimes optimistically imagined—'a cure resulting from treatment.' Sometimes the primary illness subsides, never to return; sometimes it assumes a progressive, fulminating quality; and sometimes it merges into chronicity. However, the usual course of these affections is that of irregularly phasic appearances.

. "Investigations have shown that the irregularity in the appearance of phases of crudescence is associated with the irregularity in time of disturbing or distasteful external events. Conversely the initiation of a negative phase may be related to the removal of disturbing circumstances or the interposition of favourable happenings. 'Why does he get better when he does?' is a question answered by the aetiology of natural recovery. Lastly, minor phasic exacerbations or remissions are sometimes associated with cyclic endocrine activity. It is said that menstruation usually worsens the symptoms in asthma and exophthalmic goitre, whereas the endocrine 'imbalance' of pregnancy sometimes brings about a subsidence of rheumatoid arthritis or psoriasis."

SOME BACKGROUND FACTORS
Organ Neurosis

Certain psychosomatic disorders have been spoken of as organ neuroses. From a psychological standpoint there are different varieties of organ neuroses depending upon the severity of the underlying disorder. There are very mild disturbances of organ functioning, psychosomatic dysfunctions, which are hysterical symptoms. They are spoken of as conversion phenomena—a substitute expression of an emotional tension which cannot find adequate outlet. The substitute expression is symbolic, i. e., nervous vomiting may, as part of its meaning, express unconscious disgust. There are other disorders, however, which have been referred to as vegetative neuroses. These arise not as an attempt to express an emotion but as the physiological accompaniment of constant or recurring emotional states. Here the somatic symptoms are not so much substitute expressions of repressed emotions as they are normal physiological accompaniments of the emotional state (Alexander). They are the adjustment of the organism to definite tasks which it has to face in a danger situation. They represent a utilitarian preparation and an adaptation of the internal vegetative processes (homeostasis) to a specific type of behavior which is requested from the organism. Elevated blood pressure, e. g., does not relieve anger; it appears in place of emotional tension and accompanies the emotion of rage. It may then be that the chronicity of the emotional tension (plus other factors) makes the condition morbid—psychosomatic organic disease. Any vegetative nervous system disorder deserves study of the psyche as well as the soma and often will prove to be a psychosomatic affection.

Organ Neurosis and "Organic" Disease. The emotions often exploit an organic illness and thus it is that frequently, following an infectious disease or operation, convalescence lingers and invalidism sets in. The explanation so often given is that the organic disease produces the neurosis whereas the actual mechanism is that the organic process breaks down the individual's defenses, regression occurs, and the individual's predisposition, determined by the personality structure, permits the neurosis to emerge.

An example of a contrary aspect of the relation of organic disease to neurosis is the severe neurotic disorder, hypochondriasis, in which the patient is obsessed with his neurotic symptoms and inattentive to some serious organic disorder. We have repeatedly observed patients whose only concern was with the psyche while they were dying from organic disease. Recently a patient focused all of his attention upon his heart, which was normal, while an abdominal tumor, which could be readily felt, took his life.

An important subject in psychosomatic illness is the shift from mental sphere to somatic expression. Very often in the organ neuroses the improvement of a symptom because of treatment or for any other reason may lead to mental symptoms such as mood disturbances and sometimes manic and depressive states. An important therapeutic lesson comes out of this consideration because sometimes in psychosomatic illness when we get rid of symptoms by means of medicine, surgery, or manipulation, without getting at the fundamental problem, which is emotional conflict, the difficulty is reflected immediately in mental symptoms. Jelliffe, in an article "What Price Healing" gave the history of a patient with contraction of the bladder of psychic origin, in whom dilatation of the bladder relieved urinary symptoms but was promptly followed by psychosis. Elsewhere we cite the example of the surgical removal of a goiter followed by psychosis. Such cases call attention to the necessity for psychological evaluation of the patient before surgery is attempted.

Pseudoheredity

Dunbar has laid emphasis on pseudoheredity as opposed to actual heredity in the determination of illness. This is a very important consideration to which too little reference has been made. Children identify with their parents and unconsciously imitate them in this way; patterns of behavior are laid down (which include illness as an aspect of behavior) so early in life that we often attribute a disorder to heredity when in fact it was acquired. This of course is a very involved question and we presume that the final answer can hardly be hoped for, that is, to separate constitutional and environmental factors with absolute precision. But unconscious identification with a sick parent or other member of the household in early childhood very often is the basis for an illness later in life which we may attribute wholly to heredity. When a young child is exposed to a sick parent it often shows the effect in psychosomatic illness in adult life. How often one hears a patient say that because she was exposed to a sick and complaining mother she learned to detest neurotic women and "made up her mind that she would never become one." Unfortunately this conscious resolution has little to do with the problem; it is the unconscious identification which determines illness. Without realizing it she is the "picture" of the mother in illness as in health.

Emotional Age

Emotional immaturity, which after all is the background of neurotic and psychosomatic illness, often reflects itself in the appearance of the patient, and people who look much younger than their years are often suspect as the kind of people who are apt to become ill from emotional causes. This problem will be discussed again but the emotional age is a revealing index to the kind of personality that may break down from environmental stress. If the emotional age is in harmony with the physical and intellectual and chronological ages then a person is often

said to be well adjusted and such people are usually free from psychosomatic illness, whereas those with immature emotional life as reflected
in their appearance—those in whom the emotional age is not in keeping
with the chronological, physical, and intellectual age—are the people
who provide the soil for psychosomatic sickness. Thus in medical
circles "How young you look" may be a dubious compliment.

HISTORY-TAKING

Physician's Qualifications

An important element of the doctor-patient relationship enters into
the taking of the history. We shall refer again to the qualifications of the
physician who should interest himself in psychosomatic problems. Here
it is only necessary to say that he must be so constituted that he can listen
to the patient uncritically. Sympathy for patients suffering from illness
of emotional origin is an essential part of the equipment of the physician
who would interest himself in psychosomatic problems. It goes without
saying that if he is unsympathetic it will show in his manner and will
discourage the patient from revealing feelings that are essential to an
understanding of the problem.

In addition, a physician's ability to use the psychosomatic approach
will depend upon his knowledge of psychopathology and tissue pathology
applied simultaneously. His human understanding, his sensitivity and
sympathetic appreciation of emotional factors as a cause of illness, as well
as his orientation and experience, are all important in determining his
ability to deal with psychosomatic problems.

One of the most important elements in the psychotherapeutic relationship is transference, about which we will speak later. It has to do
with the patient-physician relationship and is involved in all contacts
between physicians and patients from the moment they begin.

The Social Worker and Psychosomatic Diagnosis

We will discuss the role of the social case worker in the next chapter
but here it may be said that she can be of great help in establishing a
diagnosis as well as in treatment. This has long been recognized in clinic
and hospital practice and was clearly demonstrated during World War
II when the team of psychiatrist, psychologist, and social worker was
developed to such a considerable extent. We think that the same thing
will happen in civil practice and that not only the psychiatrist but the
internist, pediatrician, and the other major specialities will discover how
useful a well-trained medical social case worker can be in developing the
social background of illness and assisting in the management of patients
and their families. The term social and psychiatric are as interrelated and
interdependent as are the terms psyche and soma. Medicine has an im-

portant lesson to learn in the fine art of interviewing as developed by social case work (Garrett).

Criticism of Clinical Records

Some years ago Kilgore criticized the standardization of hospital clinical records. His criticism, part of which follows, still stands. "The amazing epidemic of standardization that has been visited upon American institutions in this century has not permitted our clinical records to escape. In practically all hospitals with any pretensions one finds the clinical records usually in trim aluminum covers, with some variation in charts and laboratory sheets, but with the clinical history proper invariably displayed under a stereotyped system of paragraphs, with or without the guidance of printed forms. The histories are thereby given an orderliness which is pleasing to the eye and which makes tacit claim to the admirable quality of thoroughness."

Standardized Histories. "And yet, these standardized histories are open to a very serious criticism. My criticism may be interpreted from the following illustration: In a medical ward of a class A teaching hospital I recently saw a Jewess, aged forty-five years. Five minutes of conversation brought out the facts that she had always been in reasonably good health until after the death of her husband a year ago; that she then looked hopefully for support from her eldest son; but that about three months ago she gradually experienced the final and crushing conviction that his talents were limited to the selling of newspapers, which yielded a profit of less than a dollar a day. She therefore, in addition to caring for her home and the younger children, took employment in a restaurant, standing eight hours a day washing dishes. Then came backache, sleepless nights of worry, anorexia, loss of 20 pounds, nervousness, utter exhaustion, hospitalization. Cursory examination revealed only the ordinary effects of such a life, including possibly some thyroid disturbance.

"Now, I ask of you sticklers for form and order, what do you suppose that woman's folder contained? Five and one-half closely written pages of matter comprised under twenty-eight captions, all neatly underlined with red ink and ruler! Figure out the time that probably took, and then ask yourselves how much time and energy remained to devote to the clinical problem of that woman. We toil through those five and one-half pages in search of useful bits of information. Here and there we find a few—fragmentary and uncorrelated. In the place for 'social condition' it is stated that she is a widow; under 'occupation' that she is a housewife; under 'marital history' that she has four children, but not a word about that fiasco of the eldest son. The paragraph on 'habits' speaks of weight loss but gives no hint of the possible cause. Breathlessly we work down to the captions 'complaint,' 'onset of illness', and 'course of of present illness' and find only some sketchy references to pains in the back, palpitation, breathlessness on effort, gas in the stomach, and so on, but never a word of the restaurant or the thoughts in the poor woman's head. Then comes the sacred array of paragraphs on the various systems, with reiteration of shortness of breath under 'cardiorespiratory system," of stomach gas under 'gastrointestinal,' etc., etc."

No Information on Patient as a Person. "The writer of this history was evidently painstaking and industrious, and yet what a mess he made of it! There is not the slightest doubt that if, before he ever set foot in medical school, he had been confronted with this patient and had been asked to write down what he could find out about her condition, he would have done incomparably better. And as a commentary on the teaching of clinical history-taking is not that the height of irony? The reason for this enormity is obvious. The writer of the history has been so occupied in constructing and polishing the frame in order to meet the standard specifications that he has been unable to paint the picture; indeed, he has scarcely seen the patient and her experiences at all.

"This case, to be sure, is worse than many of our hospital clinical histories, but it is none the less a good illustration of a valid general criticism of unrestrained standardization; namely, stereotypism, perfunctoriness, mediocrity."

Special Service Histories. Still another criticism of hospital histories from the standpoint of the psychosomatic approach is, that if a patient is admitted to a special ward he gets the kind of a history that the ward or service requires, namely, a history taken from the specialist's point of view, neglecting the person for the part.

It is not to be presumed that the busy physician will undeviatingly follow an outline in every case. Indeed, we realize only too well that this is an impossibility. What we rather hope is that by studying the obscure or difficult problems in his practice in this way he will gradually incorporate a psychosomatic habit into his medical thinking and into his approach to all patients. Then, very often, only a short time will be required to understand the problem.

Experience of course is important in history-taking but if one practices medicine for fifty years he will still have to give time to the patient. In other words, there are no short cuts in history-taking. While the most experienced people will quickly grasp the situation time must be taken because the patient cannot be hurried in his recital of what to him are important facts and he certainly cannot be hurried when it comes to an understanding of his illness in terms of behavior.

The revered family doctor of the small community utilized his knowledge of his patients' personal lives in evaluating their history. He knew everything that was going on and had a background of understanding gained from personal observation. Now in our elaborate medical institutions, with a lack of knowledge of the patient's background, we overemphasize the so-called scientific aspects of medicine and relegate to the background the social and emotional factors that may enter into illness. As a consequence our methods of history-taking have not kept pace with other methods of progress in medical science. Really our history forms and technics are indicative of one of the basic faults in medical knowledge and medical teaching. We have advanced very little from the teachings of Osler in our traditional concept of disease. Osler's insistence on a solid pathological foundation for medical understanding and his careful clinical observations marked an epoch in the development of medicine.

Unfortunately Osler's warmth and human understanding and his intuitive appreciation of emotional factors in illness could not become a part of our medical heritage. The body is still divided into many organs and systems; specialists look upon disease from their narrow viewpoint; and the curriculum is built up by introducing more and more special points of view. As a result the comprehensive viewpoint which is so necessary to the study of illness as an aspect of behavior can make little headway. The medical history form which we give to our medical students reflects this organic approach and this age of specialization, and as a consequence we look in vain throughout a long history for some evidence of the human being who is sick. If patients were allowed to talk more and were examined less it would probably be a good thing for medicine as a whole. As one of our patients who had been through the mill of medical investigation recently remarked, she was suffering from "testitis." How numerous are the patients who have been examined again and again by means of x-rays, chemical studies, and various other expensive and complicated methods, accumulating a sheaf of papers an inch thick, with an end result hurtful rather than helpful because the diagnosis is obscured by concentration on a part rather than on the whole.

The Person in the Patient

The majority of people who consult a general physician *wish* to find some physical cause for their ailment; hence they fall readily into the system of answering specific questions about physical health but volunteering no information about themselves as persons. Moreover, people look upon the physician as an authoritarian figure who will "do something" about their illness and they are usually quite unprepared to have to do something for themselves, in other words, discuss themselves as persons as well as "medical cases." We must look for the person in the patient. We have frequently observed that the patient who insists "that his illness is physical" is apt to be suffering from a disorder of emotional origin while the patient who is eager to blame it on the psyche often has an organic disease. Many people, seriously sick with advanced organic disease, seek to delude themselves with the idea that it may be "all mental." This applies especially to the many lay persons who have now read some of the popular writings on psychosomatic medicine.

The introduction of the psychosomatic point of view does not require a different form of history-taking; it only requires an awareness of the role that emotions play in illness, and consequently more emphasis on certain aspects of history-taking. *Thus the history need not differ in form but it must differ in substance.* In accordance with what has already been said, more attention will be paid to the behavior of the patient and to the actual words that he uses in describing his complaints as well as to the asides and apparent irrelevancies that so often give important clues to the emotional factor. Other fundamental considerations are to give the patient time, allowing him to talk with as few interruptions as possible; avoiding extensive note-taking so that the patient may feel that you are more interested in him as a person than in the setting down of the history; and showing interest and sympathy for what the patient sometime regards as trivial or silly. In addition more attention must be given to the chronological development of the life history with special emphasis on the various factors in the childhood period that may have influenced the development of the personality; with special attention to puberty and adolescence and the frequent emotional problems of that period. Interest will focus on the various epochs and crucial periods in life when psychosomatic disturbances are apt to arise, and a particular effort will be made to obtain a more complete picture of the family background.

More detailed discussion of these points and others follows.

Allowing the Patient to Talk. Although time-consuming it is important to allow the patient to tell his story with as few interruptions as possible because in this way important associations are obtained and the groundwork is laid for a good relationship with the patient. Occasionally the patient has to be led back to a discussion of the present illness but aside from such interruptions it is best to allow him to tell the story in his own way. Then one may go over the history in chronologic order with questions regarding the very first evidences of illness, which will frequently antedate the onset that the patient has first suggested. Inquiries should be made regarding the symptoms which preceded an operation because so often the history that the patient gives will begin from the time "of my operation." For example, it is important to know if the appendix was removed because it was acutely inflamed or for the so-called chronic appendicitis which often is a part of the clinical picture of psychosomatic illness. Questions regarding previous medical experiences are also important because so often the patient has picked up erroneous ideas which are harmful to him and until they are dealt with they may remain permanent obstacles to recovery.

It is usually best not to make extensive notes because then the patient feels that you are more interested in the record than you are in him. He is often vaguely irritated and thus distracted from telling his story. Often he prefers to think that some of the things he says will not be made part of a permanent record. A few notes with brief quotations of the patient's actual words will often serve as the framework on which the history later can be constructed.

In dealing with the chief complaint patients with psychosomatic illness frequently say "I hardly know where to begin." A satisfactory method is to ask the patient what is troubling him at the present time and then allow him to tell his story in his own way, observing not only what he says but how he says it, and making quotes of the statements that the patient uses. The greater the number of complaints the more likely that the illness is emotional. We often will find that the patient in his own words expresses the formula of body language to which we have already referred.

Giving the Patient Time. The essence of the psychosomatic approach in history-taking is to give the patient sufficient time to tell his story. This of course is one of the great problems in the practice of medicine. Physicians are always saying, "But how can I possibly take the time to try to understand some of these problems?" And we answer, "You must take the time; there are no short cuts." Of course, in the midst of a busy practice one cannot allow an hour for every new patient, and for simple diagnostic problems, as are the majority of cases in general practice, it is not necessary. When the problem is complicated, however, as in the case of most chronic illnesses, the kind of cases that are seen so often in the practice of internal medicine, one must find time. We suggest that if time is not available during regular office hours special appointments be made for certain patients so that sufficient time may be allotted and the interview may proceed in an unhurried fashion. Once you get to know the life situation, subsequent visits need not necessarily take up a great deal of time. Often one can put his finger on the problem very quickly, as it is realized that repetition is the key note of neurotic behavior. People get into trouble over the same situation again and again; the characters may change but the situation remains the same.

Chronologic Development of the Life History

There are two main approaches to the study of the patient with suspected psychosomatic disorder: *a cross-section study* of his personality as he appears at the time of the interview, and *a longitudinal survey* of his life from family background and early infancy to the present time. The first approach, the cross-sectional viewpoint, is represented by the story of the present illness; it is the traditional approach of the physician to his patient, and the only requirement so far as the psychosomatic history is concerned is to develop the social and psychological aspects in order to see if there is a relationship between the life situation and the medical illness.

When we approach the past history we must necessarily undertake the longitudinal study of the personality. This will be facilitated by charting the medical events on one side of the page and the life situation on the other, in the manner suggested by Adolf Meyer and widely employed by Cobb and his associates. (See the section on Arthritis for an example.) The presentation of the problem in this manner will often make it possible to see at a glance a very complicated illness from the standpoint of the relationship between medical and emotional events. It is best to employ both the age of the patient and the year of the calendar in charting medical events and life situation. Patients will often give age in relation to one medical experience, calendar year in relation to another, and "so many years ago" in referring to still other events in their medical histories. Adherence to a definite technic of chronological development is advisable in order not to become confused in regard to the timing of events.

The cross-sectional approach tries to relate the present illness and the precipitating emotional factor. The longitudinal study relates personality development and medical history. The latter gives a better idea of the personality structure and psychopathology because it shows the background and the development of the personality. One technic does not exclude the other; on the contrary, the data derived are complementary and help to establish a definitive psychosomatic diagnosis.

Explaining "Body Language" to Patients

The subject of body language which we introduced in the first chapter is a very satisfactory approach to many medical problems. Sherrington suggested that the most satisfactory way to deal with tension is by action, the least satisfactory is by thought, and in between is speech. In other words, in all people with psychosomatic illness there is some impairment of total functioning and very often a great deal of energy is consumed by thought (fantasies). If we can encourage them to get their thinking onto the surface by talking about their problems we can often understand the illness better and at the same time provide some measure of relief. Thus we often say to our patients that they are like engines with the steam up. If the wheels do not go round in productive work and the whistle is not blowing in talking about their troubles then the steam must try to get out somehow and it makes an effort to part their seams. This is almost too pat a description of the circumstances in such a case as hypertension. It is a homely explanation which people readily grasp as they realize that this short circuiting of energy is capable of disturbing bodily functions. Therefore we can say to patients that if they cannot express their tension by word or action—if they cannot say with their mouths what is disturbing them—then one of their organs will try to say it for them. Thus the patient with nausea, who has no evidence of organic disease, may be indicating that he cannot "stomach" certain situations; the patient with an itch often "lets things get under his skin." If we would only listen to our patients we would find that they express their body language in symbolic formulas.

The Case Illustration

Another very satisfactory way to get people to discuss themselves in relation to their illness is to use a case illustration. Repeatedly this is effective when other methods of trying to make people see the relation between emotions and illness fail. If one can think of an apt case illustration the patient can readily identify himself and even where there are marked divergences the patient will often see a partial application which will encourage him to talk about his personal life. Sometimes he will deny the application only to go on from that point to discuss emotional factors of importance which previously he was unable to think of.

The Autobiography

Among the technics which can be used for diagnostic purposes is the autobiography. Certain reticent people are able to express their feelings better on paper than in the interview with the physician. With such patients it is sometimes helpful, after the first or second interview, to suggest that the patient prepare an autobiography which will enable the physician "to understand the background of the illness" more readily than by spending the time in interviewing. In connection with the autobiography it must be remembered that what the patient leaves out is often more important than what he puts in. Additional information can often be obtained from corrections that the patient has made or "slips" of the pen.

We find it best not to instruct patients as to content or length of the autobiography but simply to suggest that they write their life story, including medical experiences, so that the physician may become acquainted with them as persons as well as medical cases, in shorter time than interviewing would permit. The autobiography is then used as a basis for further interviews. A slight variation which is often useful is to suggest that the patient write down any thoughts that he may have after the interview and bring them along the next time. This often produces material stimulated by the interview which ordinarily would be repressed before the next visit. Patients sometimes seem a little reluctant to place a written record of their intimate lives in any one's hands and when we sense this we suggest that we will be glad to return the record once we have had the opportunity to read it.

The Associative Anamnesis

Even when using the history form it is always advisable to allow the patient, insofar as is possible, to tell his story in his own way. This technic of letting the patient tell his own story has been developed to a fine art by Felix Deutsch, in what he calls "the associative anamnesis." He encourages the patient to talk about himself, guiding him skillfully with a question or remark formed by some of the patient's own words. This stimulates the patient to bring up material which has the most important emotional value. Deutsch notes the time and circumstances of the onset of symptoms—a correlation which cannot be emphasized too often. Physicians regularly neglect to elicit what was going on in the patient's environment when his symptoms began.

One observes whether there is anxiety, apprehension, shame, or irritability during the recital of the history. Does the patient perspire, tremble, weep, or seem agitated? On the other hand, is there too much of an air of calm or reserve or a denial of worry? The latter may be significant of a great deal of repression of emotion. It is important to note what comments are made in passing and also what the patient talks about during the physical examination. For instance, the patient with a very serious illness may insist upon talking about inconsequential things in order not to have the subject of the seriousness of his condition brought up. Contrariwise, the patient with a trifling symptom may be extremely overanxious and ask all kinds of questions pertaining to the ultimate outcome of his troubles.

Definitive Psychosomatic Diagnosis

Just as in a consideration of somatic disease it is necessary to make a complete diagnosis before we can hope to apply scientific treatment, so in psychosomatic medicine it is equally necessary. Hence just as in general medical teaching we have always emphasized etiologic, anatomic, and functional diagnosis, so in psychological medicine, as pointed out by Levine, it is necessary to make a clinical, dynamic, and genetic diagnosis before one can stand on safe ground in regard to psychotherapy.

The clinical diagnosis in psychosomatic medicine refers to the structural and physiologic deviations as well as to the underlying or associated psychological disturbance. For example, in the so-called organ neurosis, we would like to know whether we are dealing with a mild personality disorder such as hysteria or a severe personality disorder such as hypochondriasis. It is important, for example, in a functional gastrointestinal complaint, to know whether the symptoms are on the basis of conversion hysteria or a part of the clinical picture of depression in which the mood disturbance is overshadowed by the somatic complaints. When one deals with depression there is often the threat of suicide.

Dynamic diagnosis refers to the meaning and purpose of the symptoms or behavior in terms of the particular personality and its structure. Coupled with the genetic diagnosis, which is derived from the longitudinal survey of the individual life history, we are then in a position for comprehensive medical care.

In the development of the longitudinal study of the individual it will frequently be observed that psychosomatic disorders appear at epochal periods. Infancy, early childhood, later childhood, puberty and adolescence, early adult life, middle and late adult life, and old age periods, have their own special problems as indicated in the accompanying table.

CORRELATION OF LIFE SITUATION AND SYMPTOM FORMATION

LIFE SITUATION	SYMPTOM FORMATION
Oral Stage (first year of life)	
Food and love are being given to the child with no responsibilities exacted in return.	Refusal to nurse; fretfulness when nursing is over, or contentment? Protest to weaning (crying or vomiting)?
Anal Period (1-3 years)	
Responsibility of cleanliness and neatness has to be taken over in toilet habits and in other activities. This is not easy and the child needs much friendliness, understanding, and patience to accomplish it without anxiety or detriment to personality development.	Is toilet training accepted or is child stubbornly resistive, wetting and soiling beyond usual age of established cleanliness? Is there constipation, temper tantrum, stubbornness, resentment, destructiveness?
Genital Period (3-6 years)	
Period of increasing general and sexual curiosity. Period of beginning tender attachment to parent of opposite sex.	Excessive masturbation, fretfulness, disobedience, aggression, cruelty, enuresis, poor adjustment to other children?
Latent Period (6-12 years)	
Period of primary education, identification with ideals and authority.	How is social adjustment? Does he do well in studies? Does he mix well in classroom and playground? Is there sexual delinquency, truancy, aggressiveness, cruelty, poor sportsmanship, seclusiveness?

LIFE SITUATION	SYMPTOM FORMATION
Puberty (12-15 years)	
Period of maturity and beginning activity of sex glands. Extra impetus given to entire emotional life, especially emotional patterns pertaining to love and sexuality.	Are there anxiety attacks; fears of disease, of death, of harming others; nightmares, irritability, social anxiety, seclusiveness, loss of appetite, vomiting, diarrhea, cardiac palpitation?
Adolescence (15-21 years)	
Period of secondary and college education. Often the need to leave the home and live among strangers. Beginning of love relationships. Planning for life work, career, home, marriage. The fields of competition widen. Conflicts over religion or ideals and current behavior.	Are there symptoms occurring on leaving home, on beginning or ending a love affair, because of inability to compete? Is there seclusiveness and anxiety? A period in which the incidence of somatic symptoms is high!
Early Adult Life (21-40 years)	
Decisions must be made about love, marriage, work, parenthood. Parental support drops away after 21, if not before. Responsibilities of adulthood are thrust upon one. They catch up with one whether he is prepared for them or not. May be stress of military service.	Symptoms may appear in relation to engagement, marriage, pregnancy, childbirth, loss of job, failure to adjust in marriage, or new environment. "War neuroses."
Middle Adult Life (40-60 years)	
Period when anticipated ambitions are lost or realized. Children begin to leave home. Women go through menopause. Both sexes have to adjust to changing values.	Women have to cope with the menopause and loss of companionship of the children. May not be resourceful enough, become depressed and anxious. For men it is the age of business success and failure. Of divorce. Reactions to physical disease. Cancerophobia, depression and suicide.
Late Adult Life and Old Age Period (60 years plus)	
Period of retirement for men, forced or voluntary. Dependency on children for support in both sexes. Problems of physical disease (geriatrics) and the need for care by others.	Symptoms of anxiety often appear after retirement, and many symptoms are due to the frictions incident to living with children and in-laws. Arteriosclerosis and senile dementia usually make social adjustment more difficult.

In approaching the patient from the standpoint of psychosomatic diagnosis one must realize that in dealing with the emotions one cannot separate treatment from diagnosis and that really as soon as one has made an initial contact with the patient the groundwork is being prepared for treatment. There is no sharp division between the period of diagnosis and the period of beginning treatment.

The System Review

When the patient has concluded the story of the present illness it is best to review the various systems in order to round out the picture of the patient's illness, to make sure that important symptoms have not been overlooked, and thus to assist in establishing the diagnosis. Tension of emotional origin is usually reflected in more than one system of the body.

In some patients the system review may be deferred until the history nears completion. At times this part of the history can best be done while one is examining the patient. As the systematic physical examination proceeds one can inquire for symptoms regarding the parts examined. This may save some time and help the patient to relax. As one examines the genitals in men it is quite natural to inquire regarding sexual power. Women usually had better not be approached so directly on this question. Discussion of menstruation and perhaps contraceptive technics will often more readily permit women to discuss sexual feelings.

Head. *Headache*, one of the commonest complaints in psychosomatic affections, occurs either as the chief complaint or as an additional symptom. The subject will be discussed in greater detail in the chapter dealing with the central nervous system (Chapter XXI) but here it may be said that there are various kinds of headaches that may make one think of an emotional factor. Although the allergic approach has been emphasized in cases of migraine, it should always make one suspicious that an important personality disorder is present. Headaches which are described as a feeling of pressure on the head are often symbolic of problems that are weighing upon the patient. So, too, headaches beginning in the back of the head, referred from the neck region and sometimes extending down the back or into the shoulders often represent tension expressed in the neuromuscular system. When one discusses with such a patient the fact that he is always tense, that he does not know how to relax, that his muscles are taut, and consequently that the tension is expressed especially in the muscles in the back of the neck, he will understand the origin of his headache and often produce material to confirm this suggestion. To refer again to the concept of body language one may think of "tossing the head" (disdain), and "stiffnecked" (obstinacy) as well as the common slang expression, "pain in the neck."

Patients often complain of being *dizzy* or light-headed. When organic cause has been ruled out, or evaluated, as for example in patients with hypertension and anxiety, we will find that this symptom is one of the commonest manifestations of emotional tension. It is one of the first expressions of insecurity and if we think about it for a moment from a body language standpoint what better way is there to represent insecurity than for a patient to be unsure of his balance? It may become very pronounced especially after the so-called *anxiety attack*, which is so often misunderstood and labeled a heart attack, hypoglycemia, hyperthyroidism, or neurocirculatory asthenia. A patient may say that he has been perfectly well until the time of the attack and that since then he has not been himself. Not being himself often means that he is dizzy, heavy-headed, unable to concentrate, and fatigued. What he does not tell you is that he has had a fear of death and that succeeding this he has thought "he was going to lose his mind." As we shall say later in discussing treatment it is very important to get these thoughts out on the surface where they can be dealt with adequately. The most superficial rationalizations of anxiety are fear of cancer, of heart disease, and of "losing one's mind."

In connection with this last idea there are often suicidal thoughts which are very disturbing to the patient. It is always important to get these most superficial ideas out before we attempt to deal with the deeper causes of anxiety.

The anxiety attack is discussed elsewhere (p. 122). All degrees occur from "weak feelings" in the abdomen and trembling of the legs, to actual panic states. As stated above it is essential for psychosomatic diagnosis that the attack be recognized for what it is—a symptom of psychological origin which must be handled by psychotherapy. *A great deal of confusion in the management of chronic illness results from the original misinterpretation of an anxiety attack.*

Eyes. Problems regarding vision are by no means rare in psychosomatic affections. A history of many refractions; of frequent changing of lenses; of "heavy lids"; rubbing of the eyes; of pain, blurring, rings around the lights, or spots before the eyes that cannot be accounted for on an organic basis, frequently suggest that the eye is acting as a focal point for anxiety. Hysterical blindness and lesser impairments of vision of hysterical origin will usually be readily recognized.

Nose. A very frequent problem indicating a probable psychosomatic disorder is vasomotor rhinitis. In association with real or alleged sinus disease it is a major problem in medicine and neither the allergic approach nor the attentions of the rhinologist are sufficient to deal with this disorder. Almost invariably it is a part of the picture of a psychosomatic affection.

Ears. Common complaints are tinnitus, buzzing and other peculiar noises. Although rarely the chief complaint they are often associated with other psychosomatic disorders. Patients themselves frequently volunteer that when they are tense the noises grow louder and that when they are relaxed the noises abate. Even when associated with Ménière's disorder there is still the need for psychosomatic exploration.

Teeth. Elsewhere we speak of the psychosomatic aspects of dental practice (p. 725). Here we need only remind ourselves that dentistry is the most mechanical branch of medicine, and yet the teeth can no more be divorced from the rest of the personality than can any other part of the body.

There are many implications from the standpoint of psychosomatic medicine. Teeth as "foci of an infection"; peculiar sensations of the lips, cheeks, gums, and tongue; bitter or metallic tastes; and atypical neuralgias of the face for which good teeth are often sacrificed, are some of the more common problems having to do with psychosomatic medicine. Nor must we forget that psychosomatic affections frequently follow dental extractions when the loss of teeth carries special psychological significance.

Throat and Neck. The hysterical symptom of "a lump in the throat" is one of the most widely recognized indications of nervous illness. In addition to that, patients often speak of a tight sensation in the throat sometimes extending up into the ears and with this they frequently complain of "a sore throat," which is more or less continuous. This chronic type of sore throat for which no organic cause can be found is a frequent part of the psychosomatic picture. Incidentally it should be mentioned that patients who gag easily when the tongue blade is used or who volunteer the information that they gag easily, especially in the mornings, sometimes when using a tooth brush, are suspect from a psychosomatic standpoint.

Clearing of the throat is often an index of tension and frequently is associated with the so-called "post-nasal drip." This is a common symptom in neurotic patients and while it may have some actual basis in vasomotor rhinitis and sinus disease it is frequently more troublesome to patients than the findings would lead one to expect.

The question of an enlarged thyroid gland frequently enters into psychosomatic problems. Aside from the presence of actual thyrotoxicosis there is the question of the coincidence of simple enlargement of the thyroid gland with neurotic illness. So often the latter is wrongly blamed upon the former.

Respiratory System. The most frequent symptom referred to the respiratory tract is "sighing respiration" which is invariably indicative of an emotional component in the illness. Frequently spoken of by patients as shortness of breath, and sometimes mistakenly thought to be dyspnea of organic origin by physicians, one can always elicit the true nature of the complaint by discovering that it is just as apt to occur when the patient is at rest as when he is active and, moreover, the manner of the complaint—the patient placing the hand on the sternum and saying that he has trouble taking a deep breath or cannot take a deep breath— indicates its emotional origin.

When actual asthmatic breathing is present there is still the necessity for looking into the personality for other indications of emotional disorder.

Neurotic cough is not a common symptom but it does occur, very often in association with "tuberculophobia."

Cardiac System. The subject will be discussed in detail in the chapters dealing with the cardiovascular system but here it may be noted that the pain of cardiac neurosis is frequently at the apex, not necessarily related to effort, and practically always associated with sighing respirations, fatigue, and heart consciousness.

In addition one must be alert to evaluate the symptoms when actual heart disease is present in order to decide whether they are not out of proportion to the disease and therefore to be accounted for on another basis. Again and again symptoms are blamed on hypertension which are really of emotional origin.

When hypertension and arteriosclerosis both are present the differential diagnostic problems become very difficult and from the standpoint of the physician's peace of mind often the most disturbing in the whole realm of psychosomatic diagnosis. (See discussion of coronary artery disease p. 275.)

Gastrointestinal System. "The abdomen is the sounding board of the emotions" and more than any other system reflects disturbances in the emotional sphere. Hence it is that from mouth to anus occur a variety of symptoms included within the designation "functional disorders of the gastrointestinal tract." Just to list them would require much space. Peculiar or metallic tastes; burning of the gums and tongue; throat sensations already mentioned; swallowing difficulties; functional indigestion, especially to fatty and greasy foods; belching attacks; "nervous vomiting"; anorexia and chronic diarrhea; constipation and the irritable bowel syndrome with upper gastrointestinal symptoms; and pruritus of the anus are just some of the many "functional" disorders encountered. The problem of so-called chronic appendicitis has already been mentioned.

More serious psychosomatic problems are anorexia nervosa, cardiospasm, peptic ulcer, a host of disorders in connection with gall tract disease (with and without stones), and ulcerative colitis.

Not only in functional disorders of the gastrointestinal tract but in every variety of psychosomatic illness we find an extraordinary compulsion on the part of the patient to blame his illness on "something I *et.*"

To this we usually reply, especially after we get to know the patient, "No, it's probably something you *met*." So deeply ingrained is this idea that even patients who have apparently learned a good deal about the relations of life situation and symptoms will return again and again blaming new complaints on "something I et."

One of the great diagnostic problems in psychosomatic medicine is the evaluation of pain and this is especially true in the abdomen. Even to the experienced observer it is often extraordinary how an intense pain will diminish or disappear when we understand and bring to the surface the emotional background. Sometimes this can be accomplished fairly readily as, for example, when the pain reflects the fear of cancer. When patients are told there is no organic disease and, emphatically, that there is no evidence of cancer, a stubborn pain which has resisted all previous therapeutic measures, often including surgery, will immediately diminish or disappear. This is usually discovered not by asking the patient "How is the pain?" but rather noting in the subsequent visit that the patient's emphasis is now directed toward another symptom or another part of the body and that concern over pain has receded into the background.

Genito-urinary System. As would be expected symptoms referred to this region are very common in psychosomatic disorders.

Questions of menstruation and child bearing will often provide the way for a discussion of sexual adjustment. For example, how did the patient react to the first menstruation—surprised, frightened, or disgusted—and whether the patient had any preparatory information from the mother. This will often lead naturally into the question of sexual preparation for marriage. The whole problem of frigidity and impotence, as we will later discuss, is of the greatest importance from the standpoint of human behavior and illness. Frigid women and impotent men have the kind of personalities that are subject to illness of emotional origin and impairment of the sexual functions stands as a revealing index to the personality make-up that may develop psychoneurotic or psychosomatic illness. Patients frequently mislead either deliberately or unconsciously in this regard. Because of our victorian background of repression in regard to sexuality, patients tend to regard sexual problems as of no importance in relation to their illness and evade questions or deny difficulties. The simple question, "What about sexual relations?" will often elicit the response that they are normal. Sometimes the patient knows differently; more often he, or especially she, does not. There is so much ignorance in this regard that even physicians frequently confuse the terms frigidity and sterility. But, as we have stated, these are matters that are usually best understood by allowing the patient to talk freely without asking too many direct questions and the way can often be paved by discussions of such matters as menstruation, contraception, and child bearing.

Men frequently fail to confess impotence but will admit quick ejaculation which is a lesser degree of impotence and just as significant as an indication of a predisposition to neurosis.

Frequency of urination, when it occurs during the day and not during the night, is one of the most frequent symptoms of nervous origin. However, even nocturia may be emotionally determined although it is usually an indication of organic disease and calls for extensive study of the genito-urinary tract.

Menses. Dysmenorrhea is practically always an indication of difficulties in the emotional sphere. Generally speaking, the more severe the dysmenorrhea the more severe the neurotic disorder. Other disturbances of the menses also occur for emotional reasons and these will be discussed in a section devoted to the subject.

In general it may be stated that too much emphasis is placed on slight disturbances of menstruation both by patient and physician. So often the patient takes the attitude, "you can hardly expect me to be well when I have this menstrual difficulty." She thinks it is inevitable that she should be sick and often takes the same attitude with regard to having a child, dating all subsequent illness "from the time my child was born." She feels that the child has taken something out of her that she can never regain.

The physician often becomes a pathogenic agent when he approaches the menstrual problem purely from an organic standpoint, relying only on endocrine assays and endocrine products. It is true, of course, that the other symptoms of which the patient complains are often much worse in connection with the menstrual period and this is especially true of premenstrual tension but the problem is usually just as much psychological as it is endocrinological.

Musculo-skeletal System. Aches and pains, in association with fatigue, frequently referred to as "fibrositis," are very common complaints of psychosomatic origin. If slight fever is also present the differential diagnosis will have to do chiefly with rheumatic fever, tuberculosis, and brucellosis. The matter can and should be settled promptly—there is danger of invalidism in focusing too much attention on slight elevations of temperature (p. 265).

The explanation to a patient with fatigue and aches and pains that he is constantly in a state of tension, that he never relaxes, not even at night, and that his muscles are crying out in protest, will often be the first satisfactory explanation that he has had after having had innumerable physical studies. How often do we find the cause of fatigue to be emotional conflict that uses up energy which is then not available for other purposes!

People who cannot "stand a fight" and who therefore avoid situations that stir them up are usually very sensitive people, easily hurt, whose reaction to aggravation is to say, "well what's the use, it isn't worth fighting about." Nevertheless they pay in bodily symptoms, such as atypical neuralgias, for this inability to express anger.

When patients are tense, taut, and uncommunicative, they will very often begin to talk when they are put at ease and muscular relaxation occurs, and of course the reverse is equally true, that when patients can be encouraged to talk their muscle tension often diminishes.

Patients who give the appearance of being calm and who deny being nervous will nevertheless admit that they have inner tension and that they "seethe or boil within." They are "burned-up" with indignation. Patients with hypertension and coronary artery disease, or other disorders involving smooth muscle, often give this impression whereas people who tend to have accidents are often impulsive people who are highly strung and tend to act out their conflicts (p 169).

Pain in the lower back region is one of the diagnostic problems that present many difficulties and while today attention is focused on herniated disk we must not forget that the syndrome of low back pain and fatigue is often an expression of emotional conflict which frequently occurs in association with pelvic preoccupation on the part of both patient and doctor. Tired women with nagging or even "excruciating" pain in the back who are overconcerned about some slight pelvic abnormality and who are eager to have it corrected by surgery should be suspect from a psychosomatic standpoint and caution exercised before permitting such patients to be operated upon (polysurgery p. 402).

It is well known that the posture of the patient is often a gross index to his emotional attitude. He reflects, in the way he carries himself, the attitude that he has toward himself and the world. The dejected (depressed) patient shows his dejection in his posture and the confident, secure patient often reflects his attitude in the erect way that he carries himself. In this connection it may be said that the patient who is always willing to lie down has a passive attitude toward his illness, often aided and abetted by the physician who cautions rest and more rest; while the patient who insists on being up is often the individual with a lot of fight who makes a determined effort to recover from illness.

A subject which should be of great interest to orthopedic specialists is the question of supports and braces which are so often prescribed for individuals who really need inner (emotional) strength rather than a bolstering-up from the outside. They learn to depend upon these outside aids as crutches and see no need to look into their own dependent attitudes.

The social-psychiatric problems associated with rheumatoid arthritis are of great importance and will be treated in detail in the section devoted to that subject (pp. 731-743).

Skin and Appendages. Vasomotor flushing of the head, neck, and chest is probably the most frequent index of inner tension and is especially common in women. Often during the medical interview one can note the rise and fall of inner tension with the increase and decrease in the mottling of the neck and chest. We refer to this sign in regard to the psychosomatic postulates (p. 62) because not only may it be an indication of general tension but it may serve as an index to a specific problem that is disturbing the patient.

Itching without an eruption is a frequent syptom of emotional origin and as already indicated is often localized in the anal and genital regions. Patients will sometimes volunteer that the itching is so intense that they scratch "until they bleed." Less readily volunteered and therefore all the more significant is the information that sometimes orgasm occurs in connection with such scratching. While allergic factors seem more important in acute attacks of urticaria, chronic urticaria must be approached as a psychosomatic disorder.

Loss of hair, as in alopecia areata, is a common symptom of psychosomatic disorders, and overgrowth of hair, especially on the face, arms, and legs also occurs in periods of psychoneurotic disturbances. Such disorders will need differentiation from endocrine disturbances.

Seborrheic eczema of the ear, scalp, and nape of the neck often has an emotional component. Occurring as a chronic lesion in later life it is sometimes associated with acute flare-ups which involve other portions of the body. The so-called dysidroses, dermatitic or eczematoid eruptions of the hands, apparently occur in response to psychogenic factors. The emotional aspects of acne are important, but caution must be observed in subjecting young people to psychological study.

Again we must repeat that we do not think of the psychic factor as sole cause but only as one of the multiple factors in the development of these various skin disorders.

The Past Medical History

Infancy. *Birth.* Many questions regarding birth and the early infancy period cannot, of course, be answered by the patient. Sometimes the family can help to give a picture which is assuming more and more importance in personality development, that is, the first year of life. If an infant starts out as a fretful child with a feeding problem it is often so badly handicapped that the personality carries the traumatic experience as a focal conflict ready to be relighted when the experiences of adult life make their impacts.

A normal labor and a normal nursing experience in an atmosphere that provides emotional as well as physical security is probably the best insurance against psychosomatic problems later in life.

Nursing Experience. More and more we hear of the importance of a normal nursing experience from child psychiatrists. It has not been fashionable in recent years to feed babies at the breast but there is no satisfactory substitute. The formula may not differ very much but the emotional content cannot be the same. A rigid feeding schedule and a hard weaning experience frequently establish the background for functional gastrointestinal disorders.

Feeding Problems. Feeding problems are probably never entirely overcome. This statement will seem exaggerated when we think of the numerous individuals who had feeding problems in early life, changed over in adolescence and ate like gluttons to become fat and apparently very healthy people. But the difficulties of the feeding problem remain deeply ingrained in the personality and may reflect themselves in various subtle ways—if not directly in gastrointestinal symptoms later in life, then often in disturbances in character development which interfere with success and happiness.

Training Problems. Just as bottle feeding has been popular in recent years so has the effort to train children for bowel and bladder control at a very early age. As we will discuss elsewhere this often has its repercussions. A good rule to follow is for the child to receive information and training as its intellect is prepared for such information and discipline. Rarely does this happen before the second year. Frequently the story will be obtained of early training which breaks down when a new sibling appears. This regression often sets the pattern for other regressive behavior later in life.

Diseases. The various diseases of early life should be enumerated and an effort be made to judge the behavior of the individual at the time. Frequently illnesses that required much medical attention and sometimes surgical intervention, such as ear infections and tonsillectomy, are traumatic experiences followed by neurotic behavior. Tonsillectomy in early life, which we have always regarded so lightly, has been found to have considerable importance from the standpoint of the psychological development (Levy).

Childhood. It is always well to inquire whether the child was frail or strong because this will often give a clue as to the amount of care with which he was surrounded. A frail child will frequently be overprotected, surrounded with unusual care, making for dependency and passivity trends, while the robust child will be allowed to develop in a normal manner without pathological solicitude on the part of the parents.

The various diseases, operations, and injuries that occur in later childhood can be regarded from a psychological standpoint in the same way as in early childhood although the individual is usually better prepared because of his intellectual and emotional maturity to deal with these traumatic experiences.

Frequently during this period behavior which is considered normal for the small child will be remarked upon, for example, thumb-sucking, nail-biting, bed-wetting, nightmares, fears, tantrums, and masturbation. Parents and physicians often regard these matters as trivial—"the child will grow out of them" but they may represent the prototype of serious psychosomatic disturbances later in life. It is true that to a limited extent any one of these "bad habits" can be regarded as a normal part of childhood. It is when the symptom is excessive, persists for a long time, or is associated with other habits, that it becomes significant.

Questions regarding the kind of sexual education that the individual has had from its parents will frequently permit discussion of masturbation with the guilt and false ideas that are so commonly associated and that may be so distressing to the patient. We are so careful to rear our children in the proper intellectual atmosphere yet we make such serious errors in allowing their emotional education to proceed by chance. Sexual experiences of early life are very common and often serve as important screen memories for serious disturbances in personality development. In discussing sexual education or the lack of it we can often encourage the patient to talk further about his sexual development, thus providing helpful information about his behavior in adult life.

It is also during this period that questions regarding the social development may be informative. The shy child who keeps to himself and reads books instead of engaging in games is the kind of personality that often has difficulties in adult life. Even when he overcomes shyness in later years the emotional difficulty often remains within the personality to cause psychosomatic troubles. Socially poised and affable, such a person may nevertheless reflect his anxiety in the gastrointestinal tract.

It is also during this period—as the individual enters his school life—that questions regarding the social development will reveal the kind of person who adjusts well in later life or remains badly adjusted and susceptible to psychosomatic illness.

Adolescence.   Puberty and adolescence mark an important period of psychosexual development. Some of the difficulties of early life may disappear as the individual attains a better state of emotional adjustment but again many of the problems of early life are rekindled in this period. Again and again it will be found that the disorders of later life have their beginning in the adolescent period although this may be established only after repeated interviews. It is not infrequent for an illness to appear just after an individual has overcome masturbation, which had been serving as an outlet for tension of emotional origin.

A history of "anemia," for which the patient received iron, or a period of a "near-breakdown," or a questionable diagnosis of chorea, are not unusual as the early evidences of a neurotic or a psychosomatic complaint.   Bizarre behavior to which at first little attention is paid may mark the beginnings of serious mental disease.

Pain in the side in young girls is often the starting point of chronic invalidism, as we shall demonstrate by numerous case reports. Often the first conflicts that have to do with developing sexuality reflect themselves as a pain in the right side of the abdomen; then comes the diagnosis of chronic appendicitis, followed by operation. Unfortunately for the science of psychosomatic medicine the operation often does bring about relief as far as that particular pain is concerned. But the cause of the pain remains within the spirit of the individual and shows itself in another aspect of his behavior or in the production of other symptoms. Sometimes, of course, the pain is not relieved and then come operations for adhesions, followed by "polysurgical addiction" and chronic invalidism.

The beginnings of *menstruation* and the surrounding circumstances will often give important clues to the sexual development of later life. Dsymenorrhea may be first established in adolescence and may continue until the patient has had her first child. This early history, significant in regard to the emotional development, is sometimes neglected in dealing with women in their later years.

Religious conflicts, marked disturbances in parent-child relationships, and school difficulties can occur in the adolescent period and indicate emotional maladjustment that may reassert itself later in life. Questions regarding social adjustment must, of course, take account of the normal social difficulties of this period.

The work life often begins during the adolescent period and conflicts surrounding this, such as rebellion against authority, usually having to do with the influence of the parents, or sibling rivalry, are often important as precipitating factors for psychosomatic illness.

The diseases of adolescence such as tuberculosis, venereal disease, chorea, rheumatic fever, and reactions to injuries of this period, are important in relation to the emotional health.

Adulthood. Diseases, operations, and injuries assume great importance in adult life either as psychosomatic disorders or disorders with psychosomatic implications. Mention has already been made of the events leading up to operation or illness and here reference should also be made to accident-proneness, a subject to which Dunbar has made important contributions.

The *work history* will often give important clues to maladjustment because people, without realizing it, carry over in their relation to authoritative figures the attitudes which they had toward parents or siblings in early life. Thus it is that the beginnings of psychosomatic illness often will be found in conflicts surrounding work. Questions of prestige and financial reward, as well as jealousies toward other workers, are problems that frequently seem to precipitate illness.

So often we hear from patients who have illness of psychosomatic origin that they realize that "overwork is responsible." Our answer is that it is possible to work oneself into a state of illness but that the rule is "overwork plus emotional conflict." Moreover, the overwork in itself may represent the individual's effort to deal with his inner conflicts. Frequently the story is that he works hard but is in conflict with his superior or other people at work or at home, and this wear and tear plus the overwork brings about fatigue and other symptoms. Patients often will at first deny the conflict, as one of our patients with hypertension and headache who blamed his troubles on overwork and then in response to our suggestion regarding a personal problem admitted that his boss was the kind of person who said, "Now this is your department, run it" but then did not permit him to! "Burned up" inwardly, he had to "take it" with a smile.

When the family history is completed it is often expedient to inquire regarding the patient's *marital history*. Aside from the routine questions about when the patient married (year and age), number of children and their names, ages, health and emotional status, and the age and health of the *spouse*, inquiries regarding the family of the spouse, where they live, and hints as to their relation to the patient, may be obtained. Incidentally, it must not be forgotten that neurotics have a way of attracting one another and if their neuroses fit together the marriage may be successful.

Broken homes furnish soil for psychosomatic illness. The age of the patient at the time the parents separated is important but it is well to remember that long years of incompatibility probably preceded the separation.

The question of marriage is one of the most important subjects to be investigated in relation to psychosomatic illness. Marriage is an emotional hurdle that brings about illness in a great many maladjusted people. Moreover, it is almost axiomatic that the emotional maladjustment of one individual is reflected in the personality of the marital partner. As said before, neurotics have a way of attracting one another and very often their conflicts fit together like lock and key. Therefore, while it is important to inquire and derive as much information as possible about the marriage relationship it is extremely unwise to try any superficial remedies for marital maladjustment. To listen and not to talk is the best piece of advice in regard to marital situations and the same applies to matters concerning extramarital relationships, separation, and divorce. How often do physicians recommend marriage and parenthood to maladjusted people as a cure for their emotional problems! Not only does this "cure" fail but it often provides the background for additional neurotic and psychosomatic problems in the offspring. One should be extremely cautious about giving advice on the highly charged emotional problems of marriage.

Menopause has always been an important subject from an emotional standpoint and the climacteric is beginning to assume the same importance in men. One of the most frequent questions asked the physician by the woman with a psychosomatic disorder is, "Is this the beginning of the menopause?" and it doesn't make much difference what the age of the individual is because the concern may start in the thirties and the same problem continues into later adult life. Now we are beginning to hear exactly the same question in regard to men, "Is this the change of life?" and so often in regard to both, physicians are in part responsible. When a symptom is not readily explained the physician often hints that it may be the menopause. This also provides an easy if not very satisfactory solution, that is, injections of estrogen for the woman and testosterone for the man. What is so often not realized is that the responsibilities and disappointments of middle adult life have much to do with the appearance of symptoms that are attributed to ovarian or testicular failure.

While this problem—how much is hormonal and how much psychological—can be worked out with considerable accuracy in the woman, easily performed tests are not yet available for the man and, as a consequence, we are at the height of the exploitation of this subject in regard to men and their disorders of middle life. It is undoubtedly true that men do present a syndrome dependent upon testicular failure, which can be referred to as the male climacteric; still it can safely be said that most men who present such symptoms are really suffering from disorders that are primarily emotional in origin. They are in greater need of psychological understanding than of injections of testosterone.

Maladjusted people often seek their emotional satisfaction in the lives of their children. Just as the spouse frequently mirrors the emotional difficulties of the partner, so do the children of patients who present psychosomatic ailments frequently show a high degree of maladjustment and psychosomatic illness.

Feelings of inadequacy because of the failure to have children, or of guilt because of induced abortions, are often responsible for illness. Questions regarding the children, living and dead, including miscarriages and abortions, are of great importance to the psychosomatic history.

Childless couples who say that they were not very much interested in having a child or who made only slight effort to discover the cause of sterility are also very often emotionally immature people. The bachelor and, perhaps to a lesser extent, the spinster have been unable to make a satisfactory choice of mate, sometimes to be sure because of fate or circumstance but very often because of emotional difficulties. Next in order comes the childless couple who have achieved the hurdle of marriage but are unequal to the responsibility of having children. Then comes the couple with one child who felt the responsibility of the child so keenly that they were unwilling to have a larger family. It must be understood that in all of these examples there may be extenuating circumstances that nullify what has been said.

Interests, hobbies, recreations, and habits may next be inquired into. The individual who is all work and no play is often preparing the way for emotional bankruptcy which may leave him with a psychosomatic illness. On the other hand, the very "successful" person who indulges in all kinds of community activities may nevertheless be a maladjusted person, neglectful in regard to the emotional development of his or her children, while seeking an unsatisfactory solution for an emotional problem. So often patients refer with envy to the "successful" lives of these busy people little realizing what problems this "busyness" may be trying to solve.

Patients often inquire regarding hobbies, wanting a suggestion from the physician. While a suggestion is sometimes helpful, for the most part people who have the capacity to do so will find their own hobbies and the individual who can readily lose himself in avocation or recreation is indeed fortunate. Again and again we see people in whom it is obvious that this is the saving grace that prevented emotional illness.

Patients with illness of psychosomatic origin will frequently retire from many of life's activities, circumscribing and impoverishing their lives. Physicians frequently add to this problem by recommending rest to regain health. "Go home and take it easy" is probably the most frequent piece of advice in the practice of medicine. For illness of emotional origin this kind of advice is rarely if ever helpful because people do not get well by resting nor can they run away from themselves on vacation. To rest is often "to stew in their own juices" and while vacation may provide temporary help by removing them from people to whom they are "allergic," just as often it fails to take them away from the problem because they carry the conflict within themselves. It is true that when people use up energy in emotional conflict they have less left for social and work purposes but they must be made to understand that it is not rest which provides the answer but rather an effort so solve their problem.

The question of *weight* is important in regard to the psychosomatic history. Marked weight loss always makes one think of organic disease but of course it may happen for emotional reasons. A striking example is anorexia nervosa in which the individual may be reduced to skin and bones. But it is also not uncommon for people to gain weight during illness of emotional origin. "Nervous hunger," which people frequently describe as a *void* in the pit of the stomach which they try to satisfy by eating, often results in weight gain even though the patient is complaining most during that period. Obesity in itself is frequently a psychosomatic problem or has important psychosomatic implications and a weight chart can often be correlated with a chart of the life situation.

Dietary habits are important in other respects. They sometimes reflect the atmosphere of the home in which the individual was raised and suggest the amount of emphasis placed on eating and bowel habits. Constipation often has its earliest origins in childhood when the overanxious mother creates anxiety in the child regarding the kind of food and regularity of the stool.

One must never neglect to inquire regarding *sleep* because insomnia or disturbances in the sleep pattern may sometimes be one of the few clues in regard to a psychosomatic disorder. The taking of sedatives has been widely commented upon in medical and lay publications and it does seem that the barbiturates are almost as much abused as laxatives in the lives of our patients. Just as people addicted to the laxative and enema habit are apt to have illness of psychosomatic origin so people who regularly take sedatives may be placed in the same category. Poor sleep is invariably (except in the presence of grave organic disease) an indication of emotional disturbance just as nail-biting is an invariable indication of anxiety of considerable degree within the personality.

The abuse of *tobacco* is also frequent in patients with psychosomatic disorders and, of course, addiction to *alcohol* and *drugs* is even more significant of psychological disturbance. The question where social drinking leaves off and drinking to combat pathological anxiety begins is sometimes hard to decide but the real dipsomaniac is not hard to recognize. In reference to the spouse as a clue to neurotic complaints the wife of an alcoholic is frequently as easily recognized as the patient himself. She complains bitterly or assumes an air of quiet martyrdom but continues to suffer in spite of her repeated threats to leave.

But it may also be significant when people completely avoid tobacco and alcohol. Their sensitiveness and overcautious attitude are indications that they may carry the seeds of neurotic disorder within their personalities.

Family History

Probably the family history is the most important part of the psychosomatic history. Certainly it is the area in which the psychosomatic history differs most from the usual medical history. But again this is only in regard to emphasis and detail.

Simple questions, such as, "Who lives at home?" often provide the way for a great deal of information about the day-by-day activities of the patient and uncover many areas of tension that would ordinarily go unnoticed. One must often subject the family group to microscopic examination for sources of friction in the same way that the dentist systematically examines the teeth for defects. People frequently have sources of tension in their lives that they do not realize and cannot tell about in direct questioning but which come out as one surveys their life situation and gets to know the pattern of their day-by-day living. *Since it is usually the family group who harbor the emotional tensions out of which the patient's illness has developed it is very important to establish the relation of the patient to his family and to know the details about the family background.*

Parents. Age and cause of death of parents are usually noted but rarely such important factors as the age of the patient at the time of the parent's death, the patient's reaction to the death, the circumstances surrounding the death of the parent, and the anniversary of the death which often unconsciously produces a reaction years later in the patient. The question of any family conflicts following upon the death of a parent, for example, settling of the estate, and responsibilities developing upon the patient as a result of the death, are likewise important. As we learn to sharpen our observations of how the patient reacts to the medical interview one can get some idea, in the very way that the patient speaks about the parents, of conflicts that are important to him in his relationships to other people.

Siblings. Then one can discuss the siblings, noting them down in the order of their appearance, their names and ages, those who died as well as those who are alive, their health, marital status, emotional stability, where they live, getting hints about their relationship to the patient. Other people who came in contact with the patient early in life, such as grandparents who lived in the household, and other relatives and friends, may play an important part and just as we are eager to know who constitutes the household in which the patient now resides, so do we want to know the members of the household in which he lived as a child.

Family history, remote as well as close, is important in regard to various diseases and especially the emotional stability and here one often encounters a good deal of resistance on the part of the patients. They are unwilling to confess to the "stigma" of mental and nervous illness. Frequently the use of the term "nervous breakdown" will serve better in an inquiry regarding the emotional health of the family. If one member of a family is unstable the others are apt to show some instability, so that a history of mental or nervous illness, psychosomatic symptoms, a number of divorces, alcoholism, vagabondism, or peculiar behavior in the siblings or other blood relatives may be helpful in establishing the diagnosis in regard to the patient.

The Summing Up

In some instances the procedure may be varied and as the history nears completion one may stop for a moment and review the various systems, making certain that no important symptoms have been overlooked. Sometimes this part of the review can best be done while examining the patient because as the systematic physical examination proceeds one can inquire for symptoms regarding the parts examined.

DIAGNOSTIC AIDS

Casual Remarks

One of the most important points in the taking of the psychosomatic history is to be aware of the importance of asides and apparent irrelevancies because so frequently important clues are obtained in this fashion. Much anxiety may be hidden behind laughter and jokes. The middle-aged man who with a laugh "guesses that he's cracking up" is often referring to his anxiety regarding his potency and future usefulness and the middle-aged woman with her half-expressed anxiety regarding the imminence of menopause is anticipating the end of her femininity. The fear of cancer is often expressed, not at the beginning, but at the end of the interview. When the patient is informed that she has no organic disease she allows us to know how deeply she feared cancer. Apparently casual remarks, made when the more formal part of the interview is over, often express the real motive for the consultation and indicate the problem that really concerns the patient. Women in conflict over the question of having a child, or another child, frequently do not express this concern directly but introduce it casually after talking about seemingly unrelated matters.

The Patient's Ideas of the Illness

In concluding a history or after one has had an opportunity to see a patient on several occasions and has pretty well concluded the study it is always wise to ask "What have you thought about the cause of your disorder?" One is often amazed at the ideas that people have about the cause and mechanism of their illness and, quite aside from getting out the important question of fear of cancer or fear of some other serious organic disease, one sometimes can deal effectively with distorted ideas that the patient has had, some of which he has arrived at on his own and others which have been furnished to him, often inadvertently, by the physicians whom he has seen. It is impossible to make progress toward an understanding of the patient's illness until some of these distorted ideas are dealt with. They are the first rationalizations of anxiety. It is not uncommon for a patient who has had an idea regarding ulcer, cancer, heart disease, or "stroke," to accept reassurance but to hold in reserve the thought, "but if this condition continues I may develop such a disease." Consequently we often say, "You have no evidence of organic disease nor is there any indication that you will develop it."

At the same time in many patients it may be necessary to give reassurance as to the absence of any mental disease. Frequently the patient stammers out his gratitude because he has been greatly concerned about such things as cancer, heart disease, or losing his mind but has not dared to say so. This reassurance will go a long way toward making him feel better and at the same time it prepares the way for informing the patient that what he really suffers from is a disorder of his *feelings* rather than a disease of his body or mind. Then one can say that in order to confirm this opinion, certain tests should be made, arrange for them to be done, and make the next appointment, sometimes prescribing—with an explanation of what the medicine is for—sometimes postponing prescription until one knows more about the situation. It is important for the patient to realize that he is not a unique or peculiar person—that there are thousands of people who present exactly the same kind of a problem. Patients like this often imagine themselves peculiar or "different" and have a feeling of isolation. To realize that they are not unique is often very helpful to them.

Such patients are often told by well-meaning friends and physicians that they "must snap out of it" but that advice accomplishes nothing.

The War Department issued a pamphlet "What's the Score in a Case Like Mine?" to men discharged from the service because of psychoneurosis. It is a simple statement, admirable for the purpose, and ought to be useful in civil practice.

Dreams as Diagnostic Aids

One of the very great contributions made by Freud was the utilization of the dream as a means of helping the patient to understand the workings of the unconscious mind.

The dream represents the secretion of the mental apparatus and can be analyzed for diagnostic and prognostic, as well as psychotherapeutic purposes, in the same way that the urine, the secretion of the kidneys, can be analyzed for diagnostic and prognostic purposes. One must have considerable training in psychodynamics, however, before much use can be made of dream material. Interpretation requires much experience on the part of the physician and cooperation in giving associations on the part of the patient. Certain indications may be very obvious. For example, the woman who finds no interest in sexual matters but who dreams repeatedly of sexual advances by men, like the old maid who looks under the bed, is readily recognized as being more preoccupied with sexual fantasies than she thinks. Repetitive dreams have special significance and often indicate a definite personality trend. The "peace loving" person who constantly dreams of arguments and fights may be helped to recognize that there is a good deal of aggression in his make-up which he has not adequately expressed. And so it is with such dreams as those dealing with the death of relatives or friends, dreams of frustration, and dreams of semi-nudity—all may point the way toward definite conflicts in the unconscious mental life of the individual.

In experienced hands the dream can often be utilized to throw light upon the doctor-patient relationship and thus can render great assistance in helping the patient to understand his feelings. We must caution, however, that the dream is the royal road to the unconscious and that clumsy efforts to interpret may do more harm than good. A standard rule in psychotherapy is not to give information to the patient before he is prepared to take it and this is especially applicable to dream material.

Psychological Testing

Psychological tests formerly had to do only with intelligence but in the last decade, and especially as a result of psychiatric experience in World War II, psychological testing has become an integral part of personality study. While many tests have been devised, it is generally felt that no one test is adequate for total personality appraisal. An analogy might very well be made to the various tests that are used in laboratory medicine: Rarely does one test suffice for evaluating the total function of an organ. A great many tests, for example, have been devised for measuring kidney function; after long experience clinicians have pretty well agreed on a few, comprising a battery of tests, which in combination give a satisfactory pattern of measurements. The same thing is true of psychological testing for diagnostic and prognostic purposes. Question and answer technics such as the Cornell index (p. 104) have been found useful for screening purposes, that is, for a simple test, quickly performed, which permits one to say whether an individual shows evidence of gross disturbance of personality so that further study may be made if indicated. Certain so-called projective tests, such as the Rorschach method, which tries to bring to expression the psychological structure of the subject without investigating historical antecedents, have been found of great value in the more detailed evaluation of the personality.

Of all methods these two have been most widely used in the study of psychosomatic problems.

Rorschach Test. The name Rorschach is derived from the man who originated the test and pioneered in its development. Usually it requires about an hour to administer, and even a longer time to interpret. The test consists of ten bilaterally symmetrical, meaningless ink blots on cards which are presented one at a time to the patient who is asked to tell what they represent to him or what he sees in them. Half of the cards are black and white and half of them have color. The responses and comments when evaluated offer a remarkably accurate means of gaining information about the patient's reactions in terms of intellectual capacity, emotional control, quantity and quality of instinctual drive, special topics of conflict, and the manner of approach to various problems.

There are teaching centers in various parts of the country for instruction in the use and further development of the test. Both special training and considerable practice are necessary in order to use it skilfully. It has already proved of value in the differential diagnosis of psychotic and neurotic conditions since it shows the basic personality pattern, and its further usefulness is being constantly developed. The Rorschach test is also thought to be of value in helping to determine the lines along which the interest and activities of feebleminded and borderline cases should be directed.

In the field of psychosomatic medicine it should prove helpful in determining whether the personality pattern is closer to neurosis or psychosis, since very often a refractory case of psychosomatic illness is a masked psychosis. Moreover, since it measures the degree of affective control it should help us to be aware of energies which are not being utilized either socially or in work but are being dammed up or finding an outlet in a disturbance of the somatic functions. Furthermore, it may show more accurately than a history will reveal, the quality and quantity of instinctual drive which is being held in check. When one finds that a considerable amount of instinctual energy is being inhibited in the presence of psychosomatic disease we should suspect that this energy is playing a part in symptom formation. Hence, the Rorschach test may be useful not only to the psychologist and psychiatrist but also to the physician who is interested to know how misdirected emotional energies may disturb the workings of the body.

Psychosomatic Applications. Harrower used the Rorschach method in a study of the personality changes accompanying cerebral lesions and later reported on certain "neurotic signs" which occurred frequently in a group of clinically diagnosed neurotics and infrequently in the records of control subjects. Although she found nothing pathognomonic of neurosis in any one of the signs taken alone, nevertheless taken together they were of value in differentiating those maladjusted patients whose physical conditions were mainly or entirely due to psychological factors; and they pointed to the basic psychological adjustment of other patients in whom organic lesions, responsible for the symptoms, were later found.

Kemple, who has probably had the largest experience with psychosomatic cases, working with patients in the general medical wards of the Presbyterian Hospital of New York, found that Rorschach study of hospital patients with rheumatic disease, hypertensive cardiovascular disease, coronary occlusion, and fracture shows that certain distinctive personalities are associated with each illness syndrome. Patients with rheumatic disease are characteristically passive, masochistic, instinctively weak and infantile, with an underlying hysteria. Hypertensive patients are more ambitious for power; they have more conscious hostility and they experience a more constant, acute conflict between aggression and their dominant passive, dependence needs. They are more introvertive, less labile and hysterical. Obsessive-compulsive defenses, too, are conspicuous in hypertensive patients, and particularly obsessive doubts.

Patients with coronary occlusion show a distinctive pattern of aggressiveness and compulsive striving for power and prestige. Introvertive experience of creative thought is undeveloped, making them more dependent upon external achievement for satisfaction and security. They are reactive and express considerable hostility.

Fracture patients are divided into three groups: the *introvertive*, the *constricted*, and the *extratensive*, the first two groups showing the highest incidence of accidents. An effort is found among all groups to compromise between passivity and aggression, with a marked emphasis on adaptation, self-determination, independence of authority, and day-to-day pleasures. Personality constriction increases with organic damage. Neurotic conflict is evident in nearly all hospital cases, but the more limited the psychological defense mechanisms, the greater the likelihood of serious physical illness.

The Rorschach method yields no simple pathognomonic signs; a certain illness or propensity for it may be deduced only from the Rorschach picture of the personality as a complex whole. The method has proved its value not only for research, but also for differential diagnosis and for outlining a therapeutic program. Kemple states that the number of cases has not been sufficient in all groups to yield statistical validation but "the trends are unquestionably significant and agreement with the findings of previous research offers additional validity."

Ross has contributed a number of Rorschach studies on psychosomatic problems. His observations on migraine and neurocirculatory asthenia are considered elsewhere in this book under those respective headings.

An interesting consideration of the Rorschach method in regard to hypertension, arthritis, and parkinsonism by Booth indicates that the personality characteristics in chronic arthritis are reflected in some statistical features of the scores, but that this not the case in hypertension. The question then presented itself whether the responses to the ink blots had other aspects than those covered by previous methods of evaluation. Developing gestalt tendencies and kinesthetic responses to the Rorschach scoring system, Booth evolves the interesting concept that significant differences can be established between L (locomotor arthritis, parkinsonism) and V (vascular hypertension) responses, but that they are indicative not of disease but of two different types of human attitudes. In other words, form and functioning of the body, in health as well as in disease, persistently express aspects of the basic personality structure. Booth suggests that the L and V types seem to represent opposite extremes of attitudes required by western cultures; on the one hand the emphasis on competition, on the other the emphasis on the emotional dependency of a protective social environment. The psychological interpretation of the findings suggests to the author that arthritis and parkinsonism patients are dominated by an urge for individualistic, independent action while patients suffering from arterial hypertension have a tendency toward dependent relationships in the form of identification with their social environment.

Specific correlations between organ dominance, disease liability, and a form of perception were discussed, giving added insight into the physiological basis of the Rorschach method and of physiognomical understanding. The study is not only interesting from the standpoint of psychosomatic medicine but it introduces the possibility of further extending the use of the Rorschach method.

Limitations of the Test. While the Rorschach test is the most valuable single test of personality, Rapaport and Schafer state that it does not yield in all cases a definitive diagnosis or a comprehensive description of adjustment or maladjustment, which is to be expected only from a battery of tests. They find that depressions or extreme inhibitions may occur in any clinical syndrome from schizophrenia to hysteria and, by obscuring all indicators, may invalidate the test. "A second limitation is that schizophrenics with 'well-preserved fronts'—usually the paranoids—are often able to go through the test giving a conventional and acceptable set of responses. A third major limitation is that neurotic conditions are frequently indistinguishable from normal adjustments. A hysteric and a very impulsive normal, a depressive and a stereotyped and inhibited normal, an obsessive-compulsive and a ruminative or well-endowed but rigid normal, each of these pairs may give similar test records. These difficulties cannot be met by 'refining' the Rorschach test but only by using it as one of a battery of tests, since they are partly inherent in the limitations of the test and partly in those maladjustment pictures which do not project themselves in Rorschach test responses."

The Cornell Selectee Index. Mittelmann and his associates have devised a simple method of personality evaluation primarily for group study which, however, can be used for the individual. Known as the Cornell Selectee Index it is a self-administered, pencil and paper procedure which can be given to any number of individuals simultaneously. It can be completed in ten minutes and scored within one minute with the use of a simple stencil. The simplicity of this instrument makes it valuable for use in large scale surveys while the information uncovered can be used in orienting the physician giving a psychiatric interview. One must recognize that it will show only gross abnormalities and hence is useful simply as a screen test to decide upon the necessity for further study.

Narcoanalysis and Narcosynthesis. During World War II a psychotherapeutic method utilized by Grinker and Spiegel found great usefulness in the treatment of the emotional problems induced by combat experiences. It consisted of the administration of sodium pentothal intravenously, permitting the patient to relive his battle experiences with a great catharsis of feeling, and this was followed by psychotherapeutic interviews which were often very helpful in relieving the individual and permitting his return to duty. Similar methods, using sodium amytal, had previously been tried in civil practice (Horsley) and have been used to some extent for diagnostic and treatment purposes since the war.

Ripley and Wolf from an experience with 500 patients with bodily disturbances, believed to be related to problems of personality adjustment, found the method useful in distinguishing between irreversible, structurally determined disorders and functional disorders of organ systems; in differentiating neurosis and malingering; and in the study of significant situational conflicts. Sodium amytal (0.1-0.8 gm.) was used and no serious complications were encountered. The drug also proved useful in evaluating defects upon which were superimposed functional disabilities related to situational conflicts. In such conditions as migraine, asthma, hypertension, and nasal disturbances, signs and symptoms often disappeared after injection, only to be exacerbated when discussion touched on points involving emotional conflict.

Patients with pains of undertermined mechanism, notably in back or abdomen, comprised the largest group successfully managed with aid of sodium amytal. Most suitable subjects for narcoanalysis were those with disorders of personality adjustment of relatively short duration. The drug was less effective in diagnosis and treatment of subjects with rigid personalities and long-standing patterns of disability. As a therapeutic agent, sodium amytal in no sense acts specifically or automatically. Temporary symptomatic improvement must be followed up with further psychotherapy.

For a variety of reasons this technic is not ideally adapted to office practice. There is some danger in the intravenous administration of a barbiturate without anesthetic equipment (oxygen) and there is always the question whether a person should be wholly or partly deprived of consciousness in a psychiatric interview unless a third person is present, and this violates a fundamental rule in psychological study. The method would not seem to hold the same promise in civil practice, which deals with problems usually related to the whole lifetime experience of the individual and in which multiple traumatic factors have occurred, unlike combat neurosis in which the impact of a single experience was the crucial factor in determining illness. For experimental purposes in hospital and clinic it is possible that information of diagnostic and therapeutic value may come from narcosynthesis but we caution against its indiscriminate use in private practice.

Hypnosis. Much the same may be said about hypnosis, a technic which has been exploited on stage, screen, and radio. However, much serious scientific work has been done from the standpoint of diagnosis and treatment of mental and emotional problems. Hypnosis provides a quick method of influencing the unconscious mental processes in some people and therefore it is conceivable that it might be of diagnostic help in certain psychosomatic problems. It is not recommended for any but the expert.

In general it may be said regarding all tests having to do with personality evaluation that no one of them is the equal of a skillful interview conducted by a well-trained and experienced person. They may, however, furnish valuable corroborative information.

The Forces Which Favor Psychotherapy

In some cases it is difficult for the patient to see the necessity of visiting a physician when he does not get a prescription, an injection, physiotherapy, or an operation. To "just talk about himself" does not seem worth the effort, the time, or the money. There are certain forces, however, which favor psychotherapy. The first is the distress which the patient has been suffering and which has been unrelieved by the application of the traditional medical or surgical therapies. The second is the standing and prestige of the physician who tells him that he needs psychotherapy. The third may be the family, who have a greater belief in the efficiency of psychotherapy than the patient, or who may be tired of putting up with the patient's long-drawn-out illness or distressing personality eccentricities. It must be admitted that resistance to psychotherapy causes many patients to make trials in every other direction and to suffer considerably before they will accept a treatment which calls for a scrutiny of their emotions and their relations to other human beings.

The Wish to Recover. The capacity for psychotherapy can often be judged on the basis of the material which we have discussed but it is especially the individual's wish to get well or the reverse, "the unconscious desire to remain sick" that we must try to evaluate. So often the patient repeats over and over again how eager he is to get well but we recognize that unconscious forces are working in just the opposite direction to perpetuate the illness. In fact, the more the patient complains, the more we may suspect that his "unconscious wish to remain sick" is the force which will exert itself.

Transference reactions which have to do with physician-patient relationships and which we will discuss again are important in evaluating chances for recovery. We have talked about "the good patient" who cooperates but is passively defiant and with whom it is difficult, if not impossible, to bring about recovery. We must also be suspicious of people who on the surface are affable and agreeable and apparently eager to cooperate but who beneath the surface are suspicious and skeptical and really refuse to cooperate.

A rough estimate which every physician is in a position to judge daily is the degree of obsession in regard to a fear such as cancer. Many patients present a fear of cancer as the first layer of their anxiety. If they are relatively well adjusted one can abolish this fear with ease. If they have a higher degree of maladjustment the fear will quickly return or be replaced by another fear.

Age as an Index. One of the most important criteria for recovery is the age of the patient and the length of time that the illness has lasted. If an individual of middle-age has been a semi-invalid, for emotional reasons, for many years, one is less hopeful about the chances of recovery than in a young person with an illness of relatively recent origin. Young people, of course, are more malleable than old. Another estimate of value is the strength of the precipitating force. If an illness appears for a relatively trivial reason and then maintains itself it is apt to be more serious from a prognostic standpoint than an illness which appears only under great stress and then lessens as the individual makes some spontaneous recovery. It is a question of the degree of predisposition and the impact of the environmental situation. If the individual was relatively well adjusted, as many of the men in military service were, and then met an extraordinary situation he broke down but recovered on return to civil life. On the contrary, a sensitive individual with a marked neurotic pattern to his personality may break down with psychosomatic illness for reasons that may seem to be trivial.

Intelligence. One often hears patients say "But Doctor, I ought to be intelligent enough to handle this problem." Unfortunately it is not so much a matter of intelligence as of feelings. *The will and the intellect are really weak instruments compared to the emotions.* When the emotions are involved, intelligence flies out of the window. In other words, the intellect has very little to do with these problems and therefore while it is a tool with which we must work in understanding and helping these patients it is not a matter of first consideration in judging their capacity to recover. One need not be gifted intellectually in order for psychotherapy to be done. If the intelligence is normal or near normal one may work with such people. Of course, a subnormal intelligence makes the approach difficult, if not impossible.

Gain from Illness. The amount of emotional satisfaction permitted by the illness, in other words, what the patient gains from the illness, is a matter of great importance in assessing the capacity for recovery. Sometimes we must recognize that the illness is the best answer to the problem. Patients who have lived the better part of their lives, especially when they are so situated in relation to a marital or business problem that a realization of their short-comings might prove disastrous, had better not be disturbed by efforts to show a relationship between symptoms and life situation. Under such circumstances reassurance and supportive therapy are indicated rather than efforts to make the patient aware of his emotional problems. In other words, we must judge not only the ability but the capacity of the patient to face himself.

Importance of Physical Examination

As indicated in the history-taking and examination outline, physical examinations in psychosomatic illness must be fully as painstaking and thorough as when physical disease only is suspected. It must never be forgotten that the neurotic personality may develop a physical disease. If anything, physical examination may need to be more inclusive for psychosomatic illness, owing to the fact that an important symptom in psychosomatic conditions is doubt and distrust. Consequently, as the treatment gets under way and the patient resists having the emotional pain underlying his symptoms uncovered, he may question whether the physical examination was adequate enough to rule out a physical cause for his symptoms. The physician must be in a position to show that the physical examination was complete and thorough. Laboratory studies are usually indicated, with x-ray studies if necessary, and if symptoms are referable to the nervous system neurological and supplementary examinations are necessary.

EVALUATION OF THE FINDINGS

An intelligent and critical evaluation of the findings is one of the most important procedures in the management of psychosomatic illness. When there are evidences of personality disturbance and the diagnostic study rules out physical disease, or establishes how much of the problem is physical and how much is psychological and the relation between the two, then there should be no hesitancy in laying the problem before the patient. It is remarkable how many otherwise excellent physicians will postpone or delay such an evaluation of the illness or perhaps never come to a definite conclusion. Not only will the patient be benefited but the physician will add to his own reputation and enhance the prestige of medicine if he will cultivate the psychosomatic approach in his dealings with patients.

Chapter IV

TREATMENT—GENERAL PRINCIPLES OF PSYCHOTHERAPY

A point of view which we have tried to stress is that, for the most part, psychotherapy is necessary because our educational processes are confined to the intellect. In other words, our children receive scientific management from an intellectual standpoint, but for a variety of reasons —mainly constitutional and family influences—the emotional growth is stunted. It is the retarded emotional development which is fundamentally responsible for psychosomatic illness. In other words, if the intellectual age and the emotional age differ sharply, the background for illness of psychological origin exists. One might go further to say that man has four ages, first, his *chronologic age;* second, his *physical age;* third, his *intellectual age;* and fourth, his *emotional age.* For example, one can easily think of an adult who is chronologically forty, physically fifty, intellectually twelve, and emotionally only five. And it might be said that if these various ages are in harmony he is apt to be well and if they are in disharmony, he is apt to be ill. Such persons, and the world is full of them, furnish the soil for the development of psychosomatic illness. Psychotherapy, then, is a process which aims to bring about reeducation of the emotions and the psychosomatic approach takes cognizance of all factors—physical, intellectual, and emotional—in preparation for comprehensive medical care.

Emotional Growth Is Painful

But now our first difficulty enters. Emotional maladjustments are regarded by the world at large as evidences of weakness. Hence, the patient who is told by his physician that "the illness is emotional in origin" often feels that he is accused of being a weakling. In spite of the great discoveries of Freud, now more than forty years ago, the *will* is still looked upon as a supreme instrument which should control such weaknesses. By this time, it ought to be common knowledge, certainly in medical circles, that strong forces of unconscious mental origin control our behavior, including the workings of our organs, and that these forces are beyond the influence of the *will.* Therefore, the patient who is to accept the advice that he needs psychotherapy must accept the fact that while his *will* is strong and his *mind* is normal, nevertheless he does need help as far as his *emotions* are concerned, and that he cannot be expected to do this for himself any more than he could be expected to deal with his own inflamed appendix. He must consult someone who is in a position to help him readjust his emotional life.

The average patient with a pain does not need to be convinced by a physician in whom he has confidence of the necessity for a drug, physical therapy, or even an operation. But he often is unconvinced of the necessity for readjustment of the way he thinks, feels, and acts. The latter prescription is a threat to his pride and a challenge to the integrity of his personality. Physicians should be quite aware of this, as only then will they best be able to deal with their own as well as the patients' resistances to the implications that lie in the term psychotherapy. If psychotherapy is regarded as a process which attempts to influence the emotions and intellect to act in a more harmonious manner then we may recognize that it is as old as the art of healing itself. But only in the last fifty years have we had a scientific psychotherapy, a means of letting the patient know his inner needs and conflicts and of helping him to do something about them. The "rest cure" so widely popularized by S. Weir Mitchell just before the turn of the century consisted of putting the patient to bed at home or preferably in a sanitarium and seeing to it that he, or more often she, was well nursed and well fed. Essentially it was an outgrowth of the organic (neurologic) tradition and represented an attempt to cover the "twittering nerves" with a layer of fat. Such a retreat from responsibilities, authorized by the physician, often did succeed in reducing anxiety, and the nursing care and good food was welcomed by the individual's oral needs and feelings of dependency. A sea voyage, or a vacation in another climate often accomplished the same thing. Hypnotism, placebos, and electricity were used for their suggestive effect. Their use implied that a strengthening force was being introduced which would support an ego weak in structure and faltering under the strain of conflict. The physician sometimes understood what he was doing—more often he did not—and the patient, of course, understood nothing of what was happening in the "cure." Improvement was temporary and relapse occurred sooner or later when the individual returned to his former way of life.

To procure any permanent benefit the patient must be made conscious of the emotional conflicts within himself and must be helped to bring the forces which are in conflict into a more harmonious relationship. Thus an "uncovering" rather than a "covering up" psychotherapy, if indeed the latter can be dignified by that term, is much to be preferred and in the majority of patients this should be possible. It represents an effort to achieve emotional growth but *it must be recognized that emotional growth is always painful.*

Emphasis on Organic Disease

We have suggested that most physicians emphasize soma at the expense of psyche in psychosomatic illness. Several reasons have been given. *First*, the physician usually has been trained almost entirely to think of illness and disease as produced by bacteria, toxins, chemical agents, trauma, or other physical agents. He has had very little training in emotional factors as a cause of somatic dysfunction and disease. *Second*, even if he has received some instruction concerning the production of symptoms by way of the emotions he is always obsessed with the fear that he may overlook something organic which might show up in time. *Third*, he is afraid that his patient may resent a diagnosis which carries with it the implications discussed above, namely an emotional or personality weakness. So he remains on safe ground and treats symptoms, which he may suspect are of emotional origin, by the more traditional methods, comforting himself with the thought that no harm will come. That harm may be done will be demonstrated many times in the chapters to follow. *Finally*, he avoids being bothered with the tedious effort of psychotherapy and the acceptance of the responsibility that goes with it.

The Personality of the Physician

This brings us to the question of the personality of the physician himself—not only his understanding of disease but his attitudes toward the behavior of sick people. The physician who is to be successful in the diagnosis and treatment of psychosomatic illness must have a real interest in human beings as well as in human disease. To a certain extent he must identify himself with the emotional pain from which his patient suffers. There are many physicians who cannot do this. Their personalities do not permit them to understand or sympathize with suffering of emotional origin. They must get quick results and if this is not possible they do not encourage the patient to remain under their care. Such physicians ought to know themselves well enough to see to it that the patient will get to someone who will undertake the care of these problems. What happens, however, is that the physician often errs in ways already indicated. Either he does not make a correct diagnosis or he does not tell his patient straightforwardly the diagnosis he has made. He treats him medically or surgically, or, sensing the patient's personality immaturities, he may criticize him for his inadequate adjustment to life in such a way that the patient is bound to leave him. Then drifting aimlessly the patient often ends in the hands of some charlatan or, at best, in the hands of some well-meaning but incompetent person on the fringe of scientific medical practice.

We repeat that the physician who is qualified to understand and treat psychosomatic illness must not only know disease but he must also be interested in people as human beings. To put it another way, he must have as much interest in psychopathology as he has in tissue pathology. He must be one to whom the patient feels that he can reveal himself. He must have great tolerance for human foibles. He must have an open mind for all the possibilities of the effect of an idea, and its charge of emotion, upon the body as a whole or any of its parts. He must be flexible in personality and he must be willing to believe that the safe ground of accepted knowledge, often called common sense, is sometimes made up of prejudices.

Goethe said, "To the man of thought almost nothing is really ridiculous." Just because the physician does not vomit at the sight of blood he should not assume that others might not do so nor should he be intolerant of them if that is their symptom. Just because the physician himself has never known the pain and resentment of having spent his developing years with a hostile and dominating mother does not mean that he should not try to understand its effects as they appear upon someone else. It is often true that workers in psychological medicine, who are doing the most to show the relation between the emotions and body changes, are prone to overemphasize their findings. But their enthusiasm for establishing truth as quickly as possible in this new field must be met with tolerance on the part of their colleagues since their science is young and rules are not well fixed. Since the beliefs of mankind are always changing we must have the tolerance to test the validity of current ideas in psychosomatic medicine rather than to obstruct progress by condemning those ideas as lacking in common sense.

Preparation for Psychotherapy

If a physician likes people and is interested in their feelings and ideas the patient will soon come to know and feel this. He will be willing to impart his ideas and feelings to this physician. It is then up to the latter to know how to use the patient's verbal and active expressions of himself in order to show the patient the interrelation of his emotional life and his symptoms. After the physician has succeeded in showing him this relationship both patient and physician must come gradually to ignore the symptom and *treat the cause*, which is the personal emotional maladjustment. Before this process can begin, there must be some preparation for psychotherapy. This consists of a careful history, complete physical examination, including laboratory and x-ray studies if necessary, and finally a diagnostic summary and evaluation of the findings and presentation of the problem to the patient.

In the practice of medicine we have learned to treat broken bones and to prevent bacterial diseases, to influence deficiency and degenerative disease, and to remove new growths. Until recently, however, no account was taken of the strain upon the organism of growing up emotionally. The mother always has had to be a good doctor in the sense that she ministered to the pains produced by the infant's needs, to the discomforts of merely being alive and wanting many things, to the necessities of eating, sleeping, digestion, elimination; in other words, to the maintenance of enough serenity in the environment to keep the bodily functions in even balance. Thus the mother's interest, affection, and attention to bodily needs prevent the patterns of anxiety and rage which, if allowed to persist, reach deep into the organism, disturbing bodily functions and influencing even physical development itself.

The physician, as a medical scientist, must include in his studies the influence of the emotions upon healthy body physiology. When the parent has failed in the task of providing the proper degree of physical and emotional security for healthy bodily functioning, the physician must be a parent substitute and attempt to reestablish the physiological rhythms which have become disturbed and distorted. Even when permanent changes have occurred he must try to break up the pattern of disturbed function in an effort to prevent the process from going further.

The Physician as Educator

An important task of the physician as a social scientist is that of teacher as well as healer. Indeed, the original meaning of the word doctor was "teacher." Descartes said, "If ever the human race is to reach its highest practical level intellectually, morally, and physically, the science of medicine will perform that service. " If we accept this compliment and this responsibility we must look upon ourselves from a much broader point of view than as technicians engaged in the mere eradication of disease. The obstetrician has an important job in teaching the pregnant woman not only the physical facts of pregnancy and delivery but also about the child which is to come. He ought to be skilled in family counselling and qualified to teach the father something about his role in the rearing of the child and his contribution to the emotional health of the family group. The pediatrician has much to teach regarding the emotional growth which accompanies the establishment of physiological rhythms as well as to give guidance on achieving cooperation in social development. The gynecologist comes face to face with many questions and conflicts concerning the menstrual function and sexual adjustment; similarly the specialist in genito-urinary work sees many anxieties centered about urinary and sexual functions. Both should be wise in the social and emotional as well as the physical facts of sexuality.

So often the physician hears the appeal of harassed people who have struggled with the handicaps imposed by emotional immaturity, as they beg to be told how to prevent their children from repeating the same patterns of impoverished living. Something can be done for them if the physician accepts the role of educator. It is a hard job but again and again we see the benefits of emotional growth in the parent reflected in a healthier atmosphere for the development of the child.

Moreover, the physician who teaches the patient to take an interest in things outside of himself is teaching him to be a more useful citizen. The world is so much in need of teaching of this kind that to participate in it makes the practice of medicine doubly satisfying. To be both healer and educator is a rare privilege indeed.

PRESENTATION OF THE PROBLEM OF PSYCHOSOMATIC ILLNESS TO THE PATIENT

Presentation of the problem to the patient is not an easy matter. It means conveying to the patient the fact that ideas and feelings are the cause of symptoms, or are contributing to his illness, and this may not be accepted readily. Patients often feel that they are left with something too intangible to be dealt with and, unfortunately, the physician often feels the same. As a matter of fact, in a great many instances, both physician and patient can do more for illness of psychological origin than they can for purely physical disease. But both will have to realize that the personality structure, like the physical structure, is amenable to manipulation. At the present time, for the patient to be told that a feeling of fear or a feeling of disgust is causing him to vomit often leaves him dissatisfied with himself and sometimes with the physician who presents him with this explanation of his illness. This, of course, will depend to a great extent on how the matter is presented but in many instances, no matter how well presented, the implication of a personality which is not strong enough to cope with the environment remains and this may be very distressing to the patient's pride.

The Conversion of Emotion

Frequently, the physician can present the problem by giving some well-known examples of the phenomenon of conversion of emotion; for instance, blushing, sweating, loss of appetite, or frequency of urination. He can say to his patient, in substance, "Just as anyone may in the course of his daily existence show such evidences of the effects of his feelings, so it is in your case, only the feelings are not so obvious to you and the results are longer lasting. Therefore any treatment of the symptom can be only for temporary relief. What we must really treat is the emotional sensitivity and the ideas which are in the background of this illness. It will be a matter of retraining yourself in thinking and feeling toward the circumstances of life and the people around you. This will take some time but it is the only way to bring about a permanent cure." In certain cases we can add, "There will be no medicine except the emotional support which comes from our efforts in working together, plus new knowledge about yourself, and the satisfaction of living more effectually."

Discussion of Personality Disorders

Having made a survey of the life history and symptoms in chronological order one should try to arrive at an exact diagnosis of the personality disorder. This is just as important and just as possible as in the case of physical disorders. The day has come to abolish the habit of labeling a "functional" case as simply neurotic or neurasthenic. We must be able to understand the psychopathological basis of a specific personality disorder and then apply an exact diagnostic term. Treatment will thereby be facilitated, as we hope to show. The disorder usually will fall into one of the accepted classifications of psychoneuroses or psychoses or some combination of one or more of them. The term psychosomatic illness has not yet been exactly defined or generally accepted. Some physicians use the term psychosomatic illness synonymously with psychoneurosis and it is true that psychoneuroses and psychoses are often psychosomatic illnesses. Others restrict its use to disorders such as migraine, essential hypertension, and asthma, in which the vegetative nervous system seems to be fundamentally involved. We use the term in a wide sense to cover not only the physical manifestations of neurotic and psychotic disorders; the diseases of the vegetative nervous system; but also, and most importantly, the great variety of mixtures of psychological and structural disorders which make up the bulk of the practice of medicine.

THE SEVERITY OF THE NEUROSES

In the chapter on Personality Development and Psychopathology it was pointed out that generally speaking the neuroses can be regarded in degrees of severity in the following order:

1. Conversion Hysteria.
2. Neurasthenia.
3. Anxiety Hysteria.
4. Compulsion Neurosis.

Then, if we add the so-called narcissistic neuroses the list would continue:

5. Manic-depressive Psychosis.
6. Schizophrenia.
7. Psychopathic Personalities.

The term "narcissistic neuroses," as contrasted with transference neuroses, means just what the name implies, that persons suffering from these conditions are more self-centered, more indifferent to the feelings and opinions of others, and hence more difficult to influence by personal contact. They live in and for themselves and will often unconsciously seriously injure their bodies or their careers, rather than heed advice. Some even commit suicide or murder rather than yield to the pleas of another individual.

Transference

It is of course not to be assumed that all of the first group have an equal capacity for relating themselves emotionally to others. Certain patients suffering from anxiety hysteria and compulsion neurosis have great difficulty in transferring any "workable" feeling to a physician. They *doubt* the ability or the good will of the physician and continue with their illogical reasoning and behavior. On the other hand, it is not to be assumed that all narcissistic neurotics are absolutely unable to transfer workable emotions to the physician. Some schizophrenics have a capacity for transference. They may have a great deal to learn in order to live more effectively and they may take a long time to learn it, but their capacity for transference may be utilized by physicians who understand the schizophrenic. The manic-depressive personality, usually considered the least malignant of the psychoses, may be much harder to work with therapeutically than the schizophrenic. In spite of the capacity of the manic-depressive for swings to extremes of emotion during illness, between attacks he is often shallow in emotional response, stubborn, and lacking in real warmth.

Psychopathic Personality

Not often do we see the psychopathic personality suffering from physical symptoms of psychological origin. He has worked out his emotional trends in some way other than through visceral response. He may show his hate for authority by forging a check, or may satisfy his need for his mother and his sense of inferiority by alcoholic addiction. The psychopathic personality makes someone else suffer. He himself does not suffer as much as the psychoneurotic. He may even be insensitive to punishment. Society, at some point, always has to absorb the hostility and revenge of the psychopath, be it violently or subtly shown. The psychoneurotic, most psychotics, and those psychosomatically ill, are not as ruthless as the psychopath. They feel the pain of anxiety and guilt and some of their hostility gets turned upon themselves in the form of symptoms.

CONVERSION HYSTERIA

In conversion hysteria, the least severe and most easily curable of the neuroses, the conflicts have occurred at a later period in childhood, relatively speaking, than in the other neuroses. It will be recalled that the symptoms occur rather suddenly and sometimes dramatically, usually in direct time relation with some definite environmental stress. Also there is a greater tendency to modification by suggestion than in any of the other neuroses. In which area or system of the body symptoms may appear is quite unpredictable. The conversion hysteria personality is highly imaginative and passionate. They have been led to expect love and recognition and some degree of physical, sensual gratification and when it is denied them they tend to live out their wishes in symptoms or fantasies. If the latter, they may have to erect strong inhibitions to keep the fantasies from appearing in consciousness. For example, a strong urge to look at something forbidden may result in *hysterical blindness*. The blind eye cannot look and this helps to keep the idea of looking, and the wish to look, repressed. If the patient can be helped to understand his anxiety about forbidden things, usually sexual in nature, and can accept them consciously and deal with them effectively, the symptom no longer is necessary.

CONVERSION HYSTERIA

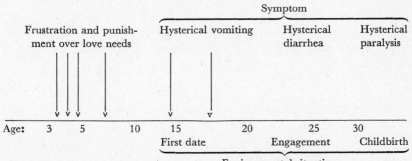

The diagram gives a very crude idea of the development of an average case of conversion hysteria. The injuries to the personality in conversion hysteria come mainly in the genital period of development, roughly between three and six years of age. The child who has matured normally feels sensual desires at this period and these desires lead to masturbation or to normal childish, though nevertheless sensually determined, overtures toward adults of the opposite sex. If punished or made to feel guilty about these the child tries to repress them but they keep cropping up and threatening her. Having the idea firmly fixed that she is sexually wicked, she is emotionally paralyzed from having her quite normal love needs gratified from then on, and later in life, at some crucial period when sexual fantasies are overstimulated, they break through in disguised form as symptoms. We have attempted to show this on the chart.

NEURASTHENIA

In neurasthenia the symptoms tend to be much more prolonged than in conversion hysteria. It will be recalled that in contradistinction to conversion hysteria, in which any part of the body may be affected, there is a tendency for a specific symptom complex in neurasthenia: fatigue, irritability and low spirits, and vague gastrointestinal complaints. To this clinical syndrome other symptoms are often added but these three symptoms will rarely be absent. As personalities neurasthenics lack the ability, buoyancy, and imagination of conversion hysteria. They are morose and irritable and can find little joy in life. It is much harder to help them to enjoy life since they have never known or were unable to feel the love or the inspiration of someone's interest in them. It takes much more effort to make the neurasthenic "feel good" than it does with the conversion hysteric. The constructive energy of the hysteric can be compared with a coiled spring which only needs some help to release it, while the neurasthenic needs to have a new spring installed.

NEURASTHENIA

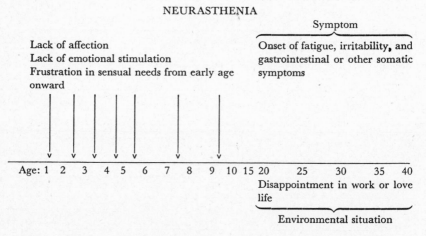

The *hysteric*, having known love, interest, and goodwill, will try to follow constructive suggestions but one has to combat a tremendous inertia in the neurasthenic. He acts as if he would say, "Why should I respond and do and think what you want? No one ever did anything for me." This inertia or negativism can be annoying to everyone and the physician is no exception. He generally reacts in the same way as anyone else, perhaps more so. It is this unfortunate characteristic of the neurasthenic, more marked than that of any other neurotic, which has prejudiced the medical profession against attempting to treat the neuroses.

The *neurasthenic* has been deprived in his early childhood and he brings to the physician his helpless, dependent, childish attitude. He presents himself and his story in such a way as to put the whole responsibility for his health, happiness, and success on the physician without himself wanting to participate in any way. He seems to say, "There's my story, doctor" (after taking plenty of time to tell it in detail). "Now you pat me and rub me and feed me medicine and take my pains away and give me a good appetite and an easy bowel movement and a good night's sleep, and give me inspiration and happiness and tell me how to be successful, and while you are about it, get my mother-in-law out of the house and I'll pay you when I get a job."

Looking for Satisfaction

The neurasthenics are asking for all of the satisfactions which they did not get in early childhood, and the request is unfulfillable. When diagnostic study has ruled out physical disease they must be gradually shown how much they want emotionally and made to see how unreasonable the request is and how it relates to early childhood. A physician who has taken the trouble really to understand this much about the patient can usually be friendly toward him, and through this friendship, make up a little of what the patient missed in childhood. The neurasthenic must be taught to work and to make friends with others and to seek help for his illness in greater enjoyment of his work and friendships. If his childhood disappointments and frustrations have not been too great, with the physician's encouragement he may be able to achieve some capacity to live in a healthier and happier fashion.

The Meaning of Symptoms

In both hysteria and neurasthenia there is value in pointing out the meaning of symptoms. What, for example, does a headache mean from the standpoint of behavior? Who or what is the cause of the headache and what does it symbolize? We have discussed this under the heading of "body language." But this must not be the sole aim of therapy. There are some symptoms which defy specific explanation but which disappear when the patient can participate in a well-rounded life without anxiety. Vomiting may express disgust, aggression, or guilt but to demonstrate what a symptom expresses should be a by-product of the therapeutic endeavor rather than an important therapeutic aim. The object is to free the patient from anxiety in his day-to-day living.

For example, a man of twenty-four complained of fatigue, headaches, and spots before the eyes. The symptoms had begun two years before when he married and moved out of his mother's home. The mother was angry at him for marrying and for reducing the amount of money he had been giving her. He felt obligated to visit his mother two or three times a week and he always had to listen to the same reproaches—what an ungrateful son he was, what a scheming woman he had married, how hard it was for his mother to get along financially, how lonely she was. Fatigue and headache were pronounced and he had to give up work completely. The aim in this case was not to speculate on the meaning of the headaches and other symptoms but to help him with his fear of his mother's hostility. The physician became a substitute authority who *did* approve of his marriage and his attempts to emancipate himself from his family, and made him feel less guilty about ignoring his mother's reproaches in his struggle for a life of his own. Thus he was helped to lead a more mature existence.

ANXIETY HYSTERIA

In anxiety hysteria attacks of apprehension occur with dysfunction of the organs which are directly under control of the autonomic nervous system. Some of the more common symptoms are palpitation of the heart, dyspnea, sweating, a feeling of great weakness and impending catastrophe. Such patients are not only very immature personalities but they have a much greater distrust of human beings than occurs in patients with conversion hysteria. They seem friendly on the surface but this friendliness will not stand the test of personal conflicts. Neither will it hold out against the feeling of anxiety which the patient develops. When the distress of the anxiety attack appears, the patient forgets the assurance that he will not die, that the heart will not stop, that there is no cancer, that he will not lose his mind. He feels sure that some calamity of this kind is about to occur and ignores everything that the physician has said.

Differential Diagnosis. The injury to the personality in anxiety hysteria is somewhat similar to that in conversion hysteria but with significant differences. Often, during early childhood, they have been stimulated to emotional response by unreliable and undependable parents. They have been spoiled children of parents who gave them a pseudo-love, in which material things have been substituted for emotional security. They have known frustration early and suffered from childish rages and tantrums over which they have considerable guilt. Spared the realities and the responsibilities of the home, the girls have been kept aloof from work and never made to plan for the management of their own home and children. They have been educated to a life of ease and luxury and indulgence (as the parent would have liked and now does vicariously enjoy through the child).

The boys have been overprotected by their mothers and have lacked the companionship of their fathers; thus they have missed a satisfactory identification to produce a strong ego and ego ideal. They have an extravagant fantasy life, especially along romantic and erotic lines, but like the patient with conversion hysteria, they fear to let it appear in open expression. Such fantasies in women often make their appearance in flashy dress, glamorous make-up, and seductive behavior while at the same time these women may be sexually frigid. When psychotherapy is attempted they may show little reaction. Instead of interest, concern, or even annoyance, they merely display indifference. The anxiety attacks and accompanying phobias give the patient a unique place in the family setting. He or she may shirk responsibility and even be waited upon and accompanied everywhere. They have difficulty in feeling close to or protected by anyone except the persons they live with: mother, husband, wife, sister. All others are aliens, who promise them no security, and are regarded with suspicion. The person with anxiety hysteria is exactly like the distrustful child of two who clings to his mother when strangers are present.

The *conversion hysteric* is ill usually only periodically and then recovers. The *neurasthenic* is ill and morose but is always a little apologetic about his incapacity. But the *anxiety hysteric* can be ill for years with the utmost nonchalance. The symptoms serve as an excuse to be pampered at the expense of others, just as in early childhood. The conversion hysteric and the neurasthenic are quite sincere in seeking cure and will make some sacrifice for it but the anxiety hysteric often will get well only when made to do so by others. If one has the opportunity of seeing such a patient in the first anxiety attack it is important to treat him intelligently.

ANXIETY HYSTERIA

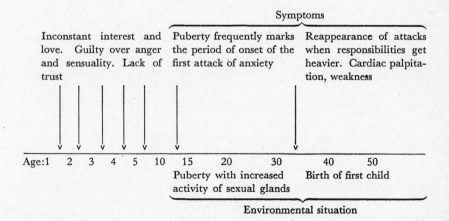

Symptoms

Inconstant interest and love. Guilty over anger and sensuality. Lack of trust

Puberty frequently marks the period of onset of the first attack of anxiety

Reappearance of attacks when responsibilities get heavier. Cardiac palpitation, weakness

Age:1 2 3 4 5 10 15 20 30 40 50

Puberty with increased activity of sexual glands

Birth of first child

Environmental situation

Treatment of the Anxiety Attack.   After carefully examining the patient and finding that he does not have physical disease he is told that he is suffering from the effects of fear and he is reassured that the distress will subside.   Frequently during an anxiety attack the rapid pulse and pounding heart engage the attention of the physician to the exclusion of emotional factors.   The physician feels the pulse and listens so attentively to the heart that doubt immediately enters the mind of the patient and he believes from that moment on that he has suffered from a heart attack. This is especially so if the physician is not emphatic in ruling out heart disease but instead suggests that the heart *seems* normal and at the same time advises rest.   Thus the suspicion of heart disease becomes confirmed. One must have the psychosomatic training and confidence to be able to say to such a patient quite emphatically, "You do not have heart disease." Then, instead of cautioning rest, we seek the emotional factors in the background of the illness.   The temptation is great to give a sedative, an "injection," or something which will indicate to the patient and family that traditional medical methods are being used.   This is immediately reassuring but ultimately harmful.   Sedatives are of very little help; if the anxiety is acute, sedation does not occur until the attack has spent itself anyhow.   To be consistent one gives no treatment other than personal reassurance.   To give drugs and do nothing about fear is to mislead the patient into feeling that his distress is due to physical pathology rather than to psychopathology.

In treating the personality for the factors which produce anxiety we must realize, as stated before, that the patient is apt to be an elusive, disinterested individual who, once over the first attack, does not want anyone to probe his feelings.   When he begins to have frequent attacks, and is afraid to go where the attack may occur (street, subway, stores, etc.), he has regressed to a position in relation to his family which unconsciously he wishes to maintain.   Hence the cooperation of the family is necessary to make him come to his physician where he can be apprised of his real troubles and learn to correct them.   For the few patients who are eager to have health and to learn the connection between anxiety and symptom formation, who have a fair understanding of what it means to be a mature person and to assume social responsibility, the prognosis is good.

COMPULSION NEUROSES

Fortunately, actual compulsion neuroses are rare.   They are very crippling states and the victims may spend their entire time in strenuous but ineffectual routines, such as washing clothes, taking precautions that no sharp instruments are about which could hurt anyone, ruminating about what keeps the world in space, and so forth.   However, many people have the so-called compulsive personality.   This is the pedantic, perfectionistic personality lacking in imagination and a sense of humor. They are annoyingly punctual, and are hostile to those who are not likewise. They worship order and neatness and disapprove strongly of those who are careless and slovenly. They are parsimonious, both in material things and in affection. They have been strongly and even cruelly disciplined as children and they avenge this behavior upon others.

Sublimation. Persons who have compulsive emotional trends directed into socially useful ends (sublimation) make good officials and supervisors of routine work. They tolerate no departure from the rules or from their own conception of orderly procedure. They see that the "i's" are dotted and the "t's" crossed on all documents, that dates tally and people come on time, and rather than hate the job for making human beings uncomfortable over trifling mistakes, they delight in being policemen and judges of petty delinquencies. The character of Javert in "Les Misérables" is a good example of the compulsive neurotic who put duty and the letter of the law above all human consideration and finally committed suicide rather than depart from his fixed code.

Childhood Background. These personalities, as children, have been shown little real affection or human tolerance. Interest they have had—yes, if they obeyed strictly. But the goodwill of their upbringers was hard to earn and they often hated and felt rebellious at such strict discipline. The parents of these people have been unusually intolerant of body excretions and sensual pleasures and have insisted upon early and thorough toilet training and no accidents allowed. They have, of course, been correspondingly rigid about cleanliness and neatness in other matters, such as clothing, books, and rooms. The anxiety instilled through such discipline may have greatly hampered sexual function, even producing impotence in the men and frigidity in women. In fact, most compulsive women are frigid and the men, if potent, function sexually in a way which precludes much happiness to self or partner. The compulsive neurotic finds it hard to "let himself go emotionally" in anything, be it love-making, enjoying a football game, or anything else.

Compulsive Actions. When the patient becomes more than a compulsive character, he leaves the realm of overpreoccupation with the details of normal living, and begins to preoccupy himself with useless concerns such as we mentioned above. There is a great waste of psychic energy in all neuroses but this is more evident in the compulsion neurotic, through his obsessive thoughts and compulsive actions, than in the neurotic with somatic symptoms. A patient who was a cook felt that he might inadvertently poison the hotel's guests by means of various chemicals used in the kitchen and would spend hours of the day and night scrubbing and rescrubbing the pots and pans and the stove, and still was in constant torment that a guest might be poisoned.

COMPULSION NEUROSES

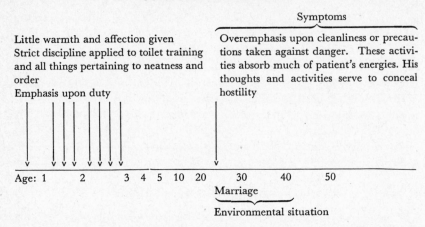

Little warmth and affection given
Strict discipline applied to toilet training
and all things pertaining to neatness and
order
Emphasis upon duty

Symptoms

Overemphasis upon cleanliness or precautions taken against danger. These activities absorb much of patient's energies. His thoughts and activities serve to conceal hostility

Age: 1   2   3   4   5   10   20   30   40   50

Marriage

Environmental situation

Treatment. The therapeutic task in compulsion neurosis is to help the patient to recognize his hostility and to replace the emotion with friendliness. This is not easy. Most cases of compulsion neurosis need intensive and major psychotherapy. The compulsive neurotic has been educated to suppress his feelings, both of love and hate, and he fears to expose either. He has been trained to behave like an unfeeling machine. It may take months of psychotherapeutic work to make him see that he has emotions of any kind. When he begins to understand that hostility underlies many of his acts and that what has seemed to be solicitude for another is merely a facade behind which lies hatred, he is often amazed and incredulous. Upon discovering such feelings of hostility one patient said, "If I love people they will take advantage of me, I know it! Love is no weapon against the meanness in this world. If I am cold and hate people I have a strength which protects me against them. If I give that up I am weak and helpless."

Special Care Necessary. The compulsive neurotic must be urged to try the friendly way of life and see what results he will get. But to reeducate the compulsive neurotic to do this is a job for a specialist, and even he fails in many cases to bring a complete cure because the patient's habits of thinking and acting are so fixed in the wrong pattern. To change the way a patient behaves presupposes that you can make him feel that he wants to change; and one may not succeed in getting a patient to feel that he wants to change. Like the hardened criminal, he feels definitely that it will not pay. He cannot see the point of trust, love, and goodwill—he has felt so differently for so long a time.

It is well to recognize the compulsive character and to know that such a person cannot be easily reached emotionally. His moroseness and lack of warmth, to be sure, is somewhat like that of the neurasthenic.

But the neurasthenic leans upon you and wants and needs something and hence he is, to put it bluntly, in a mood to bargain; he will see your point, he is willing to learn if only you give him your interest and make him feel a little better in mind or body. The compulsive neurotic, on the other hand, has acquired a sense of his own completeness—even omnipotence—so that he spurns your suggestions and proffered friendship. If, in the face of the factual evidence, he has to admit that he does not have organic disease, and if the physician says he has emotional problems, he may appear to accept this decision calmly but then takes the attitude, "Try to prove it to me." In the treatment of compulsion neurosis the *free association* technic of psychoanalysis is the best form of therapy.

WHAT PRECIPITATES A NEUROSIS?

The answer to this question has already been given in several places in this book where it has been shown that emotional growth precipitates various crises. At these points the vulnerable personality tends to break down. These crises may appear at puberty, on beginning work, during a love affair, through disappointments in vocation or financial affairs, from a death in the family, by reason of the menopause, or through some incident of later life adjustment such as having a child marry and leave home. Many people believe that a neurosis or "nervous breakdown" results only from a major and obvious catastrophe in life. It is true that these major catastrophes can precipitate neuroses. Much more often, however, the onset of a neurosis is brought about by less obvious factors.

Period of Life

Most neuroses have their onset between adolescence and middle age. This is the period of life in which increasing responsibilities have to be met. It is the period of greatest effort to establish a place in the economic and social world, as well as the period in which the individual is struggling for a satisfactory adjustment in his love life. Such a period, of course, is filled with many experiences of frustration and disappointment. If these frustrations and disappointments cannot be dealt with satisfactorily then an outbreak of symptoms will occur.

The Single Woman

Many *single* girls develop symptoms in the period between twenty and thirty if they are not making a satisfactory adjustment in their love life. For many reasons they may be unable to compete with more fortunate girls. The resulting anxiety produces symptoms and the symptoms then serve the secondary purpose of producing a certain kind of attention and at the same time excusing them from the responsibility of marriage.

The Married Woman

Often after *marriage* a woman becomes neurotically ill because her husband does not turn out to be the glamorous, attentive, and demonstrative person she had expected. She may be unwilling to exert herself to effect compatibility but instead uses tears, sulking, and inner resentment to express her dissatisfaction. Finally somatic symptoms appear.

Pregnancy may precipitate great anxiety or hostility in women who do not wish to become mothers. Emotional immaturity is usually responsible. Pregnancy to them means a distorted figure, seclusion from society, and sacrifice of time and effort when the child arrives. We have discussed this problem before. Women may not be fully aware of such feelings; consciously they may feel it their duty to have a child, but when they become pregnant vomiting may represent an unconscious effort to get rid of the fetus.

Relatives

A domineering mother or mother-in-law can be the cause of anxiety, hostility, and neurotic symptoms in either wife or husband. Well-meaning *relatives* may be a source of great conflict. They say, "I am not in the road one bit. I don't interfere with a thing that the young people want to do." And they mean it. However, they manage to make their disapproval felt in many disguises. A sigh, a raising of the eyebrow, fainting, or a "heart attack" controls the environment for them.

Career

Many women marry after having prepared themselves for a *career* or perhaps after having achieved success in work. If the marriage is unsatisfactory they toy with the idea of returning to work or to the career which they never had. Unable to adjust to marriage, too lazy or too fearful of criticism to return to work or to make a career for themselves, they suffer from a conflict which causes anxiety and symptom formation.

Menopause

If a woman with a neurotic personality manages to get through life relatively symptom-free she may still break down at the *menopause* because of the many biological and emotional factors involved in the readjustments of this period. This is discussed in the chapter on Genito-urinary Disorders and the Sexual Function.

Neurosis in Men

A man may show an outbreak of neurotic symptoms as a result of marrying, or of becoming a parent, because of anxiety over the increased responsibilities.   He, too, may be disappointed in what he fails to obtain from marriage.   The wife may not be so maternal as he would like or, on the other hand, she may be too maternal and too unromantic.   Then, too, he may develop a neurotic illness if he does not progress as rapidly as he expected in his career.   Finally, an operation or a prolonged illness may create an emotional need for being taken care of and having life made easy, and the strength necessary to resume former activity does not return.   The wise physician will emphasize the excellent physical condition and the completeness of recovery and will point out some of these psychological trends in order to prevent this "failure of recovery."   More will be said on this subject in a later chapter   (p. 180).

The Subtlety of the Onset of Neurosis

As life goes on responsibilities become greater.   If a man shows ability in his job increasing demands are put upon him; as a woman has more children her responsibilities increase.   But nothing outstanding or dramatic occurs, and often the individual is not sufficiently aware of his increasing responsibilities, and certainly not aware of his inability to meet them.   The strength of ego is related to the increasing pressure of reality just as the boy who sets out to lift a growing calf daily for as long as he can—a stunt not infrequent in rural areas—finds one day that he is no longer able to do it.   The growth of the calf is bound to outstrip the strength of the boy.   The person who undergoes the personality breakdown which characterizes neurosis often feels only slightly different with his neurotic symptoms from the way he felt a month before.   But the increasing weight of his responsibilities and consequent tensions and anxieties have been growing and he has not been able to grow correspondingly to meet them.

MANIC-DEPRESSIVE PSYCHOSES

Manic-depressive psychoses, also called the "affective psychoses," have two phases.   The *manic phase* is one of emotional well-being and overactivity, both intellectual and physical.   Many plans are made, new schemes contrived for making money, for travel, for bettering social conditions, etc.   Such people are aggressive, brutally frank, intolerant of opposition.   They may be coarse in language, sexually aggressive, and sleepless, and in a few days may become so noticeably out of control that they must be placed in a mental hospital.

Depressive Phase

The less active phase of this illness, the depression phase, is much more frequent and presents many difficult problems to the physician.

While the manic patient feels "fine" emotionally and states that he "never felt better" physically, the depressed patient feels "terrible" emotionally and has countless aches, pains, and other distresses in his body. Almost always there are gastrointestinal symptoms such as anorexia and constipation, and to these may be added headache, backache, fatigue, abdominal distress, belching, joint pains, and still other symptoms. The numerous physical complaints of the depressed person often lead the physician who is unaware of the seriousness of the emotional state to do many expensive studies and institute a great deal of physical treatment. Not only is this costly and time consuming but the serious danger of *suicide* is overlooked. Again and again we hear of tragic self-destruction under such circumstances.

Depression is a type of emotional response—a feeling-tone associated with a sense of loss, or at least a sense that something is *missing* from the self or from life. In its simplest form depression is a sense of dejection but there may be added feeling-tones of tension, worry, anxiety, agitation, and even panic. Everyone is subject to variations in mood from day to day. No one is completely unaffected by the inevitable disappointments and frustrations of everyday living. However, some people react with more pronounced mood "swings" than others do. These people have recurring attacks of depressed spirits which are part of a disturbance in personality development, the basis for which was established early in life just as in the neuroses. Some believe that there is an hereditary element in manic-depressive psychosis but much remains to be done in the study of personality factors in this illness. There has been relatively little study of psychosis from the standpoint of personality make-up and relatively little treatment by intensive psychotherapy. Still, what has been done seems to indicate that very early in the life of the manic-depressive patient the personality organization has been more severely traumatized psychologically.

Differential Diagnosis

Depression of spirits occurs in other conditions than in the affective psychoses. The phenomenon may be present as normal grief following the death of a loved one, from disappointment in a love affair, or after the loss of money. When new interests appear the depression of spirits leaves. There can be depression of spirits in all of the neuroses. But in psychotic depression the whole reaction is much more severe. There is sluggishness in speech and action, difficulty in thinking, and greatly lessened interest in the environment. There is poverty of ideas and emotion, and such as there is relates to the patient himself—his aches and pains, his sins, his unworthiness, etc. He is self-depreciative and disparaging but he cannot put forth the energy or goodwill to make a fresh start.

Suicide

The patient is hopeless about the future and may have an urge, variable in degree, toward self-destruction. As indicated previously this possibility is something to be taken seriously by every physician who treats a depressed person. There is no way to tell accurately whether suicide thoughts will be acted out or not. The suicidal tendency is not directly correlated with the severity of the depression nor with the degree to which the patient expresses his desire. It has been said that "the person who talks about it won't do it" but this is not the case. Every depressed patient is a potential suicidal risk and the relatives should be told of this possibility. *Hospital confinement* should be insisted upon when the patient has made an attempt at suicide, even in what appears to be a pseudo-attempt; or when he is too agitated; or when he cannot eat or sleep or take any interest whatever in his environment. Patients may complain bitterly over being placed in a hospital but very often, at the same time, they are glad to be relieved of the responsibility of bearing up outside. It is good for them to have the discipline and routine of the hospital environment; they find it easier to cooperate with strangers than with their relatives at home.

Convulsive Therapy (Shock Therapy)

Depressions usually last from six to eighteen months although they are occasionally longer or shorter. The matter of duration is important. In recent years this time has been shortened by convulsions induced by intravenous injections of metrazol, insulin, or by electrical shock therapy. Both methods are drastic, metrazol more so. Some brain cells must be destroyed in the process and occasional fractures and dislocations occur. But in spite of these complications the method is being used, especially electrical shock, and in three-fourths of the cases is effective in bringing an end to the depressed state. To date the convulsive therapy has been given only in hospitals by experienced operators and assistants. How the convulsion works to bring about a better integration of the psychic structure is not known. There is often a period of memory defect and even complete amnesia for a variable number of days following convulsive therapy. It is possible that the convulsion links itself up with unconscious fantasies of either punishment to the self or aggression toward others and hence guilt or hostility is more quickly dissipated. But so far as we know, no patient has remembered and hence it seems impossible to prove what takes place psychologically.

Childhood Background

This brings us to a discussion of the dynamics of the depressed state as revealed by psychological studies. The depressive reaction seems to date back to an early period when the child was deprived of affection and interest. He may have been an unwanted child or, for some other reason, normal love and security were denied to him. Economic or other emotional stress in the lives of the parents may prevent them from giving the baby what he needs in the way of interest, affection, and security. The child never received love so, as he grows older, he does not know how to give love. He pretends that he is not hurt by frustrations and rebuffs, yet their effects accumulate until he succumbs to a depression.

In this early infancy period there may have been feeding deprivations, just as well as emotional deprivations, and the results are anxiety and rage. Frustration in oral gratification leads to a wish to devour what is being withheld. Rage and guilt underlie this powerful impulse. The refusal to eat and the feeling of unworthiness in depression are thought to be due to these unsolved childhood conflicts.

Personality Structure

Depressed patients can take little and give little to others in the way of emotional satisfaction and thus there is a similarity to the personality structure of the compulsive neurotic. These ideas no doubt seem fantastic to the reader who has not been in contact with the mentally sick person. But it must be remembered that the psychotic thinks like a child and childish thinking is like the thinking of primitive man. The child starts life using his gastrointestinal tract almost exclusively to test out his environment. As he begins to build up a thinking apparatus it is not surprising that his thinking is greatly influenced by that part of himself which has been most useful as an organ of sustenance and behavior. Once having adopted the primitive animal-like gastrointestinal means of dealing with loved and hated persons (*i. e.*, devouring them), any remarks about his own worth refer to his introjected "objects" as well. Hence, in psychotherapy it is important to help the patient to turn his hostility from himself and from those whom he has psychologically incorporated, to the outside world. His aggression must be constructively externalized and his guilt must be neutralized so that he can be made free to function again. To this end the patient must be handled kindly but firmly, whether in a hospital or at home.

Treatment

It is useless to hope that a depressed patient will "clear up" by being taken on a trip or to a resort or where there is stimulation and excitement. Such attempts not only do no good but may actually make the patient worse for he is brought more frankly face to face with his emotional and social incapacities. A quiet routine, in which he may have an opportunity to work at some simple task, may be far more helpful than a trip to California or Florida. Through work the patient is able to *externalize his aggression* and to a degree absolve his sense of guilt, especially if the work is of a simple manual character. A pampered society woman in a depression may be helped to get well much quicker by being encouraged to wash dishes and scrub floors than by being sent to some expensive spa with two nurses to wait upon her every need.

Time for Psychotherapy. The best time for psychotherapy in the affective psychoses is between attacks. Then intensive therapy in the form of psychoanalysis may be tried in order to modify the existing neurosis, which drives the individual on to repeated frustrations and disappointments. Once over a manic attack or a depression the patient feels that he is well enough so that the same thing will not happen again. But it does recur all too frequently. Hence, between attacks, psychotherapy is advised since it makes for greater efficiency in the personality in any case and it may help to prevent future attacks. Psychotic persons are in love with themselves and they find it hard to relate themselves emotionally to a physician, that is, to form an effective transference relationship so that emotional difficulties can be pointed out. Nevertheless, it is worth a trial because a depression in a family is a social if not an economic tragedy; if it occurs in a parent it affects the personality growth of the children adversely, so that every means which may possibly prevent it should be tried.

The following is an attempt to point out by diagram the point of injury in the affective psychosis:

AFFECTIVE PSYCHOSES

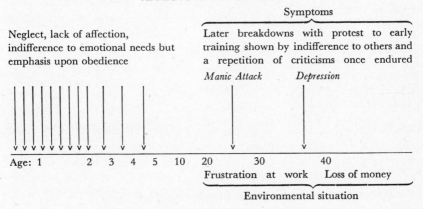

Symptoms

Neglect, lack of affection, indifference to emotional needs but emphasis upon obedience

Later breakdowns with protest to early training shown by indifference to others and a repetition of criticisms once endured

Manic Attack   *Depression*

Age: 1   2   3   4   5   10   20   30   40

Frustration at work   Loss of money

Environmental situation

SCHIZOPHRENIA

In a book on psychosomatic medicine it does not seem expedient to devote much space to a consideration of schizophrenia, one of the most complex of personality disturbances and one of the most difficult to understand. There are, of course, many pathological personality reactions which are called schizophrenia. Some need less help to establish social adaptation than certain forms of depression. However, the fact remains that schizophrenia is a disorder which does not have the same tendency to spontaneous remission as does affective psychosis. When apathy and turning away from life has occurred over a long period, when delusions and hallucinations have appeared, and confusion of thought and bizarre ideation have been expressed, there is a marked failure in social and economic functioning. To bring these people back to normal thinking and normal relations with others is a most difficult task.

Hypochondriacal Phase

There are a few general facts about schizophrenia, however, which the physician practicing general medicine should know. In the development of schizophrenia, which may occur over a period of years, there is a hypochondriacal phase—a time when the schizophrenic complains about his body. Anxiety is present and produces symptoms just as in the psychoneuroses. That a psychosis is developing instead of organic illness or neurosis may be noted in various ways. First, the schizophrenic will be even more vague in discussing his symptoms than the neurasthenic. If urged to describe a symptom he may say, "Well, let's just forget about it." Or he will describe his symptoms in a bizarre way or express strange ideas about their origin. A woman complained about distress in her chest, saying, "It's a trembling kind of pain, as if a frightened little dog were in there. I think my sister may have put it there but I don't know why." Or again the schizophrenic's talk may be rambling and he may treat every subject with equal emotional value. He comes to a physician presumably because he is ill but just as readily will talk of something inconsequential instead of describing his symptoms. Or he may laugh to himself as he discusses the possibility that he may have cancer.

Treatment

If seen early many schizophrenic patients are amenable to psychological treatment, but only in the hands of a trained psychiatrist. For the more advanced cases hospitalization and insulin shock therapy may be helpful. But the physician ought to recognize the schizophrenic patient *early*, before he is too fixed in bad habits of thinking, feeling, and acting. Medical practitioners usually have the first opportunity to see schizophrenics. Perhaps if their condition were recognized early and treated effectively we would not have such a tremendous number occupying beds in mental hospitals.

SCHIZOPHRENIA

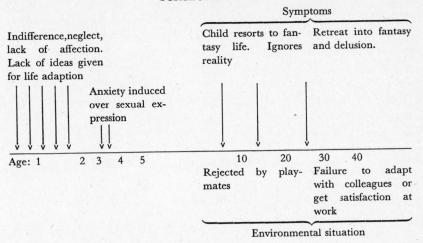

The schizophrenic, like the manic-depressive, has a great love of self. He has often been hurt and he does not trust himself to confide in many people. The one he trusts must be able to think and feel with him and must never disappoint him. The schizophrenic is willing, reluctantly so, but nevertheless willing to be led back to reality providing the leading is done slowly, kindly, patiently, and providing the real world and its values can be made more pleasant and attractive than his world of fantasy.

PSYCHOPATHIC PERSONALITY

While the general physician is not often called upon to treat the so-called psychopathic personality or what is sometimes called a *neurotic character disturbance*, he is nevertheless frequently questioned about character traits and what should be done about them. The neurotic personality, strictly speaking, is a social misfit; he does not have physical symptoms. In reality, however, the inefficiency and social maladjustment are just as symptomatic of illness as the distress of somatic dysfunction. Kleptomania may be just as much a symptom of a sick personality as a headache or an attack of diarrhea. Moreover, the psychopathic personality who does not enter a mental hospital and who does not come to the attention of a physician through neurotic symptoms, may nevertheless act as a "carrier" of emotional problems to the younger generation, particularly if he or she is a parent.

Psychopathic personalities, presented diagrammatically, lie in two areas: close to neurosis, or close to psychosis.

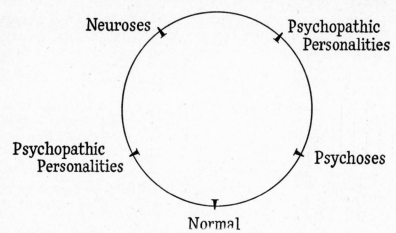

Psychopathic personality may be closely related to neurosis or psychosis.

Direct Expression of Hostility

Unless their impulses lead to antisocial conduct of such a nature that they come in conflict with the law they may be regarded as average people. Those who know them well, however, realize that "they are their own worst enemies," that they may be very unhappy individuals, starving for love, recognition, and accomplishment, but never able to achieve success because they lack the qualities of character necessary to bring the rewards of efficient and considerate living. The same instinctual forces that are found in the neuroses are at work and some of the same disappointments and frustrations occur. Whether a person falls ill somatically or socially seems to depend upon the quantity of guilt, anxiety, and hostility in his personality and how it finds expression. One guilty person may achieve punishment through a pain in the stomach and an operation whereas another will rob a store and contrive to be caught. Certainly, in many antisocial persons hostility finds a much more direct expression than in the neuroses.

Surface Friendliness

The fundamental selfishness of these people is often overlooked because they can present a surface friendliness and affability which is very misleading. This superficial attitude has every appearance of being genuine but like a fancy dress it is used only on occasions. When the psychopath's behavior is carefully studied over a period of time one finds that he makes no real contribution either to individuals or to society as a whole. Underneath his surface amiability and affability one discovers a marked coldness and indifference, even real contempt and hatred for the people with whom the psychopath comes in contact.

Clinical Considerations

Clinically it is difficult to classify neurotic character disturbances because no two personalities are exactly alike, any more than any two individuals' fingerprints. In formal psychiatry they have had various names, some of which convey the idea of an inherited etiological factor; for example, "constitutional psychopath," "constitutional psychopathic inferior," "moral insanity," and "psychopathic personality." Then they were subdivided into groups such as the pathological liars and swindlers, the eccentrics, the unstable, etc. Although these groupings have value, too much attention has been given to mere description and not enough to the dynamics of these disorders.

Personality Characteristics. When we discussed the criteria for a "normal personality" we mentioned some of the deviations from well-balanced integration. An important deviation is a predominance of immature emotional reaction to a situation, suitable only to a child or an infant. Such characters demand excessive attention; they cannot bear deprivation, and if disappointed they become sulky or depressed; they cannot restrain impulses, aggressive or sexual; and they cannot wait for the rewards of effort. There are those who pursue futile plans or activities, sometimes with some realization of their futility, but seemingly with a compulsion to carry on; there are others who seem obtusely blind to the futility of their activities. There are those with great difficulties in social contacts, with what might be called *social anxiety*. They have feelings of inferiority in any group, cannot refuse an invitation lest they offend someone, are in constant anxiety lest they say too little or too much, etc. There are those with great coldness, who are formally polite and reserved, never "let themselves go," and cannot enter into the spirit of a jolly or humorous occasion.

Sexual Behavior. Many neurotic characters have difficulties in their love life. Some long for love but cannot bring themselves into contact with those who might give it. They complain of lack of opportunity, yet they never do anything that would stimulate opportunity. Others enter into the proper social relationship but are always disappointed because this never brings them as much as they had hoped for, which is always more than the situation could in reality be expected to give. Still others enter into a series of sexual relationships, hoping to find the perfect lover and the perfect love situation. Although they derive a certain amount of pleasure, there can never be any permanence or continued satisfaction in these relationships because the individual is really in search of the love object of his childhood fantasies. In each affair he believes for a time that he has found it, but the person selected soon falls short of his unconscious ideal, and disappointed, once more he casts her aside.

Ascetics and Eccentrics

First, there are the *ascetics* who deny themselves instinctual gratification. They live a restricted, asexual life, often devoting themselves to some group activity designed to curtail the pleasures of others. Close to this type are the so-called *eccentrics* who become self-appointed combatants of some social evil, or who devote themselves to some social good in such a unique, overzealous, and often bizarre way as to nullify their efforts by the ludicrousness of their approach. Their activity represents a marked reaction formation to their own instinctual drives, which threaten to expose them if not kept under cover by this compensatory mechanism.

Neurotic Characters Who Cannot Stand Success

There are persons who display great inconsistency in behavior, who, for instance, may strive inordinately for a certain attainment or position, only to be unable to utilize or appreciate it when the goal is reached. Freud has referred to these persons "wrecked by success." For example, a man strives aggressively for a business position held by another. When the other man dies and the position is at last open, he falls ill and cannot take it. The real death has made his fantasied death wishes, hidden behind his aggression and longings, too real and perhaps too similar to death wishes held against another person in his childhood. Instead of being able to accept the position his guilt overcomes him and he falls ill.

Narcissistic Characters

Then there are those who are extremely narcissistic, who can only be loved but can give no love in return. They are like infants who demand to be nourished, cared for, and adored, but do not repay affection. If they fail to receive this adoration their self-esteem drops. It is as if they demand a compensation from the environment for something which was lacking in their childhood. Often this seems to be oral deprivation during the nursing period, or a lack of love. If persons with this type of character indulge in genital activity, they utilize the sex act as a means of promoting their self-esteem. Aggressive women and males of the Don Juan type often fall into this group.

Alcohol and Drug Addicts

Many narcissistic persons are unable to find enough emotional satisfaction and so resort to alcohol or drugs, which dull the pain of reality and give them gratification in fantasy. All *alcoholics* have some form of neurotic character disturbance. They have a longing for affection which they cannot gratify. They have social anxiety and often live a solitary life. They can love no one but themselves, so that they derive little real satisfaction from heterosexual activity. Consequently, they may renounce it entirely, and find happiness and satisfaction only in overindulgence in alcohol. When they are under its influence their self-esteem is raised to a tolerable level. Then they can be friendly, especially with those of their own sex, but because of their unusual sensitivity, irritability is likely to break through on slight provocation.

Neurotic Criminals

There are neurotic characters whose guilt, derived from early life episodes, is such a demanding force in the personality that they actually commit misdeeds in order to secure punishment to assuage this inner tension. Unconsciously they may even manage their misdeeds so clumsily as to get caught and then, as criminals in prison, bear their punishment with excessive tranquillity. They actually acquire great "peace of mind," once they have been apprehended, and have no criticism to make of justice. In this respect they remind us of the "good" hospital patient who does not rebel at chronic illness, long hospital sojourn, and even repeated operations.

The psychopathic personality has suffered great emotional deprivation in the early years of life and in a manner more similar to the psychotic than the neurotic. In later life such a person pays society back with hate and indifference and unwillingness to understand and conform.

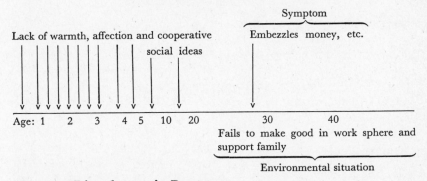

PSYCHOPATHIC PERSONALITIES

Character Disturbances in Parents

Finally there are the people whose personality one hesitates to call neurotic, and yet who act as "carriers" to produce neuroses in their offspring. Examples of such persons are the "cold" parent, the overindulgent parent, and the sexually frustrated parent, among other types.

The "Cold" Parent. Let us consider the rather grim, affectively cold parent, who has perhaps been successful socially and economically, who may have a fairly satisfactory relationship with certain adult friends, and who supplies every material luxury for his family, but who emotionally can never come down to the level of his children and can never give them the warmth of affection which their developing personalities need. The compulsion of such parents for material success has arisen out of their own childhood disappointments which have been successfully repressed. They may be devoting much time and money to public or community welfare; indeed, they may be considered full of human kindness, but as far as their own family is concerned they are cold and exacting. The lack of friendship and the inability to show affection may seriously impair the personality development of the children in such a home. Neurosis and character anomalies may develop in the children of such parents, depending upon the interaction of other persons in the home setting.

The Overindulgent Parent. Parents with tendencies quite opposite to the above, seldom considered abnormal by the general public, shower affection upon the child, overprotect him from all dangers, disappointments and frustrations, and thereby leave him ill-prepared to fight the unavoidable battles of later life. Not only is such a child protected, lest the "evil" of sexuality permeate his consciousness, but he is prevented from achieving a sense of values in other spheres. Because the parent cannot bear the child's ill will no pleasure is denied him. Since no effort is demanded, there is no incentive or capacity for effort fostered in the child's personality. How then can he compete when he has never been allowed to find out what life is about? Education to meet the responsibilities, the denials, and the dangers of life is essential for proper emotional development and must be begun early.

This type of parent personally may have made a fair adjustment to life, but he lacks the insight to see that the *good* parent is not only a *giving* parent. He has never learned that a parent who restricts and gives in proportion to effort is in the end the best parent, because such an attitude prepares the child for a life in which one's success *is* dependent upon effort.

The Sexually Frustrated Parent. The parent whose love life is not being gratified with the marital partner, will often obtain his emotional satisfaction by a bond with the child. He courts the child's attentions but excludes the marital partner and in subtle ways prevents the child from growing up emotionally. Frequently this pathological emotional bond later results in a spoiled marriage or ruined career. The responsible parent would be shocked to be told of the unconscious trends that make such a state of affairs possible, but sometimes such a shock may mean rescuing some child from later neurosis or character anomaly.

The Parent with Unconscious Hatred for the Child. Lastly, there are parents who actually have a deep unconscious hatred for a child. Their care of the child consists of a compulsive insistence on certain behavior standards, which is not at all for the child's "good," but is a defense against that parent's own unconscious personality trends. For instance, the mother who as a girl had to combat sexual tension, may insist upon such restricted conduct on the part of her daughter that it ruins her social adaptation. Some mothers cannot help but feel that a daughter is a serious rival, especially when the father shows her greater devotion. The mother may envy the girl's chances for enjoying pleasures that she missed and, as a result, unconsciously hampers the child's chances for happiness. Occasionally, but less often, does the father by similar methods hurt the personality development of a son.

The Effect on the Child. Unhappiness, moodiness, resentment, defiance, ill manners, asocial conduct, or neurosis may result from the effect of such parental personalities upon the child. To repeat, these parents are not thought of as neurotic, and yet they have a subtle disturbance in their capacity to love. The fact that they are often regarded as model parents who, inexplicably, are cursed with problem children, has led to a rejection of the theory that parental attitudes have much to do with neuroses. Those who overlook the subtle mechanisms of personality formation say, "How can that child have such a nasty disposition? His mother gave him everything. It must be glandular." Or one hears, "How can that boy be so disinterested in worthwhile things? His father has such high ideals and is so interested in public matters." Many neuroses and character disturbances, as well as psychoses, come out of such homes. But the parent, like the public, does not understand how the child could acquire this fault in character, and resents having the defect pointed out.

TRANSFERENCE

As soon as the patient and physician meet, transference begins. The term is freely used but poorly understood. It is often thought to mean no more nor less than that the woman patient falls in love with her physician. Just what takes place in the case of men patients is left undescribed. Of course, this is not the correct explanation. Nor is it enough to assume that *confidence in the physician* is all that is meant by transference. We can best illustrate the phenomenon by returning to the situation which exists between child and parent.

Repetition of Child-Parent Relationship

The child has physical needs for food and protection and emotional needs for love and security. If these needs are fulfilled he will take for granted the goodwill of the world around him. Just as he receives kindness and goodwill so he is willing to return the same. Hence we can say his transference to human beings is positive. If he does not get enough love and consideration as a child then he will not feel so kindly toward others and when he becomes an adult he may demand an excessive amount of love or he may express hostility directly. He may make his wants known in various indirect ways; for example, through gastrointestinal symptoms, or through such habits as telling a long story of his symptoms to hold the physician's attention, exaggerating his complaints or demanding excessive service. He may be suspicious that he is not being treated well enough, thoroughly enough, honestly enough, skillfully enough, etc.

In brief, the dominant personality trends, which are in part the product of the early life environmental situations, will repeat themselves in the relation between patient and physician. By carefully observing and tactfully calling attention to these tendencies at appropriate times, and then showing how they are related to symptoms, we are often able to make the patient understand and thus bring about improvement. For example, a man who has had a very dominating father may be acquiescent on the surface but hostile and defiant underneath. He may show his resentment by failing to cooperate. A woman who, as a child, was made to feel that she could never succeed at anything may continue to belittle herself until she is shown how she is repeating a childish and unnecessary pattern of behavior.

Ambivalence

Every human being is *ambivalent* in his emotions, *i. e.*, to a certain extent he will feel love and hate, trust and suspicion, for the same thing and at the same time. In the emotionally sick person ambivalence is more marked than in the average person. So while the patient may be suspicious, faultfinding, and hostile, at the same time he possesses goodwill and a hope to get well. By the same token the patient in whom goodwill and trustfulness are predominant may still have doubts and hostilities under the surface. Doubt may be in the ascendancy one day and goodwill the next.

The feelings which accompany the fantasy, "You do not love me enough," will find expression very frequently. They probably take first place among emotional trends. As we tried to show in the chapter on gastrointestinal disorders, they may be important factors in producing disturbances of tonus and secretion in the gastric neuroses.

A second common group of fantasies is characterized by the idea, "I hate you because you deprive me. You stand in my way of happiness. I would like to hurt you and make you suffer but I dare not. I must suffer instead." When we discuss headache this mechanism is mentioned. In such a case we must show the patient that his hostility has no reasonable basis but instead is carried over from some childhood experiences. We try to get the patient to reconstruct as much of these early life events as possible in order that we may help him to understand the background for his troubled feelings. Thus he may be able to relinquish the unnecessary hostility.

DYNAMIC FACTORS IN PSYCHOTHERAPY

There are three dynamic events in psychotherapy:
1. Transference of emotion to the physician.
2. Recall of childhood memories.
3. Abreaction of emotion.

The last term means not only that the patient appreciates the existence of an emotional complex, but that with such insight, he discharges the emotion, so that there is no necessity for symptoms to continue. The difference between manifesting emotion with insight, or without it, is very great. A person may be morose, weep easily and frequently, and never change this behavior if he fails to understand the real reason for his depression. Abreaction presupposes that the emotion is acted out in the presence of the physician, who is trying to help the patient with a more constructive way of thinking and acting. *In this setting* the patient can see how immature and out of place his emotion is because he can relate it to some childhood situation. Gradually he attains a greater degree of emotional maturity which helps prevent his unreasonable childish emotions from appearing again. Or if they do appear, they have less force and finally they may disappear altogether.

Case Illustrating Transference

History and Symptoms

A white man of twenty-one complained of occasional diarrhea, a bearing-down feeling in his lower abdomen, and fatigue. He said he had "colitis" and that a physician in another city had advised him to have his appendix removed. Nothing in the physical or laboratory study confirmed the diagnosis of colitis or appendicitis.

LIFE SITUATION

We learned that he was the youngest of five children of an uninspired, impractical couple who lived without joy in life. Our patient had led a very seclusive, unsociable existence. He was advised against operation and psychotherapy was suggested. He refused to heed this advice; the appendix was removed and later, during which interval he had been working and was symptomatically unimproved, he returned to us. In this interview we inquired about his symptoms and tried to question him about himself and his reactions to life and the people around him but he remained apathetic and noncommittal. We felt that we might be dealing with the early stages of schizophrenia and wrote to his parents stating that he was unresponsive to psychotherapeutic efforts.

Participation in Life

Again the patient returned, this time a little less apathetic. He said, "I know I don't talk much, I only want to listen. I have always been that way." We explained the need for participation in life in order to find its values, saying, "One must *give* and *take* emotionally in order to enjoy life. If you allow your ideas and feelings to stagnate you will not be well and happy. Furthermore, you get out of practice in how to adjust to people and when you try again you are anxious and ill at ease and this affects the workings of your stomach and intestines."

The patient answered, "I'm surprised that it matters to you what I think, say, or do. I guess it's because I just can't believe anyone is personally interested in me. I was the youngest of five children and I sometimes think I must have been an accident. All the older ones have done well and mother and father are proud of them. I never did especially well and no one ever seemed much interested in me. Sometimes it seemed that my mother and father only spoke to me to tell me that there was no money to do the things that I wanted to do. So I got into the habit of keeping my thoughts and feelings to myself."

Reestablishing Friendships

On the basis of our interest in him he soon demonstrated that he could reestablish friendships and also obtain a job. At first, he found it difficult to know what to say to his friends—"I don't know the expressions and slang used. In the three years that I have been sick and out of things I have come to feel like an old timer." He then discussed his fear of being laughed at and we assured him that "no one could be expected to know everything at twenty-one," that "life was a matter of continuous learning." His emotional development continued and soon he reported that he "hardly noticed he had symptoms any more." Occasionally he fell into an attitude of indifference for a few hours and this was a warning to him "that he must get busy and do something," rather than stay in the rut of apathy that led nowhere.

SUMMARY

Here was an example of negative feelings being *transferred* to the physician. As a child the patient had been ignored by his parents so, as a young man, he retaliated by keeping his thoughts to himself and further showed his resentment by apathy and indifference. We called his attention to what he was doing, at the same time showing our interest in him. He responded with friendliness or positive feelings, developed emotionally as well as intellectually, and became a healthier and more efficient person.

NATIONAL HEALTH PROBLEMS AND PSYCHOSOMATIC ILLNESS

Halliday, Regional Medical Officer in the Department of Health for Scotland, believes there is a definite increase in psychosomatic illness. He points out that the presence of psychosomatic illness in a community is not revealed directly in its morbidity statistics but lies concealed under a number of different medical labels. Some of these diagnostic labels are: gastritis, rheumatism, anemia, debility, heart disease. Of 335 unselected, carefully studied, insured patients it was found that approximately half of them were incorrectly designated by the labels just mentioned, when they were actually suffering from a psychoneurosis.

"Fixing" the Neurosis

Halliday stresses the need for recognition of the psychological factor and deplores a continuation of routine mechanistic treatment. He says, "If the need for supplementing the ordinary examination of the teaching schools with an investigation into psychological factors is not understood, the range of clinical observations is too narrow and adequate remedial measures appropriate to each individual cannot be taken. In such circumstances the doctor has regard only for the 'secondaries' and treatment is confined to standarized mechanistic and local interference. However, in so far as this action ignores primary causes it may be ineffective in preventing recurrences and in cutting short incapacity. Further, because of the features of innocence and increased suggestibility which are present in all patients with psychosomatic disorder, routine continuation of mechanistic treatment may succeed in fixing the symptoms for life. The risk of fixation is increased whenever treatment becomes very intensive, very elaborate, or very impersonal, and today, when ever-growing facilities are available for mechanistic diagnosis and therapy, there is a danger, if relevant considerations are omitted, of inducing 'fixation invalidism' on a scale hitherto unknown."

The Orthodox Approach to Psychosomatic Problems

With these statements of Halliday we agree. Treatment by drugs, by standardized mechanistic measures, or local interference by surgery, for an illness which is emotional in origin only leads to a prolongation of the illness and to more confirmed invalidism. "Fixation" makes cure more difficult. It increases the cost of illness enormously, to the patient, to his family, and to the community. Not only has it been noted that there is a definite increase in psychoneurosis and psychosomatic illness but also that younger age groups are being affected. The younger a patient is who falls ill with a chronic illness that is psychological in origin, the longer he is likely to remain as an expense to a family or to the community unless it is properly recognized and adequately treated. This problem is a matter of the greatest economic importance when considered in the light of health insurance plans and the Veterans Administration.

The Physician as a Pathogenic Agent

In regard to these problems Dunbar refers to the physician himself as the pathogenic agent in certain situations. She says, "It was a great step forward when we discovered that disease was also favored by elements in economic and social situations which might be traumatic. But though we now know the importance of adequate housing, education, and nutrition we still are not sufficiently aware of the fact that the physician himself is often pathogenic. He is so when he concentrates on symptoms without adequate attempt to ascertain or remove their causes. His tendency in this direction is multiplied by certain insurance measures." For example, she points out that when the insurance system does nothing more than systematize existing factors it may increase the volume of disease by increasing the volume of the wrong kind of therapy. If the psychological aspect of a disease is ignored and there is delay in monetary settlement or if payment continues over a long period of time it is likely to cause the patient to cling to his symptoms. A study made by the Industrial Health Research Board in Great Britain in 1936 concluded that "to pay a man for a psychoneurotic disability without giving him treatment in the way of psychotherapy was to push him along the downward path to complete and lasting invalidism." What a burden this has been to the United States in relation to disabled veterans!

Insurance companies often seem to be ignorant or indifferent as to the nature of psychoneurosis. When psychoneurotic illness is present they either continue to make disability payments or try to get the patient declared a malingerer in order to stop payments and invalidate his policy. On the one hand this results in fostering chronic invalidism in the client, or on the other, of creating dislike and distrust of the insurance companies. It is *an obsolete point of view that will only accept illness as "real" when it involves tissue pathology.*

The Cost of Psychotherapy

In the past few years there has been a mass destruction of human lives arising from the outward expression of hate, fear, greed, and intolerance. But the internal expression of the same emotions in the individual also causes much suffering and premature death. The physician cannot wait for the world to become more civilized in order that his patients may avoid the stress of these emotions. Rather he must work as an educator with his patients in order to bring about better emotional adjustment. The freshman is told, as he enters medical school, and the senior, as he leaves, that the profession of medicine offers a wonderful field for doing good and making a better world. This is not only through the drugs he gives, the gallbladders he drains, or the tonsils he removes, worthy acts though these may be. Much of his service to humanity lies in understanding and doing something to correct the fears and the false reasoning of the people who come under his care. When the emotions of the patient are ignored, and hate and fear are left to exert their toxic effects upon the body, then medical care, for all of its accomplishments, will never be truly scientific and the financial costs will also remain unnecessarily high. We have previously emphasized how expensive personality conflict may be in terms of somatic symptoms, inefficiency, and asocial behavior. It also costs the family, the community, and the nation large sums of money because hatred, fear, and a faulty sense of values remain beyond the bounds of medical care. Re-education of the ideational and emotional trends is time-consuming and expensive. But in the end, it is often discovered that it would have been many times cheaper from the standpoint of both suffering and expense if it had been recognized earlier.

The Cost of "No Psychotherapy"

A boy, nine years old, had cost his parents $6000 in fees to private physicians and had cost social agencies another $4000 for hospital care and clinic examinations, for what was supposedly heart disease. He was cured and remained well after ten visits to a psychiatrist in a medical center which has learned that it cannot afford *not* to have psychiatrists on its staff.

Dunbar then cites a general medical hospital maintained by a state, in which a psychiatrist was able to treat on an average of 146 out of some 3500 patients admitted annually. By doing so he reduced the average hospital days for these patients by 44 per cent, thus saving the hospital $8464.45 per year. Studies made at other hospitals indicate that such service should be extended to 80 per cent of all patients. Had this been done in the hospital mentioned the state might have been saved something like $170,000 per year. Many hospital superintendents, aware of the importance of emotional factors in illness, say they would have psychiatrists attached to their staff if they could only afford it. It would appear from the figures that they cannot afford *not* to do so. A full-time psychiatric consultant in the wards and outpatient department of the general hospital can more than make his salary from the standpoint of the saving to the hospital in patient days.

The Role of the General Physician

But once more let us emphasize that the day is here when the general physician should be able and willing to administer minor psychotherapy and recognize the criteria for major psychotherapy. Now and then there may be a patient whose inability to understand or whose reluctance to look within himself may cause him to go elsewhere in search of the more traditional therapies. But sincere patients will not do this. If we believe that personality problems are an important cause of psychosomatic disorders then it is useless to compromise, to be indirect in approach, or to try to hold the patient by giving him what he thinks he wants. The principles of management of psychosomatic disorders are outlined for the general physician in the accompanying table.

General Principles of Management of Psychosomatic Disorders

1. Give the patient time to tell his story: Listen rather than talk.

2. Get to know the patient as a person rather than just as a medical case. Look for the person in the patient.

3. Make the physical examination (including laboratory studies) as complete as necessary: Exclude or evaluate physical disease.

4. Reassure: "No evidence of cancer, heart disease, mental disease, etc."

5. Explain: Disorder and not a disease (irritable colon—not "colitis," etc.); the symptoms are real (not imaginary) and although unpleasant will do no damage to the body.

6. If disease is present explain that symptoms are out of proportion to the disease (for example, headache, fatigue, etc., in hypertension).

7. Look for (and explain) the time relationship between onset of illness and emotionally disturbing events.

8. Encourage discussion of personal problems—family setting, marital situation, work, social life, etc.

9. Ask patient to give his own explanation of illness. Reeducate on the mechanism of symptom formation. Show patient how tension of emotional origin causes symptoms.

10. Instead of cautioning rest urge patient to engage in more work and social endeavor. "Carry on in spite of symptoms." (This externalizes psychic energy—libido—and diverts attention from body sensation.)

11. If drugs are used explain their action: Avoid "mystery."

12. Try to desensitize (by repeated discussion) against noxious environmental influences (unfriendly relatives, critical employers, etc.). If desensitization is not successful and modification of environment is impossible then change of environment is indicated.

The Role of the Social Worker

Until recently, for reasons already discussed, there has been a false alignment between psychiatry and general medicine. For similar reasons social work is still looked upon with suspicion. Too often the social worker has been regarded by physicians as well as by people in general as a "snooper" or "do-gooder." People are generally reluctant to expose their weaknesses, betray their confidences, or "accept charity," and even resist militantly any attempt to get them to do these things. Nevertheless with growing prestige social work has developed as a profession with an established body of knowledge. There now exist some forty-odd schools of social work associated with universities, which furnish well-established courses in graduate work. In addition to these courses the student is required to do field work in connection with recognized private and public agencies. The opportunities are great for social workers in many fields of endeavor and medicine is beginning to appreciate the role of social case work and of medical and psychiatric social work, in their application to general medical problems.

Social case work deals with families or individuals in order to help them to lead more personally satisfying and socially useful lives. As Gayford points out, the object of the social worker is to help people help themselves and her work differs from that of the physician and psychiatrist in that she confines her efforts for the most part to current problems and environmental influences. While she may assist the physician or psychiatrist in helping the patient to release resources within himself, one of the social worker's chief functions is in changing the environment of the individual so as to reduce environmental pressures or to enrich the environment itself.

The Psychosomatic Concept in Social Case Work

From the psychosomatic standpoint Cockerill speaks of the medical and psychiatric social worker's concern with the social factors that help to make patients ill, the social problem which the illness creates, and the obstacles which may limit the patient's capacity to use what medicine has to offer.

The psychosomatic approach to illness helps social workers to recognize that the tension and anxiety created by the demands of the social environment are the outgrowth of inner as well as outer pressures.

Cockerill makes the point that the request from a physician for the professional help of a social worker is frequently on the basis that the doctor "does not have time" to explore this aspect of a patient's problem. She adds that this is an unfortunate emphasis if it means that the physician delegates this task to someone else because he is too busy. The truth of the matter is that the physician needs the help of the social worker because he does not possess her special skills and he should use her in exactly the same way that he uses any other consultant: recognizing the need, that is, the indications, and respecting her professional judgment. Only in very recent years have physicians been presented with adequate information regarding the social component in illness (a condition which is yet true of only a few medical schools) and too many physicians still think of social workers as Lady Bountiful's, priers into other people's business, or clerks in the business office who evaluate the patient's ability to pay. It is the social worker's duty to bring to the patient and to the physician an appraisal of the social component which is different from that which the physician can obtain for himself. Nor is this just a psychiatric appraisal, although the basic knowledge which permits it is an orientation in dynamic psychiatry.

In other words, the help which the social worker can give and is called upon to give has changed considerably over the years. At one time she was regarded as we have mentioned above, then she became someone who visited the home and brought back a picture of the environment in which the patient lives, and now she has become respected as a consultant in the social component of illness.

Cooperation of Physician and Social Worker

In an issue of the *Journal of Social Case Work* devoted to the psychosomatic approach both Margolis and Hertzman, among other contributors, present helpful discussion of the manner in which physician and social worker may coordinate their efforts. Margolis points out that in an effort to obtain integrated help for the patient the physician shares his professional thinking and planning with the worker, and depends upon her for an objective picture of the patient's social setting, the relationship with the family group, its socioeconomic as well as emotional resources. The social worker has her own special skills to help the patient in the interpretation of the medical problem, understanding the emotional conflicts that enter into the illness, and assisting in some of the many problems of the doctor-patient relationship. From the social worker must come the specialized knowledge of community resources for such problems as vocational guidance and other social needs related to the illness. More will be said on this subject in the discussion on arthritis (p. 737).

Hertzman indicates that when the physician is engrossed with the organic approach and neglects the patient as a person the social worker is forced to assume the responsibility for dealing with social and emotional factors. So long as the physician is not interested or is unprepared to use this material, however, it remains a separate part of the study; it is not incorporated into the total medical management. In such a situation physician and social worker operate in separate spheres. As the physician becomes more aware of the psychosomatic approach he will undoubtedly call more and more for the services of the skilled case worker.

The question is often raised, "Should not the physician himself do the work that is now considered the province of the social worker?" Our feeling is that he should have an awareness of this work and considerable understanding of it but that it remains a separate discipline to be pursued independently but constantly integrated in the teamwork of physician and social worker. We believe that not only will the social worker be utilized more and more in hospital and clinic practice but to an increasing extent in the private practice of physicians. Considerable experimentation has been done in making social work available for private patients on a fee basis and here and there one hears of a physician who utilizes the services of a social worker in his office. Soon medicine will employ psychological as well as physiological technics in the consideration of the multiple factors that enter into the production of illness, in an effort to make a definitive diagnosis, and in preparation for comprehensive medical care. Then the services of the skilled case worker will be recognized as an integral part of the medical approach to all patients, those in private as well as public care.

Necessarily there will be some overlapping and duplication in the work of the doctor and the social worker but is this not always true of the various disciplines employed by the general physician? He must be aware of the many specialities and points of view that bear upon the medical problem and be prepared to utilize each to a certain extent, meaning that in a limited sense he can use the special skills (minor surgery, minor psychotherapy, and some of the skills of the social worker) but he must be able to recognize the point at which he will call for special help from each of these specialists.

From our own experience with social workers we are prepared to say that their understanding of the social and emotional factors can be of inestimable value to the physician. He cannot do the work of the social worker any more than the social worker can do his job, but both are essential in the psychosomatic approach.

Practical Suggestions

A practical suggestion to the physician is in order. If he has been reared in the organic approach he may be unable to accept the help of the social worker. He may even look upon her as a meddler in personal affairs, one who is capable of interfering with the doctor-patient relationship. But this is far removed from modern social work, which is designed to help the patient to understand the social aspects of the life situation which has prepared the way for his illness, and to recognize the social problems it creates.

The social worker is very often sensitive to a condescending attitude on the part of the physician and leans over backward in her efforts not to antagonize him. This is not a healthy relationship. If the two are prepared to work together much can be accomplished.

Social case work has stated that one of the important considerations in dealing with the client is to find out what he wants for himself; this is the important issue, and not always easy to fathom because what he says he wants is often not what he actually wants. Just as in social work sometimes the patient is not fully aware of his difficulties, sometimes he does not know that there is any help for them, or that it is the function of the doctor to assist him in this regard, so medicine could well utilize this lesson in realizing that so often what the patient complains about is not in reality what is troubling him.

Social Work as a Career

There is an intimate relation between medical illness and social breakdown. Surveys of the case load of private family agencies will show that an important medical problem exists in the background of social breakdown in a large number of cases and the reverse, of course, is equally true: Social problems help to create medical illness. Therefore there is a real need for physicians and social workers to understand each other's problems and to have considerable awareness of each other's training and qualifications. This means that more medical information must be introduced into schools of social work and more knowledge of the technics of social work must be introduced in the schools of medicine. When this is done on a broad scale we will finally break down the false alignment between the two professions and find more mutual help. The social worker in any field requires a better body of medical knowledge than the average person and of course this is especially true of the medical social worker. Too often in the past the medical social worker has been a clerk juggling the finances of the patient in the business office of the hospital. This is a prostitution of the profession of social work.

Along with the many opportunities which now exist for a career for the social worker we believe that more and more they will be used in private offices and clinics. Indeed social work permits a very satisfactory career from a professional standpoint. We often recommend both to young women and young men who find it difficult to get into medical school, that they may be just as richly rewarded from the standpoint of a professional career in social work. The financial returns will not be large but the opportunity for helpful and interesting professional work should yield its own satisfactions.

Chapter V

TREATMENT—"NORMAL" PROBLEMS IN PSYCHOTHERAPY

If we recall that our definition of psychotherapy stated that the emotional attitude must be modified for more efficient and happy living then we naturally turn to the years of childhood as the most satisfactory period for psychotherapy—perhaps it would be better to say, the most satisfactory period in which to *eliminate the necessity for psychotherapy*. The word *therapy* implies that there is a disease to be treated but one might also add that every child has a disease in the sense that he has many physical and emotional discomforts which require alleviation.

PROBLEMS OF GROWTH AND ADJUSTMENT

The natural distresses of children are too often overlooked or deliberately ignored. Physical diseases get prompt attention. Fever or a rash sends the mother to the telephone for the physician; but as long as the child suffers only the pain of frustration and emotional neglect nothing is done. If physicians and parents recognized the symptoms of emotional illness as promptly as they do the symptoms of physical disease and if they were as concerned about emotional development as they are about physical and intellectual development then we would not need so much medical and psychiatric care as we do today, nor would our mental hospitals and penal institutions be so overcrowded. Psychotherapy connotes reeducation as opposed to the general idea that the child's life is one of education. Reeducation is necessary only if education turns out badly. The truth of the matter is that the child is being constantly educated and then reeducated: he is taught to pick up and hold things and soon afterward he is taught not to pick up and hold things just because the articles are valuable or belong to someone else. He is educated to walk freely and then he must be reeducated not to walk in certain dangerous places. He is educated to retain control of his bowels and bladder and then a few days later he is reproached because he does not urinate or defecate upon command. All growth is a matter of obtaining and then relinquishing—it is an experience of new attitudes and changing values. This brings us to a consideration of the so-called "problems" of infancy and childhood, often regarded by distracted parents

151

as the inherited traits of the queer relatives on the other side of the family. Really they are only problems of growth and adjustment to a complex and often ignorant environment.

FEEDING PROBLEMS

Most of the feeding problems encountered in infancy are of emotional origin. An increasing number of women do not want to nurse their children at the breast. They selfishly do not want their social or work life interfered with or they are neurotically prejudiced against the nursing experience as "messy" and disgusting. People generally give the infant no credit for reacting to the attitudes of those around him but anyone who has studied the early problems of the child knows that he reacts with tension and fretfulness to a reluctant and impatient nursing experience. The mother "who is giving up something for her child," or who never wanted him in the first place, makes her hostility felt and the child shows it. The mother who wanted her child and wants to nurse him is usually rewarded with a healthy infant. The child of the impatient, disinterested mother, even if she has plenty of milk, may be anxious and nurses poorly, and such milk as he does take causes indigestion, vomiting, and diarrhea. We admit that the general practitioner or pediatrician who discusses these problems is flirting with unpopularity. However, if he is tactful and sincere and can give good reasons for his advice to nurse the child then it can usually be managed. It may not be accepted at once as an important consideration but if followed up it can be made convincing. To the mother who quite consciously rejects nursing it is well to point out that her attitude is one that will not only cause trouble at present but will cause more trouble later on. She can be told that the patience and interest which she shows for the child will pay dividends later on in placidity, happiness, and ease of management. This makes the appeal partly to her own selfishness but it is better this way. In effect, it says, "You had better be kind to the child now and treat him well or he will pay you back in bad behavior later on." It seems a pity to have to hold such a club over the heads of parents but it is often necessary.

It should not be difficult to explain to parents that vomiting or diarrhea may be due to an unfriendly environment. There are many adults who suffer from indigestion, flatulence, and sometimes vomiting or diarrhea when confronted with an environment which they sense to be unfriendly. It is small wonder that the child's digestive system should be upset under similar circumstances.

The Importance of Nursing

It is recommended that, when possible, infants should be nursed at the breast for about eight months. Aside from the question of any virtue which may be in mother's milk, this is an important procedure from the standpoint of emotional adjustment and personality structure. To be held close to the mother, to feel her warmth and to have the oral satisfaction of nursing on a human rather than an artificial nipple, establishes emotional security for the infant during crucial months of his development. Such an experience may pave the way for later health and happiness.

If the nursing experience has been satisfactory a gradual change from the breast to other feedings will offer little difficulty. It is the insecure, anxious child who fears what is new and different and may rebel at changing from breast to bottle. If he does rebel, tact, patience, and a calm, soothing manner will help in time. The mother who quickly grows pessimistic about the ability of her child to make the normal transition, and who runs to the phone to call the physician at the slightest sign that the child does not wish to conform, adds to the problem.

Treatment

The physician who deals with a feeding problem often feels that he must do something "scientific" such as changing the formula or suggesting a new procedure. Often he doesn't care to run the risk of the ill will of the mother by discussing her responsibility for the child's anxiety. Nevertheless, the cause of many feeding problems lies in the attitude of the mother or nurse and the treatment of such problems is *the management of the one caring for the child*. The physician would learn much if, instead of concentrating on the discussion of symptoms, he would ask, "Are you enjoying the care of this baby? Does he worry you? What are the things you concern yourself about regarding him?" When the child's care assumes too great an importance and becomes too much of a "problem" to the mother then the mother becomes too big a problem to the child and symptoms result. High-strung mothers have created many life-long gastrointestinal invalids. *Psychotherapy for the mother rather than a new formula for the baby is the proper answer*. In this connection, it may be said that if the atmosphere of the home is not right it is impossible to keep the child from absorbing it, no matter how many books on child care and child psychology the mother may read. On the other hand, if the parents love each other and love their children they may break a few rules of psychology without harming their children.

To *summarize*, in cases of vomiting, diarrhea, or refusal to take food in children:

1. Examine for physical disease but always have in mind the fact that the gastrointestinal tract may be disturbed by unpleasant emotional stimuli which the child cannot "swallow," "digest," or "assimilate."

2.   The mind of the child is just as much in need of emotional nourishment as the body is in need of physical nourishment. This emotional nurture should begin just as early in life and be supervised every bit as carefully.

3.   The meaning of weaning to the child's emotional life should be explained to the mother. The following can be emphasized:

(a)   Breast feeding of the infant should be a mutually enjoyable experience to mother and child.

(b)   Be flexible in nursing schedule.

(c)   Indigestion (colic) will occur in fretful, insecure babies just as in fretful, insecure adults.

(d)   Do not make the weaning process too rapid. Some babies take longer than others. Think of what your particular baby seems to need rather than worrying about whether he conforms to the book.

(e)   Make new foods palatable, of the right temperature, and attractive.

(f)   Do not let your interest become so seriously focused on the weaning process that you forget to play with the baby. The baby needs more mothering and more play at this time. It will help him to accept weaning.

THUMB-SUCKING

Sucking the thumb or the fingers is a habit which has aroused considerable controversy. Once this behavior is understood there is no further cause for alarm on the part of either mother or physician. We have explained that the infant derives pleasure and relieves tension by sucking. When the child is hungry, tense, lonely or tired, and no one feeds him, plays with him or otherwise pleasantly distracts him he will comfort himself by sucking his thumb. Any child, even the most well-adjusted, will occasionally resort to the practice but it will not become persistent or excessive if the child is well fed, weaned carefully and slowly, and if he is played with enough. When encountered as a persistent habit the following points should be kept in mind in advising the parent:

1.   Do not forget that the activity of sucking is normal. In the first year to eighteen months of life, sucking is one of the chief pleasures.

2.   If thumb-sucking is excessive do not interfere directly with the activity. Avoid scolding and pulling the thumb out of the mouth, avoid mechanical restraints, avoid foul-tasting applications and above all, avoid shame, criticism, and ridicule.

3.   Play with the child more often and use play materials suitable to his age. Encourage him to play with other children.

4.   See that he has opportunity (space) to be active and to explore.

5.   If the home atmosphere is not one of happiness, ease, and friendliness the adults should strive to make it so rather than to concern themselves only with the baby's problem.

BOWEL AND BLADDER TRAINING

The achievement of bowel and bladder control is a very important phase of human personality development.   Instead of being recognized as such it is usually regarded as an unpleasant stage of childhood to be hurried through as quickly as possible and without regard for the child's feelings.

Moving the bowels and bladder at will is normal for the child.   He cares nothing for cleanliness. Society is doing itself a favor, as far as he is concerned, when it asks him to assume the difficult responsibility of controlling his excretions.   Even under the most favorable circumstances he is thrown into conflict.   He is forced to choose between two pleasures. He cannot have the comfort of evacuation at will and still retain the friendship of his mother or nurse.   He must endure the distress of bowel and bladder control in order to have the love and good will of his parent. Under the best circumstances (a good relationship between mother and child) this should take considerable time.   If the mother scolds and punishes instead of understanding that time, patience, kindness, and praise are necessary, the child may be trained quickly but at great cost to his emotional development.   Moreover, such early training is very apt to be broken later on.   Since the motor tracts of the spinal cord are not completely myelinated until the child is one year old the futility of attempting toilet training much before this time is evident.   Some ambitious mothers, eager to have a clean child, will begin toilet training long before one year.   Normally complete cleanliness and dryness is not achieved until between the ages of two and two and a half.   Therefore, it is apparent how much patience and tolerance must be exercised in order that the child should not get the unfortunate opinion of himself that he is dirty, stupid, bad, and inferior.

Management

The ability to control bowels and bladder increases gradually with the child's ability to talk and express his feelings in regard to toilet needs, and also on his corresponding ability to understand the speech of parents and what they expect of him.   The mother will notice at what time of day the bowels usually move and begin placing the child on the toilet at these times.   If after five to ten minutes no results are obtained he should be taken off.   There is no point in keeping him there for long periods of time.   Give praise freely if evacuation is accomplished.   Often the child will move the bowels just after being taken off the toilet. Probably it is deliberate and for a short time he may do the same thing. He is merely getting used to the method and making his own decision about whether to accept it. If he is a little slow to accept it the mother should be patient and kind, and if she does not make too much fuss, it will take care of itself. Such behavior in the beginning does not necessarily mean stubbornness or indifference. But stubbornness can be aroused if the mother is too impatient for quick results. Many constipation, colitis, and even character problems in adults can be traced to the mistakes in training of this period of life. If more women knew these simple facts and trained children accordingly instead of trying to regulate toilet habits in relation to their own prejudices against dirt, there would be fewer anxious, inhibited, and rebellious children. The truth of the matter is that a well-adjusted, intelligent child will quickly become clean, with little training, once the proper time has arrived.

Enuresis

Enuresis is the term applied to bed-wetting and inadequate bladder control beyond the age when bladder control is usual in the average child. While occasionally there are physical reasons, in the majority of cases this represents a defect in personality development. It means that the child has not formed an emotional bond to his mother of sufficient strength to enable him to exert the necessary control. If he loves the mother enough—which means the mother must have loved him enough—usually he can accept this responsibility. His resolve to please the mother permeates into the deeper layers of the mind, and leads to an acceptance of the mother's desire, whereupon control of the nervous mechanism of the bladder is maintained. If insufficient desire to please the mother (nurse or other person) has not been awakened the child concerns himself only with his own comfort and empties the bladder when tension causes the slightest discomfort.

In the months when control is being established (around the age of two or even later) *the arrival of a new baby* in the home may cause a return of enuresis. This comes about because the child is envious of the attention the new baby gets and he resorts to this earlier means of drawing attention to himself. Of course, it may mean more than a simple bid for attention. It may also express resentment toward the new baby or resentment toward lack of attention for any other reason. Enuresis may persist to the age of puberty, sometimes into adolescence, and rarely into adulthood.

Treatment. It is bad medical advice to assure the parents that the enuretic child "will grow out of it." It is true that in time most enuresis disapppears. But this may be after years of bed-wetting, shame, embarrassing situations, and painful scenes, each leading to further crippling of the personality.

1. Enuresis, aside from some rare physical disease, means a personality defect.

2. Explain the nature of the defect to the parent.

3. Point out that scolding and shaming are not only useless but actually harmful.

4. Advise the mother to make consistent efforts to win the child's goodwill. Make bladder control a by-product of friendly cooperation between mother and child.

5. Give approval when the bed is dry. Do not disapprove when it is not.

6. Rewards (candy, trips, etc.) are not contraindicated but such bribery should not be necessary or, at least, should not be in the foreground of the picture. Consistent goodwill and pleasant day-to-day living between mother and child with a simple explanation of what is expected should be enough to solve the problem.

7. Care should be taken not to make the enuretic child feel that he is dirty. First, it contributes to a feeling of inferiority and secondly, since the child cannot distinguish between the organs of sex and of excretion, in later years he may find it difficult to avoid transferring the idea of dirt to the natural sexual functions.

TANTRUMS

Rage reactions in children are common and, within certain limits, are not abnormal. They may be simple reactions to a feeling of helplessness, for example, when the child is learning to manage new toys. This fact should be kept in mind by parents who have the urge to buy toys which may be beyond his power to use. If the toy is right for him and he merely gets angry once in a while no attention need be paid to this burst of rage. However, these rages may relate themselves to his discipline, and if he has rages too frequently over trivial matters, or if he tries to force those around him to yield to his whims in this way, he may need special management.

Treatment

If the rage (or *negativism*) is prolonged and does not respond to kind reasoning the child may have to be ignored while the rage spends itself. He may be reasoned with afterward. Try to inject understanding into the discussion, a sense of humor if possible, and help the child to save face. Avoid lecturing and moralizing but instead try to encourage better control by understanding and friendliness. Here, as in so many other problems of child training, it is most important that the parent does not get side-tracked into intellectual discussion of what is "good' and "bad" to do. Just as children gradually win control over their bodies so do they over their minds and the parent must convey to the child that he (the parent) understands selfish, egoistic behavior. Such a parent is better able to retain a friendly feeling between the child and himself, which will enable the child to give up selfish emotional releases. The parents should concern themselves more about what the child feels regarding them and the world in general than how *they* (the parents) feel about the child's "bad" habits.

SEXUALITY OF CHILDHOOD

There is a growing healthy tendency for parents to include education about sex with the rest of the child's education. Certainly there is no need to isolate sexual education—to give it only at a certain time and under certain conditions. This idea has always been naive because often the "proper time" never arrived at all, or if it did, the embarrassed parent, finding it difficult to put in words what he did know, and afraid that the child already knew more than he, made a very bad job of the lecture. Moreover, if the child actually was untutored concerning sexuality, he could not listen and absorb much in one lecture anyhow. Therefore, with increasing knowledge parents are beginning to give their children information about sexual matters *as they ask for it*, and answering what they ask in a straightforward, simple manner. Children are usually first interested in genital differences and they can be told that boys and girls are constructed differently. If they ask why this is so they can be told the function of each organ in reproduction. Usually a child will be satisfied for some time when told that boys and girls *are* different. He thinks this over for a time before wanting to know *why* they are different.

Genital Differences

There *is* some tendency for children to be uneasy about the fact of genital difference, the girl often feeling that she has had a penis and lost it—the boy feeling that if people exist without a penis his, too, might be taken away. Such ideas in children should not be laughed at. The girl may be told of her future role as a mother and the boy can be reassured that one does not lose the penis.

Many parents find it especially hard to explain the act of sexual intercourse itself but the question of "How does the seed get into the woman?" must be answered factually some time. The best time is when the child wants to know and the best person to give the information is the parent.

Parents who are afraid that information about sexuality will result in premature sex play or experimentation should not be so naive as to assume that the uninformed child will escape this desire. The truth is that "knowing" from a trusted source tends to reduce curiosity and the desire to experiment. The quiet child who asks no question is not to be regarded as disinterested in sex; all children who are normal are interested in sex just as they are interested in everything else. If interest is lacking it is most regrettable, for the fears which induce such inhibitions are going to interfere with socialization and marital happiness later in life. In such an instance some opportunity should be taken to open the subject so that the parent and child can share some knowledge of sexuality. Conservative people say, "Why not let well enough alone?" But a child who shows no interest whatever in sexuality is not "well enough" to avoid some form of maladjustment later in life.

Infantile Masturbation

The tendency to manipulate the genital organ for the sake of the pleasure is present in all human beings. It is quite common as a natural phenomenon from the ages of one to six but occurs both before and after these ages. Masturbation is not a sign of innate moral depravity on the part of the child. Like thumb-sucking, masturbation increases or decreases depending upon other ways of satisfying inner emotional needs.

Masturbation, as such, should be ignored. Efforts should be made to turn the child's attention away from seeking pleasure upon his own body by encouraging him to seek pleasure in the world around him. *Do not* advise mechanical restraint, scolding, punishing, or humiliation. Such actions ignore the real challenge, which is to make the child happier with life around him so that he does not fall back upon this egoistic form of satisfaction.

Environmental Responsibility. As with other behavior problems, in a home where there is a problem of chronic masturbation in the child, the parents are not happy in their own adjustment. They have not been able to bring happiness to each other and this lack of inner contentment finds expression in the child. As Eben Holden said of the man and his horse, "Got t' judge the owner as well as the hoss, and if there's anything the matter with his conscience it'll come out in the hoss somewhere." The same thing is true of parents and children. If the parents have a disturbance in their emotional lives, it is almost certain to show up as some defect in the personality of the child. Masturbation has often been preceded by insufficient emotional satisfaction through the nursing, weaning, and sphincter training period. Finding the genital organ a source of pleasure the child resorts to self-gratification in masturbation. The lack in the emotional life needs correction; otherwise, the habit may continue or, because of fear or shame, it is suppressed only to be replaced later in life by some other sensual gratification such as addiction to drugs or alcohol. *Finally it should be remembered that masturbation is not a "cause" of anything.* What threats have not been made to stop it—feeblemindedness, insanity, weakness, etc.! When excessive, it is a "result" of a defect in the emotional life and to make threats about its supposed evil consequences does nothing to relieve and does much to complicate the problem.

NIGHTMARES

A common problem of childhood and one not to be taken lightly is the matter of night terrors. Probably no child escapes having an occasional nightmare. He cries out in his sleep, usually wakes up crying, reports his frightening dreams and with a little reassurance goes to sleep again. However, this phenomenon of growth may become too frequent and the intensity of the anxiety too great. The anxiety and the terrifying dreams grow out of fears and threats of punishment which have been exaggerated. Fear of punishment is usually the result of the child's own aggressive or sexual impulses. He fears that he cannot control these impulses, that they may break loose and then bring punishment. It is especially during sleep that the forbidden impulses are permitted free play. Games which involve ideas of war, destruction or other catastrophe, sex play, motion pictures depicting cruelty, fairy stories of the same content or exciting radio programs may stir up the impulses of hostility or sexual fantasies which result in guilty feelings, and these, in turn, produce fantasies of punishment. Hostility toward a parent or sibling may create an anxiety dream. The children may be afraid to sleep alone or in the dark or their fears may be expressed during the day as fantasies of harm coming to themselves or someone close to them.

Treatment

Anxiety of this degree requires attention. How often we meet the statement regarding the child, "He will grow out of it." It is true that in time the behavior pattern changes but unless the basic cause of the fear has been removed the anxiety merely becomes repressed, *i. e.*, stored up in the unconscious mind, ready to cause some future trouble—a real phobia or a disturbance in organ function. Anxiety, expressed in nightmares, may be as dangerous to future health and efficiency as a focus of pulmonary tuberculosis—probably more so. Therefore, if night terrors are frequent and intense, the physician should (1) not ignore them or allow the parent to ignore them, (2) make an effort to elicit the content of the dream. Is it robbers, war, a threatening parent, an animal, a fear of murder, or other catastrophe? To the boy the threatening figure will often resemble the father and this may be obvious to him. This occurs when the father has been too severe or when the mother has portrayed him too often in this role. To the girl the threatening figure will more often be the mother. (3) Try to help the child link up the "scary picture" of the dream with the actual events which have stimulated the dream. Help the child to understand what he is afraid of. If the mother is a strict person explain to her the necessity for less discipline. If the anxiety is growing out of horror stories remove their source and give the child more friendship and reassurance. (4) Help the child to feel safe and loved during the day and, in most cases, he will rest more comfortably at night.

OTHER "NORMAL" PROBLEMS OF CHILDHOOD

During infancy and childhood there are many other problems such as truancy, lying, stealing, cruelty, indifference to studies, etc., the basis for which lie in the same factors which have been discussed so far. These likewise are to a degree normal reactions of childhood. When, or perhaps before, they become disturbing to parents or school authorities advice from the physician is needed. However, since this volume is not primarily devoted to childhood problems we have briefly discussed only some of the most important. At the end of the volume we will refer the interested reader to other books which discuss the many problems of child behavior. One cannot stress too much the necessity for study of the early years of emotional development in order to understand the psychopathological trends which produce neuroses and psychosomatic disorders.

ADOLESCENCE

Puberty, with its sudden increase in activity of the glands of internal secretion, marks the beginning of adolescence. This extra impetus to the psychic sexual organization may precipitate *anxiety attacks*. Those occurring at night take the form of frightening dreams in which the dreamer is falling from a high place, or is being pursued, shot at, pinioned and held down, etc. Daytime anxiety may take the form of unpleasant bodily sensations, a feeling of faintness, fear of being ill, fears of developing cancer, tuberculosis, heart trouble, venereal disease, etc. Youngsters may remain at home because they fear for their own safety or for the safety of some member of the family.

Treatment should be in the form of factual enlightenment on the causes of anxiety and reassurance and friendliness on the part of the parents or other adults with whom the young person is in contact. This has been discussed. But we can repeat that the anxiety attack means, "I fear that I cannot control my sex impulses or my aggression" and the pursuing, threatening figure in the dream or the fear of disease in the waking state means, "I should be or I am being punished or attacked." Explain to the adolescent that his impulses do not differ from those of others; discuss them with him and assure him that all will be well if he will trust himself and carry on his usual activities. He may have to be seen frequently for further reassurance and further discussion before the anxiety is brought under control.

While clumsy psychotherapy can be especially harmful at this period the tactful physician will know how to cultivate in the patient an understanding of his anxiety about sexual impulses. Such feelings that are poorly understood or sexual drives which are inadequately harnessed to wholesome ideas are generally the basis of anxiety attacks during adolescence. It is important for the physician to know what to look for in these cases just as he knows what to look for in the urine of a patient with symptoms of kidney disease. One need not fear "putting sexual thoughts" into the mind of a young boy or girl. They are already there, often unrelated to healthy social thinking and conduct, and it is the job of the physician to relate them. If they are not the cause of the difficulty no harm has been done. Every child of this age should have a knowledge of healthy sexual functioning and if the parent has been unable to impart it the physician should be able to take over the role of the parent in this regard.

Masturbation in Adolescence

Adolescents frequently are openly or secretly distressed about their masturbation activities. They may come to a physician to discuss the matter directly or they may come under the pretext of some other complaint to see if the interview will make it easy for them to introduce the subject. In fact, symptoms of fatigue, indigestion, headaches, etc., may occur following a sudden breaking off of the habit of masturbation. The physician should be able to lead up to the question tactfully by taking a personal as well as a medical history. If masturbation is a matter of anxiety the physician should stress that masturbation (1) is a normal phenomenon, (2) that in itself it has no bad effects upon health, either physical or mental, (3) that to reduce its frequency the young person must strive to live a healthy and well-rounded social life, (4) if anxiety and guilt persist after these efforts a serious neurosis may be the underlying factor and this will require psychiatric care.

Prestige

Adolescents are often unhappy over their lack of popularity either with their own or the opposite sex, or both. When this is the case to a serious degree it usually is the result of shyness and timidity (anxiety) dating back to early childhood. It may mean that the adolescent was never taught to play with other children or never had the opportunity to do so. It may mean that he was shamed, frowned upon, or punished for manifesting sexual interest. It should be realized that the social life of adolescence requires the manifestation of a certain amount of sexual interest. The boy who goes to dancing school and is supposed to ask girls to dance with him, perhaps after he has previously been shamed for his interest in girls; and the girl who is nagged by her mother because she is not more popular with boys but who had always been told that boys were dangerous (sexually aggressive) creatures, are both under a considerable handicap.

Social Anxiety. Parents who want their adolescent children to mingle socially in a happy way must begin early in the child's life to make him comfortable with other children. If the adolescent is afraid of the opinion of other boys or girls he must have the opportunity to discuss his fears about himself and then be helped to enter social situations and prove that his fears are groundless. Adolescents often worry about their appearance—that their nose is too long, their eyes not the right color, their legs not symmetrical enough, their hair unattractive, their teeth not straight. If an obvious defect is present and can be corrected it may be done. If it is not an obvious defect then it is likely the necessary help is in the realm of emotional acceptance of one's self and suggestions for more normal activities toward socialization.

The presence of *acne* upon the face or back may be a real source of emotional distress to the adolescent. Its relation to the emotions is not well understood but psychotherapy is part of its management. It is frequent in emotionally disturbed adolescents and, by its very presence, adds to the emotional problem.

The aim in management must be to help the adolescent with his struggles of this difficult life period. He can be neither child nor adult. The physician may be a very important person in whom he is to find security and counsel and the physician who can be a wise counsellor at this period may be doing a very good job in preventive medicine.

Emancipation from Parents

Adolescents often develop a strong resentment against parental restrictions of any kind. They resent being advised to come in at a certain hour, they resent having to account for their spending money, etc. Any real difficulty of this kind is usually due to a failure on the part of the parents to give the child a proper perspective upon living. The child has not been made to feel that the time spent with his parents was a preparation for living apart from them, or he has not been made to feel that supervision was aimed at making him able to discipline himself. If this philosophy is carried out with goodwill the adolescent will usually accept it. If trouble arises it is generally because the child has been disciplined too much according to the parents' own whims rather than according to a consistent pattern.

Prohibitions. It is probably safe to say that in the home where comradeship and generosity of spirit have existed between parents and children there is no special resentment of authority or impatience for emancipation. The frequent cry of the adolescent is, "They do not trust me." Too often his protest is justified. The parents do not trust him especially in relation to sex. They often suspect the worst when the adolescent's plan of conduct is on a higher plane than they realize. The parent fears and prohibits rather than shares something of the young person's activities by a friendlier, accepting manner.

Of course, even in the best of homes the adolescent swings between a feeling that he is completely ready for the world one day and a fear that he is still quite young and dependent the next. Parents must understand this vacillation and be flexible enough to deal with it.

Struggle with Religious and Ethical Concepts

Some adolescents come into conflict with their religious teaching and the prevailing codes of behavior. They become concerned about the actual difficulties that human beings have in being kind and just. They wonder if they have not been misled by an impractical philosophy of life or if they are not too weak within themselves to combat the world as they find it. They have misgivings as to how they are to hold the ideal relationship with God and still maintain a satisfactory working relationship with man. Such conflicts are usually not serious. If the adolescent has an opportunity to discuss his concern now and then with an older person who understands his dilemma, the problem will usually take care of itself. An over-concern or constant rumination about the nature of God and the place of religion, however, to the exclusion of a normal interest in adolescent activities, may mean compulsion neurosis or early schizophrenia and calls for psychiatric advice.

Codes for Sexual Behavior

Some adolescents are relatively untroubled by sexual fantasy and sexual desire while others have great preoccupation and much emotional unrest in this sphere.

The adolescent with a strong sex drive usually has some psychological problem superimposed upon his normal sexual desire; for example, a need for reassurance that he is loved. He seeks for comfort and reassurance on this score much as a child does when it asks to be taken in its mother's arms. The sexual relationship in the adolescent, therefore, may serve an excessive need for this kind of reassurance—the proof that he or she is attractive and lovable can only be attained by a sexual relationship. Of course, there are many other motives, such as the necessity for proving himself potent or sophisticated. The usual advice offered is that work and physical exercise will diminish sexual desire. To explain that sexual desire has other motives capable of satisfaction, without the sexual act itself, may help some. A boy who insists on sexual intercourse as "proof of affection" can often be shown that such affection exists without the necessity for his indulging in sexual play. Modern adolescents are not much impressed by arguments that sexual relations are contrary to religious teachings, dangerous to health, or harmful to social prestige. Relating their thinking on the subject with responsibility to society as a whole is probably more effective.

The Necessity for Cautious Management

We have suggested that adolescence needs a guiding hand, and here and there a friendly suggestion. But we must not disturb the adolescent with clumsy psychotherapeutic endeavors. In general we do not try to probe too deeply; we do not try to settle all of his affairs at once. We must understand his needs, be his friend, give him the proper perspective and often he will work out his own destiny satisfactorily. Patience, tact, and time are important. If, after a reasonable period of friendly supervision, he becomes *more* involved with somatic symptoms, fears, obsessive ruminations, and failure to adapt socially, then referral to a psychiatrist is indicated.

We must remember that adolescence is the period when habits in thinking and behavior are formed which may lead to mental disease, particularly schizophrenia. An adolescent does not have to be too withdrawn or too "queer" to be thought of as a potential schizophrenic. He may be going through the motions of living and yet be very lonely and unhappy. The physician is often in a position to have something to say on these matters. His advice is often asked by parents, or by adolescents themselves, and even if his advice is not sought he may still, as a friend, be able to drop a useful hint. The physician must be aware of these emotional problems because crucial time may be lost if the assumption "he'll snap out of it" is the only attitude adapted toward these problems.

Parents' Concern over Adolescents

It not infrequently happens that an individual in middle life, particularly a woman, becomes distressed at the behavior of her adolescent children. Up to this point she has kept them well dominated "as her babies" and they have not shown any inclination to get out from under control. However, as the adolescent comes in contact with the ideas and opinions of others he may not remain as passive and yielding as before. Then it is that his parents become concerned over the late hours, the company he keeps, the interest he shows in dancing, dates, or foolish and time-wasting hobbies. He, on the other hand, remains unconcerned; he seems to have no interest in any future occupation and is quite indifferent to the opinion of his elders. He may be irritable, moody, truculent, and even though he lives under the parental roof he shares nothing of himself with the parents and comes and goes as a stranger. They do not know what he is thinking and often feel they have "lost" their child. The youngster may even insist upon an early marriage as one means of getting away from home. Or he may form what parents regard as very undesirable friendships and social connections, and may even go so far as to become involved in delinquent behavior.

Making Friends Early in Life. We have discussed the necessity for the parents to begin making friends of their children at an early age and to try to keep up the friendship. If this is done with understanding no insurmountable problems should arise. However, when an adolescent does become a real problem to himself or to others it is a pretty safe assumption that in some manner the parents are to blame. The parents may have acted with good intent but their good intentions have disregarded the feelings and wishes of the young person and hence misunderstanding grows through the years. The adolescent may quite frankly state that it is not he but his parents who need advice and he will often be right. So whatever the problem is, the management does not consist in dealing with the adolescent alone but the parents must be taught to understand the adolescent just as he is brought to understand them. The adolescent who is merely "lectured to" by the physician is not likely to show much change. He has already been lectured to, too much, and having developed a lack of respect for authority he is not likely to pay much attention to a physician unless the latter really tries to understand his point of view. The physician should try to act as an intermediary between him and his parents and an honest effort should be made on the part of everyone concerned to understand and remedy grievances.

WORK ADJUSTMENT

(Some Psychosomatic Aspects of Industrial Medicine)

There are a great many people who find their jobs unsatisfactory. Such a situation is often a source of conflict and anxiety and, therefore, is of interest to psychosomatic medicine. In the first place there are many people who do not want to work at all if they would only admit it. Some will admit the fact to themselves but not to anyone else. Others are not conscious of how strong their desire is to live in complete idleness. They have never been taught the necessity for nor have they experienced the satisfaction to be gained from work. They have not been indoctrinated during the years of growth and education with the idea of holding a definite job nor with a feeling of community responsibility. This is by no means limited to the families of the well-to-do. Parents who have a difficult struggle to provide for themselves and their families will often allow their children to grow up quite unaware of the fact that work must be done if the individual and the nation are to prosper. The result, too often, is that the human product of such a home does not seriously plan for a career of work. If by twenty-one or thereabouts the girl hasn't married a rich man or if the boy hasn't been called for a "big job" then "you take what you can get." "What you can get" is often not very satisfying to this young person so lacking in a sense of reality. He or she wants a great deal for a minimum of effort and becomes unhappy if progress is slow or if his ambition is never realized.

Work Plus Conflict. Other young people may realize the necessity for work and be anxious to do their job but fear their superiors and even their fellow workers. They imagine that they will be disapproved of, scolded, held up to ridicule, demoted. Without being aware of the fact, the necessity for going to work each day under the stern authority of the boss makes the person unhappy and may even induce such symptoms as morning anorexia, nausea and vomiting, or depression and fatigue. The self-explanation often is "I'm overworked" but our experience is that overwork is not so common a cause of illness as *work plus conflict in personal relationships*. In such a person it will often be found that the relationship to the parents was poor; the child may have demanded too much—the parents may have been nagging and fault-finding or at least very stingy with their praise and goodwill. Since no enthusiasm was shown for a job well done he can develop no enthusiasm for *his* job later in life. In cases in which there is conflict centering around work the physician should try to unearth the different factors that have to do with the negative attitude toward work and then help the patient to understand that the situation may be related to his childhood experience. The physician often can help by assuming, to some extent, the parental role and improving upon it by showing an interest in the patient's work and his progress. Such ego-bolstering may help greatly to keep the patient on the job.

Changing Jobs. Sometimes a change in job will have to be considered. Vocational tests may indicate unusual ability for some other work. But very often it will be found that it is better for the dissatisfied and unhappy individual to try to make himself over to fit his job rather than to wander around trying to find the job to fit him. In this respect work problems resemble marriage problems, which we are soon to consider. Often the individual needs to change himself instead of changing partners.

Counseling in Industry

As a result of greater knowledge concerning the social and emotional factors in disease, in absenteeism, and in the morale of workers generally, the physician finds it necessary to know more about the complex interrelations of the worker, his colleagues, and the job. To use such knowledge can forestall serious emotional illnesses and physical disabilities. This is an important part of preventive medicine.

The Stages of Employment. The subject has been developing since the first world war but the greatest strides have been made in recent years. Giberson speaks of five crucial stages of employment. The first is the *novice* period, in which many employees, while anxious about making good, offer youth, eagerness, enthusiasm, and alertness. Obviously, a friendly reception and a help in getting started right pays big dividends in morale later on. The second phase occurs *after about five years' of service*. The employee has grown to be part of the organization, but at this period is vulnerable to certain dissatisfactions. He may be impatient of progress; promotions do not come up to expectation; and discontent, unhappiness, and a spirit of unrest may creep in. This employee needs a shock absorber, someone to listen to complaints and to be tactful, patient, and offer a guidance which will prevent the useless floating from job to job which is so unprofitable to both employer and employee and represents, in many cases, a neurotic struggle on the part of the individual.

Another critical period concerns *the age of thirty*. This is particularly a period of unrest for the single woman. Shall she stay on in the working world, or should she try to do more about marriage? Dissatisfaction over not being married is unconscious, and she displaces this "wrongness" onto trivial frustrations on the job. However, the man likewise can be very impatient at this time. It is a period of keen competition when a man feels that he should be building a reputation for himself. Moreover, the dependency of parents at this period may interfere with plans. The resentment which is felt because of this situation may be carried directly to the job.

The *menopause* can usher in a period when irritability, depression, fatigue, malaise, insomnia, and other symptoms appear. The psychopathology of the menopausal period is discussed elsewhere (p. 453). It is advisable for the industrial physician to know this period well and to be able to assure women that a normal physiologic process is going on which they may face without fear of physical or emotional ill health. It would probably be a most helpful procedure to have all women of thirty-five attend a series of lectures and discussions about the menopause. It could be entitled "Common Sense for Ten Years Hence."

A fifth group is made up of *older employees*, primarily those who have spent most of their working lives in the same organization. They feel that they have given years of faithful service without having accomplished much. Often they have failed to keep pace with new developments. Instead of being able to look within, they blame the organization for not having had the proper consideration for them. Inflexible, they become unhappy and sick.

The Accident Problem.   Giberson also refers to the accident problem, which we discuss elsewhere (p. 748). "Fear, worry, illness, psychologic unrest, fatigue, and boredom cost many lives. Anger, irritability, bravado, perverseness, and childishness all take their toll in human accidents." She feels that two basic factors contributing to accidents are *lack of physical coordination* and *inattention*. "If we are to prevent accidents and not merely mop up after them, these two factors must be detected and remedied upon their first appearance. Physiologic fatigue from undernourishment and too long hours of work; mental fatigue arising from long periods of concentrated work; and "nervous fatigue" caused by monotony on a job, poor industrial relations in a shop, dissatisfaction and lack of adjustment to conditions—all these contribute greatly to accidents."

Morale.   As far as morale is concerned the lessons of military service could with profit be carried into industry. Giberson says, "Morale does not happen; it grows out of a personal identification with the nation's destiny. Good industrial morale is dependent upon good mental and emotional health; normal behavior cannot be expected from sick people. There are always a few mentally ill persons in every large group; a considerably larger number of people whose thinking and emotions are out of balance because of physical disease; and a great number of people whose emotions are temporarily upset. Sick people cannot, despite their willingness, exhibit high morale. Mental and emotional ills are no respecters of persons; they may affect the top executive as readily as the day laborer. Wherever there are emotional ills there is a threat to the general morale and all steps must be taken to discover these danger points."

In particular the *supervisor* must be educated regarding social and emotional factors. In most instances the supervisor has been taught to handle the machine but not the man. The supervisor, in his limited sphere, is an executive charged with the handling of people. The extent of his production can be measured by his ability to correlate man and machine. Never in the history of industrial development, says Giberson, has there been greater need for complete understanding between medical advisors and personnel people.

COURTSHIP AND ENGAGEMENT

Courtship and engagement often precipitate psychosomatic illness. Marriage is an emotional hurdle that some people cannot take while others may stumble in the effort. Such persons, particularly women, are unhappy at the idea of leaving their own parents, dread sexual relations, and do not want the responsibilities of a home and children. To some women these ideas are partly conscious while to others they are completely unconscious. Whether partly conscious or wholly unconscious they can produce anxiety and this anxiety may be expressed in symptoms. Many women have postponed engagement or marriage time and again because of "poor health," not realizing that the "poor health" represented their anxiety about marriage. Hence the physician should be alert to these possibilities and when a young person has symptoms suggesting psychosomatic illness it is important to discuss the problem of marriage. The physician may then discover that the patient is planning marriage because it is "high time," "the thing to do," "a smart move," "an escape from home," "an easier way of living," "to please mother and father," or one of a number of reasons other than the mature one of making a home in the real sense of the word.

Emotional Immaturity

A young woman who had been overprotected by her parents was courted by a devoted young man. As his intentions grew more serious and he talked of marriage our patient lost her appetite, slept poorly, complained of weakness and fatigue, became irritable and depressed, and cried a great deal. She spoke of her reluctance of moving to another city and of leaving her parents, even though the distance was not great. Her parents thought that she had a physical ailment and were surprised when it was pointed out to them how they had pampered and babied this girl until she was totally unprepared to face adult responsibility. When the meaning of her symptoms was made clear they promptly disappeared. However, this did not mean the cure was complete. Inquiry revealed that prior to this time she had had symptoms during periods of emotional stress and therefore it was important to continue her reeducation. To be satisfied with the mere removal of symptoms in such a case, particularly at this age period, is like giving rest and sedation to a patient with pulmonary hemorrhage, and when the bleeding stops, having no further concern as to where the bleeding originated.

Invalidism. Woman's most important responsibilities are bound up in the marriage relationship but she is often woefully ignorant of these responsibilities because her parents either would not or could not educate her properly. So many parents would rather have their daughters innocent and useless than informed and capable. This may be all right for a mother's peace of mind but it is difficult for the husbands and children of these "child-women." Emotional immaturity naturally cannot be changed in one session with the physician. This the patient and family must learn. But the physician too must learn to recognize the special importance of this phase of emotional immaturity. Too often he has prescribed sedatives and rest and allowed one more childish person to continue on the road of chronic fatigue and chronic illness when the everyday responsibilities have proved too burdening. Education for better adaptation will often have lasting good results and will make the difference between a fairly efficient person and a chronic invalid.

MARITAL ADJUSTMENTS

Marriage as a source of conflict has many implications for psychosomatic medicine. Physicians have always known that marriage and medicine had something in common; from ancient times to the present the advice to marry and have children has been a frequent prescription for certain ailments. But, paradoxical though it may seem, many illnesses arise from the marriage situation, and this fact has not been so clearly appreciated. Marriage is a social institution into which one should bring his best capacities. Human beings should be trained to make it an important part of their living to marry, to share life harmoniously with someone else, and to provide a setting in which children may grow up happily and learn to be of use to themselves and others. Instead of this attitude one finds girls growing up looking for "a good catch," someone "to support them," to give them "a good home," "to take care of them." We find men fearing that they will be "caught," avoiding the "ball and chain," rebelling against losing their "freedom," and declaring that "no woman is going to make a sucker out of me." Even though these attitudes may be thought of as extreme and unusual, less pronounced but similar ideas are all too common since very few men and women have had any systematic or scientific preparation for marriage. A woman may drift along until advancing age frightens her into accepting an offer of marriage which is not especially attractive or a man may be drawn into marriage because in flight from loneliness he has sought the company of a woman and then marries because "she or her parents sort of expect it or take for granted" that he will.

Incompatibility

With as little thought as this given to the positive aspects of marriage it is little wonder that dissatisfaction and strife arise. Many small misunderstandings and annoyances come from the simple, lazy unwillingness of men and women to consider some of the fundamental differences in the habits and personality of each sex. For example, a man will be annoyed and scold because his wife takes longer to dress than he, yet he would be equally angry if she did not look well. A woman will be greatly annoyed because her husband plays golf with the boys on Saturday afternoon, yet she will not take the trouble to learn to play with him and she would be unhappy if he was not popular with his friends. If the wife does a good job of decorating a room, preparing a meal, or arranging a party, she likes and needs appreciation. A man, too, after working hard to achieve a desired position, needs his wife's appreciation. But her only expression of satisfaction may be that "at last" they will be able to have a new coat, a trip, or a private school for Junior. Men and women in marriage should respect each other's goals and ambitions. The capacity to do this is an evidence of maturity and of the capacity for love.

If either party gets the idea of changing the other "for his own good" or is no longer able to feel that the marriage is a constructive partnership then it is time to see the physician, a psychiatrist, or some person skilled in marriage counseling. The longer a man and wife continue to hurt each other or "get on each other's nerves" the harder it will be to make a fresh start with new ideas.

Hostility in the Marriage Relationship

People are thought of as marrying and living together because they are in love but, unfortunately, it is also true that people often live in hate rather than in love. Sometimes this hatred and hostility for the marital partner is outspoken; at other times, it is hardly conscious, and still more often it is deeply buried.

A middle-aged woman presented herself with a clinical picture that first was thought to be cardiovascular-renal disease. However, we were unable to discover any evidence of a cardiac disorder and the urine, blood pressure, and kidney function were within normal limits. After vainly trying to understand the obscure illness, it finally became clear that the patient had a great deal of repressed hostility for an alcoholic husband but could not bring herself to leave him. The husband suddenly died and we were amazed at the transformation that took place in this woman immediately afterward. Instead of grief, she had relief and her symptoms were immediately abolished.

A young woman, recently married, complained of generalized aches and pains and fatigue. While some of her symptoms had appeared soon after marriage, the fatigue dated from the birth of her child, two and one-half years previously, at which time, as she expressed it, "she gave all of her physical strength to her baby." She had been remarkably healthy during the period of pregnancy but had been sick since that time. Physical examination and laboratory studies failed to disclose any evidence of organic disease and the patient herself suspected an emotional cause. She stated that she was revolted by her husband and almost since the very beginning of her marriage had carried on an extramarital affair with a much older man. She was completely frigid with her husband and had fantasies of hostility and hatred during intercourse, but managed to have sexual satisfaction with her extramarital partner. Her reasons for dissatisfaction with her husband did not seem well-founded, and it was clear that even before her marriage she had had great difficulties in her relationship to other people, especially the members of her immediate family.

While she recognized the psychological origin for her symptoms, she nevertheless was unwilling to do anything about it, *i. e.*, anything decisive. She could not bring herself to leave her husband even though she despised him; she felt guilty over her extramarital affair, yet would not give it up; and she would not make any real effort to get at the source of her difficulties by psychotherapy. She contented herself with the partial solution of having another child, because "she was so well while she was carrying the first." This happens very often. *Certain neurotic patients enjoy a sense of well-being during the period that they are carrying a child, only to have symptoms recur after the baby is born.*

Marriage for "Therapeutic" Reasons

In the kind of immature personality now being dealt with, marriage and children do not offer any help. On the contrary, they really only add to the problem. This last patient is a very good example of the kind of person that physicians ought not to counsel to get married in order to solve emotional problems. In fact, it may be added as a rule that it is unwise to give advice concerning marriage. If people are capable of accomplishing marriage for themselves, they will do so without urging, and if they are incapable of achieving marriage, to urge them to do so places a responsibility that the wise physician should be cautious about accepting. The same thing is true about the advice to have children. The fear of having a child is very common in neurotic women. It may be very slight or it may be very pronounced. The unwillingness of a newly married young woman to have a child during the first year of married life may be looked upon as almost normal for this day and age. It is one of the reasons why good *contraceptive* advice is a distinct aid to marital adjustment. But to women who have pronounced fears of having children, contraceptive advice is only a partial answer or no answer at all to their deeper psychological problems.

Education in Marriage

When marriage is going badly and is producing resentment or illness let us counsel the partners, aid them in taking more mature attitudes, and thus try to make a more constructive institution out of marriage. We believe that often a marriage of two serious-minded persons need not end in divorce if they seek help early enough and each will take suggestions and try to do his part.

An intelligent couple who had been married for eight years and had had children sought help because of marriage difficulties. The husband complained that his wife was nagging, unsociable, frigid, neglected her appearance and was unappreciative of his efforts to advance himself and to become successful. He made an excellent impression and one got the feeling that marriage had given him a raw deal. No comment was made, however, and a desire was expressed to meet his wife and get her observations on the situation. She reported that this handsome, fine-appearing man had been dogmatic and dictatorial from the beginning of marriage. He took the attitude that since the man made the money he could make all the suggestions and give all the orders. On many occasions during the marriage he had walked out and stayed away a day or two in order to make her yield upon some small point. She was sensitive, came from a proud family, and had given up a good position to marry and she resented the "high-handed methods of her husband." As for her lack of sociability and indifference to appearance she said, "He is obsessed with the idea of getting ahead. I want to get ahead too but I can't make a social life alone. He says 'make friends.' But I can't go to a country club dance by myself when he just has to see some man from out of town. I can't make dates for an evening and break them, at a moment's notice, just because he concludes at four o'clock that he has to work that night. We haven't had a vacation in four years. Sex has come to mean little to me. I don't think I was ever especially highly sexed but such feelings as I had, have been pretty well cooled by his running out on me to discipline me, and by his faultfinding that I do not come up to his expectations as a wife."

After each had had the opportunity to express himself freely we felt that it was important to begin with suggestions to the husband. Fortunately he was the one who had come for advice and had expressed himself as ready "to do anything to improve conditions." We pointed out that he was overlooking his wife's personality make-up and, in fact, was overlooking certain things that are important in the make-up of any woman.

We pointed out that he was expecting her to create a home and social life which could never become a reality without his cooperation.

We suggested that the only way to win back his wife's interest for greater emotional participation in the sexual relation was for him to act more like a lover than a faultfinding and harassed business man. It was a significant fact that the patient's father had been separated from his wife and while she had been willing to try to save the marriage the father always cruelly denied her any such opportunity. With this example of indifference to women's feelings before him it was understandable how our patient had been influenced in regard to his attitude toward women. We informed the wife of the necessity for being responsive to any new changes in her huband's attitude and in a short time we received an appreciative note about the improved state of affairs.

The Sexual Relationship in Marriage

We have discussed in a preceding chapter the various factors that have to do with impotence in the man and frigidity in the woman. A few more words will not be amiss on this important phase of marriage counseling which, by the way, is coming to be more and more a part of the physician's duty. It is a widely accepted fact that women are entitled to equality of sexual enjoyment with men. Man no longer uses his wife simply to gratify his own sexual desire without taking the time or trouble to gratify hers. By the same token it is now recognized that a wife is frigid who grudgingly or condescendingly acquiesces to the sex relationship without being able to participate emotionally. Such attitudes on the part of man and wife will do much to drive away possibilities for pleasure, and when mutual enjoyment fades from the sexual relationship a deterioration of other relationships is sure to follow.

Education in Sex Matters. Investigation shows that the cause of marital disharmony and failure is due in most instances to failure in the achievement of a happy sexual adjustment in early married life. Studies on marriage also show that the failure to achieve this happy sexual adjustment has often been due to inadequate education in matters pertaining to sex. For instance, it is clearly stated by many authorities that women may not achieve orgasm with the first intercourse, in fact, that it may be some weeks or even months before it is achieved. If the man does not realize this and becomes impatient, reproachful, or condemning, he may permanently prevent the achievement of this pleasure.

Most women are slower to become sexually aroused than the men, both in love-making before the sexual act begins and in the sex act itself. The man should control himself accordingly and will be rewarded by his wife's gratitude and his own sense of accomplishment. Both parties should educate themselves to be frank in expressing their individual desires. Each should come to know what acts or caresses give the keenest pleasure. Sexual intercourse with orgasm should bring about relaxation. If it does not, anxiety is present. The physician should help the patient to understand that shame or anxiety are acquired; they are not natural inheritances.

Pamphlets or books may not lead to a happy sexual adjustment but they do help to clarify thinking, to awaken certain emotions and to provide the way for further help. There are no rules in regard to frequency of intercourse but if the couple accomplish a satisfactory adjustment the question of frequency usually solves itself.

Contraceptive Advice. In women fear of unwanted pregnancy may hinder the enjoyment of the sex act, but men, too, are affected by this problem. Both can be helped by trustworthy advice on contraception. Only in Massachusetts and Connecticut have laws been enforced regarding the dissemination of birth control information. Many larger communities have marriage counsel centers where engaged or young married couples may go for advice. Courses on marriage and family relationships are given in a few colleges. We believe that increasing demands will be made upon the general physician as a marriage counselor and therefore he should be prepared to give advice on all phases of the subject, including contraception and the fitting of contraceptive devices.

DIVORCE

The physician's advice is frequently sought regarding the problem of divorce. The management of such problems requires the same scientific preparation and detachment as the management of a case of pneumonia or appendicitis. In other words, divorce is a *major operation* in personal and social relations and one which the physician must try to view scientifically rather than in the light of his personal prejudices. There seems to be an instinctive attitude in all human beings, and physicians are no exception, that at the mention of divorce the first reaction is to think of doing everything and saying everything which will keep the couple together. Some people cannot believe that there is ever anything salutary, helpful, or constructive about divorce. However, it would seem self-evident that the institution of marriage itself can only be improved if people will take a more open-minded attitude toward divorce and, by trying to ascertain its cause, learn how to prevent it.

Research on Divorce

An early divorce may mean strength in both parties rather than weakness. Divorce is regarded as a social evil and is disapproved of and those who take part in it are sometimes not supposed to have the right feelings for society. But some of the people who stay married out of fear, shame, laziness, or because they do not have the courage to make an attempt to improve marital conditions are less admirable than some who seek divorce. There has been research into the causes of divorce just as there has been research into the causes of crime and delinquency. What has been found is not unrelated to crime and delinquency. It is that divorce grows out of emotional immaturity in one or both parties. If divorce is a social evil then just disapproving of it will not cure it any more than just locking up the delinquent will cure him. Let us start by educating children in preparation for marriage.

Marriage Counseling

When a physician is confronted with a marital problem one safe rule is "never take sides"! Do not even make suggestions until both parties have been seen and the story of each heard at length. There may be an occasional exception to this but on the whole it is a good rule.

It is generally fruitless for either married partner to attempt to conceal what he feels about the other. If there is anything short of love, acceptance, and cooperation in their attitude it will show itself in some way. One couple, married ten years, who had grown apart, agreed, after some of their problems had been pointed out, "The trouble with us is that we never told each other the truth in the beginning. We tried to protect each other's feelings only to find out that this was useless as we have hurt each other just the same." The man had a poor relationship with his mother and had married his wife because she was ill and "he felt sorry for her." She had married because he asked her to but she had had no particular desire to marry; she had been overprotected by her parents and would have been perfectly content to go on in the same way indefinitely. The husband disapproved of her inadequacy from the beginning. She was emotionally immature and sexually frigid. She had little interest in his work and friends. She was always too fatigued to be a companion to him in sports or recreation. "His energy made me tired." Every time he asked her to do anything for him the thought ran through her mind, "If I were home with mother I wouldn't have to do this." She disapproved of his management of money and the friends he brought to the house. Both thought it "the sporting thing to do" to go on and say nothing. Although they could not keep their disapproval of each other hidden they did not consider professional help until another woman entered the picture. In this case divorce was the solution for both parties, for each wanted it and agreed upon it, but it was regrettable that they came to this decision so late when it was not easy for either to make a new life and new attachments. There were no children so that phase of the problem did not have to be considered.

8

Constructive Elements. We believe that strenuous efforts should be made to educate, counsel, strengthen, and hold a marriage together if there are constructive elements in it. But we also believe that neither the law, the church, nor the medical profession should blindly and arrogantly frown upon divorce. More possibilities for neurotic illness and social maladjustment arise in a family where marital discord exists than from any other source. Much as children need two parents for ideal personality formation they need peace, security, and affection more. Better one parent and peace than two parents and an atmosphere of hostility, bitterness, and reproach.

Advice to Have Children. It is true that a certain number of immature people enter marriage thoughtlessly and get out of it in the same way. However, this is by no means the rule. On the contrary many intelligent, well-meaning people, after having made real efforts to make a success of marriage, and after serious consideration of all factors, may still want a divorce and their conclusions therefore may be entirely sound. A man and woman, who may have thought that they had something in common before marriage, but who, in a reasonable time afterward, find they do not and, furthermore, find that they are hurting each other every day in their relations together, may be proposing an entirely constructive social act when they contemplate divorce. If the couple have not been married long, friends and relatives are apt to say, "Oh, they are young yet. They have not settled down. They do not know what they want. They have to learn to make sacrifices." Lastly and worst of all—and unfortunately often by the advice of a physician—they are told, "What you need is a child—then you will have a common interest." We condemn this as stupid and dangerous advice. While it may succeed in holding a marriage together, who can say how many children are thus sacrificed on the altar of incompatibility?

In *marriage counseling* the physician should try to help people to think clearly on the following questions.

1. Did you have a common goal or goals when you married? What happened to them?

2. How have you been hurting each other? Has it been through neglect, indifference, nagging, argument, infidelity, disagreement over the matter of children, religious or educational differences, differences regarding friends, recreations, vacations, or lastly but not least, sexual incompatibility?

3. Why have you been hurting each other? Has the hurt one protested too much or not at all? Have you failed to be frank with each other?

4. Do you listen to each other and really try to understand what the other is saying when discussions arise? Has an honest attempt been made to understand how the other person is being hurt?

5. How will children fare as the result of divorce? Has any plan been made for them which will give them reasonably healthy home conditions in which to grow up?

6. How will the other partner of the marriage manage if divorce is desired by only one member of the marriage? Usually this is more important in the case of the woman than in the case of the man, although not always. If young, the woman may wish to marry again and may have an opportunity to do so. Herein lies good argument for early divorce if it is going to take place. It gives both parties a better opportunity for rearranging their lives than if divorce is postponed ten or fifteen years.

7. Would either party be interested to try to change himself under the guidance of a physician or psychiatrist? If sexual incompatibility or other evidence of emotional immaturity is present would the person in question try a treatment period, to see what results might be obtained before going through with a divorce?

If these points are taken up with each of the marital partners and also discussed jointly and they still feel there is no hope for reconciliation or compatible living then it is likely that the decision should be for divorce. If both parties agree, no suggestion should be made about having a child or having another child, or trying a separation for a while, or any of the wishful-thinking suggestions which are so often made under these circumstances.

Psychotherapy

If there is some obvious personality maladjustment consultation with a psychiatrist should be urged. Sometimes skillful psychotherapy saves marriage. Again let us emphasize, however, that there should be no wholesale condemnation of divorce, since many times the people who carry it out are acting in better faith toward each other, toward their children, and toward the community at large than well-meaning friends and physicians who urge them to stay together at any and all costs. Few physicians realize how much mental pain and suffering may result from a marriage in which a disappointed, unhappy, frustrated individual is acting out his dissatisfaction upon the marital partner. It leads to neurosis, and even to psychosis, and aggravates existing somatic disease, not to mention the manner in which such an unhappy atmosphere warps the minds and careers of children. Those who would force two people to live together under such circumstances are more guilty of bad faith with society than the couple who would try to remedy their situation by divorce.

PARENTHOOD

Parenthood is highly charged with emotion for both sexes but, of course, more so for the woman. How often the physician hears the comment, "I was perfectly well until my first child was born," or "I haven't had a well day since the birth of my youngest child." What does this mean? Certainly, in the great majority of instances it does not mean that pregnancy has produced or aggravated heart, lung, or kidney disease. Usually it means that the woman in question was emotionally weak and unconsciously did not want the child in the first place. Then pregnancy and parturition probably stirred up false ideas which had been lying dormant within her. These ideas run something as follows. "Children spoil your figure." "Children tie you down." "Children sap your strength." "Nursing a child weakens one." "Giving birth to a child tears you to pieces and you are never the same 'down there.' " Many women, after giving birth to a child, feel as though they have done their bit for the rest of their lives. From that point on this type of woman believes that others should take care of her. They "never get their strength back" because they never wanted to assume very much responsibility in the first place. By means of their invalidism they avoid further pregnancies, avoid marital responsibilities such as sexual intercourse, and are able to live a thoroughly self-centered life. In a word, they control their environment by illness.

Emotional Background for Invalidism

Because knowledge of body functioning preceded knowledge of psychic functioning it has been common practice for the medical profession to think only along the line of physical dysfunction. When a woman says, "Having a child sapped my strength," physicians are inclined to think in terms of anemia and glandular inadequacies, uterine displacement, lack of vitamins, etc., and ignore the fact that the woman is really referring to a lack of emotional strength and to a lack of enthusiasm about her job as a mother.

Children draw their energy for later life responsibilities from the love, attention, information, imagination, and zest for living of their parents. How can a child become very enthusiastic about the joy of living when all she had heard was, "Don't bother mother, she's not well." "Don't make too much noise, dear, mother isn't strong." Or worse still, "Mother had such a hard time when you were born. She never had her health since."

The Father as a Contributor to the Child's Emotional Growth

It is a refreshing sight to see a young woman enthusiastic about having a child, leading an active, healthy life during her pregnancy, and planning in an intelligent way to see that the child has what it needs both physically and emotionally. But the matter of caring for and being interested in children should not be left to the wife alone. Children need a father as well as a mother for the best results in personality development. In other words, the father is important not only as the provider but also as a contributor to the child's emotional growth. Modern life makes it rather difficult in some cases for fathers to spend a great deal of time with their children. This being so it is all the more important that the quality of the relation between father and child should be exceptionally good. Wolfe discusses this problem in detail. Modern machinery and appliances, both in urban and rural areas, have taken away the opportunity for father and son to work side by side. Men, to some extent, have ceased to be the head of the house in the sense that the mother makes decisions about clothing, school, hours of going to bed, and summer vacations. She does not have to work very hard to get this authority, as many men are quite willing to hand over all decisions while they concern themselves only with business and making money for the family support. Such a division of labor is of doubtful value. Wolfe says that when the moral education of children is taken over by women the conscience tends to be formed by a female. Children growing up and constantly taking orders from women do not develop the kindly feeling toward the female sex which they should have. It leads to passivity in men and aggressiveness in women and this is not conducive to the best kind of relationship between the two sexes. *The father and mother should share the various decisions that come up regarding the child, whether the child is boy or girl.*

The father must learn to give his family more of himself in time and comradeship. This is particularly true when the father's work is far removed from the family atmosphere. On the farm the children work with the parents and know the meaning of the work. In the shop this same state of affairs may also prevail. The children take an active part in the work and through this close association they come to know each other in a wholesome way. In other cases children grow up without having any real idea of what the father does to earn a living. He has never thought it important to explain his work and they have never thought to inquire about it.

Education

One of the great problems with adolescents is what they are going to do with their lives. This problem is more frequent with children who have not been associated with the parent's work. The parent works hard to bring home the money to provide for the child's education but gives little consideration to the question of what this education is for.

No father can safely put off becoming acquainted with his child until some time when the child is half grown. A parent who wishes to have the comradeship of his son or daughter at the age of fifteen must begin to cultivate the child's friendship when he is a baby. No grown child, for instance, can suddenly become friendly with a parent who has neglected him. The child will not feel that the parent's interest is genuine and he will probably be right in his supposition. The boy needs a friendly father as an example. A girl too, needs a father's interest, for through this interest she will develop a natural relationship with men. No girl who has been neglected by her father or who has been treated unkindly by him will be able to achieve the best kind of relationship with a husband. The same holds true for a boy and his mother. The mother must protect him as a baby and encourage increasing independence as he grows older. A husband and wife who have found happiness for themselves need only to share their lives generously with their children to fortify them for the problems of later life. *Slavish devotion to books on bringing up children is not a substitute for a wholesome family atmosphere in the preparation for living.* In general terms it may be said that when young people consult a physician about these problems his attitude should be that of a friendly parent rather than that of a detached scientist.

CONVALESCENCE AFTER ILLNESS OR OPERATION

Physicians often observe that physical factors alone cannot explain why convalescence after illness or operation is so long in some cases and so short in others. After an acute febrile illness some patients are soon up and back on the job. The same is true after operation. Others are very slow to "feel well" and convalescence is long drawn out. Some patients actually "never recover" from a certain illness or operation. The illness or operation is a crucial turning point in their lives. A state of semi-invalidism is maintained indefinitely; little or no work is done and former responsibilities are never taken up again.

Unconscious Wish to Remain Ill

To understand this phenomenon we have only to remember that all human beings have an unconscious urge to return to the state of early childhood in which they had no responsibilities and were well cared for. In a severe illness or operation the emotional interest of the patient is withdrawn from the outside world and centered upon himself. An emotional regression to this infantile state is furthered by a general anesthetic or by unconsciousness which has been brought about by any other cause. The first few days after operation have been compared to the very early days of the child's life. The patient awakens from anesthesia usually to find a nurse who takes care of his every wish and need in the same way as the mother once did. The patient likes this and, in fact, may be as fussy as a child about having anyone but his nurse do things for him. He resents being left alone for any length of time and resents any interest on the nurse's part in anyone but himself.

The Authority of the Physician

The surgeon or medical man often takes the place of the father, whose authority is accepted without question. The patient is in a very suggestible frame of mind and the physician or surgeon must be cautious in his comments regarding the patient or his illness. Many patients like to dramatize their illness or operation and a physician who intimates that the patient is lucky to have recovered or who implies that a long convalescence will be necessary from such a serious illness or operation may be suggesting something which the patient is all too ready to accept and to a much greater degree than the physician intended. It is natural for the physician, who is human, to want to appear as a benefactor in the eyes of his patient, but he should remember the patient may unconsciously want to be a chronic invalid, and in emphasizing the seriousness of the illness from which he has saved his patient, the latter may reach the conclusion that he is now a very delicate organism whose whole future existence is precarious. The patient may unconsciously use his illness or operation as a means of gratifying a need for dependence and inactivity, or if he does make an inadequate effort to carry on he will blame everthing that happens to him on the results of that certain illness or operation. *Therefore, a very important consideration in the mind of every physician and nurse should be that it is part of their duty to combat the self-absorption which to some extent occurs in every patient.* This being the case physicians and nurses should encourage independence as soon as the physical circumstances permit in order to help the patient return to normal health. Often the nurse, in her eagerness to give "service" to the patient, brings about an abrupt change when she leaves, which is difficult for the patient to manage. It is better for the nurse to encourage the patient to be independent before she leaves rather than to cater to the desires of the patient up to the last moment.

It is so easy for the well-meaning physician, after an illness or operation, to show sympathy and goodwill by warnings of "be careful," "take it easy," "get back into things slowly," without differentiating between the patient who needs such warnings and the patient who *must not* have them. The physician who would be most kind must recognize this difference in people and act accordingly. Much chronic invalidism can thus be avoided.

PSYCHOLOGY OF PREGNANCY AND PARTURITION

Vomiting of Pregnancy

A frequently encountered psychosomatic problem is the vomiting of pregnancy. Physical factors are undoubtedly concerned but there is also a large psychogenic component in the vomiting of pregnancy. As we have pointed out before, there are many women who for various reasons do not want to become pregnant. This wish may be quite conscious or quite unconscious. If the latter, it may be masked by conscious ideas of wanting a child but this is the kind of patient in whom the vomiting of pregnancy is especially apt to occur. Such patients unconsciously feel that being pregnant indicates that some sin has been committed, or they feel that pregnancy may spoil their figure, interfere with their pleasure or add some unpleasant responsibility to their lives. Consequently, quite unconsciously of course, they would like to rid themselves of the offending fetus. Their childhood fantasies suggest that pregnancy has taken place by way of the gastrointestinal tract and they conceive of the expulsion of the fetus in the same way. The education of later life on the anatomy of the internal organs does not change their vague, childish concepts of babies growing in the stomach and, therefore, unconscious mental forces vainly attempt to get rid of the baby by vomiting.

It is impossible to say to what extent the vomiting of pregnancy is due to a physical (hormonal) factor or how much is due to a psychological cause. As in so many other psychosomatic problems both factors probably operate in most cases, their relative proportion depending upon the psychosomatic structure of the individual. Kroger and DeLee report using hypnosis successfully in seventeen of nineteen cases of nausea and vomiting of pregnancy, in which little or no relief had followed a wide variety of symptomatic treatments.

Treatment for the psychological aspect of the vomiting of pregnancy can be approached as follows:

Prophylaxis

1. Healthy emotional development for children.

2. Proper sexual instruction of children, including emphasis on the dignity of pregnancy and motherhood.

3. Sexual hygiene and marriage courses in schools and colleges.

4. Avoidance of the concept of morning sickness or any other gastrointestinal upset as an inevitable complication of pregnancy.

Immediate Treatment

1. If the vomiting of pregnancy is severe the patient should be put to bed in a quiet room, with nursing care, and relatives and friends excluded.

2. Present the problem to the patient as one of resistance to the pregnant state. Explain the mental mechanisms detailed above. Do this even though it is felt that other factors are playing a role. To regard vomiting in pregnancy as a physical ailment and to neglect it as a problem in behavior is to fail to do justice to the patient.

Pseudocyesis

The enlarged abdomen and amenorrhea of false pregnancy are well known. The classical case usually involves a neurotic woman, near the menopause, who has had no children and strongly desires a child. Other cases occur in younger women who have had illicit intercourse and, fearing pregnancy, are convinced that they are pregnant. In addition to the amenorrhea and enlarged abdomen, the patients present all the symptoms suggestive of pregnancy, including morning nausea and vomiting, enlargement and tingling of the breasts, areolar pigmentation, and even milk secretion. Sometimes the symptom complex is carried through so convincingly that the patient apparently comes to term and the error is not realized until labor is unproductive.

A recent study of three cases by Steinberg and associates indicates that pseudocyesis is not only accompanied by subjective and superficial appearances of true pregnancy but that the urinary excretion of gonadotropins and estrogens is increased in this condition as it is in normal pregnancy. Although the output of gonadotropins and estrogens was far above normal, it was not sufficient to result in a positive Friedman test. After the patients manifesting pseudocyesis had been convinced of the nature of their condition, the signs and symptoms disappeared and the excretion of hormones returned to normal level.

The authors conclude that in view of the absence of pregnancy or abnormality of the pituitary or ovary, it appears that this increased hormonal output must be attributed to the influence of the psyche on the endocrine system.

Delivery and Convalescence after Delivery

Fear of giving birth to a child is almost universal. Ideas from childhood or even later life which concern themselves with the notion of great pain and suffering, being cut open, being torn, being split apart or dying at the time of childbirth cause great anxiety. Many women are not consciously aware of such ideas but suffer anxiety during pregnancy which increases as the time for childbirth arrives. The patient hears from other women, "You are never the same after having a child." "The loss of blood makes you weak and sometimes you never get your strength back." Many women feel that "they have given their all" when they have had a child, in return for which they should be adored and pampered the rest of their lives. This kind of thinking is related to that which was described as failure to recover from illness or operation. It is responsible for a state of passive dependency that may last much longer than it normally should. With good prenatal and postnatal care childbearing is a normal experience from which there should be quick and easy recovery and no unpleasant after-effects.

Treatment. Here again, as in the vomiting of pregnancy, a proper mental hygiene concerning pregnancy and childbirth should be given to female children and carried on in the school system.

Physicians should be aware of the anxieties which may attend pregnancy and childbirth and should encourage the patient to talk about her fears. He should frankly explain the processes of pregnancy and delivery in a truthful but reassuring way.

Just as we discussed with regard to illness and operations, physicians should be careful in their use of terms and not emphasize to their patients that they have had a "hard" or "difficult" labor. This is especially true for certain personalities.

The physician should encourage the mother to nurse her child at the breast.

FAILURE IN ACCOMPLISHMENT

At some period in middle life it often happens that the anxiety underlying a psychosomatic disorder is due to a sense of personal or economic failure. A man may have failed to advance in his work or in his profession to the point that he had hoped or he may not have achieved financial security. A married woman may not have fulfilled her hopes to have a child or children, or her children have failed to fulfill her hopes for their accomplishments, or they may have "grown away" from her, or she may not have achieved her social aspirations or a career outside the home. Another woman has failed to acquire a husband, a home, or children, or has failed to achieve her ambition in her career.

The physician should be aware that *spinsters* suffer the greatest emotional deprivation because they may not only be frustrated in their love life but also in their careers. They will often attempt to deny any sense of frustration or failure; they hasten to assure the physician that "everything is all right," "they are perfectly satisfied," "they wouldn't have had it any other way." However, such statements usually mean that the patient cannot bear to face her disappointment.

Acknowledging Frustration

If a sense of failure is suspected and this is pointed out to the patient he may ask, "Well, suppose I haven't accomplished all that I would have liked? If I dwell upon it won't it make me worse?" The answer to this is that it may cause more mental suffering but that if the patient is seriously ill it is better for him to become conscious of frustration in order for him to realize that it may be the cause of his symptoms. In the second place it is only by acknowledging failure that he can analyze the causes and attempt to modify his attitudes and efforts for a more successful approach to the remainder of his life. The business man may thereby be helped to attack his problems more efficiently. A woman may be helped to become a more companionable and a more stimulating mother to her children. The spinster may be helped to deal more constructively with the problem of marriage and if marriage is not possible, perhaps she can be helped to plan a career or extend her circle of interests.

PSYCHOSOMATIC PROBLEMS OF AGING

The nation is aging rapidly. In 1900 only 17 per cent of the total population of the United States were forty-five years old or more. In 1940, 26.5 per cent were over forty-five, and conservative estimates are that in 1980 more than 40 per cent of our population will be over forty-five years of age. Therefore, gerontology, the science of aging, becomes an important study. This has been recognized in the development of a division on gerontology in the National Institute of Health. Much of the following material has been taken from the excellent writings of Stieglitz, who has done so much to develop this subject.

The two terms, gerontology and geriatrics, must not be confused. Geriatrics is a special field of medical practice which deals with disease in aged individuals, and gerontology is the science of aging. Senescence is that part of the aging process which occurs after the peak of development. Although the changes of senescence are largely involutional, they do not represent solely decline. There are important compensations in certain functional capacities. Hence the unutilized potentialities of the aging are worthy of serious consideration.

Stieglitz states that the problems of aging with which gerontology is concerned, are divisible into three major categories:

1. *The biology of senescence as a process.*
2. *The clinical problems of senescence in man.* Here questions are divisible into those relating to normal senescence and those relating to abnormality due to disorders associated with advancing years. Normal aging brings many changes, some obvious, others obscure, but all insidious

and progressive. Chronologic age is not identical with biologic age. This we have already discussed. The common concept that senescence implies decline is erroneous for there is considerable compensation in certain functional capacities. Loss of physical strength and speed of reaction is often counterbalanced by increased skill and judgment. The popular phrase, "You can't teach an old dog new tricks" had done great harm. As a result many older people admit defeat before trying and opportunities for adult education are suppressed. Recent studies reveal that once this resistance to adult learning is overcome the capacity to learn is really very slightly diminished by aging. It would be better to say, "It is never too late to learn." This has a considerable bearing upon the psychosomatic problems of the aging. To distinguish certain phenomena of disease from those attributable to aging is most difficult. As we have tried to stress, the phenomena of disease are in many instances only exaggerations of normal reactions and do not imply new mechanisms. The most significant of the geriatric disorders are cardiovascular-renal disease, arthritis, diabetes, cancer, and certain syndromes of the climacteric. Of all these the cardiovascular-renal group, which includes hypertensive arterial disease and atherosclerosis, is the most significant. Arthritis also plays an immense role in disability, although its mortality is low. Not only are these disorders usually insidious in onset, but they are chronically progressive and bring about greater or lesser degrees of invalidism.

3. *Social-economic and psychological problems.* The sociologic problems produced by increased longevity and greater life expectancy and the rising median age of the population are immense and complex. Industry is just awakening to the implications of the fact that the average age of employees is increasing at a surprising rate. Problems of placement and retirement, utilization and conservation of the health of older men in positions of great responsibility, the complexities of the workmen's compensation laws in relation to occupational exacerbation of preexistent disease, and many more questions are becoming increasingly important.

The Role of Chronic Disease

Important also in regard to these considerations is a contribution by Ernst Boas on "The Unseen Plague—Chronic Disease" in which he says, "Society has assumed responsibility for many of the acutely ill, as well as for the tuberculous, the insane, the epileptic, and feebleminded. If a person is stricken with pneumonia, acute appendicitis, or with tuberculosis, or mental disease and is unable to obtain medical care, the community provides it at public expense. For the chronically ill, this principle has not as yet received acceptance as a public policy. It is natural that first attention should have been given to diseases that are immediately menacing. Rehabilitation of the chronic sick, and the prevention or postponement of disablement is to the public interest, for it prevents dependency of their families and the consequent tax on the public treasury. The community must act to provide the benefits of modern medicine to sufferers from chronic disease. Methods of diagnosis and treatment have made such progress in the past twenty-five years that many persons with chronic disease may now be restored to comparative health, to an extent not thought possible in the past.

"Private philanthropy cannot be relied on to shoulder the greater part of this responsibility for the chronic sick, as public authorities have assumed in the past. The care of the chronic sick cannot be left to the accident of philanthropy. Voluntary agencies find it increasingly difficult to obtain funds for permanent or long-continued institutional care, and in the future, the greater part of the burden must either be distributed among the entire population through an insurance system, or met by a tax supported program."

Relation to Unemployment and Dependency. "There is a reciprocal relationship between chronic disease and poverty; prolonged illness leads to destitution, and want breeds disease. The treatment of many of the chronic sick is ineffectual unless decent housing and adequate food are available. It is not the individual sick alone, or even they and their families alone who suffer because of the close link between chronic illness and poverty and economic dependency. Chronic illness is responsible for most of the 'unemployables' on relief; it fills homes for incurables and almshouses with crippled invalids; it accounts for a large proportion of the population of hospitals, and of homes for the aged.

"Chronic illness is a great, destructive force in society. It carries in its wake unemployment, destitution, neglect of home, neglect of children, disorganization of family life and dissipation of community resources. Control of the inroads that chronic illness makes on the individual and on society can be made effective through comprehensive study and social planning."

A public health representative has recently discussed the problem in the following manner:

"You will recall Lincoln's statement that the country could not exist 'half slave and half free.' The possession of slaves enslaves the possessor. In the last decade we have come to recognize that the country cannot exist half prosperous and half starved. When millions of people lack food the security of the fortunate few who are prosperous is constantly menaced.

"What we have been slow to recognize, however, is that the country cannot endure half healthy and half diseased. We know that if a festering slum exists in a city, no part of that city is secure, because germs do not respect social stratifications. But a larger, more important yet at the same time more insidious problem in regard to public health and social security, is the question of chronic degenerative disease. It is an essential but undeveloped aspect of social security.

"The public assumption of responsibility for the chronically sick has been limited chiefly to the crippled, the tuberculous, the syphilitic and the mentally diseased but beyond this are many other chronic diseases, the social consequences of which are masked by unemployment and dependency. It is not only a humanitarian proposition; it is a wise economic investment to discover and, where possible, correct the chronic disease that stands behind dependency and unemployment. As we teach social workers something about the disease background of social problems and at the same time teach medical men something about the social background of illness, we will realize that our problems are indissoluble."

Old Age and Industry

In addition to the physical changes that occur with advancing years there are various sociological factors involving the adjustment of the individual to his environment which often result in emotional conflict. In our society old age is often regarded as an affliction and any skill and judgment acquired through years of experience is pushed aside for the energy and new ideas of youth. Old age receives little of the veneration so often accorded to the aged in such parts of the world as China or even in various parts of Europe. It is common practice in industry to view the man of forty-five or fifty as being too old to learn or physically incapable of measuring up to certain standards of production. In an industrial world where speed and precision are so important the older person is usually thrust aside in favor of the greater speed, agility, and endurance of youth. On careful thought it seems clear that the wisdom of experience, the mature judgment, the emotional stability, and the capacity to teach the young would compensate for speed and endurance. Nevertheless, it is true that a marked preference by industry for younger men leads to insecurity on the part of the man who nears fifty.

Mental Changes in Old Age

Of course, it is true that many human beings are unable to retain emotional and ideational flexibility as they grow older. They adjust badly to new ideas, they resist change, they are slow to make new friends, they have difficulties in memory, and what begins as a mild uneasiness often goes on to irritability, insomnia, and a general apprehensiveness and restlessness. To Overholser's recent excellent discussion of this topic we are indebted for many helpful suggestions.

What part cerebral arteriosclerosis, which interferes with nutrition of the brain, may play is difficult to determine. What begins as pessimism and mild mental depression often goes on to fears of death and delusions of persecution, and the afflicted individual becomes a menace to himself and a responsibility to others. He may wander aimlessly about the house or into the street. He may be careless with matches and fire, and, because of the breaking through of earlier repressed sexual impulses, he may make improper sexual advances to women or to young children.

Aging judgments may become so bad as to necessitate taking the man from his business. Sometimes such a person is permitted to harm a business because relatives and partners are afraid to hurt his feelings or are afraid to arouse his anger. It is often difficult to say when the memory defects, irritability, and querulousness of old age have merged into actual psychosis. However, evidence of intellectual defect, the presence of marked insomnia, restlessness, delusions, and hallucinations or other evidences of lack of control usually enable one to make a diagnosis of mental illness even though some parts of the personality are still intact. If cerebral arteriosclerosis is marked, or if an intracranial vascular accident occurs, the progression of mental symptoms may be greatly accelerated.

Treatment

Prophylaxis. In the disorders of old age, no less than in any other psychosomatic problem, there should be some thought as to prevention. The child who is taught to be sociable and adaptable and resourceful will usually continue so in adult life and even in old age. But education must not stop in childhood. _Adult education_ is being looked upon with increasing interest. Community high schools are instituting classes in all kinds of subjects. Hobbies are discovered, as well as new forms of recreation, not to mention instruction in many subjects which contribute to intellectual improvement. People should be encouraged to attend these courses. They are of inestimable value as emotional investments against the impoverishments of later years.

Friction in the Home. Aging people are often problems in the homes of children. The differences in points of view cause frictions. The aging person may want to be a good sport and not get in the way but he or she cannot help giving unwanted advice. If there are children in the home they often try to supervise them—by an outmoded standard of values. The family physician often is reluctant to take part in family differences of this kind.   However, if he wishes to relieve the emotional strains which are causing anxiety and producing symptoms, he may have to get acquainted with the two points of view, usually of daughter and mother-in-law, and suggest ways in which they can be reconciled.   The aging parent or parent-in-law will often listen to advice from a physician when the same thing coming from a son or daughter would be rejected. The same is true when the son or daughter needs advice.

The Interests of the Children.   When excessive irritability or attitudes of suspicion create too much friction in the home and cannot be corrected, it may be best to place the older person in a *nursing home* where he or she is associated with other people of the same age.   If this can be afforded it usually makes life much more pleasant for everyone concerned.   Often sons and daughters are reluctant to do this, fearing the older person may not like it, or may reproach them for having been pushed out, or that neighbors, friends, or other relatives may accuse them of disloyalty.   As a consequence an otherwise happy family life may be disrupted.   In such cases the physician must try to think of the greatest good to the greatest number.   A consideration of first importance must be the children in such a home.   They must not serve as a buffer between the conflicting interests of different generations.

Mental Hospitals.   Placing the psychotic aged person in a mental hospital is usually a last resort.   When restlessness and insomnia can no longer be controlled by sedatives and hypnotics and when the aged person has lost control of himself in other ways, he must be given closer supervision and control than is possible in the average home.   Sometimes depression of spirits is so marked in aged people that they contemplate and actually carry out *suicide*.   It is not uncommon for the aged person to have such impairment in judgment and emotional control as to make sexual advances, and when this happens to small children it may have very unfortunate consequences.   Certainly this demands the supervision which mental hospitals can give.   When the mental state is one of slow progression, occurring in a person who has shown emotional and social limitations during most of his lifetime, it usually means a steady development toward greater dementia.

Chapter VI

TREATMENT—SPECIAL PSYCHOTHERAPEUTIC PROCEDURES

From what has been said in previous chapters regarding psychotherapy it is evident that one of the tasks of any psychotherapeutic technic is to reduce the amount of energy which enters channels unprofitable to the welfare of the patient. This energy then becomes available for useful purposes. Normal amounts of energy are an individual's birthright but the energy soon becomes attached to such emotions as the need for dependency, the desire for sensual gratification, the need for affection, prestige, love, and security. If a man's need for security has been adequately met during his early years it is not likely that he will develop an hysterical paralysis of the legs when danger threatens on the battlefield. If a woman's craving for affection has been met satisfactorily during her childhood she is not likely to become overweight or to develop gastrointestinal symptoms when her turn comes to give affection to others or when she is deprived of it herself. If sexual curiosity has been satisfied and some normal outlet for sensual indulgence has been permitted in childhood a patient is not likely to suffer from hysterical blindness after witnessing a sexual scene. Emotions and ideas press hard for an outlet and if they are denied free expression through normal channels they are shunted into some organ or organ system, or find release in childish rather than adult behavior. "Every psychic tendency seeks adequate bodily expression." Hence, psychotherapeutic technics hope to release energy being used in symptom formation so that it can be used in more constructive ways.

Resistance to Treatment

Since no human being likes to admit that he is childish or weak or that he differs too much from his fellows, he resists facing these facts. This *resistance* has always to be reckoned with in treatment. It grows out of the natural reluctance to discuss or relive unpleasant experiences. The more unacceptable the patient feels his emotions and ideas to be, the more he tries to avoid or circumvent any treatment which tries to bring them out. Treatment then can be approached from two directions. The therapist can help the patient to *suppress* his unacceptable ideas or he can help the patient to *bring them into the open.* By the latter technic he encounters resistance. It might be compared to treating a boil by sprinkling it with powder, thus hiding it, or opening it with a knife, which the patient resists. The dissimilarity here is that the boil will eventually open spontaneously, thus leading to recovery, whereas spontaneous recovery in most illnesses of psychic origin does not occur. Karl Menninger speaks of the principle of *suppression* and the principle of *expression.* The physician, in the suppressive method of psychotherapy, assumes an active attitude toward the patient's conflicts and endeavors to push them into the unconscious. In expressive psychotherapy the physician endeavors to bring the conflict into the open, where it can be viewed by physician and patient alike, so that an effort can be made to modify the faulty emotional trends. Under suppression Menninger lists terrorism, placebos, rest, hypnosis, suggestion, exhortation, persuasion, command, and religious assurance. The methods using the principle of expression are mental catharsis, psychiatric counsel, and psychoanalysis.

SUPPRESSIVE THERAPY

Terrorism

Terrorism seems out of place as a psychotherapeutic technic and yet this method is used relatively frequently in an attempt to cure psychoneuroses, particularly of the hysterical type. An example follows. A physician was called to see a farm hand who had been discharged and who suddenly developed trembling and an inability to walk. The physician decided that the condition was hysterical. He ordered that the stove poker be heated red hot, stating that when this had been done he would apply it to the patient's back. When the red-hot poker was removed from the stove, and the physician advanced toward the patient, his trembling ceased and his paralysis disappeared.

While this "treatment" brought about normal functioning for the time being it did nothing to help the patient understand why he had to behave in such a manner and so, of course, it did nothing to prevent a future recurrence of the same symptom. Such therapy must be regarded as both unscientific and inhuman, and is only to be compared to the barbarous treatment accorded the insane a century ago.

Placebos

The most frequent method of psychotherapy is the giving of placebos. These take the form of harmless drugs or hypodermic injections of sterile water combined with promises of improvement or cure. The physician implies that the medicine has great virtue and the patient, feeling that he has received some potent drug, is sometimes relieved of symptoms. The administration of the placebo is at least a recognition that the patient is suffering. This the patient appreciates and probably, in many instances, he gets well out of gratitude to the physician for the recognition. Certainly, the giving of placebos is far more satisfying to the patient than to be told that there is nothing wrong and that he need not worry about himself. Whether, in the long run, one method has more worth than the other is debatable. Strictly speaking, a placebo means an inactive or inert drug given to produce a satisfying effect upon the patient. But certain drugs of medicinal value are also given for their suggestive effect, without being specifically indicated. A timely example is _vitamin therapy_. This great advance in our understanding of health and disease has been prostituted by the placebo philosophy. Not only are vitamins administered in the relatively few conditions for which it has been proved that they are specifically indicated but in addition every obscure illness, physical or psychological, gets its complement of vitamins. The eagerness of the profession to find a physical answer to all medical problems and the gullibility of the public, which also wants to swallow a magic pill to abolish any and all ills, find a common answer in vitamins. The _vita_ part of the term is not without significance in this connection. Drug houses and department stores, candy stores and slot machines, peddle vitamins to the extent of millions of dollars annually—money which would go a long ways toward real disease prevention. Apparently we must complete the swing of the pendulum as we have with "focal infection."

The physician who prescribes placebos, in whatever form, is not consciously dishonest. He wants to help his patient. He knows his patient expects drug treatment. He is aware of the resistance of the patient to the idea that his symptoms are the result of emotional conflict. He has seen the beneficial effects of suggestion by placebos in other cases and hopes that the same thing will happen again. When he runs out of placebos the patient runs out on him. The answer to this problem lies in an appreciation of the need for correct diagnosis of psychogenic illness and the adoption of an expressive type of psychotherapy rather than a suppressive one.

Rest

Rest and vacation are the first things that a physician thinks of in dealing with illness of emotional origin. He recognizes that the symptoms are due to external pressures of work or family life (which induce emotional conflicts) and he thinks first of reducing the pressures. It is felt, and rightly so, that in many instances rest will have a salutary effect. To be given permission by an authority like the physician to leave one's daily duties and go to bed does much to reduce anxiety and remove symptoms. In fact, about the turn of the present century, S. Weir Mitchell achieved fame for himself by prescribing the "rest cure." Believing that weakness and nervous exhaustion were responsible for illness of emotional origin he prescribed a definite regimen of rest and forced feeding. It worked very successfully because it catered to some of the most basic needs of the psychoneurotic individual. The patient was removed from the struggle of life; he was nursed and massaged, pampered and well fed. In short, he was treated as an infant and all of the infantile longings, called forth by the illness, were satisfied. Symptoms disappeared and in many cases the improvement continued for some time. In others, a frequent repetition of the rest cure was necessary. But a great many patients continued to be invalids for life and their characters were not improved by a treatment which provided so much secondary gain from illness. Rest has its value in relieving symptoms, but it does nothing to make the patient understand himself better. It does not show him what has made him ill nor does it cure emotional conflicts. The truth of the matter is that a "rest cure" or even a recommendation "to take it easy" does a positive disservice to many neurotic patients. A great many of these patients have to be told to "carry on in spite of symptoms," while the neurotic mechanisms underlying the symptoms are being worked out.

Suggestion and Persuasion

Suggestion and persuasion are closely allied. Persuasion is added to suggestion in order to convince the patient that the suggestion is a good one and that in following it he will be benefited. In the same way command is combined with exhortation. If a patient suffers from paralysis of the legs it is suggested that there is no disease in his legs and that he can use them. This is repeated to him in various ways in order to persuade him of the truth of the suggestion. Then follows the command to use the legs. The aim of these methods is to make the patient cooperate by overcoming the forces which seek dependence and disability. Sometimes the method succeeds but very often the forces which seek dependence and relief from responsibility are too powerful to be overcome by any combination of suggestion, persuasion, command, or exhortation.

Hypnosis

A special and intense form of suggestion is utilized in hypnosis. The patient is asked to relax and is told that he is going to sleep. The hypnotist repeats his command in a low but firm voice. Sometimes he asks the patient to look at a bright object such as a ring, a coin, or some other small object. Or the hypnotist may stroke the forehead or the arms of the patient, repeating in a monotone some such formula as the following. "You are going to sleep. Your eyes are getting heavy. You feel very drowsy. Your eyes are getting heavier and heavier. The lids are closing.

You are going to sleep." After a matter of seconds or minutes the patient enters a trance-like state of varying depth. In this sleeping state the patient will carry out commands, either during his trance, or after waking. This latter phenomenon is called *posthypnotic suggestion.*

Under hypnosis it can be suggested that pains will diminish, paralysis will disappear, that memory for certain events will be restored, in fact, almost any suggestion can be made, providing it does not conflict too much with the patient's training and fixed beliefs. It is said that patients who are hypnotized will not commit immoral or illegal acts, especially if their training has been highly moral.

Experimental Value. Hypnosis has been known and used since the first part of the eighteenth century and has enjoyed popularity from time to time. It was used extensively by an Austrian named Mesmer and at time takes his name as "Mesmerism." It was also used by Charcot in Paris in the treatment of hysteria about 1870. Theoretically interesting, it has little practical value in treatment. It has had great value in psychological experimentation, especially from the standpoint of its contribution to psychopathology. The effects of hypnotism are not lasting. Through its use temporary dissociations of mental phenomena can occur and for the time being resistances can be overcome. For instance, dissociations can be brought about which will prevent the registry of pain impulses. A traumatic event which has induced paralysis can be dissociated so that function can once more take place. Painful affects which have produced defective memory can be dissociated so that memory returns. In other words, parts of the mind can be made to function without the knowledge of another part of the mind.

Temporary Cure. Normal people under hypnosis can be made to laugh, to feel strange sensations in their bodies, to make ludicrous statements and to carry out ridiculous acts without remembering what took place. In emotionally ill people that part of the personality which disturbs normal function can be influenced by hypnosis. However, since this does nothing to bring about an understanding of the factors which produce the symptoms, the "cure" is only temporary, or the conflict takes some other form of expression.

Psychoanalysis has shown that it takes a conscious reliving of the unpleasant experiences to produce any permanent discharge of the unpleasant affect which is producing symptoms. This requires much time and effort. So hypnosis remains a therapy of suggestion, uncertain in its results and limited in its possibilities. At best it can cause a temporary shifting about of conflicts but it does not actually cure them. Furthermore it brings about a greater dependence upon some outer authority (the hypnotist).

A therapy which *reveals* rather than *conceals* the emotional pathology has greater value!

Religious Assurances

Undoubtedly many cures, more temporary than permanent, have taken place through religious assurances. These may take the form of affirmation, blessing, anointing, ingestion of consecrated bread, utilization of the sign of the cross, visit to a shrine, or reassurance by a religious personage. When we attempt to explain this phenomenon scientifically we should bear in mind that love has a beneficial effect upon disturbances of emotional origin. The suffering child is helped by the security which he feels in the presence of his mother and father. Religion has much to do with mother and father figures. It is the childish parts of the personality which are in great need of love and reassurance in illness of emotional origin. Hence, when conflicts produced by guilt, hostility, and sexuality produce pain and suffering, contact with a religious force may do much to bring relief. Physicians recognize the spiritual values of religion for themselves and their patients but they possess neither the religious training nor the desire to utilize religious assurances psychotherapeutically. A rare exception may be made; occasionally a patient is so inaccessible to psychotherapy that religion must be called upon to perform a function for which it is not intended. In the great majority of patients, however, as we have repeatedly emphasized, it is the direct working with the patient's emotional conflicts by the physician himself, based on his knowledge of the personality structure, which will have more controlled and more lasting results.

There is only one large religious order which specializes in healing the sick and its method of doing so does not deviate from the principles mentioned above. Christian Science has undoubtedly made many people feel better and function better, but it has also delayed scientific help to thousands of people until it was too late to be of any value. We feel that there is no power in Christian Science which is not possessed by clergyman, priest, or rabbi, none of whom attempts to heal the sick. They comfort and help the sick but the cure of disease is left in the hands of the medical profession.

EXPRESSIVE THERAPY
Psychoanalysis

Psychoanalysis is founded upon the psychobiological development of the individual. It is a medically orientated psychology; it is a psychology related to physiology. It teaches that physiological processes and psychological processes are indissolubly related in their development. It is a psychology of instincts. It shows how some of the most important emotional trends and ideas in the life of the human being are implanted in early childhood. It recognizes that these early life experiences and the resulting ideas and emotions are registered in the unconscious mind as forces which influence behavior. A psychology so intimately related to the functioning of the human body is obviously the best suited to the physician's use.

Psychoanalysis as a treatment aims at the redistribution of psychic energy. This means that when emotional trends are directed into wrong channels psychoanalysis attempts to make the reasons clear to the patient and thus help him in redistributing this energy into more constructive channels.

There still remains a misconception as to the nature of psychoanalysis. Some use the term to cover a single psychiatric interview which attempts to evaluate the existing personality disturbance. Others use the term to designate a few interviews in which the attempt is made to modify surface anxiety and correct a few faulty ideas. Psychoanalysis, however, is a major psychotherapeutic operation and it must take a long time. It follows a definite technic, as outlined by Freud, which consists of several sessions weekly over a number of months or a year or more, depending upon the severity of the illness.

Special qualifications are required for those who practice psychoanalysis. In fact, it was one of the first medical specialties to require certification of its members. They must have experience in psychiatric hospitals for a year or more. They must be trained in neurology. They have to undergo a *personal psychoanalysis* in order to be aware of their own personality difficulties. They must begin the practice of psychoanalysis under the control of those more experienced in the field and must have supervision in the treatment of at least two cases. They must attend lectures on the theory of psychoanalysis and on psychoanalytic technic, and they must attend seminars in which the clinical aspects of the neuroses and psychoses are presented. The discipline is arduous and the preparation may occupy five or six years. In this country most psychoanalysts are first physicians and psychiatrists, who then add to their psychiatric knowledge the training in psychoanalysis just outlined.

It is sometimes surprising how uninformed students of medicine and physicians are regarding the differences among neurologists, psychiatrists, psychoanalysts, and psychologists. The *neurologist* is trained in the structure and function of the nervous system. He studies neuropathology, neurophysiology, and the clinical phenomena of organic disease of the nervous system. The fields of neurology and psychiatry have become so extensive that it is practically impossible to be a first-class neurologist and at the same time a first-class psychiatrist. However, since there is a dearth of practitioners in these fields it is necessary, in many communties, for the specialties to be combined as neuropsychiatry. Nevertheless, the tendency toward separation should be encouraged.

The emphasis in the training of the *psychiatrist* has been on the psychoses. He has usually spent long years working in mental hospitals. Just as the neurologist has spent some time with psychotics in order to have some acquaintance with mental illness, so the psychiatrist has spent some time in neurology in order to be able to recognize some of the more common and more evident neurological disorders. However, the psychiatrist does not pretend to make a refined neurological diagnosis and usually refers such work to his neurological colleague.

The *psychoanalyst* is a psychiatrist who has received special training in the psychopathology of the unconscious mind, originated by Freud, and his work with patients is usually confined to the practice of this particular psychotherapeutic technic. *Psychoanalysis is related to psychiatry as microscopic anatomy is related to gross anatomy.*

The *psychologist* is not a physician and does not treat sick people. Psychologists can be divided roughly into three main groups composed of (1) the experimental psychologist who studies animal as well as human behavior; (2) the clinical psychologist who concerns himself with measurements of intelligence, tests of vocational aptitude, and is now attempting to develop some satisfactory measurement of personality values; (3) the consulting psychologist who uses his knowledge of mental life in personnel work and counseling with normal groups.

During World War II the psychologist became an important member of a team composed of psychiatrist, social worker, and psychologist, and fortunately in many instances this teamwork is continuing in civilian practice.

Harrower has said that the psychologist with his personality tests must do more than establish a diagnosis. He must assume the more positive role of assessing the dimensions and depths of the personality and exploring the individual's potentialities and resources. Thus his task would lie not simply in the diagnosis of a neurosis, but rather in a description of the type of personality in which neurotic symptoms were finding expression. In this way he can be of greater help to the psychotherapist who can then make use of this knowledge in planning for the patient's welfare.

Academic psychology, for the most part, has been very critical of psychoanalysis, but in embracing the Rorschach technic of personality evaluation, it has moved a little closer toward accepting the basic concepts of psychoanalysis. An appreciation of the workings of unconscious mental forces, as revealed by the Rorschach method, has made the depth psychology of Sigmund Freud a little more acceptable. Indeed, the Rorschach test has done for psychology what the psychosomatic concept has done for medicine, that is, provided a bridge of understanding between the organic tradition and a dynamic explanation of human behavior in sickness as well as in health.

Indications for Psychoanalysis. Having tried to make clear what psychoanalysis is, we must say something about the indications for its use. For the most part, at present, patients only come to psychoanalysis when all other methods have been exhausted and all treatments have failed to help them. In brief, it is indicated in most severe neuroses. It is indicated in some cases of psychopathic personality such as alcoholism, sexual perversion, kleptomania, and other character disturbances, providing that the patient has a strong desire to get well and there can be some cooperation and support from the family. Kubie summarizes the indications for psychoanalysis as (1) treatment for a fully developed neurosis, (2) to prevent neurosis from developing, (3) to prevent development or recurrence of a psychosis, (4) to find out the cause of some unhappy maladjusment in the personality. To these we would add: (5) to prevent a mild neurosis from becoming a severe and crippling illness as age advances and frustrations increase, and (6) to cure or alleviate the symptoms of psychosomatic disorder.

Treatment by psychoanalysis is preferable early in life. Aside from the psychoanalysis of children, which is done for severe personality maladjustments, the next period of choice is early adult life. Clinical experience has shown that the adolescent period is not satisfactory. Since psychoanalysis means an inevitable change in certain fundamental attitudes toward life it is highly desirable that such a procedure be undertaken before too many irrevocable commitments have been made. A great many people make choices of career, marriage, parenthood, and other crucial decisions, in an effort to solve neurotic conflicts. In other words, these decisions are often symptomatic of their personality disorder. Therefore, if they are to be treated by psychoanalysis it had better be before, rather than after, these decisions have been made. Most analysts prefer patients under the age of forty, although the procedure may still have value after this age. It is especially important for a woman to solve her problems as early in life as possible, for if she wishes to marry and have children her time is limited, not to mention the limitation in opportunities.

The Technic of Psychoanalysis. Psychoanalysis is usually conducted with the patient lying on a couch while the physician sits behind him. In this position it is usually much easier for a patient to talk. As Alexander expressed it, "in the relaxed and matter of fact atmosphere of the psychoanalytic sessions the patient is encouraged to express himself in intelligible language instead of in the distorted language of his symptoms." The patient is instructed to say everything that comes to his mind, regardless of how inappropriate, irrelevant, or personal it may seem to be. As the patient follows this rule certain trends of thought are manifested. Hostility, fear, feelings of dependency, sexual fantasies, ideas of suspicion, jealousy, and so forth, weave themselves into a pattern which expresses the patient's total personality. The material appears slowly—a little each day. As the material comes up its influence on the daily life of the patient is observed. Observed, too, is the reverse of this situation, that is, the influence of the daily life happenings on the material from the unconscious mental life. As Kubie puts it, "The patient's present life is a screen on which the past throws its shadows."

Relation of Patient to Analyst. As these ideas and feelings are expressed a certain relation to the analyst is noted. Again to quote Kubie, "The analyst becomes a storm center of highly charged emotions." Hostility, fear, anger, and the like, which arose in other connections, are often expressed in relation to the analyst, whose own analysis permits him to tolerate their expression. After a variable time the patient begins to understand how unjustified these emotions are in relation to the analyst, who has tried to be entirely objective in his explanations, and he also sees that they have had their derivation from earlier life experience, usually the experiences of childhood. The reliving of the emotional experience, and the insight gained thereby, permit the mind to discharge the pathological material. This process is called *abreaction*. Psychic energy, which no longer has to be expended in repressing the pathological material, is now free to be turned into more constructive channels.

The Study of Emotional Trends. In coming to the analyst several times a week, the patient has an opportunity to study his most basic emotional trends. Physician and patient focus their attention upon the feelings expressed toward the world in general and the analyst in particular, and the result is often most surprising to the patient. Having assumed that he was decisive he finds himself vacillating; having thought himself courageous he finds that he is timid; in his own eyes generous and magnanimous, he finds himself petty and parsimonious. On the contrary, he may have considered himself stupid only to find that his ideas have merit. He has been handicapped by a feeling of inferiority and finds that his capacities are equal or superior to those of his associates. The opportunity offered by psychoanalysis to speak frankly and fearlessly about one's self reveals many things which the person has never before known about himself. Some people will fairly readily assimilate these facts and make some rearrangement of their lives. Others have so much hate, resentment, bitterness, and distrust built up within them that they find it difficult to bring about any change in attitude.

Transference. The relation of patient to physician is a phenomenon which has been given particular attention by Freud and his followers ever since psychoanalysis began. This tendency for emotion from another time and situation to occur in the psychotherapeutic session and to express itself in relation to the therapist is known as *transference*. The transference situation has many important implications for medicine in general and the management and utilization of this phenomenon is a most significant feature of psychoanalysis.

Alexander defines the transference as merely a projection of the past into the analytic situation and the tranference situation, in reality, as nothing more than the relation between patient and physician. The transference manifestations occur under the continuous control of the ego and the patient is aware of their unmotivated nature. "The essential point is that in the transference, the adult with his stronger and more resistant ego faces in reduced quantity the same kind of conflict which as a child his weak ego could not solve. The solution of the reduced emotional conflict effects an increase in the resistance of the conscious ego, which becomes able to face mental conflicts and situations which were previously unbearable. This principle of analytic treatment can be compared with that of active immunization, by means of which the resistance of the body is partially increased by fighting small quantities of toxin."

In the setting of the psychiatric interview (when the attentions of the patient and the physician are not focused on the physical aspects of illness) there is time and opportunity for the patient to express his feelings and that is when we are in the best position to see the basic emotional trends in action.

While the patient exhibits emotional attitudes which he has held toward a parent or someone else who has played an important role in his life, he is, of course, still able to react to the doctor as he really is. The doctor may be conscientious, kind, and considerate, and this may be felt by the patient if he has some capacity for reality testing. In fact, some degree of being able to react emotionally to the present is essential to therapeutic progress. However, it is an important part of therapy to help the patient understand that some of his emotions are those of childhood and are now no longer necessary or useful. He must not only appreciate this intellectually, he must feel it emotionally. Indeed this should be stated in reverse, because what the patient feels and exhibits in his behavior is then explained intellectually.

When the patient's childhood attitudes are especially prominent he may see the physician and his role in a distorted way, but the physician must maintain his objectivity and allow full freedom of expression in order that the patient may get the necessary understanding of his problem.

Many people in their day-to-day living have different moods, exhibit petty jealousies, become unreasonably angry over trifles, feel themselves exploited, blame others for lack of consideration, and they never change. In the controlled patient-physician relation, however, the setting is different: (1) The patient acknowledges that he is ill for emotional reasons;(2) he asks the physician to help him; (3) the physician remains objective and is neither critical nor punitive as (4) he explains how the mind functions and how to correct harmful attitudes.

The Use of Dreams. Freud was the first to utilize the dream as a means of helping the patient to understand the workings of the unconscious mind. Some patients dream freely, one or more dreams every night, while others dream rarely. There is mental activity going on during sleep whether it is remembered as a dream or not. Some patients immediately accept the dream as meaningful while others have great resistance to "seeing any sense in dreams." Some dreams are very clear and understandable as *wish fulfillments*. A child dreams that he owns and rides a pony, or the business man, who must remain at work every day, may dream that he is attending a ball game. Other dreams, however, may be much more difficult to understand, as for instance a dream that a relative or friend is ill or dead or a dream in which one is in an embarrassing state of semi-nudity. Then there is the dream of being in a dangerous situation and great anxiety is felt. However, when the patient learns to associate freely to the various details of his dream it can be shown that they do make sense—that they attempt to reveal his forgotten experiences, his repressed desires, and his unconscious fears and dislikes.

To the psychoanalyst the dream represents the secretion of the mental apparatus, which can be analyzed for diagnostic and prognostic purposes, just as the urine, the secretion of the kidneys, can be analyzed by the general physician for diagnostic and prognostic purposes.

Now just as the patient transfers his emotions to the analyst so the analyst cannot avoid transferring certain feelings toward his patient. This phenomenon is called *countertransference*. But by his own analysis, made in preparation to practice psychoanalysis, the analyst is in a much better position to remain detached. The psychoanalyst, being human, does not relish being criticized, condemned, and berated for months on end, but his insight and understanding make it possible for him to endure this without efforts to retaliate. So also the psychoanalyst is naturally pleased by his patient's gratitude and admiration but he does not allow this to deter him from pointing out his patient's shortcomings, when this is necessary. In short, the analyst has tried to obtain through his training as great an objectivity as possible, concerning human emotions. Thus he can maintain an objective attitude toward the emotionally sick person in his attempt to help him to achieve emotional stability.

Psychoanalysis, therefore, is a process of emotional reeducation. Emotions and ideas which have been unconscious are made conscious, with resulting better attitudes and more efficient living.

Hypnoanalysis

Within the last decade efforts have been made to combine hypnosis with psychoanalysis, for example: (1) in suggesting the recall of infantile experience or events surrounding the onset of illness or any other relevant associations, (2) in the recall of dreams and their interpretations, (3) to promote the analysis of the transference and (4) to make whatever interpretations seem necessary to insure the goal, a goal not only of symptom relief but of a better functioning ego.

This alliance between the hitherto dynamic but unwieldy hypnosis and the slower, tedious but better controlled psychoanalysis has been called hypnoanalysis (Wolberg). It is for a skilled psychiatrist to use and not for the average physician.

Transference and the Physician

Transference and countertransference are not solely the concern of the psychoanalyst. Fortunately (or unfortunately) the average patient-physician relationship engenders these same problems and they are even more difficult to understand because they are unconscious. For this reason the physician should be as free of mental conflict as possible in order not to confuse his patient's thinking any further. The less insight the physician has into his own emotions, the less likely he is to present the best attitude for the patient's recovery.

For instance, a physician may believe that women are by nature frigid; if he does, he will be of little help with the neuroses in which sexual difficulties enter strongly into the picture. He would, likewise, be a relatively useless counsellor in most marital problems. Or the physician may be unable to stand anxiety in his patients without dosing them with sedatives. Or he cannot tolerate their displeasure and so will try to please them rather than doing what is best for them. He may not like neurotic people and, being unaware of this, may mistakenly and sometimes cruelly subject them to painful, useless, and expensive medical and surgical procedures. He may hold on to certain patients too long and fail to refer them for the expert help which they need. This may arise from his own insecurity represented by the necessity for a large income. Or, overconfident, he takes chances which are not scientifically justified.

Some pediatricians, feeling that children are "spoiled" by too much affection, teach the mothers to be frustrating rather than to give their affections freely. The obstetrician's inability to deal with the anxieties, questions, and discomforts of the mother, may result in so much anxiety and suffering during pregnancy and delivery that the number of children is limited. A surgeon with a great deal of unconscious hostility toward women cannot understand them, and when they come to his office unhappy and complaining, and very willing to attribute their distress to some bodily disorder, he, having the tools and knowing the technics of cutting, thinks he may remove the discomfort (which often represents childishness, dependency, and hostility) by surgery. He tries to remove a pain from the body which really resides in the spirit, or psyche.

Although these attitudes on the part of the physician are not ordinarily thought of as *transference* reactions the truth is that every physician gets into a transference situation with every patient the moment they meet, regardless of the problem. Each immediately brings many unconscious attitudes into the relationship, and these attitudes, of which both may be completely unaware, have great influence on the outcome of the illness.

The psychoanalyst has the kind of training which tends to reduce to a minimum these unfortunate attitudes. He does not claim to be completely objective. He merely claims to be relatively so, and he is always on the alert to keep his own immature attitudes and prejudices out of the picture, in order to give the patient the best opportunity for self-development. He also tries to pass on to his colleagues in the other areas of medicine some of the insight into interpersonal relations that will keep destructive countertransference reactions at a minimum.

Mental Catharsis

Mental catharsis is self-explanatory. It means talking to someone about your troubles. The one who talks usually feels better afterward even though the listener says nothing. He feels that someone has shared his trouble with him and hence he has less of a burden to carry. The listener, by withholding criticism, is usually regarded as having said, "I do not blame you. I understand why you feel as you do. You need not feel guilty. I might have done the same thing."

Such psychotherapy, of course, has distinct limitations. In the first place the patient talks about his conscious troubles, whereas neurotic symptoms have their roots in the unconscious mind. Hence the patient might talk endlessly because he is not discussing real issues. Nevertheless, listening to another's troubles is a first principle in psychotherapy and such value as it has should not be lost sight of. A well-trained and experienced psychotherapist can accomplish great good simply by directing a conversation, listening carefully and saying little, while a poorly trained and inexperienced psychotherapist can do real harm by talking instead of listening.

Psychiatric Counsel

The most common form of psychotherapy is psychiatric counsel. Only a limited number of patients can be psychoanalyzed and, of course, all patients do not need such long and intensive treatment. In psychiatric counseling the physician attempts to learn as much as possible about the patient's ideas and trends of thought, in order to help him.

For this purpose the physician should have a background of psychoanalytic understanding. Every physician cannot be psychoanalyzed but information is readily available to acquaint him with the nature of unconscious mental processes. *Such knowledge is just as important for the practice of medicine as a basic training in anatomy and physiology.*

Psychosomatic history, thorough physical examination, laboratory and perhaps special studies, prepare the way for psychiatric counsel in psychosomatic illness. With negative physical examination or symptoms out of proportion to the physical disease we are in a position to say to the patient, "I believe your illness is of emotional origin. Worry and anxiety can influence the function of the body and I think this is so in your case."

The patient may readily agree or may be skeptical. As a rule the patient says, "But there must be something the matter," meaning, of course, something physical. "This is not my imagination. I can't believe I'm neurotic. I hate neurotic people who do nothing but complain."

Illness Not Imaginary. In the first place the physician must explain that he *did not say* the illness was imaginary. On the contrary, he has said it was just as real as though it were a physical disease. Patients must be taught to have as much respect for emotions as for bacteria. Pain in the abdomen from anxiety is no more imaginary than pain from appendicitis.

The physician can go on to say, "To have symptoms as a result of emotion is not a sign of weakness. Very capable people, doing the world's most important jobs, have emotional conflicts. Those who try to avoid conflict by assuming no responsibility are the weak ones. To be 'nervous,' to have anxiety, is only an evidence that energy is not being expressed in the proper channels."

Approximating Facts. The patient then may say, "All right, if my symptoms are due to my emotions what can I do about it?" When we come to the point of helping the patient to "do something about it" we should think a moment of what the patient may be feeling. We must never be too eager to "tell," to "educate," to "advise." Learn to know what the resistances are to the patient's self-education. Much of what a patient "learns" in psychotherapy is self-evident truth except that the patient has not been quite aware of the situation. In fact, many times the physician has been surprised to hear his patient say, after being told about himself and what to do, "Why doctor, I knew that already." The point is that the patient has often known "that two and two were in his mind but he did not put them together to make four." The facts were there; the patient was aware of them; but they were isolated. The physician helps to approximate them.

Understanding Emotional Problems. But the physician must understand the emotional problems of his patient before help can be given. Sometimes the patient's greatest suffering is from immediate deprivations; sometimes from childhood deprivations. In still other instances it may be a combination of the two. An example of the first is a woman who develops insomnia, indigestion, and mental depression. Her husband is cold and unromantic; there are financial worries; and they live in an uncongenial neighborhood. The feeling of deprivation and the anxiety aroused by these immediate problems make the patient ill. Had the environment been more favorable she might have remained well.

Another woman, the oldest of eleven children, married happily at twenty-three. She remained well until the age of twenty-eight and then became ill with indigestion, fatigue, and dizziness. Her husband was devoted to her and tried to get her the best medical care. For three years she was subjected to much medical and surgical treatment but continued to grow more depressed and disinterested in living. She had known many deprivations in childhood. For one thing she had been a feeding problem. Then when she was a year and a half old a sibling was born and when she was three years of age another came. Later the mother suffered a nervous breakdown and was very self-centered for a period of months. Our patient had to help with the other children and, being the oldest, had to assume much responsibility. Her own wants and desires were neglected. Falling ill at twenty-eight, with depression and lack of interest in her home and husband, meant that she was overcome once more with the same emotional emptiness as in her loveless childhood. In this case the childhood forces were more important in causing illness than any immediate deprivations.

In a third case a man wanted to enter a business project of which his father disapproved. He needed his father's financial as well as his moral support. When this was withheld the patient developed headaches, fatigue, and constipation. There was obvious conflict over an immediate problem but his childhood fear of his father made the solution to the present problem doubly difficult and this had to be dealt with to give him relief.

Necessity for Cooperation. After we understand the patient's life situation we can make suggestions for help but the patient must cooperate as an active participant. Keeping in mind what has been said about passivity and the need for dependence in emotionally sick people, it is not difficult to understand that the patient does not relish the necessity for taking an active part in working out his cure. This dependent attitude of "letting the doctor do it" plus the physician's urge "to do something definite" accounts for the frequent submission, on the part of the patient, to operations, baths, electric treatments, diets, and so forth. The patient does not have to think or take much initiative. He submits and waits for results. In psychotherapy the patient must act. He may talk and define his problem but there always comes a point when he must do something about it.

In the *first case* just cited, the woman suffered largely because her husband did not understand her need for affection. This brought up the question of whether the physician should see the husband. The patient was, of course, informed that this would be done tactfully, on the basis of a discussion of her health. Having received the wife's consent the physician informed the husband that her symptoms arose from unhappiness and anxiety rather than from tissue pathology and that it was to his advantage to understand the causes so that he could help her to recover. The husband was able to see the necessity for a more sympathetic interest in his wife's feelings.

We then explained to the patient that her neighborhood could not be completely unfriendly and that she could certainly find some people with common interests if she would only look for them. We said, "Make it your job to visit a neighbor this week and do not leave until you have found that you and she have at least two interests in common." She took up the challenge, found a neighbor who liked a certain radio program which they discussed, and also found that each had contemplated attending a night-school hobby class but had not wanted to go alone. And so they arranged to begin together. Considerable improvement in her symptoms followed.

The *second case* was more difficult to approach. Psychotherapy would have been easier if it had been done early. A long fixation on the physical aspects of her illness induced the patient to center a great deal of atttention upon her body and she had grown distrustful that anything could be done for her. The first task was to have her accept the emotional basis for her illness. She had complained bitterly that no one understood her but when someone tried to understand her she turned once more to her somatic distress. We said, "You obviously have needed someone to interest himself in your feelings. Directing attention to your body has not helped. Now why do you try again to draw attention to your body when you have admitted that the trouble is in your feelings?" The patient replied, "I don't know. When I find what I want I don't seem to know how to use it."

She continued, "I love my husband so much. I'd give my soul to be well and be able to enjoy my life with him." We said, "You speak as though you cared but actually you seem compelled to give your thoughts and feelings to your own aches and pains. If you will turn your energy toward other interests and other people perhaps you will have less bodily discomfort." The patient would answer, "I don't see how you can take pain away without medicine." We said, "Perhaps you cannot see that far but let us proceed one step at a time. Use your goodwill and such effort as you have, to direct your attention outward instead of inward." She then complained of lack of appetite and we explained that just as she had no appetite for living so she had no appetite for food—that the symptoms represented behavior and not disease! On her next visit she reported a better appetite and began to show an interest in the emotional origin of her illness. In a short time she began to do her own housework again. In our interviews we continued to instruct her to dismiss the thoughts and feelings she had centered on her body and instead to direct them toward other people and other interests. Improvement was slow but, under the circumstances, satisfactory.

In the *third case* the patient could readily see that his symptoms arose in direct relation to his problem with his father. He felt thwarted by an insurmountable hurdle. When asked if he could not borrow the money elsewhere and go ahead with his venture he declared this was impossible. However, discussion showed that it seemed impossible only because he feared his father's disapproval of the venture. We asked him, "Does your father not want you to succeed? Does he not want you to use your own judgement and have the satisfaction of accomplishment?" He answered in the affirmative. We said, "Then why not go to your father and discuss your plans as man to man?" The patient still had anxiety about following this advice so we asked him to discuss his childhood relation to his father. He said, "I never asked favors of my father. I never dared press an issue. I couldn't bear to have him grow impatient or angry with me or refuse me anything. Yet I now know that he likes me and trusts me to a considerable extent. I've heard mother and his friends say so." We again pointed out that he was laboring under the same anxiety that he felt as a boy and that this prevented him from taking a convincing attitude with his father. He permitted his anxiety to convey the impression that he did not fully believe in the project, whereas the thing he was really afraid of was not the success of the project but the success of his appeal to his father. Finally after a third interview he saw his father, enlisted his interest and support, and his symptoms disappeared.

Understanding the Background of Anxiety. From these examples it may be seen that successful psychiatric counseling depends upon understanding the background of the patient's anxiety—whether the conflict is chiefly a product of the impact on the patient's specific emotional make-up of the present, or the past external situation, or as is usually true, a combination of the two. For this purpose we must have some understanding of personality structure and psychopathology. Then to a large extent, we must ignore the symptoms and attack the basic sources of the conflict. When we say "ignore the symptoms" we mean "Teach the patient to carry on in spite of symptoms." Only in this way can improvement be brought about.

The Use of Dreams. Dreams can be utilized in psychiatric counseling although they cannot be as useful in this form of therapy as in psychoanalysis. In the latter treatment more time and attention can be given to associations to the dream and, with frequent repetition of ideas, there is a greater opportunity to see certain personality trends of thought or action. Thus understanding of the nature of his unconscious activity will more surely come to the patient.

Patients are often skeptical regarding the significance of dreams but some dreams are so clear that even the most skeptical person must admit that they have meaning. The woman who maintains that she has no sexual interest but dreams repeatedly of sexual advances by men, should admit, when the opportunity is afforded of calling her attention to the idea, that a certain part of her mental life must have some interest in the subject. The man who insists that he has no resentment against his family, friends, or employers but who repeatedly dreams of arguments and fights with them, may be helped through his dreams to see an aggressive side of himself which he is repressing. One says to the patient something like this, "Mental activity goes on during sleep and some of the things you wish, some of the things you fear, and in fact anything that you feel strongly about may present itself in your dream pictures. The ideas may be disguised, they may appear in symbolic form, or they may be contained within what seems to be a lot of meaningless action. But, after all, dreams are a product of your mental activity and perhaps we can use them to help in understanding you."

Thus the willingness or ability to understand dreams varies greatly among patients. Some patients are annoyed to have the physician try to see meaning in them. They require the actual feelings which they experience in daily living to convince them of the psychic forces existing within them. Other patients may volunteer dreams and ask to have them discussed. Often it is helpful to question as to whether there are dreams with a frequently recurring theme. *Repetitive dreams* have special significance. They clearly indicate a definite personality trend.

Keeping Material Suppressed. Sometimes a patient will ask, "If I do not like the people I am supposed to like isn't it better not to bring it out—won't it make our relations more strained?" Or a patient with greatly repressed erotic trend, especially if single, may ask, "If I have these tendencies won't it make a greater problem for me to become more aware of them?" The answer generally is "No," since we must not forget that we are treating the cause of symptoms and symptoms should be no more respectable than the emotion they represent. Secondly, when unconscious wishes are made conscious, with the exception of potential psychotics, there is still the healthy part of the personality to help solve the problem raised by hostility or sexual tension. The hate, jealousy, and sexual tension in psychoneurotics are just additional facts of life which they must face and find a solution for, as other people try to do.

Their problems do not differ in kind from those of average "healthy" people—only the solution is more difficult and they need help. If a physician accepts such patients he should be aware of the sort of "trap" which these emotionally immature people set. They talk and act as if to say, "I'm just a little child. How can you expect me to struggle with those powerful forces?" With such an attitude the physician must be sympathetic but he must also try to avoid giving direct advice. He should give his patient the chance no one else has ever given him, that is, to think and express himself freely about what may be socially taboo. If undesirable thoughts or feelings are in the mind they are better managed when made conscious than when left unconscious. When the dream helps to make the unconscious more understandable it should be used as an adjunct in understanding and counseling the patient.

Something Less than Cure. Now we must say something of the other side of the picture. Physicians attempting psychotherapy sometimes must curb their zeal to accomplish too much. There are severe neurotics and potential psychotics to whom some information, especially if it is given carelessly, only serves to increase their anxiety. Unless they can be seen frequently so as to gain friendly support and work over their thoughts, they become worse. One should proceed carefully in the first interview and see what his patient can tolerate. It is better not to probe too much or attempt to enlighten too much at one time. This is particularly true in adolescents. A physician who is meticulous in administering digitalis or insulin will tell a neurotic patient that he is lazy, cowardly, doesn't love his family, hates his father, cannot face life, etc., and then wonders why the patient is not better the next day.

Removing a Symptom that the Patient Needs. Even the physician who proceeds more slowly and more carefully may try too hard to remove a symptom which the patient needs. Remember that the symptom often represents the answer to a psychological conflict and in taking the symptom away something must be given in its place or, stated better, the patient must be helped to find something in its place. This takes time, patience, and resourcefulness. It can rarely be done by one or even several "pep talks." The external situation may be impossible to solve or even when a solution exists the patient may not have available the potential resources for the solution. Fortunately some modification of the external situation or the patient's inner life, or both, can usually be effected.

In an article entitled "What Price Healing," Jelliffe strikingly demonstrated that serious emotional illness may result when a symptom is removed by medicine or surgery, without attention to the underlying emotional make-up and the life situation. When psychosomatic illness has become definitely "fixed," its pattern "set," it must be realized that the emotional needs of the patient are being partially satisfied by the illness itself and it may be necessary to allow him to keep his illness as the best answer to his problem. For example, a woman of fifty-five suffered from pains in the back and legs and occasionally in the joints. She was carefully studied over a period of three years for evidence of physical disease and none was found. She had had a barren childhood, a loveless marriage, had raised two children, and both refused to live with her. Her husband was dead and she was painfully lonely. But she had always prided herself on her self-sufficiency. She could not be told that she was lonely or that she needed friendship. To accept the idea that she was lonely would be an admission of weakness which she could not tolerate. To tell her that she needed friends was to make her realize that she had never cultivated friends and was too rigid at this point to learn how. She would keep a nurse for a while and either the nurse would leave because of her constant complaining or she would find some excuse to discharge her. Of course, she also changed physicians frequently. Since she had money to spend for what she wanted, her son was advised to cease concerning himself about her and permit her to live the only pattern of existence which was possible for her to live.

In other words, as physicians we sometimes have to admit that the illness must be allowed to continue—that, under certain circumstances, it is the best answer to a life problem.

GROUP PSYCHOTHERAPY

The time that must be devoted to each patient in individual psychotherapy has led various workers to attempt treatment in groups instead of singly. The procedure had been carried out with some success even before World War II. During the war, the larger numbers of patients made group psychotherapy a greater necessity than ever before, and it was used on an extensive scale. Although it will probably continue to be used since it can benefit a large number of persons at one time, it lacks many of the benefits of individual therapy and of course can never completely replace it. While the technic varies to some extent, the following plan is generally followed:

Technic

Instead of talking with one patient, the physician brings together a group with common problems and talks with them. From eight to twelve patients gather in a room of appropriate size; preferably the chairs are arranged in a circle, for this facilitates discussion. The physician acts as a leader and the relation of the emotions to bodily changes (the conversion of conflict into symptoms) may be simply stated. Tact and ingenuity are required to bring the patients into the discussion. The interest of the physician must not stray too far from the group to individuals or the therapeutic value becomes lost to the others. Yet, he must be able to recognize and to call upon the more articulate members in the beginning to ask questions, express opinions, recount their symptoms, cite experiences which have produced symptoms or even those which have relieved symptoms. If a group shares fears of being alone, then the mechanism of helpless anxiety is discussed. Here are some of the consequences of the procedure:

1. There is expression of emotion (ventilation) which, plus the fact of recounting of experiences in the presence of others, reduces anxiety.

2. Personal problems seem less personal when it is learned that others have felt the same way, hence there is relief from guilt and feelings of inferiority.

3. The patient benefits from the experience of socialization in the group setting.

4. Inspired to offer a solution for another person's problem, a patient may find that he is offering the solution to his own.

While the physician is a member of the group he is at the same time its discussion leader. He may be consulted on a point of specific information or he may find it necessary to bring the subject back so that it may prove profitable to the majority. Frequently he presents a summary in concluding the discussion.

Some advocates of group therapy find it best to permit no additions to the group once it has started, carrying the same patients through the various sessions to a conclusion. Others feel that the introduction of new members does not impair the efficiency of the group and indeed has certain advantages to offer the new members.

No large-scale application has yet been made to specific psychosomatic problems but Ackerman reported some experience in psychosomatic disorders with such symptoms as headache, insomnia, and fatigue.

Heath, at the same meeting, described his experience in the treatment of merchant seamen, among whom was a group of alcoholics. Here the group meetings resembled the Alcoholics Anonymous meetings and after discharge the members of the group joined this organization.

Because there is little removal of infantile amnesia, and because the working out of transference phenomena is impossible, real depth understanding may not be reached in group therapy. Nevertheless the group method has much to offer and undoubtedly will find wide application, especially in a period when there are so few psychiatrists.

Group Psychotherapy as a Community Experiment

An attempt has been made to examine how far a continuously changing population of patients and staff could develop its form of community within the framework of a military psychiatric hospital in England. Referring to the "Northfield Experiment" Lt. Col. T. F. Main speaks of the hospital as a therapeutic institution. He describes the demoralizing effect which the usual hospital may inadvertently have: "By tradition a hospital is a place wherein sick people may receive shelter from the stormy blasts of life, the care and attention of nursing and medical auxiliaries, and the individual attention of a skilled doctor. The concept of a hospital as a refuge too often means, however, that patients are robbed of their status of responsible human beings. Too often they are called 'good' or 'bad' only according to the degree of their passivity in the face of the hospital demand for their obedience, dependency and gratitude. The fine traditional mixture of charity and discipline which they receive is a practised technic for removing their initiative as adult beings, and making them 'patient.' They are less trouble thus to the staff. Hospitals which follow this orthodoxy are usually designed for the individual treatment of the individual patient by an individual doctor, not in a real social setting, but in a state of retirement from society. So, isolated and dominated, the patient tends to remain gripped by the hospital machine even in the games or prescribed occupations which fill in his time between treatments.

"Within such a setting, health and stability are too often bought at the excessive price of desocialisation. Sooner or later the patient, alone and unsupported, must face the difficult task of returning to the society in which he became unstable, and there regain social integration, and a daily sense of values and a purpose. This task is no light one for a desocialised man, however healthy he may have become . . . Treatment of the neurotic patient who suffers from a disturbance of social relationships cannot, therefore, be regarded as satisfactory unless it is undertaken within a framework of social reality which can provide him with opportunities for attaining fuller social insight and for expressing and modifying his emotional drives according to the demands of real life. In any case, the fact must be faced that radical individual psychotherapy is not a practicable proposition for the huge numbers of patients confronting the psychiatric world today. It is doubtful whether the hospital can usefully remain a building within which individual treatment is practised. Perhaps it must become a therapeutic institution. The Northfield Experiment is an attempt to use a hospital not as an organization run by doctors in the interests of their own greater efficiency, but as a community with the immediate aim of full participation of all its daily members in its daily life and the eventual aim of the resocialisation of the neurotic individual for life in ordinary society."

In continuing the description of the Northfield Experiment, Major Bridger describes the program of admission, the natural way in which the patient meets the psychiatrist and the social worker; how the patient himself selects his activities; the opportunities for joining in recreation, which means more than just being shown a "good time"; and the introduction to the treatment ward where a democratic self-government obtains, and where "he can now embark on a secure but flexible program, involving not only the life in his ward and his selected activity, but also the social opportunities inside and outside the hospital." In these social relationships, individually and in groups, the psychiatrist has an opportunity to observe the behavior which will be of the greatest value in treatment. It is the integration of the patient into the hospital as a community which is important because, as Bridger concludes, "for all groups, whether founded spontaneously or not, whether large or small, it is true to say that the individual contribution has a value only in so far as it has a significance to the community; it is equally true to say that the individual can only experience full freedom and satisfaction in a society that recognizes his worth, and gives him the opportunity to develop in a spirit of warm human relationships."

The Northfield Experiment as described by Lt. Col. Main and his associates is social medicine in the finest sense and carries an important lesson for the future development of civil medicine.

Chapter VII

TRAINING IN PSYCHOSOMATIC MEDICINE

This subject can be introduced by some very interesting observations by Romano on ward round instruction. Staff physicians often fail to recognize that ward or classroom teaching can be either a harmful or a helpful experience for the patient. The patient may hear things said or absorb ideas which will concern him anxiously for the rest of his life or he may learn something about himself in a way which will prove helpful. Whichever result is obtained will depend upon the physician's manner of preparing the patient for the experience, how he is dealt with during the teaching period, and how his remarks or questions are managed after it is over.

Romano reports the study of 100 unselected patients from the Medical Service of the Peter Bent Brigham Hospital before, during, and after teaching rounds. These rounds consisted of the presentation of patients to a group of from fifty to seventy persons composed of members of the hospital staff, visiting physicians, students, and nurses.

Ward Round Instruction

All patients were seen by the senior house officer of the ward the preceding afternoon or evening. Each patient was told that he was to be presented before a large group of physicians and that he was chosen because his problem presented certain difficulties which would be better understood and treated after general discussion. Before presentation the patient was studied for an evaluation of his personality structure and the emotional significance of the illness. Pulse, respiration, and blood pressure were determined both before and after the presentation.

The patient was again interviewed from one to three hours after the presentation and an effort made to elicit a spontaneous discussion of his reactions. This was supplemented by questions related to various phases of the procedure.

Some patients were distressed by a recitation of the history, usually by historical data that were unfamiliar to them; for example, a patient with hypertensive encephalopathy had not realized before that he had had convulsions. The presentation of material related to past or present personality difficulties led to resentment, anger, and humiliation in

217.

certain cases; for example, in one patient who had attempted suicide a few years before. Social data also, especially if it concerned prestige or security factors, provoked resentment.

In the majority of cases, however, the patients were not upset by the historical data and many said that it was comforting to know that the doctors had taken such pains to learn all about them.

Physical Examinations. Several patients were annoyed by physical examinations during the procedure. In this connection two factors seemed to be of considerable significance. The first was sensitivity and embarrassment of the patients to being disrobed and examined before a group. Some were sensitive about obesity or hair growth or body contour. The second factor was that examination of a particular organ might take such a long time or receive so much attention that the patient would become alarmed. A boy of fifteen said, "I wondered why they examined my heart so long. I haven't got heart disease, have I?"

The Reaction of the Patient. Sixty-nine patients were present throughout the discussion and eleven of these would have preferred to have been removed when the discussion was going on. Thirty-one of the patients were removed before discussion and sixteen of these would have rather remained for the complete discussion. They said they did not want to miss anything concerning themselves and that they would have been reassured by the group discussion. Some patients were made anxious by removal, the patient sometimes wondering if this meant that his condition was getting worse or if there was something that was too alarming for him to hear.

Romano speaks of the "final explanation" in which the program of treatment and the probable period of disability are explained to the patient. This gives an opportunity for the patient to ask questions and for the house officers to correct any misunderstanding which the patient may have concerning his illness.

The Physician-Patient Relationship. Romano recommends what is so often forgotten—that care should be taken to avoid presentation of details of personal and social data in the patient's presence. When psychogenic factors are considered, the presentation and discussion should be conducted in the patient's absence. With proper understanding and preparation the whole procedure of ward round teaching may be utilized in a psychotherapeutic way.

It is noteworthy that many patients were more impressed with how the discussants spoke and behaved than with what they said. This is an important lesson regarding the physician-patient relationship.

The Psychosomatic Approach in Teaching

An important contribution to present methods of teaching has been made by Deutsch, Kaufman, and Blumgart. They deplore the diagnosis of psychological illness by exclusion: "It must be demonstrated to the student that he may make the diagnosis of psychoneurosis only in the presence of certain positive information. He must be able to demonstrate an actual conflict between environmental factors and the individual needs, or a conflict arising from internal forces. Furthermore, he should be able to demonstrate the patient's attempt at solution and relate the current conflict-solution to an earlier situation in which similar mechanisms were utilized. He should also be able to demonstrate that the symptom complex has a definite conscious or unconscious significance and represents a partial, though unsatisfactory, solution. In addition, he should be cognizant of the secondary gain involved."

Physician-Patient Relationship. They discuss the physician-patient relationship as follows: "The physician-patient relationship, based as it is on reciprocal emotional attitudes, is a very important element in the art of medicine. Too little attention has been paid to the multiple factors which enter into this relationship. It is often not realized that the physician plays a psychological role which is not altogether determined by reality. This is evidenced by the devotion of many patients to the family practitioner, not because he is a better scientific physician, but because he is a combination of father confessor, authority, and arbiter in the solution of family difficulties.

"The physician, as a rule, is accustomed to expect only favorable reactions and tends to accept himself at the patient's overvaluation. The emotional attitudes of the patient to the physician are based upon earlier experiences. The physician may be identified with figures, such as the father, which played an important role in the early life of the patient. In addition the role of the physician is determined by many other factors, not the least of which is the expectation of a cure. As a rule the positive aspects come to the forefront rather early. Sooner or later the patient, either because of disappointment, frustration, or identification of the physician with earlier figures, may acquire certain hostile reactions. The physician on his part may also develop certain emotional reactions toward the patient. 'Good' patients are those whom they can cure easily, and 'bad' patients, those they cannot cure. Or the attitude of the physician may depend upon the type of illness presented by the patient; whether the illness is understood in terms of organic etiology, or is to some degree of neurotic origin and therefore not evaluated properly."

Ambivalence. "The ambivalence of the patient's emotional attitudes may be conscious or unconscious but the physician unless he understands these phenomena, to which one school of psychology has given the name of 'transference,' may fail to comprehend the illness and the patient's problems satisfactorily. Instead of realizing that, to a great extent, the patient's attitudes towards him are a repetition of earlier attitudes he tends to accept them at their face value and reacts as if he were the object of overvaluation or of hostility.

"The therapeutic values inherent in this relationship are considerable and should be emphasized to the students. Many physicians unconsciously create such positive relationships. One hears of doctors who have extraordinary therapeutic results because of a 'wonderful personality.' But it is not sufficient for the doctor to have such a personality. He must also attempt to understand why his personality is effective with some patients and fails with others; he must evaluate his success and failure not only in terms of the technical medical skill, but also in terms of the emotional relationships involved."

Plan of Teaching. The plan of teaching evolved by these authors was to assign the patient to a student who studied him in the routine way. He formulated the problem as he saw it and then presented his findings to the psychiatrist who also examined the patient. The problem was then formulated in the light of the teacher's experience and the special psychosomatic approach. Attention was directed to those aspects of the material which revealed the patient's emotional attitudes, especially as they related to his symptoms. The student then returned to the patient, either with the teacher or alone, for further examination and study. The problem was reformulated by the student in the light of his new knowledge and findings, and prepared for the conference presentation.

This presentation consisted of a differential diagnosis, an evaluation of the psychosomatic and therapeutic problem involved, and consideration of the necessary steps for further study of the situation. The psychiatrist discussed the psychological findings and interrelations in terms of the personality organization, the presence or absence of conflict situations, the structure of the psychoneurotic symptoms, and the psychological reaction of the patient. At the end of the conference, it was the function of one of the authors to synthesize the data.

One important aspect of the teaching conference was the exploration of the gaps in the material elicited by the student. The appropriate method of obtaining adequate material was discussed. The role of the recent conflict in relation to old conflicts, the factors of environmental influence, family constellations, social factors, and the patient's attitude toward the illness were discussed. Emphasis was laid upon the physician-patient relationship, as it presented itself during the interview. Finally the prognosis, therapeutic problem, and plan of treatment were formulated.

Agreement in Findings. Our own teaching experience in psychosomatic medicine, from which most of the cases in this book have been taken, has been carried out almost identically with the above plan and we are in complete agreement as to their conclusions. Deutsch, Kaufman, and Blumgart found that a knowledge of formal psychiatry, which often centers around psychotic syndromes, was not enough to acquaint the student with the rather intricate psychophysiological relationships of psychosomatic medicine. They believe that a successful program for the teaching of psychosomatic medicine should begin in the preclinical years. With this point of view we are heartily in accord. Like these authors we feel that the medical psychology of psychoanalysis is unusually well fitted to accompany studies of the body's physiological functions. By correlating physiology and medical psychology in the preclinical years their clinical relationships are better understood. Moreover, if the student does not begin his training in psychosomatic medicine before the last two years the time is too short to give him satisfactory instruction in the subject.

Attitude of House Officers. An important point is stated as follows: "One of the major problems involved in a well-rounded course of psychosomatic teaching is the attitude of the house officers and the attending staff. A teacher of psychosomatic medicine is in an even unhappier position than the psychiatrist in a general hospital. The house officer is perfectly willing to let the psychiatrist put a diagnostic label on a patient whom he himself has already recognized as psychotic. The teacher of psychosomatic medicine, however, deals directly with medical problems. As a rule the resident staff, by background and training, is not particularly interested in psychological factors except in very general terms. In the rush of an active clinical service, the house officer has relatively little time to spend probing into the intricacies of personality organization. A diagnosis arrived at by laboratory techniques seems safe and sure. Psychological investigation is looked upon as dealing with imponderables 'not subject to the ordinary criteria of scientific investigation.' The student, to a great extent, takes his cue from the house officer who is almost a contemporary in clinical experience. Our experience has been that it is essential, in so far as possible, to have the house officer attend the teaching conferences and, in addition, to conduct special seminars dealing with psychosomatic problems for the resident staff and the junior attending physicians. The importance of this step cannot be overemphasized, since it requires sustained teaching effort to familiarize the staff with the concepts involved and to demonstrate, preferably on the ward-patient and in the routine problems that arise, the validity of these concepts."

The "Organic Tradition" in Teaching. Again our own experience is the same as theirs. Medical teaching is heavily weighted on the organic side and the impact of psychosomatic instruction is apt to be slight unless it can have the continued support of the house officers and younger men men of the staff. For example, our psychosomatic conferences for senior medical students are given during the first third of the teaching year. During this period clinical clerks, supervised by house officers, are apt to be very alert to the psychological and social background of illness and this is shown by the medical histories which they take. When the teaching is over the majority of the class no longer give the same attention to these factors. A small number of the students remain permanently interested in psychosomatic medicine.

It takes a long time and constant effort to bring about a change in point of view as fundamental as that required for the acceptance of psychosomatic medicine. An adequate approach to the concept of the relation of the emotions to bodily illness will only be achieved when psychopathology is recognized to be a scientific discipline, entitled to an equal place with tissue pathology in medical teaching.

Pre-clinical Training. To obtain this standing it will be necessary to begin training the student before he enters medical school. In his college education equal emphasis must be placed upon such studies as sociology, anthropology, and philosophy as upon biology, embryology, and chemistry. The tendency has been to neglect the former in favor of the latter. Studies having to do with the cultural aspects of man are regarded as luxuries, whereas biology and chemistry are regarded as more scientific and therefore necessities. They are necessities, but the studies dealing with the cultural aspects of man are no less necessary in the premedical education of a physician. Psychology, of course, should be added but at present most college courses in psychology have little to do with human behavior as it presents itself to the physician and as it has to do with disease. Premedical psychology has been even less influenced by the discoveries of psychoanalysis than has medical psychology.

Early in his medical course—we think during his *first year* in medical school—the student should be brought in contact with the behavior aspects of illness. He should be shown that there is an application of psychology to illness just as physiology applies to disease. Instruction in *psychobiology* should parallel his study of physiology and anatomy. He must learn that as physical growth of the human being progresses, ideas are registered upon the mind and emotional development occurs. He must realize that physiological processes such as eating, sleeping, and eliminating all have psychological aspects. He should learn that mind growth follows a pattern just as body growth does. He must know that the mind needs a balanced diet for each age period, just as the body does, and that unless the emotional nourishment is well balanced deficiencies may result later in life; deficiencies that take the form of poor social adaptation, mental suffering, and bodily symptoms, alone or combined. When emotional nutrition is accorded the same respect as bodily nutrition we will have less "mental avitaminosis."

Personality Study of the Student Himself. At this point it should be emphasized that an emotional evaluation of the student must become a part of the requirements for admission to medical school. We are very careful to study our students for evidence of physical disease, tuberculosis, for example. But we are not sufficiently concerned about their emotional health. If a medical student breaks down with tuberculosis we feel a heavy responsibility for having failed to detect it in its incipiency. If a medical student has a "nervous breakdown" or commits suicide, how much more we should feel that we have failed in our duty for not having detected the personality background that permits such a tragic occurrence.

Just as important is the question of whether his personality is suited to the practice of medicine. Since he so often touches the lives of people in times of stress and discouragement it stands to reason that he himself should not be in a state of psychological conflict. Unfortunately our tests of personality fitness are not as well developed as tests to determine physical fitness. However, a beginning has been made in such a program.

Second year instruction should cover psychological problems of adolescence correlated with physiological and endocrinological information. These lectures should deal with psychological aspects of menstruation, sexual problems, and also courtship and engagement, pregnancy, marital relationships, the climacteric and senescence. They should consider the matter of work adjustment. The personality structure of the psychoneuroses should be discussed and cases presented.

Clinical Training. Entering *the third year* with a background of personality study the student is prepared to understand the major psychoses. This teaching is done by combined lecture and case presentation. It has been our practice to have students prepare the case for presentation. Such history as is possible is taken and then a visit is made to the home for a talk with relatives and friends. Consultation with the psychiatrist follows. The actual case presentation is made by the students themselves under the supervision of the psychiatrist. They develop a closer emotional relationship to the patient during this study than they could possibly gain by being onlookers. *In this way the students learn that a psychotic individual is not just a person bereft of his senses, with grotesque behavior, who is put on exhibition to entertain them.* Instead they learn that psychotic patients usually retain many feelings and ideas and some of their sanity and that this can be worked with. Rather than rejecting mental illness from their spher of interests they learn to view it with sympathy. They learn that many patients who finally arrive at an institution for psychotics have been under the care of general physicians during the period of the development of the psychosis and they see that many of the symptoms which were treated as organic disease were the complaints of a man or woman emotionally ill. From visiting the homes they see more clearly what social and environmental conditions and what family undercurrents of emotion may contribute to mental illness.

During *the fourth year* the student has an opportunity to apply the medical psychology which he has learned to the patients in the general wards and outpatient departments. Ward, class, and clinic presentations of patients showing the interrelationship of personality and physical illness are rapidly becoming a part of the curriculum in most medical schools. We have already discussed our conferences which permit internist, psychiatrist, and students to discuss the diagnostic and treatment problems of psychosomatic cases. In addition to these presentations in psychosomatic medicine the student has an opportunity to enter the psychiatric outpatient department and there, under guidance, follow the treatment of a case. Here he receives instruction in the management of the transference relationship and other dynamic factors of psychotherapy. Such training should equip interns and house officers with a good start in understanding the influence of personality factors in illness and disease. Instruction in psychosomatic medicine should be continued with interns and residents by showing them how they can correlate their psychological understanding with the physical studies which are being made during the patient's stay in the hospital.

FURTHER TRAINING IN PSYCHOSOMATIC MEDICINE

The Specialist

As we have stated before, it is essential for the development of the psychosomatic concept that divisions of psychiatry be established in general hospitals, in other words, not only a psychiatric staff and outpatient department but a ward or division for the study and treatment of such patients. Psychiatry can no longer lead an isolated existence. Until we bring it into physical proximity with general medicine we cannot hope for a real integration of the two.

Many young physicians are asking how they can obtain more training in psychosomatic medicine. If they have a deep interest in psychological medicine it will probably be better for them to become psychiatrists. They can pursue the same studies as if they were in general medicine and occupy a less ambiguous position. But it is possible that among internists there may be some who will wish to perfect themselves in the study of psychosomatic problems just as is now done with regard to cardiology, gastroenterology, and other studies. This will require, in addition to regular medical training, a fellowship in psychosomatic medicine. The essential feature of this fellowship will consist of a personal psychoanalysis. The reasons have already been stated in the discussion on psychoanalysis. Such opportunities now exist in a few of the large medical centers. More are badly needed. During this period they will attend lectures and seminars on the theoretical as well as the practical aspects of the psychoses, psychoneuroses, and psychosomatic disorders.

It is even more important that residents in medicine and the other specialties shall have the opportunity for psychiatric training. This will require a good department of psychiatry and real cooperation on the part of the other departments. Saslow discusses such an experiment in comprehensive medicine. When we have homogenization rather than stratification of psychiatry in our medical institutions, as Margolin puts it, we shall have achieved the psychosomatic goal.

In general we agree with Barr, who says, in speaking of specialization in psychosomatic medicine, "Such an attitude may have some justification in expediency to meet existing conditions, but can do little toward the final solution of the problem. Psychosomatic medicine is medicine itself. The role of humanist cannot be assigned to any one group, whether its members be called psychiatrists, psychosomaticists, or priests. The study of man and his values is at least as much a part of internal medicine as is physiology, chemistry, or anatomy. *Fundamental concepts which involve or modify our understanding of all disease can never be regarded as clinical specialties.*"

The General Physician

For the physician who has already established himself and would like to know more about psychosomatic medicine we recommend that he study his patients along the lines that we have indicated and that he supplement his study by additional reading. Some references have been given for the chapter on psychopathology; additional selected references will be found at the end of the book. If the physician lives in a city that has a psychoanalytic society he will probably have the opportunity of attending lectures and seminars on the psychopathology and the clinical aspects of psychosomatic problems.

To meet a growing demand on the part of practitioners and to explore the possibilities of postgraduate teaching in this field, intensive courses of one month duration were given at the Temple University Medical School on two occasions (1945 and 1946) for a small group of carefully selected internists and general practitioners. Under the sponsorship of the Commonwealth Fund, a course in psychiatry for general physicians was conducted in April 1946 at the University of Minnesota. A description of the project was published by the Commonwealth Fund.

Even more important than study, however, are the physician's feelings for the patient as a human being and the realization that illness is an aspect of human behavior.

Part Two

SPECIAL APPLICATIONS TO GENERAL MEDICINE AND THE SPECIALTIES

Chapter VIII

THE CARDIOVASCULAR SYSTEM

In spite of the enormous incidence of cardiovascular disease, *the majority of patients who have symptoms referred to the heart region do not have evidence of organic heart disease.* The reason is not hard to find. From time immemorial the heart has been the traditional seat of the emotions and hence acts as a focal point for anxiety. No other body organ is used so frequently in a symbolic way to refer to love and to hate, which, as W. C. Menninger pointed out, should lead us to think of the emotional significance of disturbances involving the heart. As a symbol of love we are familiar with the universal use of the heart as a valentine and the colloquial expression of "warmhearted," "loving with all my heart," "heart-felt." We speak of being "light-hearted" and of the heart "bounding with joy." But we also speak of being "heavy-hearted," and of "the heart growing weary." Then, too, we refer to the "faint-hearted" and the "chicken-hearted"; or think of the heart "racing with fear" or "fluttering or trembling." Hate and hostility are expressed in such terms as "hard-hearted," "heartless," and "cold-blooded" instead of "warm-hearted." The injured person is spoken of as suffering from "heartache," or of being "heartsick." All of these expressions have significance from the standpoint of *body language* as discussed in the previous chapter.

ANXIETY AND THE HEART

Do the expressions enclosed in quotation marks have any real meaning from the standpoint of psychopathology? Is there any actual relation of anxiety and the anxiety attack, also described in the previous chapter, to disorders of the heart and the cardiovascular system? Anxiety neurosis stands in close relation to physiological changes and is therefore of utmost significance to all branches of medicine. This relation to physiological changes is especially close in the cardiovascular system. Moreover, anxiety neurosis, in its varying degrees, is probably the most frequent disorder of civilized life. The various forms of the anxiety attack were described by Freud more than forty years ago. Not only did he call attention to such disturbances of cardiac function as palpitation, arrhythmia, and tachycardia, but he also spoke of the disturbances of respiration and a host of physiological changes that are so often today regarded as evidences of vasomotor instability or autonomic imbalance. Furthermore, Freud emphasized the fact that these attacks are not always accompanied by recognizable anxiety. This, of course, is one special reason why they are so often regarded as indications of physical disease. We agree with Wolfe that in more than forty years clinical medicine has taken practically no cognizance of anxiety neurosis except perhaps by adopting the term, devoid of its meaning, for all possible states of fear and anxiety.

From the standpoint of psychosomatic medicine we can discuss the effect of the emotions upon the cardiovascular system from the following standpoints:

1. The effect of anxiety upon the normal heart, including the syndrome spoken of as neurocirculatory asthenia.

2. The effect of anxiety upon a diseased heart.

3. The relation of the emotions to the problem of hypertension.

ANXIETY AND THE NORMAL HEART (CARDIAC NEUROSIS)

Precipitating Factors

Cardiac neurosis* arises in predisposed persons who have been subjected to a precipitating factor. Such persons carry an unusual amount of anxiety in their make-ups. Then, under special circumstances, that anxiety is attached to the heart largely because the heart is regarded as the all-important bodily organ and is associated with the idea of sudden death.

This anxiety or even the personality predisposition may be anything but obvious and yet in reviewing the histories of patients with cardiac neuroses, it is interesting to note how frequently one obtains the story of some "nervous breakdown," either during the period of school life or in the course of some later period of stress. In an excellent paper on this subject Conner called attention to the following four groups of causes which may act as the precipitating events for the development of cardiac neurosis:

1. *The statement of some physician or life insurance examiner that the heart shows some abnormality such as a murmur or irregularity of rhythm; or the rejection of the applicant for life insurance on the score of some heart disturbance or of "high blood pressure."* Sometimes it is the mere assumption on the part of the applicant himself that the heart must be diseased because two or three examiners were called in to listen to it. In a person predisposed, the slightest suggestion that the heart is not right may be enough to start

---

* It is hardly necessary to say that we consider the designation "neurosis with cardiac manifestations" to be much more satisfactory, but because of tradition the term cardiac neurosis will probably continue to be used.

the whole train of reactions that lead up to the development of cardiac neurosis. As will be stated in the discussion on neurocirculatory asthenia, this problem is of the greatest importance in the examination of young men for army service. Unusual attention to the cardiac examination or some casual remarks may be the starting point for later disability.

2. *The occurrence of some dramatic case of heart disease, perhaps with sudden death, among relatives or friends of the patient.* This is a frequent precipitating factor for cardiac neurosis particularly if the patient has been in close contact with the relative or friend or has actually nursed such a person. The continual emotional stress plus hard work and often lack of sleep prepare the way for the development of the first heart symptoms.

3. *The appearance of some symptom which calls the attention of the patient to his heart and leads to doubt as to its integrity.* This may be a sudden skip, a flutter or a twinge of pain, or it may be merely what is regarded as undue palpitation or dyspnea after some special exertion. Such disturbing symptoms are often first noticed during convalescence from an illness, such as an attack of grippe, or they may appear as a result of the excessive use of tobacco or coffee.

4. *Some profound and protracted emotional disturbance*, such as deep grief or prolonged anxiety, in which, however, there is at first no element of doubt concerning the state of the heart. This was strikingly illustrated by the innumerable instances of the condition known as "irritable heart of soldiers," "effort syndrome," or "neurocirculatory asthenia" which developed in military service. As a result of the profound and long-continued emotional disturbance incident to the process of volunteering or being drafted into the army, such cases were encountered in great numbers (see chart, Chapter II, p. 55).

Symptoms

Under circumstances such as those that have just been discussed, pain in the heart region, fatigue, sighing respirations, insomnia, ringing or pounding in the ears, and faintness, dizziness, nervousness, irritability and flushes are apt to make their appearance. At first, there may be only discomfort in the heart region with the later development of other symptoms, particularly fatigue, which may be overwhelming and lead to complete invalidism.

The chief symptoms group themselves under the headings of (a) pain and distress in the heart region, (b) dyspnea and fatigue, (c) palpitation or heart consciousness, (d) tachycardia and other disturbances of rhythm, and (e) a group of symptoms which include all of the above in addition to evidences of vasomotor instability. This is often looked upon as a special form of cardiac neurosis, occurring especially in military life, and referred to as effort syndrome, neurocirculatory asthenia (N. C. A.) or "disordered action of the heart" (D. A. H.).

George Wolf and Harold Wolff made an important study of symptoms referable to the cardiovascular and respiratory systems occurring in patients with and without structural disease of the heart. A detailed, day-to-day physiological and psychological investigation was made of the way these persons responded to a standard exercise test as determined by cardiovascular and respiratory measurements.

The investigators took especial note of the reactions to persistent low-grade stresses and strains which are part of "everyday" living. Their results indicate that in a setting of adverse life circumstances and associated emotional reactions, performance in terms of respiration and work of the heart is costly. This high cost may manifest itself in cardiovascular symptoms which are not dependent alone upon gross structural heart disorder. This uneconomical performance may also manifest itself in impaired total efficiency of the individual. (See chart, p. 238).

Pain. It has been estimated by Bishop that 25 per cent of all patients visiting the office of a cardiologist have cardiac pain as a primary complaint. It need hardly be said that all pain in the cardiac region does not originate in the heart. The long controversy that raged in regard to angina pectoris and its relation to coronary vessel disease and coronary thrombosis has been pretty well settled. Most authorities agree that the pain of angina pectoris is of heart muscle origin due to actual interference with the blood supply. Nor is there often much question regarding the differential diagnosis of *angina pectoris* and *coronary occlusion*. The typical syndromes are now well recognized. Indeed, in regard to coronary occlusion it might almost be said that it is too well recognized because of the frequency with which the diagnosis is made when it fails to exist. This is especially true of acute upper abdominal emergencies such as acute cholecystitis, ruptured peptic ulcer, and acute pancreatitis.

Harrison, in a valuable study to which further reference will be made, estimates that pain in the chest is present in from 15 to 25 per cent of all adult patients who need hospital care.

Other conditions not so well known may cause severe pain and are occasionally mistaken for coronary occlusion or angina. *Pulmonary embolism*, giving rise to the syndrome of acute cor pulmonale, may be confusing. It occurs especially after operation or fracture. The symptom picture, characterized by pressure over the chest, breathlessness, cough and bloody expectoration and sometimes shock, with accentuated pulmonary second sound, and confirmation by x-ray and often by electrocardiogram, is rapidly gaining recognition. *Rupture of the aorta* and *dissecting aneurysm* are other causes for severe pain in the cardiac region so frequently mistaken for coronary occlusion. Pain in the back which may extend down the legs and an interference with the pulse in one or more extremities are often present. *Spontaneous pneumothorax* and *interstitial emphysema* both may be responsible for pain in the heart region but the former is accompanied by displacement of heart and trachea and pronounced dyspnea and the latter frequently gives rise to a peculiar auscultatory crunch which assists in diagnosis. *Pericarditis* is another cause of pain but the surrounding circumstances assist in diagnosis. With this brief mention of some of the important organic causes of severe pain in the cardiac region let us go on to the more difficult cardiac pain problem of angina pectoris and the so-called pseudo-angina.

Angina Pectoris and Pseudo-angina. When characteristic effort pain with its peculiar distribution occurs in a hypertensive arteriosclerotic individual there is no problem of diagnosis—angina pectoris is present regardless of other findings. But under many other circumstances the problem may be a most difficult one. Intercostal neuralgia and spinal disease, hiatal hernia and cardiospasm, gallbladder and ulcer syndromes, as well as tobacco poisoning, are causes for pain in the cardiac region that must be borne in mind in regard to the problem of so-called pseudo-angina. The diagnostic problem is often difficult but if these various conditions are thought of the problem can usually be solved after careful study. Unfortunately the diagnosis of the anginal syndrome not infrequently must rest solely on subjective phenomena. Abnormal physical signs, x-ray, and electrocardiographic evidence may be absent. It is important to recognize that the discomfort of the anginal syndrome appears, with few exceptions, when additional work is imposed on the heart. The abnormal sensation is usually of relatively short duration; it rarely lasts for more than a few minutes. It frequently disappears promptly when the patient rests and in the majority of instances after the administration of nitrites. The discomfort usually is described as being beneath the sternum. The distribution of the pain is variable; it may appear in the left arm; sometimes the pain extends into the abdomen, at times, but less commonly, into the back and occasionally into the jaws and face.

In Harrison's study of seventy-seven patients with angina pectoris the pain was in the substernal region in only about 50 per cent of the cases, and the discomfort was only mild or minimal in about the same number. He also found that aggravation by recumbent posture, improvement after eating, and nocturnal attacks occur more frequently than is commonly believed.

Harrison regards the most important features in the diagnosis of angina pectoris to be: (1) the history of relationship to effort, (2) the short duration of pain, and (3) the demonstration that the amount of muscular effort required to induce the pain is increased by glyceryl trinitrate. A very important aspect of this matter is that a large percentage of patients with angina pectoris also suffer from chest pain due to other disorders and that these disorders may be either related to the angina pectoris (as in myocardial infarction and reflex disturbances of the skeletal system) or unrelated to it (as in gallbladder disease, hiatal hernia, esophageal spasm, and the like). Owing to the frequent coexistence of two causes of chest pain, one of them may be overlooked unless unusual care is employed in obtaining the history, which Harrison finds is the one most important method of examination and in many patients more important than all the other procedures combined.

(See case report, H. G., p. 300).

The same writer finds that when electrocardiograms are taken following muscular effort, changes of the S-T segments and of the T waves of such a nature as to be specifically suggestive of the presence of angina pectoris may be encountered in 50 to 60 per cent of patients. This was true not only of his study but of other studies that have been reported.

A word should be added regarding the relation of emotional factors to electrocardiographic changes. Wendkos has shown alterations in the T wave in the precordial lead in patients with neurocirculatory asthenia to be indistinguishable from those associated with structural heart disease. Mainzer and Krause, in their study of the effects of fear on the electrocardiogram, showed that on the operating table immediately before induction of general anesthesia an abnormal electrocardiographic record was found to develop in roughly two fifths of fifty-three cases, when compared with the tracings of the previous day. Not only were these alterations observed in persons with cardiac disorders, where they merely accentuated the pathological character of the cardiogram already existing, but they occurred frequently in patients whose cardiograms had been normal. Although in a number of instances the changes disappeared when the patient was under anesthetic, or at least by the next day, in some cases they were still encountered twenty-four hours after the operation.

Therefore in *pseudo-angina* careful analysis will usually show evident differences from true anginal pain. Rarely is the pain referred directly to the retrosternal region. Friedman found that patients suffering from functional cardiovascular disease experienced two separate and distinct types of precordial pain, which were not due to the same cause. The more common type was a sharp, piercing, transient pain at the left nipple which appeared to penetrate into the chest itself. The patients described it as a sensation of being "stabbed with a sharp needle," or being "torn" or "cut with a knife." Many patients became aware of irregular heart action in connection with this pain; others noted only the forceful heart action. Friedman believes that this particular pain originates from the nerve fibers in the heart muscle in association with arrhythmia or excessively forceful cardiac contraction.

The second type of precordial pain was a dull, aching, persistent discomfort, a combination of fatigue and pain, frequently described as "soreness." It was not so sharply localized as the other type of pain; it lasted for hours rather than minutes; and it was related to effort but did not come on immediately following exertion.

Some patients experienced both types of pain. Friedman confirms the observation of Wood, that patients with the dull type of precordial pain almost invariably used only the upper third of their chests in breathing. When such patients were asked to hyperventilate the majority complained of this dull precordial pain. When adhesive tape was applied to the chest in order to reduce the upper-chest breathing, forcing the patients to resort to abdominal breathing, the pain was abolished. Casts, too, were applied and kept on for a longer period but it is significant that when the casts were removed the patients reverted to upper-chest breathing and the pains returned. It is also interesting to record that when Friedman bound the chests of normal persons in the manner described (so that they had to breathe with the upper half of their chests) and then instructed them to exercise, the same kind of precordial pain appeared in these normal subjects.

Friedman concludes, therefore, that the dull type of precordial pain is primarily due to the excessive use of the intercostal muscles in respiration. But this pseudo-angina may have the characteristic features of true anginal pain and occasionally the recognition of its real nature must rest on the other factors present.

For example, let us refer to the frequent problem of the obese woman of menopausal age with a labile blood pressure who complains of severe lancinating pain in the precordial region, breathlessness, and fatigue. Has she or has she not angina pectoris? If we remember that the pain of cardiac neurosis bears no definite relationship to effort, is frequently described as sticking, needle-like, or soreness; that it is often associated with inframammary tenderness and hyperalgesia, so that the pressure of the stethoscope sometime elicits it; and that it may be accompanied by a sense of choking as well as sighing respirations, we shall have *no difficulty in the differential diagnosis particularly when we associate these symptoms with the whole picture and life situation of the individual with cardiac neurosis.*

Willius referred to a common error resulting from misinterpretation of the pain and soreness of inflammatory disease of the wall of the chest due to *fibromyositis* or *intercostal neuralgia*. Ordinarily, the painful sensations arising from this source are of rather long duration, often lasting for hours at a time; they occur when the patient is resting as well as when he is active and are likely to be exaggerated by deep breathing, coughing, and sudden movements of the upper extremities and body. At some time during the course of the trouble, regions of localized tenderness may be found on application of firm pressure over the ribs or sternum and in the intercostal spaces. Severe and fairly continuous pain occasionally is followed by the typical skin lesions of *herpes zoster*.

Another erroneous diagnosis of anginal syndrome to which Willius referred is due to *spondylitis* of the thoracic portion of the spine. Distribution of pain in the thorax and over its anterior surface is not uncommon as painful impulses are caused by impingement and irritation of spinal nerves by the hypertrophic arthritis. Under these circumstances, the pain is likely to occur on motion of the spine and when the patient is recumbent, particularly when considerable relaxation of the spine occurs and certain degrees of abnormal curvature result. Careful x-ray examination will permit the recognition of spondylitis.

Sometimes it is very difficult to exclude the *esophagus* and *upper digestive tract* as the source of pains which simulate angina. Special x-ray technics and esophagoscopy studies have helped a great deal. It is a pretty safe rule to regard with suspicion any substernal pain that comes with effort regardless of whether the gastrointestinal tract seems to be responsible. *Tobacco* is a frequent offender in regard to pseudo-angina and had better be withheld whether or not the diagnosis of true angina is established.

The differential diagnosis of pain in the chest may be a most difficult problem and is never to be regarded lightly. In any patient with pain in the chest, no matter how closely it may seem to be related to emotional factors, very careful physical studies must be made. In closing this discusion of cardiac pain, we cannot emphasize this point too strongly.

Dyspnea. Shortness of breath is the most common symptom of heart disease, but it also occurs for a variety of other reasons; for example, in lung diseases such as emphysema and bronchial asthma, in anemia and obesity, and in the air-hunger of acidosis. But the dyspnea of actual heart disease occurs either directly as the result of exertion or in attacks of cardiac asthma. The dyspnea is determined by the vital capacity, which is reduced in patients with cardiac disease as a result of pulmonary congestion brought on by back pressure from the left side of the heart. Harrison referred to other factors, such as respiratory stimulation, the result of impulses arising in the moving muscles and in the distended great veins, as important in the production of dyspnea on exertion. Contrary to former beliefs alteration in the blood gases is of much less significance in the pathogenesis of exertional dyspnea.

In the study by Wolf and Wolff, observations upon the respiratory function of patients and normal individuals showed that increase in the tidal volume and minute ventilation occurred in the setting of adverse life situations and associated emotional responses. They point out that increase in tidal volume may be brought about by such means as diminished oxygen capacity of the blood (anemia), impairment in alveolar oxygen transport in the lungs, increased oxygen demand in the tissues, acidosis, and obstruction in the air passage.

For our purpose we may conclude that cardiac dyspnea is in the main a reflex rather than a chemical disturbance and that its most important cause is congestion of the lungs. Therefore it seems strange that dyspnea of functional origin, which has nothing to do with congestion of the lungs, should be so frequently mistaken for the shortness of breath of organic heart disease. Here the dyspnea is due to anxiety even when the anxiety is not recognized. Indeed the shortness of breath often has a symbolic meaning. Although the patient describes "shortness of breath" careful questioning often will reveal that what he really has is a sensation of a weight on the chest—"a load on the chest"—which he can get rid of by talking about his troubles. It is an inability to obtain a deep breath plus a sensation that the air taken into the lungs is insufficient and does not enter deeply into the lungs. When an effort is made to overcome this sensation it leads to periodic sighing or "sighing respirations" and frequently the patient will demonstrate this in the course of an examination. For example, if he is asked to explain what he means by shortness of breath, he will place the hand on the lower sternum or epigastrium, take a deep sighing respiration and then often describe the feeling that the lungs seem insufficiently filled with air. Occasionally it is true that if the patients are suffering from severe emotional strain or anxiety, hyperpnea develops to the extent that hyperventilation tetany or syncope may result. Indeed, the test of hyperventilation in such subjects will frequently bring about such evidence of tetany as a positive Chvostek sign. It is of the greatest importance to differentiate this sighing respiration from dyspnea of cardiac origin.

A study of dyspnea and hyperventilation associated with sustained conflict, anxiety, humiliation, frustration and anger (in the paper by Wolf and Wolff already referred to) is illustrated in the accompanying figure.

The experiments indicate that the efficiency of the organism as evidenced in cardiovascular function was impaired (that is, the work of the heart was increased) under circumstances of conflict which resulted in reactions of anger, frustration, humiliation, and anxiety. Respiratory inefficiency was apparent (that is, oxygen utilization was diminished) and was shown to be dependent upon impairment of the ventilatory rather than the respiratory mechanism of respiration.

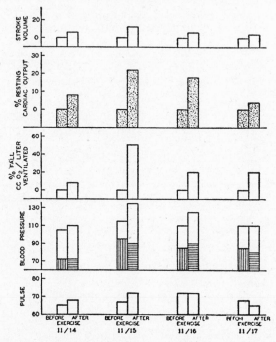

Fig. 1. Dyspnea and palpitation after exercise caused by hyperventilation and increased cardiac output in association with anxiety, frustration and anger. The per cent fall of ccs. of oxygen per liter ventilated is equivalent to per cent increase in air ventilated per cc. of oxygen utilized.

(Wolf, G. A., and Wolff, H. G., Studies on the Nature of Certain Symptoms Associated with Cardiovascular Disorders, Psychosom. Med., 8:293, 1946.)

Palpitation. "Heart consciousness," which comprises either tachycardia or arrhythmia or both, is a very frequent symptom in the cardiac neuroses and often leads to a mistaken diagnosis of organic heart disease. But it is also true that just as the heart may be speeded up by emotion so may it be retarded, and occasionally during anxiety attacks, especially in nightmares, great slowing of the heart occurs, apparently from vagal stimulation. More frequently, however, the heart is speeded up in its action and this together with premature contractions may lead to heart consciousness. Sometimes this is apparent only when the patient is lying on his left side or it occurs only in certain periods but occasionally the patient is aware of the heart all of the time. When organic disease of the heart has been eliminated and when significant arrhythmias have not been demonstrated one can feel quite certain that the awareness of the heart action is to be explained psychologically. Instances of actual auricular fibrillation occurring during periods of emotional stress, which did not seem to have an organic basis, have been encountered. Palpitation is sometimes the very first symptom of a cardiac neurosis. In the patient who has been prepared from the standpoint of his psychological make-up, certain life situations, such as prolonged emotional stress, plus such other factors as overindulgence in coffee and tobacco, will make a slight twinge or a skipped beat a sufficient stimulus to call attention to the heart and from that point on he may suffer from palpitation. Then, as Oille pointed out, if the physician gives medicine "to help prevent the irregularity" or makes the statement "the missed beats are not important if they don't get any worse," a cardiac neurosis has been established.

Wolf and Wolff suggest that changes in the intensity of frequency of stimuli caused by the beat of the heart may be associated with (a) increased stroke volume, (b) displacement of the heart or of tissues around it so that tissues ordinarily not stimulated by the beating heart are in a position to be stimulated, (c) occurrence of a beat out of phase with preceding and succeeding beats, and (d) rapid beating of the heart.

From their data they inferred that "significant change in stroke volume or in heart rate will cause mechanical disturbances such as traction and displacements within the chest, thus constituting adequate stimuli for the sensations interpreted as palpitation. It is, however, also apparent that the subjects' attitudes toward these sensations may become of major significance and be a factor in a chain of circumstances which accentuates or perpetuates the symptom. This may explain the frequent occurrence of palpitation in anxious patients with cardiac "neuroses," with or without structural cardiovascular disease. It may also indicate why patients who have apparently adequate stimuli such as occur in auricular fibrillation do not always experience palpitation. . . ."

In other words, certain attitudes as a result of conditioning in conjunction with minimal mechanical stimuli may pave the way for palpitation. Either alone may produce no symptoms. Having once suffered the experience of palpitation, should the patient develop anxiety or fear of heart disease, increased attention to this area of the body plus a stimulus in the form of exaggerated recoil of the heart or rapid pulse, associated with fear and anxiety, may potentiate the "vicious cycle" and the troublesome symptom of palpitation will prevail. It is generally known that palpitation associated with premature contractions will disappear upon reassurance that heart disease is not present, although the premature contractions may persist.

Murmur. Probably no single objective finding leads to more false diagnoses of cardiac disease than a murmur. A systolic murmur can be found in a large number of healthy young adults if they are examined in various postures, in different phases of respiration, before and after exercise. These functional murmurs are also much more common during fevers. They are rather faint, but sometimes moderately loud, and are heard in the apical or pulmonic areas. Kilgore feels that if they are not very loud, not high pitched, if they are markedly changed by respiration and posture and not accompanied by other signs of heart disease (especially enlargement of the heart), by deficient heart function, or by a history of rheumatism or chorea, these systolic murmurs should not be regarded as pathologic. And in the case of borderline systolic murmurs—some of the louder ones, less clearly dependent on posture or respiration—the diagnosis of valvular disease, if suspected but not confirmed by other physical signs, should in general be held in abeyance until radiographic and electrocardiographic studies have been made.

The first point in the prophylaxis of cardiac neurosis enters in regard to this problem. If there is any question regarding the significance of the murmur the patient had better not be apprised of the fact or even made suspicious of heart disease until one can marshal his evidence in order completely to exonerate the heart. This is of special significance in regard to present-day recruiting of young men for military service. The beginnings of a cardiac neurosis can often be traced to the indiscreet remark of an examining physician who detects for the first time a systolic murmur at the apex of the heart unaccompanied by other evidence of organic disease.

Treatment

Separate chapters will deal with treatment both of general and special problems in psychosomatic medicine but cardiac neurosis is so common and important an illness, with such individual characteristics, that some discussion of treatment will be considered here.

Prophylaxis. The first thing to consider is prophylaxis. This means that in people predisposed because of their neurotic personality structure the physician must be particularly careful not to focus attention upon the heart in the course of a general physical examination, such as for insurance purposes, for military reasons, during recovery from infectious disease, or more important still, during an anxiety attack. In the last instance, especially, our behaviour must match our words and when we tell such a patient that he does not have evidences of organic heart disease we must not say hesitatingly, "I do not *think* you have heart disease" but we must on the contrary say very definitely, "You do not have heart disease" and then instead of cautioning rest or giving "heart" medicine, which of course increases the patient's suspicion that we are not telling the truth or that we don't know, we must make the recommendation to "carry on in spite of symptoms."

Once cardiac neurosis has developed the problem of eradicating the idea of heart disease from the patient's mind and reestablishing health becomes more difficult. In some instance it is relatively simple and a tactful explanation of the situation and reassurance may be all that is needed. But depending upon the severity of the underlying neurosis and the length of time that the cardiac symptoms have persisted, the problem may be very difficult. Under such circumstances the service of a trained psychiatrist may be necessary, but generally it is the attending physician who must assume the responsibility and care of such patients. We will discuss this question later.

Importance of History and Physical Examination. It goes without saying that the first requisite is a careful history and physical examination. Often it is wise to carry out additional studies because a casual announcement after a hasty and superficial examination that "there is nothing the matter with the heart" will almost certainly fail to carry conviction. But there must be a point at which examinations stop and at that point one must say with conviction, "There is nothing the matter with your heart." Then if the patient can be persuaded to accept without resentment the idea that his symptoms are of emotional origin the battle is half won. From that point on, the liberal application of reassurance and encouragement will often accomplish a great deal. But the reassurance must be not simply that of the spoken word; the patient must be shown how to reassure himself by a demonstration that his symptoms can be made better rather than worse by the exercise and effort which he has been afraid to take.

Therefore we plan a program for the patient, of course using common sense in what we ask him to do. We do not ask a patient who has been incapacitated for months to go out and do a full day's work. On the contrary, we set an easy task at first. But we do say, "This much we know you can do and you must do it regardless of how you feel." That means that if you ask the patient to walk a block he must do so regardless of whether he feels faint or whether he feels that he will die before he gets back. It is kind of specious reasoning but we often say, "We will accept the responsibility for anything that happens to you" and this seems to be very persuasive to this type of patient.

Kilgore, in an excellent paper on the subject, emphasized the fact that once we have eliminated the idea of organic heart disease we must then tell the patient his slogan must be, "Carry on in spite of symptoms." This is a very successful way of handling such patients, and of course, their confidence mounts in proportion to the degree of accomplishment.

Drugs. If medicines are used the patient must have a definite under-standing that they are palliative rather than curative and that they have nothing to do with the heart itself. For example, if small doses of sedatives are used it is wise to explain to the patient that "they take the edge off his nervousness." The use of digitalis is, of course, a blunder. No intelligent patient could possibly be persuaded that his heart is sound if at the same time he is asked to take digitalis. If any rest in bed is to be recommended, and sometimes the patient will have to resort to some rest in the beginning, he must understand that this has nothing to do with his heart; that it is simply a question of having used up energy and that "his storage battery needs recharging." But for him to believe that the cultivation of a horizontal philosophy of life is going to cure him is erroneous because too much rest simply plays into the unconscious tendency to remain sick. In the final analysis it is the cultivation of an *erect philosophy of life* that is going to accomplish cure. The use of massage, hydrotherapy, and gymnastic work must be looked upon not only from the standpoint of possible beneficial results but the unhealthy suggestions that can come from such sources must be considered Again and again it has been our experience that people who do not work directly with physicians, but rather in institutions that are developed solely from a commercial standpoint, are very prone to give the patient suggestions that are bad for him, not necessarily del berately, but by taking the pulse and commenting about it, taking the blood pressure and telling the blood pressure figures, referring to the muscle tone as bad or the circulation as poor, and so forth, they work harm rather than good. Subjects who develop cardiac neuroses usually do not tolerate coffee or tobacco well and we have found it useful to limit coffee and stop tobacco. This need not be an undeviating rule because some patients can tolerate both but the point is that many tense people find momentary relaxation from the nervous cigarette habit but the end result is a bad one and the only way they can stop it is to quit rather than to cut down.

Psychotherapy. All of this, however, only leads to a consideration of psychotherapy, which is the fundamental method of treating the cardiac neuroses. Such management is very often rewarded by results that are just as satisfying as any in the field of internal medicine. We said before that this is usually a problem for the general physician. Certainly we cannot send all such patients to psychiatrists, not that there is anything reprehensible about sending patients to psychiatrists, but these problems are so numerous that general physicians must learn to deal with them. We have already pointed out that just as there is a minor and a major surgery so is there a minor and a major psychotherapy and many of the cardiac neuroses can be helped by minor psychotherapy. However, if a major disorder exists we must be able to recognize it and send such patients to psychiatrists. Furthermore, we must do our best to educate our patients and the medical profession to look upon psychic ailments in exactly the same way that they look upon organic ailments, that is, that there is no stigma to be attached to an illness simply because it is of emotional origin and hence there is no disgrace and certainly nothing to be ashamed of in consulting a psychiatrist.

Explaining the Illness to the Patient. Having determined then that we are dealing with cardiac neurosis (anxiety neurosis with cardiac manifestations) we first of all examine our patient as carefully as we can in order to rule out an organic disease but also, as mentioned in the beginning of the discussion, for the purpose of establishing a basis for psychotherapy. There is nothing so valuable as a thorough history and a complete physical examination in establishing a good relationship with the patient. It is then that you can say to the patient, and the statement carries conviction, "You do not have organic disease; this illness is of emotional origin." We use the latter term, emotional origin, advisedly because we find that it is the best way to explain to an intelligent patient that the illness is psychogenic. Patients often resent the term "just nerves" and they certainly resent the implication that the illness is "imaginary" or the impression that they sometimes gain from an unsympathetic physician that they are malingering. To say that the illness is functional does not offer sufficient explanation and patients frequently do not understand. To apply to the illness a term such as neurocirculatory asthenia, effort syndrome, or hyperthyroidism is simply to delude yourself or to delude the patient. And yet this is frequently done just because the physician feels that he must give the illness a name and because he does not know how to approach the patient from an emotional standpoint. Hence the illness gets the name of a physical disease and often the unpropitious treatment that goes along with it.

One thing that we will have to discuss later is the unfortunate circumstance, as far as scientific psychological medicine is concerned, that no matter what you call the illness, if the patient has sufficient confidence in the physician, any kind of treatment may cause an alleviation of symptoms. Hence many physicians build up great reputations without really understanding the nature of such illnesses. What we are suggesting is that we call a spade a spade but attempt to do it in a way that the patient will understand. This, of course, is taking a chance with certain patients because do what you will they may resent the implication that the illness is emotional, largely due to the belief that because we have "will power" and because we have intelligence, we ought to be able to handle "our nerves." But, of course, it is true that without help and without enlightenment a patient cannot handle anxiety of unconscious origin any more than he himself can handle an acutely inflamed appendix.

Organ Language. To go on with our method of handling such patients once we have told them that the illness is emotional we may use illustrations of how the emotions influence the functions of our body in order to show them that their emotions may be responsible for symptoms. Such examples as blushing, gooseflesh, vomiting, and diarrhea, as well as pallor, racing pulse, and palpitation, occurring for various emotional reasons, are usually convincing. We say to them that if they have an emotional problem which they cannot express by word or deed the tension arising from the emotional situation must express itself somehow and the organs of the body may take over the function of expression by a language of their own. ("Every psychic tendency seeks adequate bodily expression.")

Thus, if an individual finds it difficult to swallow it may not be that there is an obstruction in the gullet but it may be some situation in the environment that the individual cannot swallow. If the person "cannot tolerate something on his stomach" it may be something in his life situation that he cannot tolerate and the stomach is simply expressing it because he, for some reason, cannot; and if he has "a load on his chest" that is represented by sighing respirations or a "weight on the heart" that produces discomfort, the relation to his own illness is brought even nearer.

This kind of illustration will often permit a patient to talk freely about some problem that has been disturbing him perhaps more than he knew. Indeed, it is the very fact that such things are unconscious that makes it necessary for the body to express the emotions in such a primitive fashion as "organ language." Therefore we must strive to make the matter conscious and if we succeed it is likely that the particular symptoms will disappear. The problem is not quite so simple as this illustration seems to make it but we will try to expand this point later. In other words, we must encourage our patients to talk about their "other troubles" in order to find out about the present trouble. To put it another way, *the more we can persuade our patients to talk about themselves as human beings rather than as medical cases the sooner we will come to understand their symptoms of emotional origin.*

This is usually best done by skillfully and tactfully *directing the conversation* rather than by asking direct questions. In regard to the latter point a word of caution is in order. It is often better to allow the patients to discuss matters of an intimate nature such as sexual problems without asking direct questions concerning sexual matters. If the patient has confidence in his physician he will frequently introduce these matters of his own accord but if it is necessary to ask questions it must be done in a way to indicate that such matters are perfectly natural, like any other natural function of the body, and that you are not asking as a matter of morbid curiosity; in other words, that you are scientifically and not morally interested.

Another point which may now be stated is that it is much better to listen than to talk. In other words, to give advice about important personal matters (such, for example, as marriage and divorce) is a distinctly dangerous matter for the physician to attempt. It is much better for him to listen, to direct, to allow the patient to see his problems, perhaps in a slightly different way, and then to come to his own conclusions about highly charged emotional matters.

Practical Suggestions

We often say to patients who complain of palpitation that it is like the question of the horse and his rider. If the horse is whipped he will run but it is not the horse that is responsible—it is the rider. And so it is with the patient and his heart: It is not the heart that is at fault, it is the person himself, that is, his attitude and his feelings that are "making the heart run."

An important point is that the patient often seemingly agrees with the physician regarding the integrity of his heart but his skepticism prompts him to think (although he rarely tells the physician), "all right, the doctor says my heart is normal but if this keeps up, surely something will happen to it"; in other words, he hangs on to the notion that he is in for trouble, "that his heart will wear out"; "that he will develop angina or high blood pressure"; or that some other trouble confronts him which the physician cannot know about *even if he is telling the truth*. Therefore we often try to forestall this kind of thinking by telling the patient that his heart is normal and there is no reason why anything should happen to it.

The following case of typical cardiac neurosis occurred in an uneducated servant girl. It illustrates points which will be discussed in the treatment chapters, namely, that the poor develop neuroses as well as the rich and that the uneducated, if possessed of normal intelligence, can be treated by psychotherapy as well as the educated. Superior intellectual attainments are not necessary.

Cardiac Neurosis

CASE 1

A single, white girl, age thirty, was first seen in October, 1939. She complained of *pain in the precordial region* and *fatigue*.

History and Symptoms

Her trouble had begun during the preceding spring. She felt tired and run down and then following a slight cold developed a sticking pain in the heart region. Her physician had found "a slight murmur, probably not important" and had recommended rest and a tonic to "strengthen her." Finally the pain and fatigue had become so pronounced that she could no longer work.

She had been a healthy child. The appendix was removed at the age of twelve because of an acute attack of appendicitis. Menses were established at sixteen, occurring every three weeks and usually attended by severe cramps. Because of the severe dysmenorrhea she had submitted to an operation at the age of eighteen and one ovary was removed. On this occasion at the hospital the physicians "seemed very interested in her heart" and she then became suspicious that something was the matter.

Family History. The mother died at the age of forty-three from "heart trouble." The patient was fifteen at the time. She nursed her mother and helped look after the house during the period of her mother's illness. The father was living and well and one brother, younger than the patient, was well. There was no other evidence of heart disease in the family.

Physical Examination and Laboratory Studies

The patient was fairly well-nourished. She seemed under considerable stress at the time of the examination. There was pronounced flush over the neck and upper chest; the blood pressure was 150/80; the heart was overactive but seemed normal in size. A slight systolic murmur was heard at the apex, but there was no shock or thrill. Palpitation over the apex area elicited tenderness. The remainder of the physical examination was negative.

Routine laboratory studies including the urine, blood count, blood Wassermann, and sedimentation rate were within normal limits. Basal metabolism was normal. Fluroscopic examination disclosed a normal sized heart and the electrocardiogram showed a normal tracing. Gynecological examination was negative.

LIFE SITUATION

Since her mother's death the patient had been employed in the house of a "well-to-do but stingy family" The patient was a passive person with a good deal of repressed hostility which was awakened when her mistress made what she considered unusual demands upon her. Discussion developed that the onset of the precordial pain had occurred just prior to housecleaning time. Then she remarked that each year she became ill right after housecleaning was over and this year she had become ill just before and, therefore, had been unable to do it because of the pain. Brief discussion brought out the fact that she considered that the housecleaning was too much for one person to do and that she resented the fact that her mistress, who could well afford extra help, insisted that she alone must do the work. Although she had never actually remonstrated before, she always became sick after the housecleaning was over (a belated and passive complaint) but this year her illness interfered with the job. Her manner indicated her deep resentment against her mistress and the simple expression of her unexpressed hostility, plus the suggestion of heart disease because of the mother's death, was enough to indicate to her the cause for illness. When she was assured of the absence of heart disease and reassured as to her ability to carry on, and the explanation of the emotional background of the illness was made clear to her, she promptly recovered. A short time later she found another position and has remained well since.

The following is an instance of a rather more complicated problem which also yielded a good result to superficial psychotherapy.

Cardiac Neurosis

CASE 2

A white man, thirty-nine years old, was first seen in the spring of 1938.

History and Symptoms

He complained of *pain around the heart* and *down the left arm* to the finger tips which was "deep and touched the bone." His left hand felt hot, "as though it had fever in it."

Trouble had begun about ten years before, first with a sense of discomfort in the heart region on occasions but later occurring constantly.

There was no relation to effort; on the contrary he felt better when he exercised. He thought that indulgence in tobacco made the pain worse.

He had had a great deal of medical attention, many studies had been done, and he had taken a number of long rest periods but nothing had helped him. He stated that his constant preoccupation with his pain interfered with his work and happiness.

Past History. He had been a healthy child and had never had a serious illness. At about the age of twenty-one he contracted gonorrhea and inadequate treatment resulted in "a residual infection of the prostate" according to a later medical advisor. He continued under the care of a urologist, receiving prostatic massage at regular intervals, and this had become so much a part of his routine that he failed to mention it when his medical history was first taken. Wassermann tests were negative but, as developed later, to him one venereal disease was as bad as another and just as capable of producing irrevocable damage to the vital organs.

Several years later, during the height of the depression, stomach trouble began. A diagnosis of spastic colon was made but it was not until a physician prescribed bismuth that he began to improve. Then came the pain around the heart which has already been described.

Family History The father died suddenly of heart disease at the age of fifty when the patient was eighteen. The patient felt that he resembled his father closely The mother died of cancer of the stomach several years later. Two older brothers and a younger sister were in good health.

Physical Examination and Laboratory Studies

Although the patient had had a careful examination by physicians of good reputation we felt it necessary to repeat his studies under slightly different circumstances. Therefore, after a careful history and general physical examination, including routine laboratory studies, showed no evidence of organic disease, we informed the patient that (1) we would repeat the electrocardiogram both before and after exercise "in order to prove the absence of even latent disease," (2) that we would require not only a blood Wassermann test but a spinal fluid Wassermann test after a provocative dose of neosalvarsan in order absolutely to confirm the absence of syphilis, and (3) that we would ask for another urological opinion in order to decide whether there was a residual infection of the prostate. All of these studies were done and all proved negative; in other words, the electrocardiogram was normal before and after exercise, the Wassermann tests after provocative therapy were negative, and the best urological opinion that we could obtain decided that the prostate was normal and massage was no longer necessary.

LIFE SITUATION

A study of the life situation revealed that the patient had always been in mortal terror of venereal infection and that having been infected with gonorrhea he arrived at the conclusion, following the statement that his prostate was infected, that the infection would persist and would affect his vital organs. Either in casual contacts or through reading he had decided that the gastrointestinal tract as well as the heart was susceptible to the influence of such infection. After developing gastrointestinal symptoms he did not improve until a medicine which he knew was used in the treatment of syphilis (bismuth) was given to him. Later he developed the "heart symptoms" and as will be recalled from his description "the pain touched the bone," which was an indication once more of his ideas about the effects of venereal disease. Then in the course of his studies he was told by one physician that the aorta, under the fluoroscope, was somewhat enlarged and this confirmed his idea that the heart had been invaded by the venereal infection. All of this information, however, was very difficult to obtain, largely because the patient was so unwilling to admit it even to himself. It was only from hints such as those already mentioned and the further fact that the patient took his vacations at a spa well known for its attention to venereal diseases that we were able to conclude that a number of false ideas existed in this young man concerning the effect upon his vital organs of a venereal infection long since cured.

TREATMENT

When we combined this explanation with the reassurance of absence of organic disease, following studies which appealed to him as being much more thorough than any he had undergone, his pain quite quickly diminished and he was able once more not only to work effectively but to enjoy life, which he hitherto had been unable to do, because he considered himself morally as well as physically diseased. One year later he reported himself well and no longer needed medical attention.

SUMMARY

A young, white man with pain in his heart region held the erroneous belief that an attack of gonorrhea years before might have damaged his heart. An indication that this was the mental mechanism responsible for the cardiac neurosis was derived from hints in his history. A more than usually thorough study plus the explanation of the emotional background of the illness resulted in a very satisfactory recovery.

LOW BLOOD PRESSURE (HYPOTENSION)

The problem of low blood pressure will be discussed again in relation to other conditions (pp. 505 and 656). At this point it is only necessary to say that, if anything, the concept of low blood pressure is even more open to criticism as an explanation for certain symptoms of unknown origin, than is high blood pressure. When a patient speaks of weakness and fatigue it is so easy to say that "the blood pressure is low" or that "he is anemic," or both. It is much more difficult to examine the personality and study the life situation than it is to slap a cuff on the arm or have a technician do a blood count. A great many people go through life considering themselves victims of low blood pressure, with inadequate energy, easily fatigued, resting a lot and taking great care of themselves, often on the basis of a diagnosis of low blood pressure that really is unrelated to their symptoms. Their energy is low because it is consumed by emotional conflict and often it can be liberated by appropriate psychotherapy. Instead of cautioning these people to rest, and urging them to husband their energy, we ought to encourage them to do more instead of less. If for one reason or another, we cannot undertake psychotherapy, at least we will not play into their unconscious fantasies regarding inadequacy and incapacity.

It is true, of course, that there is such a thing as essential hypotension but it is remarkably infrequent and has nothing to do with the thousands of inadequate people who limp through life leaning on the crutch of "low blood pressure," that has been furnished by some physician. We can say to these people, what has been proved by long observation, that low blood pressure is not a disease—it is more likely to be an indication of longevity.

One hears frequently that the problem of neurocirculatory asthenia was of less consequence in World War II than in World War I. While this may be so the incidence was really greater, as shown in chapter II (page 55).

"NEUROCIRCULATORY ASTHENIA"

A special form of cardiac neurosis, met with chiefly in military life, has come to be known as neurocirculatory asthenia (N. C. A.), effort syndrome, or disordered action of the heart (D. A. H.). J. M. DaCosta recognized the "irritable heart" of soldiers during the American Civil War and the chief contribution to heart disease during the first World War was the reemphasis of this syndrome by Sir Thomas Lewis. Since that time the term has been applied very widely, not only to the functional cardiac disorders met with in military life, but also to an increasing number of such disorders in civil life. Whether this has been a healthy development in medicine will be discussed shortly.

Incidence in Military Service

Speaking of heart disease in the military service, Kilgore stated that studies based on service and later hospital records, when subjected to a review and examination of the persons concerned, call for caution in accepting the results. "The fact is that many diagnoses of mitral insufficiency, myocarditis, angina pectoris and the like were mistakenly entered in the records and have been carried forward as grounds for disability ratings, long after the passage of years and accumulating evidence should have removed any doubt about the original diagnostic errors. Thomas Lewis, in reviewing the studies at Hampstead from 1914 to 1918, estimated that *about five-sixths of the British army diagnoses of organic heart disease were erroneous,* an estimate probably not far from the truth of our own past performance. And for the practical conduct of medical service for our armed forces of the future we may safely assume that real heart disease, infrequently encountered, will usually receive adequate recognition and treatment, while other things with the superficial appearance of heart disease will require special care if we are to avoid the costly mistakes of the past."

Clinical Picture

Wittkower and his associates, who made a study of the effort syndrome in the British military service, stated that the patients are not fakers or malingerers and have no conscious intention of escaping from the service. From a careful study of fifty selected cases with clear-cut effort syndrome they emphasize the fundamental importance of emotional factors in the etiology. (Of every ten patients admitted to cardiac hospitals in World War I, nine were suffering from functional disorders, most commonly effort syndrome [Lewis, 1940].) They describe the disorder as characterized by disproportionate breathlessness and fatigue on effort, and a varying degree of undue disturbance of the pulse rate on exercise. There may also be dizziness or fainting attacks, blurred vision, thoracic pain of the left inframammary type, palpitation and tachycardia, indigestion and constipation, headaches, insomnia and nightmares, "nervousness," undue sweating, tremor, cramps and numbness of the limbs. In addition there may be blueness or mottled coloring of the hands, dermatographia, and a variety of neurovascular phenomena. The pulse at rest and in sleep is normal but is easily accelerated by motion or exercise and is abnormally slow in its return to normal after exercise. Blood pressure is as a rule normal at rest but exhibits the same exaggerated response to exercise and emotion as does the pulse. The electrocardiogram does not reveal any structural changes. The differentiation from organic disease of the heart ought not to present great difficulties. The diagnostic problem at times likewise involves the differentiation of diseases such as pulmonary tuberculosis, undulant fever, and exophthalmic goiter. Wittkower's experience showed that soldiers suffering from effort syndrome, unless very mild, were unfit for military service. There is little tendency to spontaneous improvement, and methods of treatment so far employed, though temporarily beneficial in some cases, have failed almost completely in restoring fitness for full service.

The Development of the Syndrome

Given a neuropathic predisposition based on hereditary and constitutional inadequacy, many factors can assume the role of exciting or initiating agents. Among these, infectious or physical agents, and the psychic strain of war, are most important.

Kilgore said that candidates for the effort syndrome are those with poor posture, flabby muscles, and often poor nutrition; those with tachycardia, labile blood pressure, cool, moist and bluish extremities, marked dermatographia, and dripping axillas; those who have avoided strenuous athletics and sought light work; often those who eschew tobacco and alcohol, perhaps after experiencing poor tolerance, and those who are given to worry and to the study and adoption of diets and other health fads. Men with such poor natural stamina may break down in ordinary military training; and then, despite the best of treatment, they are apt to continue in a state of pensioned disability, from which it is difficult or impossible ever to wean them. Others, better endowed by nature, stand vigorous training exercises but fail when sufficient physical or nervous strain follows infection, prolonged fatigue, insufficient food and shelter, anxiety, and the like. In the latter group disability is more often temporary because its chief causes are removable.

"Neurocirculatory Asthenia" in Civil Life

Most patients thought to be suffering from effort syndrome or neurocirculatory asthenia are in reality psychoneurotics with cardiac manifestations. Perhaps some few cases in congenitally defective or constitutionally inferior persons—those poor postured, flabby muscled, poor nutritioned people, who show evidence of pronounced vasomotor instability, and who may present a postural defect in the electrocardiogram and difference in pulse rate and blood pressure in standing and recumbency—might be referred to as neurocirculatory asthenia but even here the psychic factor is the most important and is the only one that is really amenable to treatment. Medicine as a whole and cardiology in particular would be benefited if the term were dropped altogether. In its place we could speak of cardiac neurosis with or without evidences of vasomotor instability.

Neurocirculatory asthenia seemed to be less of a problem in World War II than in World War I, probably because it became recognized for what it is, namely psychoneurosis with cardiac manifestations, and was classified as such rather than as heart disease. Then too, in the latter instance there was probably better selection at the time of induction into service. One of the reasons the British made so little headway with the disorder from a psychotherapeutic standpoint in the first war (returning only 20 per cent to front-line duty) is that in their management of the disorder valuable time was lost and the neurosis was permitted to consolidate; then of course it became more difficult to treat.

These deductions received recent confirmation in a large experience with so-called "effort syndrome" at the Mill Hill Emergency Hospital of London, England: 2,323 cases treated at the Effort Syndrome Unit of this neurosis center, which permitted a number of studies on the functional responses of such persons. From this study the belief is stated that effort syndrome is largely a question of neurosis, and that the problem is one for the psychiatrist rather than the cardiologist. Three groups are made:

Group 1. Poor physical endowment is the primary factor in producing symptoms. Here one is dealing with a poor machine which shows excessive response to physical effort; the patient has effort intolerance which has been present since his earliest recollection.

Group 2. Similar to Group 1, but the patient responds in a neurotic manner to his constitutional inferiority. In this sense there is a psychological etiology but the constitutional factor is the basic one. The emotional reaction may take any form, depending upon the personality makeup. The patient feels that he has an effort intolerance but his disability may actually be less than he believes it to be. Such patients usually give a history of effort intolerance since childhood, whereas the mere disability of Group 1 frequently changes under stress to the neurotic attitude of Group 2.

Group 3. Primarily neurotic. Here the usual etiological factors determining a neurosis will apply. The form may be selected by the constitutional physical inferiority which, if present, colors the whole picture but is of only secondary importance; or it may be selected wholly on a psychogenetic basis. Such "illness" tends to be of comparatively recent origin and is particularly prone to result from the emotional and physical stresses of wartime.

A comparison of oxygen uptake, lactate rise, and pulse area made after exercise in normal subjects, in patients suffering from anxiety states, and in effort syndrome patients, showed that the patients with anxiety states and those with effort syndromes had a significantly poorer exercise response when matched with normal controls.

If there is a postural circulatory defect the blood pressure drops and the pulse rate increases as the patient arises from recumbency to the upright position. For a proper test eight minutes should be permitted to elapse after the patient assumes the erect posture. Sometimes the blood pressure will not change so much as the pulse rate. Sometimes there are electrocardiographic changes to correlate with pulse and blood pressure changes. Voltage of T waves tends to be lowered in the erect position and P deflections in leads 2 and 3 show a higher voltage. This can be referred to as the electrocardiographic evidence of what has been called the postural syndrome.

It may be quite true that the vasomotor instability and the psychological disorder are parallel manifestations of the same basic fault. In one instance the poor physical endowment may be the chief problem, in another instance the personality disorder. It is largely a question of where the emphasis is placed: We believe that placing the emphasis on the "constitutional inadequacy" is a mistake. In the first place it is so often not true, and in the second place nothing can be done about it anyhow, whereas one can usually do something about a psychological disturbance.

In this connection Friedman found that most patients suffering from functional cardiovascular disease experienced transient giddiness. It usually occurred following rapid or abrupt change from the supine to the erect position. Experimental studies revealed that the symptom was most likely due to cerebral anemia arising from the retardation of the forward flow of blood. When giddy patients arose, it was observed fluoroscopically that a sudden, abrupt decrease in the width and pulsatile excursion of the pulmonary artery (conus) took place and the force of cardiac contraction was observed to dwindle although the rate increased remarkably. No such change was observed in normal individuals. A schematic representation of the probable mechanism underlying the giddiness of functional cardiovascular disease is shown in the accompany ing diagram.

CHART 1—THE PROBABLE MECHANISM UNDERLYING THE GIDDINESS
OF FUNCTIONAL CARDIOVASCULAR DISEASE*

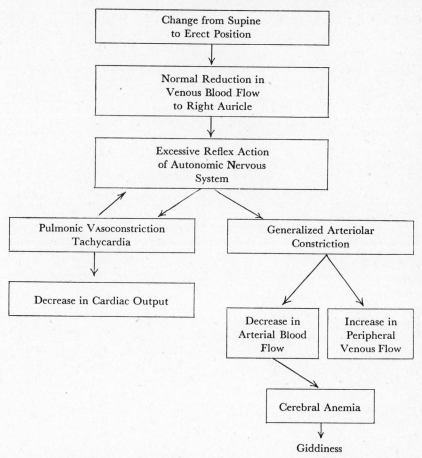

* Friedman, Meyer: Functional Cardiovascular Disease, Williams and Wilkins
Co., Baltimore, 1947.

In the constitutionally normal individual, whose problem is purely
psychological, it is certainly a great mistake to label him neurocirculatory asthenia, effort syndrome, or, worse yet, disordered action
of the heart, because it places emphasis on the cardiovascular system
and away from the psychological cause. Certainly here, at least, the
term must be dropped and in its place we should speak of cardiac neurosis
or neurosis with cardiac manifestations. Call psychosomatic illness by
the name of a disease, and you foster neuroticism. Call it by the name of
a disorder and explain it in terms of behavior, and the patient is im-
measurably better off. No great objection can be found to the term
"effort syndrome" because it leaves the way open for further investiga-

tion, while the phrase "neurocirculatory asthenia" often closes the subject—it gives the physician the feeling that the condition is understood and that nothing more than physical treatments are called for.

Margolin* has well stated that "the syndrome which in 1917 was named 'neurocirculatory asthenia' was originally observed in military combat situations. Anxiety neurosis, on the other hand, is a syndrome that was defined in a civilian environment. With the establishment of these two terms in nosological practice to cover a relatively unclassified group of somatic and psychic symptoms, anxiety neurosis and neurocirculatory asthenia began to appear as diagnoses in both civilian and military settings. It is important to realize that neurocirculatory asthenia as a term stresses the pathophysiological manifestations, whereas anxiety neurosis calls attention to the psychopathological phenomena. The significance of this distinction becomes apparent when the psychiatrist diagnoses anxiety neurosis in a patient who, according to the internist, exhibits neurocirculatory asthenia. In addition, this difference may be expressed by the patient's choice of his presenting symptom which may be psychological or physical. In fact this unconscious selection may determine whether the patient will be referred to the psychiatrist or to the internist.

"In addition to the psychological and somatic aspects of these conditions, an environmental aspect must be considered. In military combat, reactions may be evoked which must be regarded as appropriate and normal, in spite of the fact that they would appear abnormal in a civilian setting."

Differential Diagnosis

The great difficulty has been that, in keeping with our terminology referable to the cardiovascular system, our whole attitude and all observations have been limited to the cardiovascular system instead of including an approach to the subject from a psychosomatic standpoint. As to how these patients are classified, all depends upon the point of view. For example, some physicians think of them as endocrine problems, especially from the standpoint of the thyroid, and treat them as instances of hyperthyroidism; others think of them from a metabolic standpoint and speak of them as suffering from hypoglycemia or hyperinsulinism; others, impressed by the psychic disturbance, refer to them as instances of chronic nervous exhaustion, anxiety neurosis, or neurasthenia, but the latter two terms are used devoid of psychic meaning and no psychic studies are made. Still others have been impressed by the slight fever that occurs

*Margolin, S.: Presented before the Psychosomatic Forum, New York City, 1950.

in many of these cases and have studied them from that standpoint. A case will be cited in which this problem is encountered. Hamman, in two papers devoted to the "Diagnosis of Obscure Fever" and speaking of the *effort syndrome*, said, "The fever may persist for years and the most thorough investigation fail to discover any acceptable cause for it. The character of the symptoms and their long duration force us to look upon effort syndrome as a neurosis of obscure mechanism and origin. Unexplained, slight fever is so frequently present in this condition that we regard it as an important element of the clinical manifestations."

Friedman found low-grade fever, rarely exceeding 100.5°F, in more than 30 per cent of patients suffering from "functional" cardiovascular disease. He could detect no evidence that the fever was a manifestation of infection, either acute or chronic.

Among thirty patients only two were found whose serums when diluted forty times were able to agglutinate Brucella melitensis, but both exhibited a negative reaction to the skin test. Otherwise all the patients were negative to the above examinations. The average basal metabolic rate was minus 5 per cent.

Friedman cautions reservation in the diagnosis of undulant fever in any patient who exhibits manifestations of functional cardiovascular disease, including fever, for over six months. Incidentally, Friedman holds that the presence of fever in this syndrome is a definite indication of hypothalamic involvement. Our own feeling is that unfortunately this brings us no closer to an understanding of this disorder.

Again and again focal infection has been thought of and "foci of infection" have been removed. There is not the slightest reason for believing that "focal infection" bears any relation to this disorder. Tobacco poisoning, tuberculosis, brucellosis, and colitis are frequent terms used in connection with such patients. Altogether neurocirculatory asthenia seems to be a catch-basket into which are thrown a great variety of ill-defined conditions.

The chief differential diagnostic problems have centered about early tuberculosis—"spot on the lung"—undulant fever, and focal infection; thyrotoxicosis, because the basal metabolism may be slightly increased; colitis, because of the frequent slight bowel disturbance; and neurasthenia or anxiety neurosis as an emasculated concept, that is, a "nervous" name without any attempt to study psychic mechanisms. A chart summarizes some of the differentiating features.

TABLE 1.—DIFFERENTIAL DIAGNOSIS IN "NEUROCIRCULATORY ASTHENIA."

	Cardiac Neurosis	"Neurocirculatory Asthenia"	Hyperthyroidism	Chronic Infections (Tuberculosis—Brucellosis)
Family History	Unstable (epilepsy, neurosis, psychosis)	Unstable	Unstable	Stable
Past History	Poor adjustment (childhood neurosis, nervous breakdown)	Poor adjustment	Poor adjustment	Well adjusted
Precipitating Cause	Emotional stress, psychic trauma	Stress of military service	Emotional stress, psychic trauma	Sufficient exposure to specific organism
Clinical Picture	Precordial pain, fatigue, breathlessness, palpitation	Precordial pain, fatigue, breathlessness, palpitation	Goiter; exophthalmos; fine tremor; emotionalism	Febrile features conspicuous; anxiety features absent or inconspicuous
Physical Examination and Laboratory Studies	Normal cardiovascular system, rapid pulse while awake	Evidences of neurocirculatory instability — cold, sweaty and cyanotic extremities; flushing of face and neck; postural change in pulse, blood pressure and electrocardiogram; slight elevation of temperature	Rapid pulse, awake and asleep; plus basal metabolism; response to iodine	T.B.: plus x-ray; plus sputum Brucellosis: plus skin, agglutination tests, and blood culture
Treatment	Psychotherapy	Psychotherapy and medical measures	Surgery plus psychotherapy	Medical measures
Prognosis	Depends on severity of underlying neurosis	Poor	Good	Good

Treatment

Prophylaxis. Undoubtedly the most important phase in the treatment of this condition is prevention. So far as military service is concerned prophylaxis should begin at the time of induction of the recruit. The faulty examinations in World War I are clearly illustrated, as pointed out by Lewis, by the fact that nearly half the patients invalided for effort syndrome or heart disease developed the symptoms before joining the orces and more than half developed them before their training was complete. "There is not the slightest doubt," stated Lewis, ' that adequate examination would have eliminated most of these men, would have kept them in useful employment, would have spared them much suffering, would have saved hospital space and large funds of the M nistry of Pensions. Such men were six or seven months in training, five months in hospital, and gave in return 2.2 months of full and 1.5 to 2 months of light duty."

Everything that was said regarding the treatment of cardiac neurosis applies equally well to this special form. As far as military service is concerned Kilgore stated that the medical officer, "who finds a murmur or arrhythmia or who hears the complaint of syncope, palpitation, or precordial pain should be aware that he carries a responsibility comparable in importance to that involved in a delicate surgical operation. If he is sure of his ground, the task should be easy. If the heart is diseased he will frankly state the case and advise accordingly, being careful not to implant an exaggerated idea of the gravity of the condition. And if he is sure the sign or symptom in question does not mean heart disease, he will be equally frank and decided. In doing so however, he should remember that words are often discounted and that attitude is more convincing. Reassuring statements may be nullified by merely calling an associate to listen to an interesting murmur or by cautioning the patient to be a little careful."

Diagnosis by Exclusion. It is under such circumstances that the physician often plays an unfortunate role because if he indicates any doubt as to the integrity of the heart he may add to the neurotic problem. The error can be attributed to two factors, first, the desire of the physician to find something "tangible' to explain the illness, growing out of the organic tradition in medicine, and second, the unfamiliarity of the physician with heart diseases and hence his insecurity in dealing with such problems. But the fault lies not so much in his unfamiliarity with the physical problems of heart disease as in his inadequate psychological training. He tries to establish the diagnosis simply by the exclusion of organic disease rather than by the simultaneous examination of the body and the personality of the patient. The latter examination should tell if the patient's psychological structure is such as to predispose him to the development of cardiac neurosis. When one approaches the subject of heart disease solely on the basis of exclusion of organic disease, and is so deeply rooted in the organic tradition as to be unwilling to make a diagnosis of cardiac neurosis, he subjects such patients to an unnecessary amount of physical examination and laboratory investigation, thus fastening attention more than ever upon the heart.

Errors in Diagnosis. Chief among the physical signs often responsible for mistaken diagnosis of cardiovascular disease are benign murmurs and arrhythmias, simple tachycardia, and temporary elevation of blood pressure from the excitement of a medical examination. Some with the last-mentioned condition may be candidates for essential hypertension later in life, but they should not be regarded as abnormal without repeated observation under conditions of quiet and reassurance. More will be said on this subject in the chapter on hypertension.

Kilgore found that "cardiac arrhythmia in young recruits is chiefly sinus arrhythmia—alternate acceleration and retardation in heart rate —usually but not always timed with respiratory cycles. It is always benign and, as a rule, easily recognized. But at times the transitions from faster to slower rhythm and vice versa are very severe and abrupt, and create the impression of heart block. Premature contractions are also not uncommon in the young. They sometimes result from damage to the myocardium, especially those of atrial origin (usually recognizable by the fact that the pulse intermission is shorter than two normal intervals); but they are more often benign and should be so considered unless other evidence of heart disease can be found. They may produce but faint sounds, sometimes only a faint first sound, especially when occurring early in diastole; and if this is missed in auscultation, the compensatory pause may cause the mistaken diagnosis of heart block. In general no such diagnosis should be made in young soldiers without electrocardiographic confirmation."

In a thorough review of this subject, Dunn concluded that the majority of patients with neurocirculatory asthenia show a psychological disturbance; that neurotic traits are commonly found; and that the family setting and early life experience of the patient seem of more significance than the constitutional and hereditary factors.

Personality Studies. Wittkower and his associates stated that none of the patients suffering from *effort syndrome* was found to be emotionally well adjusted. Five *personality types* were found:

The majority (group 1) conformed to the obsessional type, possessing, as their most obvious characteristics, an overkeen sense of duty and overrigid morality. In this group, conflicts over fear of showing fear after severe fighting experiences, problems related to responsibility and overrigid morality, and breakdown after obsessional overwork, were common findings.

In group 2, in addition to overconscientiousness and a rigid moral code, there was less repression of aggressiveness and at the same time a deep-seated attitude of resentment, obviously arising from experiences of early childhood. Here strained parental relationships, sometimes resulting in problems over subordination, were predominant.

A third much smaller group was made up of open rebels who were overtly overaggressive and whose conflicts were related to overaggressiveness.

A fourth group was infantile in build and asthenic or generally of poor physique. With this was combined emotional and instinctual immaturity. Endowed with inferior physique they struggled in vain against this handicap.

A last small group was made up of hysterical quitters. They were individuals who had apparently given up the struggle for existence before it had properly started. They escaped into dependence in the face of apparently insurmountable tasks.

Systematic psychotherapy was indicated in group 1. In groups 2 and 3 there was a response to psychotherapy which released aggressiveness and reduced conflict. Group 4 gave some response to graduated exercises and superficial psychotherapy, while group 5 could not be trained as soldiers.

Personality Differences. Obvious differences in the make-up of the personality were encountered in effort syndrome as compared with those in other psychosomatic disorders. In patients suffering from colitis, peptic ulcer, and effort syndrome Wittkower found the common factors to be overconscientiousness and overscrupulousness. But, whereas the gastric ulcer patient is often concerned with economic security (problems of bread and butter) and the colitis patient with overtidiness, overcleanliness, and hoarding carried to irrational extremes, the effort syndrome patient is preoccupied with problems of morality, self-regard, religiosity, patriotism, duty, responsibility, and self-sacrifice. The overcleanliness of the colitis patient compares with the sublimated puritanism of the effort syndrome patient.

Phobias. In all, eighteen patients exhibited gross nervous symptoms prior to the onset of effort syndrome, most commonly of a phobic nature. Later experience suggested that the breathlessness of effort syndrome is the physiological correlate of what appears in the psychological sphere as fear of suffocation (*claustrophobia*). On close inquiry most service patients disclosed the existence of overt or latent claustrophobia before the frank onset of effort syndrome; for example, they had uneasiness when traveling by subway, or they complained of having felt faint or uncomfortable in warm rooms, or in rooms without an open window. Difficulty or discomfort in wearing a respirator was also common and often could be demonstrated by a pulse or respiration rate which rose unduly when the patient was wearing the respirator.

Rorschach Study. Ross studied neurocirculatory asthenia by the Rorschach method (fifty cases compared with fifty controls). He confirmed the following findings:

(*a*) Certain personality features are associated with neurocirculatory asthenia to a greater degree than would be accounted for by chance.

(*b*) These personality features include several which have been previously reported from clinical psychiatric study, namely, features characteristic of psychoneurosis, in particular a tendency to give up easily under stress ("hysterical quitters") and obsessive-compulsive traits.

(*c*) Sexually disturbing stimuli do not appear to cause as great difficulty for these patients as they do for miscellaneous civilian psychoneurotics, but other anxiety-producing stimuli are handled with even greater difficulty.

(*d*) When the neurocirculatory asthenia patients are divided into two groups, the more long-standing cases are found to possess the neurotic features to a more marked degree, while those of more recent onset show a stronger similarity to cases of migraine with persistence toward success and "ambitious perfectionism."

Many of the points mentioned in the discussion are illustrated by the following cases.

Neurocirculatory Asthenia
Induced by Military Service; Paranoid Character; Poor Prognosis

---

CASE 3

History and Symptoms

A white man, thirty-six, was first seen in April, 1945.

He complained of irregular heart action, weakness, and fatigue, and said he felt unable to work. There was a sudden sensation in his chest that felt like "a balloon inflated." The condition had developed in the army and he had been discharged because of it with 60 per cent disability.

The illness began in October 1944, while he was in military training. He had to row upstream against a swift current until he felt exhausted, then the boat got stuck in the mud and everybody had to get out and push the boat to the river bank. Following this there was a "double quick" march for nine miles. When he reached camp the heart action was very rapid. Medical service was not immediately available, and when he did get to the dispensary "nothing was done for him." The rapid heart action and shortness of breath prevented him from sleeping. Finally an army physician told him that he had auricular fibrillation and kept him in bed for four days. Following this he was put through a thorough and "strenuous" physical checkup. Then he was discharged as physically unfit because of his heart. An electrocardiographic tracing was reported as auricular fibrillation with an occasional premature ventricular contraction.

The patient was bitter about his treatment in the service, referred to the army doctors in disrespectful terms, and felt that he had been given a "bad deal" because of the "excessive strain of the physical examination on top of 'what he already had.' "

After he had been discharged from the service his civilian physician reported that he had been well before he entered the service and that his work often required him to lift packages of 100 pounds in weight which he could do without ill effect. He told the patient that he suffered from heart-muscle strain, that rest and relaxation would help him, and gave him medicine containing digitalis.

Past History. In a more detailed investigation of his past history it was learned that he often showed fits of temper as a child and would get very angry at members of the family on the slightest provocation. He had suffered from headaches and fatigue beginning in high school and these had continued for about ten years. Then he became involved in a tempestuous love affair that "nearly drove him crazy." This broke up in 1940 at a time when "his nerves gave 'way." Gradually he recovered and was inducted into the army in January 1942. After his discharge he returned to his home and to his father's business. He reported much aggravation with his father, who conducted the business in a way of which the patient did not approve and would accept no suggestions from the patient. A younger brother and sister were unsympathetic to the patient's illness and only the mother, who was described as hard-working, intelligent woman, "had any consideration for him."

Physical Examination and Laboratory Studies

Physical examination with special attention to the cardiovascular system disclosed no evidence of organic disease. The blood pressure was within normal limits; the heart was normal in size according to orthodiagram; and the electrocardiographic tracing was also within normal limits. Eye-grounds were physiologic. Routine laboratory studies were normal and glucose tolerance was normal.

LIFE SITUATION

Each time the patient returned he was encouraged to talk about his home situation and the burden of his complaint was always the same. He was disgusted with his father, whom he described as a stupid and obstinate man who refused to accept the patient's modern ideas about how to run the business. The son openly threatened the father with violence and on occasion was told "to get out if he didn't like it." But he felt unable to work and therefore was dependent upon his father for assistance. He was "humiliated" by the necessity of "borrowing" money from his father. This yielding to his dependency of course only infuriated him the more and while he recognized that the aggravation at home "exaggerated his condition" he continued to believe that his heart had been weakened by the overexertion and bad treatment which he had received in the army, that he was unable to undergo any real physical exertion, and that if he did so it would set him back for a matter of months. Thus, he was caught in the conflict of his impotent rage—acknowledging his depenence upon the father whom he hated. He would refuse to help in the store and would try to absent himself from home "to escape the aggravation." Finally he tried a succession of jobs as a salesman but they always involved more exertion than he felt he could undergo.

Hostility

It was impossible to convince him that his heart was sound and that the whole problem was one of a disorder of his feelings rather than of his body. Although he expressed his feelings freely in the interviews this was so far from modifying the fury of his murderous impulses that he obtained very little relief. The family physician reported that both the mother and father were very much afraid of him because of his threats to the father. Moreover, the family physician also reported that any disturbance in the home was not the fault of the father and mother, but that they were kind and amenable people who would do anything for their children.

Finally the patient was called by the Veterans Administration for a resurvey and his disability was reduced from 60 to 10 per cent. He was more furious than ever with the injustice meted out to him, felt that we had conspired with the V. A. physicians, and broke off his treatment. During the time he remained under observation (April 1945 to November 1946) the only indications of improvement were his acknowledgement of somewhat lessened heart consciousness and his efforts to work, which he did for short periods of time.

SUMMARY

A young man developed the syndrome of neurocirculatory asthenia following an episode of physical exhaustion during military service. He had had previous neurotic difficulties and the illness was perpetuated by a home situation that gave rise to impotent rage. The paranoid character of the patient indicated the poor prognosis and constituted a real threat to his family.

Neurocirculatory Asthenia
Long-continued, Low Fever of Obscure Origin; Questionable Endocarditis;
Markedly Neurotic Person

CASE 4

History and Symptoms

The patient was a rather attractive American-born Italian woman, twenty-eight years old. She complained of fatigue, shortness of breath, and pain in the precordium. She was well until September 1938, when she noticed a gradually increasing fatigue and was ordered to bed by her physician, where she remained for two weeks. Then she was somewhat improved until about Christmas time when she again became tired and "was in and out of bed for the remainder of the winter." In June 1939, her physician again ordered her to go to bed because she was so fatigued and because he thought that she had a "leak in her heart." At the same time she discovered that she had slight fever and from then on, following the physician's orders, she took her temperature four or five times a day. The temperature was never above 99.4° or 99.6°. In spite of a vacation at the seashore during the summer she failed to regain her strength, finally changed physicians, and was then referred to the hospital for further study.

The shortness of breath had been present for about four months. She described the shortness of breath as coming with slight exertion and demonstrated by placing her hand over her lower sternum and then stating that she felt as though she would like to take a deep breath but felt herself unable to do so. Thus she described the typical sighing respiration so common in functional problems. The pain was felt over the whole heart region and extended into the back to the angle of the left scapula.

Past History. The patient said she was a healthy child. Her father died when she was six, and the mother remarried two years later. The patient continued at school until the eighth grade, then worked in the store that her stepfather had established and also helped around the house. The menses began about eleven and had always been very painful until her baby was born. Since then they had not been painful. About the age of sixteen she developed indigestion which was said to be due to "stomach ulcer," but the diagnosis was never proved. She herself felt that it was nervous indigestion. It continued until the baby was born, that is, for five or six years. At seventeen she became engaged. Her fiance "had a heart lesion, which necessitated some care at the time but did not bother him afterwards." She married at twenty and became pregnant one year later. She had some nausea and vomiting for a short time during pregnancy but then remained very well. She had a hard delivery and a prolonged convalescence and was unable to nurse the child. During the hospital stay, following labor, she had slight fever. She had not had any indigestion since. Shortly afterwards she had to work very hard, taking care of the household as well as the child, looking after and cooking for six people.

Physical Examination and Laboratory Studies

The patient was referred into the hospital as a case of neurocirculatory asthenia or possible endocarditis. The general physical examination showed a well-nourished. young white woman, who did not appear ill. The temperature was slightly elevated, reaching about 99.6° in the afternoon, and at the lowest point in the morning was 97.°, which gave the temperature chart a quite irregular appearance. However, later it hovered about the base line and tended to fluctuate less. The pulse and respiration were not increased. Aside from a slight systolic murmur at the apex of the heart, after the patient had exercised and was placed in the left lateral position, there were no physical findings to suggest organic disease. Moreover, the heart seemed normal in size and this was corroborated by the x-ray examination. The lungs were clear and resonant and the x-ray likewise confirmed normal lung findings.

The urinalysis was entirely normal; the blood count was within normal limits, both as to red and white blood cells, and differential count; and the Wassermann test was negative. The sedimentation rate was slightly increased but it was done during the menstrual period (the rates were 19 and 23 mm.) and this might have had some bearing upon it. Several blood cultures, both ordinary and massive, had been negative, and agglutination tests, especially for undulant fever, were negative.

Fatigue More Important than Fever. For the above reasons we felt certain that the patient did not have subacute bacterial endocarditis. It was, of course, difficult to rule this out with certainty at first. However, the normal heart size and the normal electrocardiographic tracings, together with the other clinical features, impressed us that the cardiovascular system was normal and while we were not sure at that moment, we believed that a little more time and observation would prove the point.

The clinical feature which seemed to us most important to work out was the cause of the fatigue although the patient and her previous medical advisors had focused their interest upon the slight elevation of temperature.

LIFE SITUATION

Here was an illustration of the fact that children need more than bed and board in order to grow up to be healthy and happy individuals. This patient, for example, was born in America of Italian parents who enforced old world standards in bringing up the child. She was not permitted the freedom of playing with the other children of the neighborhood. The mother thought the other little girls in the neighborhood were badly behaved and would teach her bad things. When she became an adolescent both parents felt she might get into "bad company" and hence they would not permit her to associate with friends of her own age. "I was always with older people," she told us. We know how often this produces problems in later life adjustment to recreation and sexuality.

Lack of Education

The stepfather was especially strict and inconsiderate in raising this patient and her younger brother. Moreover, it seemed that her mother did not take her part, being interested only in establishing her own security in her second marriage. "Mother was one of those women whose aim was to keep her husband satisfied no matter how much the children were sacrificed." For example, the stepfather was always critical and would choose the meal time especially to voice his criticism of her. Then "food would stick in my throat," an indication that she was unable "to swallow" her environmental situation.

The patient had few friends and was allowed no freedom during her adolescence. She left school at the eighth grade, although she wanted very much to go on with her education, and she was made to work in in the store and in the home with little opportunity for recreation. There was practically no social life, the family living very much within itself. She resented deeply the fact that she could not go on with her schooling and pictured herself as a person who would have derived much benefit from further education. She felt that she might have been able to go to college and "make something of herself." These were the thoughts which were disturbing her during her adolescence and during the period when she developed what she later looked upon as "nervous indigestion." It was also interesting that during this period she was very fatigued although this was brought out only by questioning—she did not remember it in connection with the story of the present illness. Any individual with the amount of anxiety and conflict that his patient had must suffer extreme muscular tension and consequent fatigue.

Birth of Child

Shortly after the baby was born it became ill, had repeated colds, frequent slight elevations of temperature, the cause for which physicians could not discover, and then developed a running ear which caused the patient a great deal of distress. This state of ill health had continued. She had been criticized for being so fussy about the child and so insistent upon cleanliness in bringing it up. In fact she was very meticulous as a housekeeper and according to her statement things had to be done just so and if they were not she was much upset and felt that things were in an uncompleted state.

Stepfather's Illness

About three years ago her stepfather had an illness which was reported to be encephalitis, and then developed a change in personality. He began "to stare at the patient," especially at the table and then made accusations to the mother that the patient was being untrue to her husband. He insisted that she was carrying on with men in the neighborhood and this caused her a great deal of concern. She insisted that there was no foundation in truth for these accusations, nor could she think of any possible reason why he should make these statements. Finally matters reached such a point that the stepfather threatened that she must either leave the house or he would. Without warning he carried out his threat one day in August, 1938; shortly, however, he had a change of heart, returned and suffered the patient to remain in the house, stating that he would change his attitude. It was true that he no longer made the accusations but the patient still felt that he stared at her and of course that he was thinking evil thoughts. *This period of emotional stress immediately preceded the beginning of her illness in September, 1938.*

Hostility Toward Parents

Here in the ward we noted that the patient was a very sensitive person who was very resentful of any discussion of her private life. After winning her confidence, however, we found that she really appreciated the interest taken in her and that she burned with resentment against her mother and stepfather. She felt, and we thought with justification, that she had had a raw deal in life and so she carried a great deal of hostility within her toward fate in general and her parents in particular. Nevertheless, she did not dare to establish her own home which, of course, was what she wanted and could afford to do. She said "that it would be too hard on her mother and stepfather" who needed her financial help. Thus, she could not retaliate in any active way for the bad way in which they treated her. Nor could she tolerate any evidence of this hostility within herself.

TREATMENT

Approach to Treatment. In regard to treatment we thought it important to evaluate the fever and heart murmur in relation to the patient's activity. If there was not sufficient evidence to warrant a positive diagnosis of heart disease then it was advisable from the standpoint of psychosomatic treatment to stop taking temperature readings and have this patient resume normal activity. In other words, she had to be treated as a psychoneurosis of the neurasthenic type to see what effect could be produced upon the symptoms through an education toward a more normal way of life. Instead of considering her as an invalid we would have to encourage her to move into a home of her own where she would not be exposed to a psychotic stepfather and an unsympathetic mother. She had to be helped to make new friends of her own age and to join in their interests. She had to learn that resentment about the things she had missed was only natural and that no reason existed for guilt over this resentment. To be helped to express her hostility more directly and to find people with whom she could live comfortably we believed would affect her symptoms favorably.

Difficulties Presented by Question of a Heart Lesion. This patient presented a difficult psychosomatic problem. If it had not been for the question concerning the actual presence of a heart lesion we would not have found it so difficult to understand or to deal with. It was obvious that we were dealing with a person who was emotionally quite ill and since we know that *the commonest cause of fatigue is not infection but emotional conflict*, we felt that the explanation might apply here. If so it would have been simple to say to this patient—"The important symptom in your case is not the slight fever, which is insignificant and only a phase of your disturbed constitutional make-up; the important symptom is fatigue and that is related to your emotional problems." Therefore, instead of ordering her to go to bed we would do quite the opposite and instruct her "to carry on in spite of symptoms." Then we could follow the suggestions already made that the proper treatment for her would be to encourage her to establish a home of her own, to remedy her educational defect, perhaps by going to night school, and to expand her social life, all of which would give her greater assurance and furnish her with the things which would give her satisfaction.

Just so long as there was a question of a heart lesion, however, we could not do this and while we believed that there was no definite evidence of organic heart disease we felt that we would have to wait a short time in order to prove this conclusively. Thus in dealing with patients of this kind we must map out a program of investigation and prosecute it actively and then within a certain limited time, having assured ourselves that there is no organic disease present, say to the patient—"You do not have organic disease, the slight fever is not important, throw your thermometer away and let us get after the cause of fatigue because that is your important problem."

Insignificance of Slight Fever. The question is often raised as to whether there is such a thing as *fever of psychogenic origin.* In cases just like this that we have previously studied, in which low fever of obscure origin seemed at first sight to be the central problem, we were able to demonstrate over a period of time that no organic disease was present and none developed. Such patients are often thought to have early tuberculosis and frequently spend long periods in sanatoria (p. 615). The patient and the physician focus all of their attention on finding the cause of the slight fever and the problem becomes very much like that of essential hypertension in which so much anxiety is centered on the blood pressure figures. It seems to us that it is not important whether we term the fever itself psychogenic. What is more important is that in such patients we realize that the fever is not the most important part of the problem but simply represents one phase of a disturbance in the constitutional make-up of the individual of which the disturbance in the emotional life represents another and more important phase—more important because the patient frequently derives great benefit from an improvement in the life situation.

Final Conference Before Leaving Hospital. Further studies showed the sedimentation rate varying from 10 to 19 mm. The electrocardiogram, repeated in the upright and recumbent postures, showed no evidence of postural circulatory deficiency. Sinus x-rays were negative and x-rays of the teeth were normal. The chest x-ray was negative and massive blood cultures were negative. All agglutination tests were negative and the Addis count on the urinary sediment showed nothing abnormal. During the last week in the hospital the temperature curve was somewhat closer to average, varying between 97.2 and 99.6. There was some evidence of allergic rhinitis.

We then felt secure enough regarding the absence of organic disease, and a heart lesion in particular, to go over the situation with the patient in the following manner.

Crucial Emotional Factor. We sketched her problem for her as we saw it, that is, that the slight fever was inconsequential but that the fatigue was the important problem and that the cause of fatigue was emotional conflict; that she had had a very difficult childhood and adolescence, resenting the fact that she could not be educated and had to work, that she really had no chance for a good time like other young girls but immediately became interested in a young man whom she married. Then came the baby and lots of difficulties with it and then the episode with the stepfather. After we had sketched this outline of her history she said, "I did not tell you before but during the last year I have been afraid that he would come in during the night and kill me." When questioned as to why she had this thought she would give no answer and only after several months did she finally relate an episode of attempted seduction on the part of the stepfather which had been responsible for her great fear of him. She, of course, had always been too ashamed and too fearful of his vengeance to tell anyone about it.

Follow-up in Outpatient Department. The patient was seen every two weeks in the outpatient department and at the end of a year she was much improved. It took considerable persuasion to get her to establish her own home but this she finally did and improvement was more rapid from that point on. Another source of tension with which we were able to help her was in regard to her son whose enuresis and soiling during the day was a great annoyance to her. We persuaded her to bring the boy to the children's outpatient psychiatric department and as a result of his treatment there he had been much improved. Gradually she was relieved of anxiety regarding the possibility of heart disease and no longer took her temperature. The most important phase of the treatment, however, had to do with a personal contact which was established between a social worker, who was attached to the psychiatric department, and the patient.

Social Worker. The worker was able to furnish an important link between the patient's visit to us and her behavior at home. By acting as an intelligent and sympathetic friend she was able to help the patient see the relationship between her illness and her life situation and, moreover, was able to provide her with sustained support and a feeling of security at times when her anxiety arose. She was an invaluable help to us in the management of this patient and we felt certain that recovery would not have advanced so far if it had not been for her help.

Preventing Chronic Invalidism. When we thought back upon this case we felt sure that a very sick person had been saved from chronic invalidism. It is true that great effort was required on the part of everybody concerned—the physicians, the patient, and the social worker. But the lessons learned in the care of this patient will be applicable to the many other patients who, fortunately, do not present quite so complicated a problem.

SUMMARY

A young white woman presented a clinical picture thought to be neurocirculatory asthenia. Slight fever also suggested endocarditis. The absence of a heart lesion was finally established. Too much attention was focused on the fever and not enough on the fatigue, which was emotional in origin. With the help of a social worker the emotional problem was handled and the patient restored to fairly satisfactory health.

Chapter IX

THE CARDIOVASCULAR SYSTEM—EMOTIONAL FACTORS IN ORGANIC HEART DISEASE

As indicated in the previous discussion, many contributions have been made to the subject of the cardiac neuroses and it is quite generally appreciated that such disorders are psychogenic in origin and that psychotherapy is essential in treatment. But it has not been recognized that psychological factors are even more important in organic cardiovascular disease. In her comprehensive study of emotions and bodily changes Dunbar made particular mention of the work of Fahrenkamp and other foreign authors who have dealt with this problem, and both she and Wolfe in America have made notable contributions. The subject, however, needs repeated emphasis. For while a neurotic with a normal heart may suffer a great deal subjectively and may even have a disturbance of cardiac function marked by various forms of arrhythmia, the heart, certainly in the majority of such patients, remains structurally healthy. We are not considering the involved psychosomatic question of whether long-continued emotional stress can produce structural changes in the cardiovascular system. That is a problem for future determination. We are dealing here only with what are generally acknowledged to be unequivocal psychosomatic relationships.

IMPORTANCE OF EMOTIONAL FACTOR

The neurotic patient who has organic heart disease may add a real burden to the work of his heart, either through constant tension of psychic origin or, more especially, by means of acute episodes of emotional origin. This may hasten a cardiac breakdown which might be indefinitely postponed if there were no psychic stress. Thus the psychic factors may be even more important that the physical in producing incapacity. This is the problem which Dunbar and Wolfe have dealt with so effectively.

Wolfe called attention to the fallacy in medical thinking that if organic disease of the cardiovascular system is present, the physician is satisfied to let the matter rest without seeking to discover the psychic factor. The physician thinks "there is plenty of pathology present" to account for the trouble and looks no further for disabling factors. Hence, when such physicians examine a patient, no matter what his personality or complaints, if a physical defect is found the illness is apt to be attributed to that even if it is only a pathological curiosity. As far as the heart is concerned this is especially the case in instances of congenital lesions and well-compensated mitral stenosis, and in many patients with essential hypertension. Repeatedly in nervous children with insignificant congenital lesions, in neurotic young women with mitral stenosis and normally functioning hearts, and in emotionally unstable women at the menopausal age with hypertension, the error is made of attributing the symptoms to the heart itself. We have already stated that this is one way for a physician to add to the neurotic problem. Both his organic training and his insecurity in dealing with cardiac disorders have been responsible for this attitude. But even better trained and more sophisticated clinicians make errors of a similar kind in many of the more complicated psychosomatic cardiac problems, especially those that occur in the hypertensive-arteriosclerotic group. In an effort to throw light upon this problem a number of cases will be cited. Here again the fault lies in the inadequate psychological preparation of even the better trained clinician. His diagnosis of a functional disorder depends upon an exclusion of the organic factor which is really almost as fallacious as though one attempted to exclude appendicitis by a psychiatric investigation.

EVALUATING THE EMOTIONAL FACTOR

The discussion as to whether emotional factors influence organic disease occurs especially in regard to coronary occlusion. Here some physicians take it for granted that a psychic event may precipitate the occlusion but the proof that is advanced is usually only on the basis of a time relationship, that is, it is pointed out that just before the occlusion occurred something of an emotional nature happened. Opponents point out that everybody is subject to emotional stress; they insist on the greater importance of the physical changes and minimize emotional circumstances as purely coincidental or, at most, as having slight influence.

The debate if stated in these terms can never be settled, because it overlooks the structure of the personality and the reaction of the whole organism, which is at the same time both physical and mental. A person with physical disease, though its apparent "cause" may be an external agency of some kind, is likely to be affected emotionally as well. Emotional crises may have an influence on the progress of the illness. Therefore, psychiatric intervention may hasten convalescence or retard degenerative processes, whereas a burden of repressed anxiety, resulting in prolonged muscle tension or other bodily changes, may place too heavy a strain on some organ or organs, which later develops a disorder that is diagnosed as functional. Such a case, if taken in time, may be rendered symptom-free by adequate psychiatric treatment. Whether the activating agent be physical or mental, the disease process itself has both aspects. *The mere discovery of unpleasant circumstances in the life situation of an individual is no indication of emotional complications and still less of the psychogenic origin of the difficulty.* As Dunbar has stated, the significant questions concern the patient's ability to adjust to such situations, his pattern of reacting to them, the degree of anxiety in his make-up, the nature and seriousness of his conflicts, as well as upon his physical defects and patterns of physical behavior.

The Wolf and Wolff study, to which frequent reference has been made, called attention to the fact that "heart pain in the presence of anatomical narrowing of the coronary arteries may result from increased work of the heart attendant upon prolonged elevation of the blood pressure and cardiac output in association with rage, resentment, anxiety, fear and tension." But those writers also note that "heart pain in the presence of anatomical narrowing of the arteries may result from a fall in the cardiac output and coronary blood flow in association with desperation and defeat."

They refer to this as the "hypodynamic response." Even though coronary thrombosis occurs frequently in persons with hypertension, this does not minimize the possible importance of the hypodynamic reaction in coronary thrombosis. They say, "Although it is generally accepted that a rise in cardiac output and subsequent increase in the work of the heart are more effective in producing myocardial ischemia and pain, a fall in minute volume would also decrease the coronary blood flow; and in addition, given a preexisting occlusive disease of the coronary arteries, could present an optimal state for the development of myocardial infarction. Such a set of circumstances would explain some instances of anginal or coronary thrombosis occurring in individuals during inactivity or immobilization in bed and accompanying surgical shock."

PROBLEMS OF CORONARY OCCLUSION

In a thoughtful paper on "Mental Adjustment to Heart Disease," Sprague, speaking especially of coronary thrombosis, stated that the factors which determine disability may be considered under the following heads:

1. Physical incapacity as evidenced by congestive or anginal failure, or circulatory disturbances due to abnormal heart rhythms.

2. The character of the patient's work, which by necessity may keep the manual laborer from being able to carry on his trade.

3. Fear of heart disease as an incapacitating or fatal ailment. In such fears there is the normal human reaction to an unpredictable menace, but there is often the terror fostered by the gloomy predictions of the patient's medical advisers. In these predictions we recognize too commonly an attempt on the part of the doctor to protect himself if the patient suddenly dies, or to attribute to himself some virtue in his therapy if the patient does well while suffering from such a serious disease.

4. The influence of *disability insurance* in making it unnecessary to work in order to live, even though the income from this source may be too meager for the patient to maintain his standard of living.

5. The attitude of industry, largely mediated by the industrial compensation laws, which tend to be interpreted as holding employment responsible for any cardiovascular failure while a man is at work, thus making the cardiac patient unemployable. Sprague added illustrative cases to show two sides of the disability problem. One group consisted of patients who carried on their labors for years with grave heart disease, often with symptoms, but refused to give up to wait in terror for death on some indefinite future day. The other group, with similar disease, often of less marked degree, confessed defeat and devoted their lives to fear and worry over their eventual demise.

PSYCHOSIS IN CARDIAC DISEASE

In order to complete our consideration of emotions and heart disease we ought to discuss the frank psychoses, of exhaustive or toxic nature, which occasionally accompany grave heart disease. This phase of the subject, however, is well treated in many textbooks of medicine and cardiology. Other than to say that the psychosis sometimes occurs very insidiously and that the form which it assumes depends upon the underlying personality of the individual we will deal no further with this subject. *One must be aware of the fact, however, that just as the emotions may influence the working of the heart so may advanced disease of the heart aggravate or precipitate emotional disorders.*

The following cases are not presented with any purpose of throwing light on the somewhat irrelevant controversy of physiogenesis versus psychogenesis, but to illustrate that in many cases of disease ordinarily diagnosed in its physical aspects only, psychological study is of the greatest clinical importance.

Congenital Heart Disease and Anxiety Neurosis

Non-progressive, Asymptomatic, Congenital Heart Lesion Plus a Crippling Anxiety Neurosis Focused on the Heart. Anxiety Attacks. Insomnia. Impotence of Psychological Origin. Good Response to Psychotherapy.

CASE 5

History and Symptoms

A white man, aged thirty-seven, first seen in March 1938, complained of "a heart condition," insomnia, tiredness and dizziness, inability to relax, rapid heart action, missed beats and sweating. According to the physician who referred him, he had suicidal tendencies.

The heart murmur had been discovered in school at the age of twelve. He did not recall that any particular attention was paid to it at this time, but in high school he was taken off the ball team because of "an athletic heart." Thus he grew up with the idea that there was something seriously wrong with his heart.

At the age of twenty-nine, while swimming in an indoor pool, he had a sudden attack of palpitation, which was called a "heart attack" by his physician, and several days of complete bed rest were advised. On two subsequent occasions he also had the same kind of attack; one attack terminated in a vomiting seizure. The other symptoms mentioned above had also been present since that time. He had seen many doctors, had limited his activities considerably and, according to his statement, had not wanted to marry because of his heart condition.

Just before coming to us he had suffered much from insomnia and, at lunch the day before, he had had rapid heart action and sweating, had felt dizzy and faint, and had a very heavy feeling in his chest. He had been nervous and jittery since. He became so desperate that he threatened suicide.

Physical Examination

Physical examination showed a robust man with perhaps slight cyanosis of the lips but no dyspnea and no clubbing or jaundice. The heart action was forceful. There was slight scoliosis which was responsible for some displacement of the heart to the left; the organ did not seem enlarged. The sounds were well heard and seemed normal except for a slight systolic murmur in the third left interspace. There was no thrill. The remainder of the physical examination was negative.

Laboratory Studies

Ordinary laboratory studies were within normal limits. There was no evidence of impairment of cardiac function and the response to effort was normal. We concluded that we were dealing with a congenital lesion, probably ductus arteriosus, which had not affected the working of the heart.

Notes on Cardiac Condition

In 1934, and again in 1936, the patient was studied by Dr. Hugo Roesler to whom we are obliged for permitting us to use the following notes:

"1934: Mild cyanosis of the lips. Heart not enlarged. The apex is rather diffuse and a double wave short systolic retraction is noted. The first apical sound is split; no thrill. In the third left intercostal space there is a low, soft, deep-seated systolic murmur. The pulmonic second sound is hardly audible. The murmur is not influenced by respiration. Blood pressure systolic 138, diastolic 95. Rate 80 per minute. Roentgen-ray: the heart is normal in size; there is moderate prominence and increased systolic pulsation of the pulmonic arc.

"*Electrocardiogram:* Regular sinus rhythm; normal auriculo-ventricular conduction time. Moderate slurring of the initial deflection in Leads II and III. The T-waves are positive in all three leads. A Q-wave is present in Lead III.

"*Discussion:* Congenital cardiovascular malformation, most probably patency of the ductus arteriosus; other malformations may be present but cannot be proved. The patient has had attacks of either sinus or auricular tachycardia and also attacks of what seemed to be auricular fibrillation. But these disturbances are not in connection with the anatomical malformation. There is no evidence of disease or dysfunction of the myocardium. Personality study is advised.

"1936: General findings, fluoroscopy, and electrocardiogram unchanged (see illustration). Blood pressure: standing, 120/60; recumbent, 130/80. Conclusions as before."

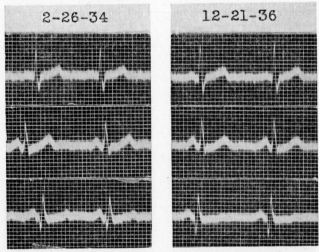

Fig. 2 (Case 5). Electrocardiographic tracings showing no change from 1934 to 1936.

LIFE SITUATION

The patient was the next to the youngest in a family of nine children. His mother had died at the age of forty-seven, when the patient was thirteen, of some "kidney condition"; she had been sick for years. The father had married again shortly and the patient then made his home with the father and step-mother; all of the siblings had married and lived away from home.

Father's Illness

A short time before the patient became ill his father had had a stroke of apoplexy and had been a cripple but not an invalid since. At the age of seventy-two he was found to have high blood pressure. The patient supported his father and step-mother, receiving no help from the rest of the family; this he very much resented, although he did not readily admit it. Conversations regarding his inability to marry indicated that not only his "heart condition," but the fact that he was responsible for the care of his sick father and his stepmother was a deterrent. In other words the patient felt that he was sacrificing himself for his invalid father. His feelings, therefore, were mixed. On the one hand he felt that it was his duty to support his parents but on the other he resented the restrictions imposed on his own life.

Psychic Traumatic Event

Another circumstance that seemed important was that, following his father's stroke and just before the patient's first "heart attack," a man had been suddenly killed at his place of business and he felt that he had given the order to this man which had resulted in his being in a certain spot at the moment that the accident occurred which resulted in his death. He could not forgive himself "for sending this man to his death," although it was obvious that it was a routine order in the ordinary conduct of the business. Nevertheless, guilt and self-accusation persisted. Further study indicated that this episode had reminded him of his father's stroke and had energized his conflicting feelings in regard to his father, for it it became clear that the excessive solicitude for his father covered unconscious hostility. Therefore, whenever he was reminded that his father's welfare might be threatened it was as though a burden might be lifted from his shoulders and at the same time guilt over the thought awakened his anxiety. This anxiety not only disturbed his heart action, but resulted in insomnia and excessive urination as well.

Anxiety Symptoms

When he was disturbed, the patient's "chest" (heart) would feel "solid, heavy and hot"; the left arm would "ache and feel numb"; the left hand was "cold"; the head "felt swollen," the hair "stood on end," he would "drool saliva" and "urinate large quantities at frequent intervals." *These were clearly the symptoms and signs of his pronounced anxiety.* Insomnia seemed to disturb his efficiency as much as concern over his heart. His attitude was a determination to go to sleep which, of course, resulted in just the opposite effect. He could not understand that one must be philosophic about insomnia—that sleep must be gently wooed rather than fought. He gave the impression of being not only a vigorous but a violent person, with no outlet for his *aggression.* Thus he would dream a great deal about fighting and became much disturbed in witnessing athletic contests. When he visited us he would stomp in and jerk the office chair before seating himself.

Impotence

A symptom to which he apparently paid little attention but which was significant as a further indication of his neurotic difficulties was impotence which he said came on gradually shortly after he became ill. It was obviously of psychological origin because the physical examination was negative and the impotence would assert itself only at certain times and with certain women.

TREATMENT

Reassurance

We explained to the patient that he had a congenital lesion of the heart that in no way inconvenienced the working of that organ and we assured him that his symptoms had nothing to do with this "pathological curiosity." Gradually we succeeded in convincing him that his heart was not seriously diseased, that he was able to engage in many activities that he had denied himself, and that no harm would come to his heart as a result.

The anxiety attacks became less intense and came at greater intervals and his sleeping was much improved. Occasionally an attack would occur and when it did all of his doubts regarding his heart would return. This would necessitate further reassurance along the lines already indicated.

Psychic Background for Illness

At the same time an effort was made to show the patient some of the psychic reasons for his illness. Attacks would frequently occur when family situations arose which stirred up his aggression. Because of this throttled aggression he was checkmated in all directions. His solicitude for his father and step-mother would not permit him to express any indignation to them or to his brothers. He was afraid to work hard or to engage in any athletic activities because of his heart, and even his sexual function was impaired. Hence, it was obvious that we were dealing with a severely inhibited individual whose normal aggression could find no outlet. Nevertheless, as he gained confidence from reassurance and some insight into the emotional background of his illness he became a more effective and a more contented person, engaged in longer hours of harder work and indulged himself in other regards. However, his attention had been so fixed upon his heart that the slightest recurrence of symptoms would bring some of his old doubts back again. Once more, reassurance, like a dose of medicine, would improve his condition. That is, he would be told once more that his heart was not responsible for his symptoms, that they were due to anxiety and that the anxiety was related to his family situation. Always the effort would be made to take his attention away from his heart and turn it onto his personal affairs. Mention of his work or his family would usually accomplish this.

SUMMARY

In a young man with a congenital heart lesion but normal cardiac function, the advice of physicians to rest and to limit his activities had played into his unconscious need for illness. Just the opposite kind of tactics—teaching him to ignore his heart, so far as it was possible for him to do so, to carry on his activities in spite of symptoms, together with the effort to show a relationship between his attacks and his emotional life—resulted in a considerable degree of improved health and happiness, so that he became more efficient in his work and more effective in his social contacts.

Mitral Stenosis and Anxiety Neurosis
Organic Heart Disease; Possible Thyrotoxicosis; Psychoneurosis

---

CASE 6

An Italian woman, age thirty-three, married, was admitted to the Temple University Hospital November 16, 1938.

History and Symptoms

The patient complained of palpitation of the heart and a tight, "pulling" pain in the back of the ears.

Present Illness

The patient stated that she was well until a year and a half before when this curious sensation in the back of the ears began. She was told that her tonsils were responsible and about seven months before admission they were removed but without relief from pain. She also suffered from easy fatigability and had lost considerable weight. She felt so weak that she spent most of her time in bed. Loud noises or jars increased the discomfort behind her ears. This was worse during damp weather and also during the menstrual period. Constipation had been present, for which rough foods had been recommended, but these caused pain in the abdomen. Palpitation of the heart was continuous and at times kept her awake.

Systemic Inquiry

The systemic inquiry revealed many symptoms. She had a dull headache especially around the nose and eyes; blurring of vision; a rash as well as pain behind the ears; a tight feeling in the upper chest and shortness of breath with slight exertion; nausea and occasional vomiting.

The menses had always been normal but during the last year had become scanty and there was some dysmenorrhea which, however, was not very disturbing. Her best weight had been 114 pounds; later she was reduced to 90 but had then gained back to 106.

Past History

The patient had jaundice at the age of eight and inflammatory rheumatism at ten. She had been married for fifteen years; her husband was living and well; she had never been pregnant.

Family History

The mother was seventy-five and living and well. The father died at thirty-two of pneumonia. Two younger brothers and two older sisters were living and well.

Physical Examination

The examination showed a well-nourished young white woman lying comfortably in bed but with some appearance of apprehension. *The heart action was very forceful and there was definite evidence of mitral stenosis.* The thyroid gland was not enlarged and there was no exophthalmos, stare, or other eye signs of hyperthyroidism. No tremor. The pulse varied between 80 and 90 and the temperature was normal. There was slight seborrheic dermatitis behind the ears. While being examined a pronounced vasomotor flush appeared on the neck, chest, and abdomen.

Diagnosis

A tentative diagnosis was made of rheumatic heart disease with mitral stenosis; possible hyperthyroidism and/or psychoneurosis.

Laboratory Findings

Cardiac consultation confirmed the diagnosis of mitral organic disease and also suggested hyperthyroidism. Blood pressure readings varied from 158–150 systolic and 98–105 diastolic. The first basal metabolic rate was 22 per cent and the blood cholesterol 107 mg. A subsequent basal metabolism was minus 3 per cent, and still another was minus 8 per cent, both considered reliable.

Circulation studies by Dr. Kleinbart were normal—saccharin time, 8 seconds; ether time, 5 seconds; venous pressure, 3 cm. The saccharin time was repeated the same day and found to be 11 seconds. The sedimentation rate was within normal limits. The urine analysis was negative. The blood count was good and Wassermann test negative. Biliary drainage showed cholesterin crystals suggesting cholelithiasis but cholecystogram showed normal gallbladder function and no stone shadows were seen.

LIFE SITUATION

The patient was first interviewed by Dr. Brody, to whom she gave the following information:

Early Life

Her father died when the patient was quite young and she remembered nothing concerning him. A sister and maternal cousin were stated to be very nervous. The mother remarried at the age of sixty-four, more than thirty years after the death of her first husband. As a girl the patient had few friends. She finished one year of high school at the age of fifteen and then worked for the next three years as a telephone operator. She felt that it was at this time that she became nervous. After one and one-half years of courtship she was married at the age of eighteen. Not long after marriage, during a mild attack of influenza, she was told by a physician that she had a "bad heart and that she should never have children." This was a great shock to the patient and she preferred not to discuss the topic, not even mentioning it to her husband. Instead she turned her attention to pets, a cat and a dog, but both were killed and this also was a great shock to her. The patient later volunteered the information that she had no sex desire and that she rarely had intercourse with her husband.

Diagnosis of Ménière's Disease

She added to the story of her illness by stating that after six months she began to feel weak and dizzy, and "lost everything from the body" indicating that she lost control of her bowels and vomited. A physician told the patient she probably had Ménière's syndrome. At this time her tonsils were removed but symptoms persisted until finally she was admitted to the Temple University Hospital.

Realization of "Nervousness"

In discussing these difficulties with the patient she said that she was nervous and realized that many of her symptoms, such as cold feet, moist hands, perspiration and flushed face, were all due to nervousness; "even the thumping of her heart, trembling of her hands, and quivering inside were all due to this nervousness." The patient claimed that when she ate rough foods she had a pain as though a knife were being stabbed into her abdomen, coming out at a spot directly opposite in the back. This, too, she thought was due to nervousness.

Subsequent Observations

Based upon personality study, further study of the basal metabolism, and further clinical observation, hyperthyroidism was ruled out so that we could conclude that this patient's symptoms were of neurotic origin and that her incapacity was out of proportion to her physical disease.

Traumatic Effect of Medical Opinion

If the question of hyperthyroidism had not arisen this would have represented a fairly common problem, that is, undoubted evidence of organic heart disease but, and this is the important point—symptoms out of proportion to the organic disease, which were due to an added cardiac neurosis. And in this case it would seem that the statement of the physician when the patient was eighteen (that is, that she had serious heart disease and should never become pregnant) served as a point to which she attached her anxiety. We cannot, of course, censure her medical advisor because he may not have placed the emphasis on the statement that she alleges. *Moreover, in patients of this kind almost any medical opinion may be misinterpreted.* Their anxiety and indecision on such matters as becoming pregnant leads them to a conclusion which the physician may not have intended and a suggestion from the physician is interpreted as a categorical statement. Therefore, the special necessity for tact and the careful use of terms in dealing with neurotic patients.

Caution Regarding Physical Examination

The same suggestions for caution apply to the physical examinations of neurotic patients. It is not unusual for a suspicious hysterical woman with fantasies of being seduced to misinterpret an ordinary movement in the physical examination as an amorous advance. The presence of nurse, office assistant, or some member of the patient's family is therefore to be recommended.

SUMMARY

A patient with mitral stenosis presented "symptoms out of proportion to the disease." At first thought to be due to hyperthyroidism they were later proved to be of neurotic origin. A physician's statement regarding the heart lesion probably had traumatic effect.

Coronary Occlusion
Apparently Precipitated by an Emotional Factor in a Patient with Anxiety Neurosis; Difficulties of Management

---

CASE 7

History and Symptoms

A white man, forty years old, had his first hospital admission in 1931. At that time he complained of severe pain in the lower middle part of the chest which radiated into the left arm. It had come on following a large meal. He was treated for "acute indigestion" but was told by his doctor that he had a heart condition. The pain, unlike previous attacks of indigestion, lasted a number of hours and was finally relieved by morphine. There were no special findings recorded so far as the heart was concerned.

The blood pressure was 130/100. The temperature was not elevated nor was the pulse. The white blood cells were 8700. The urine showed a trace of albumin and some hyaline casts. A diagnosis of coronary artery disease was made.

Second Hospital Admission. The next hospital admission was in 1935; the following is an abstract of the hospital record:

On June 27, 1935, the patient was operated upon for bilateral hernia. This was successful and recovery occurred in two weeks. Then about a month later, he experienced marked dizziness especially when lying down or trying to get out of bed. At times he became dizzy while walking and would find it necessary to hold on to something. He was unable to continue with his job. Then early in September, 1935, dizziness was replaced by periodic headaches. The headache was present on arising and very often was relieved upon reclining. For two weeks before admission it had been constant. The headache was worse at the back of the head, going into the neck and shoulders, and at times radiating into the forehead and face on each side of the nose. The patient had also experienced an earache, seemingly concurrent with the headache. In October, 1934, the patient had three upper teeth removed under the supervision of a physician who also x-rayed all sinuses and gave a negative report. His eyes were then examined and new glasses were ordered which the patient acquired. Later he experienced some precordial distress; this he felt was due to "gas." He described this pain as "prickling."

Physical examination and routine laboratory tests were negative.

Cardiovascular report—X-ray, entirely normal findings; electro-cardiogram, essentially normal (there was a rather deep Q wave in lead III which was not considered significant). Conclusions: No definite evidence of cardiovascular disease.

Diagnosis. The patient was discharged on January 2, 1936. The final diagnosis was "psychoneurosis; anxiety state."

Third Hospital Admission. The next admission was in October, 1936, when he complained of pain in the chest, weakness and nervousness. The pain had been almost constant and he also suffered from attacks of crying spells. The patient was depressed and nervous and stated that he had been a semi-invalid since the hernia operation. The attacks of pain in the chest occurred half a dozen times a day often accompanied by nausea and belching. The pain would come on after a heavy meal and also awaken him at night. He had been constipated and suffered from headaches.

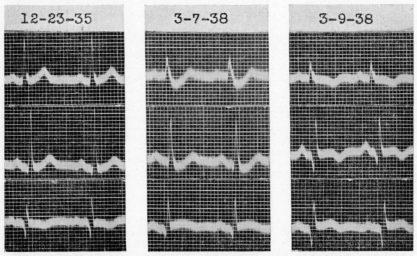

Fig. 3 (Case 7.) Electrocardiographic tracings before and after coronary occlusion.

Automobile Accident. In May, 1936, the patient had a narrow escape from an automobile accident which was followed immediately by a "severe heart attack" requiring morphine. Since the automobile accident the patient has said that all of his symptoms had increased in severity.

The electrocardiogram was essentially the same as the year before. A chest lead was taken in addition and was normal. The Q III was not so pronounced as in the previous electrocardiogram. The patient was studied by the psychiatrist. He was regarded as neurasthenic and hysterical. Psychiatric treatment was recommended.

Coronary Occlusion. The final admission was March, 1938. The patient had been riding downtown in a bus, developed a pain in his chest, got got off in front of the hospital and made his way to the receiving ward. He showed definite evidence of coronary occlusion! This was confirmed by the electrocardiogram.*

LIFE SITUATION

The patient was shown to the senior class in clinical psychiatric conference and the point was made that there is no reason why a neurotic patient should not have coronary artery disease and develop coronary occlusion; that it is not a question of either a medical disease or a psychological disorder but rather a question of how much of one and how much of the other and the intimate relationship between them. It seemed clear that an emotional situation related to his personality had immediately preceded the actual coronary occlusion. Here attention was called to the ordinary medical history which recounted only the fact that the patient was riding downtown in a bus when the pain occurred which necessitated his getting off and coming to the hospital. What was going on in the head of this patient, however, while he was riding in the bus, was the important thing. The patient had been having considerable trouble at his place of employment and just at this time was very angry with his employer. Although ordinarily meek and passive, he had made up his mind to defy his employer and he was going downtown "to tell him where to get off" but instead of that he was "laid low with a pain in his chest."

Unexpressed Hostility

As in many other psychosomatic disturbances, anger, especially that which cannot be appeased, is turned in upon the individual. It seemed that this patient for many years had had a neurotic personality, an anxiety neurosis, and that he now had in addition coronary occlusion, precipitated by emotional stress.

TREATMENT

The point also was made that the presence of this actual coronary artery disease and occlusion in a patient with an anxiety neurosis makes treatment most difficult. If the patient has only a cardiac neurosis and absolutely no evidence of organic disease, then one can say with great certainty, "You do not have evidence of organic heart disease," and use

* Several of the house staff were impressed that here at last was an "explanation for the whole illness." In other words, here was a patient who had been considered hysterical and all the time he was suffering from coronary artery disease and now there was definite proof—actual coronary occlusion!

that as the basis for subsequent psychotherapy. However, when the patient does have evidence of organic heart disease and especially when he has had coronary occlusion, then one cannot use this reassurance as the background of treatment and in some cases, as in this patient, the problem that is presented is almost unsolvable. Because such a patient cannot be encouraged to be active when he has actual coronary disease and so long as he is cautioned to rest, anxiety regarding his heart will increase. Our follow-up on this patient demonstrated that he will in all likelihood remain a real cardiac invalid. However, we have known patients with neurotic personalities who suffered coronary occlusion and by skillful handling did not become invalids. In one such patient whose personality was known to carry a heavy burden of anxiety the physician in charge did not volunteer the terms angina pectoris or coronary occlusion in discussing his illness with him, but referred only to the muscle change which had occurred. He was then able to reassure the patient regarding the healing of this muscular lesion. Following ten weeks of rest in bed and then gradual resumption of activities, the patient was able to reestablish a useful and energetic life and died six years later, at the age of sixty-eight, of an intracranial vascular accident. It goes without saying that it is much less difficult to deal with the patient who has coronary disease and who is not neurotic because here one can educate the patient correctly regarding his heart and the amount of exertion that he may safely undergo.

SUMMARY

A neurotic patient with coronary artery disease developed coronary occlusion coincident with an emotional situation in which he was unable to express hostility. The difficulties of the management of neurosis in a patient who has suffered a coronary occlusion are described.

Coronary Occlusion Preceded by Psychic Trauma

CASE 8

The subject of the patient's attitude and behavior in ward-round teaching has recently been thoughtfully dealt with by Romano. It was discussed in a previous chapter. The subject is of great importance, though none of his experiences were so unfortunate as the following.

History and Symptoms

A middle-aged, Italian woman developed coronary occlusion while she was a patient in the hospital. She had been a diabetic for years.

Her husband had had very little work for several months preceding her admission to the hospital and she could not afford the special food that she needed. She developed palpitation and finally asked the physician who had taken care of her for many years to send her into the hospital. He reported that "there was too much red tape and that she wouldn't like it—that she would come out and curse him for sending her." Finally she entered the hospital on her own initiative. She was told that it would take a few days to standardize her but this was not accomplished until the tenth day. She then prepared to go home.

A few days before, she had witnessed general ward rounds and had been very much upset by the demonstration of patients to a group of physicians and students. She told the nurse and interns that it must not happen to her. However, on the particular day in question she was resting in the sun parlor preparatory to going home when the nurse came for her and asked her to come into the ward. She said immediately, "What is it, class?" The nurse said "Yes," and the patient became very nervous and angry. She told the nurse it would be impossible, that "she would get sick—she knew what her heart could stand," but the nurse persuaded her to return to the ward. As she approached the ward she felt a pressing pain under the sternum, which she described as a "lump," and again she remonstrated with the intern as she entered the door. She was so upset that when the attending physician, who had known nothing about her feelings, asked her several questions, she found the strength of voice to answer only two and then could talk no more. She said, "I could not remember what happened after that." Then she added significantly, "I am like a child. If I am disappointed, it breaks my heart." When the class left she went into the bathroom thinking that she might be able to cry and that this would relieve her. She was unable to cry, came back to the ward, but finally "cried her eyes out." As she did so the pain became sharper. She called for the nurse and insisted upon having the intern. Then she urged that her own physician be called and she reported that she was very sick "and was going to die." The intern later reported that she was having an "hysterical attack," saying that the patient had been one of the most difficult personalities that he had ever handled in any ward work. Nevertheless an electrocardiogram was ordered. It showed coronary occlusion! It is probably significant that everybody, from that point on, remarked how docile she had become. The patient made an excellent recovery. Serial electrocardiograms before and after the coronary occlusion are shown in the accompanying diagram.

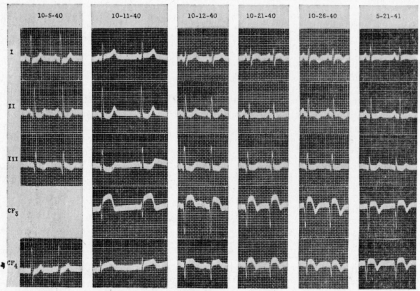

Fig. 4 (Case 8). Electrocardiographic tracings showing findings prior to coronary occlusion (10-5-40) and serial studies following the occlusion.

LIFE SITUATION

She was born and brought up in Italy in a peasant family with ten children. She had worked very hard but considered herself healthy. She married at nineteen and very shortly afterwards had a miscarriage. The following year she came to America. At twenty-one she had a pelvis operation and both ovaries were removed so that a surgical menopause ensued. She resigned herself to not having children and "her husband did not care." At times she spoke about bringing some children over from Italy but he said, "No, if we can't have our own, we won't have any." Her husband had been very good to her and they had led a quiet life in America. He had been employed as a laborer and always made a satisfactory living up until the few months prior to hospital admission, when work was scarce and their income was much reduced.

She was a meticulously clean housekeeper and could not tolerate dirt or disorder. She was very religious and had gone to church every day. During the last three or four years she had felt herself becoming quite nervous. She was always fearful that auto accidents might occur because they lived near a large boulevard where accidents were frequent. She could not stand to see people hurt. Two years before she had a bad fright when a burglar attempted to enter a house across the street during the night. She felt it "as a shock in the heart" and was paralyzed with fear. She went back to bed without waking her husband and "shook all night."

Since then she had not felt right and her physician said that diabetes "was due to the shock."

SUMMARY

A middle-aged, neurotic, and diabetic female felt humiliated and enraged by being presented to a class of students. Substernal pain developed which was thought to be part of an "hysterical attack" but the electrocardiogram showed coronary occlusion. Recovery occurred.

> ### Cardiac Neurosis with Bundle Branch Block
> Psychic Shock; Clinical Picture of Cardiac Neurosis; Electrocardiographic Evidence of Bundle Branch Block

CASE 9

A white woman of thirty-five years was first seen in February, 1942, She complained of fatigue and pains around the heart, palpitation and breathlessness.

The trouble had begun about a year before when, because of complete exhaustion, she had remained in bed for several months. It was during this period that pain in the heart region first occurred followed by palpitation and breathlessness on slight exertion.

She had conidered herself a healthy child. The menstrual history had been normal. About ten years ago the appendix had been removed because of severe pain in the right side of the abdomen and since then she had had occasional bowel disturbances marked by alternating attacks of constipation and mucous diarrhea which she referred to as colitis.

Family History

The patient was one of six children; all of the others were healthy. The mother was living and well. The father had died quite suddenly of pneumonia about the time the patient was preparing to marry. While she was devoted to her father, she found herself unable to express her grief and often wondered about her peculiar reaction to his death. She was the middle one of the large number of children and as she stated it, "I'm always in the middle of everything."

Physical Examination and Laboratory Studies

The patient seemed a reserved and depressed person. She was rather pale but fairly well nourished. There was no dyspnea or cyanosis. The hair was prematurely gray and the nails were somewhat brittle. The heart seemed normal in size and position but there was a low-pitched systolic murmur at the apex. No shock or thrill could be detected. The remainder of the general physical examination was negative, and routine laboratory studies were normal. Blood pressure was normal. There was no evidence of impairment of cardiac function. Orthodiagram showed the size of the heart to be within normal limits but the electrocardiogram, which is reproduced, showed evidence of bundle branch block. Repeated electrocardiograms over a period of six months showed the same findings.

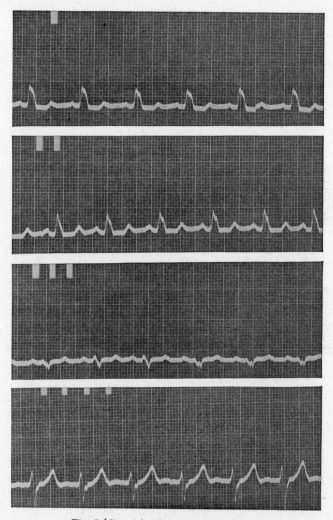

Fig. 5 (Case 9.)   Bundle branch block.

LIFE SITUATION

Immediately before the onset of the present illness the patient lost her only child in an automobile accident. When the news was brought to her the shock was so great that from that point on, she was "a completely changed person." She was so overwhelmed and so exhausted that she was forced to go to bed, where she remained for about two weeks. Then when she attempted to resume her activities she developed pain in the heart region followed by the other symptoms which have been described and her physician recommended a more prolonged rest. This time she remained in bed for about three months and during this period she insisted that there must be something the matter with her heart, which the electrocardiogram apparently confirmed.

There had been nothing remarkable about her previous life history except that she had always been a rather shy and retiring person. There were frequent digestive disturbances for which she would seek medical attention, but for which there seemed to be no organic basis.

Follow-up

The patient was informed that the heart was normal in size and function and that no particular significance need be attached to the electrocardiographic findings. She was urged to talk about the loss of her child, instead of refusing "to allow herself to think about the tragedy" and in this way, some of the feelings attached to that lamentable occurrence were brought to light and, at the same time, partially discharged. She was further informed that the exhaustion was the result of the loss of energy that had been consumed by the shock and the resulting loss of interest in her everyday life, and that her efforts must be to take up her activities once more and to lead as nearly a normal life as possible. On this basis her recovery proceeded although the electrocardiographic findings remained.

SUMMARY

A young white woman sustained an overwhelming psychic shock and then developed exhaustion and the clinical picture of cardiac neurosis, but the electrocardiogram demonstrated unmistakable evidence of persistent bundle branch block. Whether this lesion preceded the psychic shock or followed it, was impossible to say, but it indicates the necessity for equal attention to physical and psychological factors in the study of illness.

Hypertensive-Arteriosclerotic Disease
Repeated Attacks of Pulmonary Edema; Progressive Heart Failure;
Coronary Thrombosis

CASE 10

History and Symptoms

A white woman, age forty-four, was admitted to Temple University Hospital February 22, 1937. She complained of attacks of pain and a heavy sensation in the heart region with tingling sensations in the left arm and hand. The trouble had begun about ten years before when, following some kind of nasal difficulty, a physician discovered high blood pressure and sugar in the urine. He ordered the tonsils removed, which was done under local anesthesia. She was very nervous—"the nose and throat man couldn't work right"—but the operation was done without any serious consequences. She was very heavy at that time, weighing 210. By dieting the weight was reduced to 143 pounds.

Prior to that time she had been well except for irregular menstruation and following the weight reduction the menses became regular. After having been married twelve years she became pregnant for the first time at the age of forty. About the sixth month of pregnancy, the legs began to swell and in the seventh month she was taken to the hospital for a "uremic condition" and at eight and one-half months the pregnancy was terminated by a cesarean section and a living child obtained.

At the same time the patient was sterilized by cutting and cauterizing the tubes. Following the puerperium she was treated for "high blood pressure and bad kidneys." A sensation of ringing in the head continued from time to time, especially when she was nervous. She was studied from the standpoint of possible gland disturbance because of marked hirsutism. She had always had a lot of hair on the body but at about eighteen it began to grow on the chest, face, and back. Some of this was removed from time to time by "electric needle." A sister also had a lot of hair but not so much as the patient. X-ray treatments of the left side of the patient's face left a bad scar.

Present Illness. About three or four years ago while still at the hospital clinic and shortly after the baby's birth, she began to have nocturnal attacks of pain in the teeth. These attacks would wake her up; the pain would shoot down the sternum and into the back "like a thin-bladed knife." The pain was accompanied by heavy breathing, "a moist chest," and she was referred to another hospital for study and there it was found that nitroglycerine gave marked relief. The blood pressure was still 200 and the blood sugar was 280. She remained in the hospital thirteen weeks and then went to a convalescent home.

Then five months before admission to Temple University Hospital she had an attack of "grippe" and the arms and the left hand felt as though they were asleep. She had been practically invalided since.

The attacks began with a "sensation of numbness in the left hand, a noise in the chest, with pains in the chest and the back, a terrible beating starts in the chest and goes down to the bottom of the spine where the coccyx was removed." At other times she spoke of a quivering in the chest, especially on the left side, associated with a pain in the back. But the attack usually started with pain in the teeth and might go into the ears. The hands became cold and she often perspired freely.

Past History. Scarlet fever and measles in childhood without complications. Menstruation began at thirteen; irregular and usually late. In 1935 following a fall the coccyx was removed without much relief from discomfort.

Family History. The mother died at fifty-three from uremia; the father died at seventy from unknown cause. A brother died at twenty-one from pneumonia. One brother and a sister were living and well.

Physical Examination

An obese woman with masculine appearance and a general physical structure that was rather masculine. There was a pronounced x-ray burn of the left side of the face; the skin was coarse and oily and there was a heavy hirsutism of male distribution.

There was questionable slight cardiac enlargement to the left. The apex beat was forceful; the heart sounds good; A2 plus. The blood pressure was 168/108 on both arms. No other findings of importance were noted except that the gynecological examination showed very large labia majora, masculine distribution of hair, and markedly enlarged clitoris and a male type of pelvis.

The following questions suggested themselves: 1. Was this ordinary essential hypertension or was it connected with an endocrinopathy? 2. Had she coronary artery disease or was the precordial pain of another origin? 3. What was the significance of the history of sugar in the urine and the hyperglycemia?

Course in Hospital. The patient had attacks of precordial pain in the hospital. The intern reported that they were relieved by nitroglycerine. The blood sugar during an attack was 119, the pulse 100, the blood pressure 204/140, and there was profuse perspiration.

Laboratory studies made during an interval of freedom from attacks showed—urine, normal; blood count, good; basal metabolic rate, plus 2 per cent; blood Wassermann, negative. Blood chemistry: urea, 10.5 mg., sugar, 125 mg., urea clearance, 89 per cent; glucose tolerance: fasting 155 mg., one-half hour 157 mg., one hour 200 mg., two hours 219 mg., three hours 199 mg.; serum clacium 12.7 mg.; serum phosphorus, 3.9 mg. Two-hour specific gravity test was 1004–1018. Fasting blood sugar just before discharge, 98 mg.

The temperature was normal in the hospital and the pulse averaged 80 and regular. Blood pressure records, during freedom from attacks, were between 160 and 180 systolic, and between 100 and 120 diastolic. Weight, 150 pounds on discharge.

Electrocardiogram. Left axis deviation. Low S-T take off in leads 1 and 2. T wave diphasic in lead one. One month later there was a deep S-T depression in lead 1; inversion of T in lead 2; S-T segment closer to the base line and absent Q in lead 4. Coronary artery disease with the possibility of healed infarct was suggested but it was felt that both tracings were compatible with the findings which one sees in the course of hypertension.

The *neurological* examination was negative.

The *gynecological* examination showed the vulvar abnormalities previously noted, which were considered congenital; otherwise the examination was negative.

Eyegrounds. Fields grossly normal. Fundi—retinal arteriosclerosis, grade two, of the hypertensive type with evidence of previous retinitis.

Consultation from an *endocrine* standpoint suggested the following possibilities: 1. adrenal cortex hyperfunction. 2. pituitary basophilism, or 3. arrhenoblastoma of the ovary. Hormone assay and x-ray studies were requested.

X-ray showed the cardiac silhouette to be within normal limits as to size. "Heart area by careful measurement well within normal limits for patient's predicted heart area according to height and weight." The skull was normal and no demineralization of long bones was noted. *Urinary tract* after injection of uroselectan showed no evidence of disease and nothing to indicate renal or perirenal tumor.

Air Injection of Adrenal Area. March 18, 1937, an air injection of the right adrenal area was attempted but was unsuccessful. The patient had an attack in which she became pulseless, cyanotic and unconscious for a moment. On March 22, 1937, it was noted that since the attempted visualization of adrenals the patient had complained of pain in the left chest, especially in the heart region. She described it as a sensation which she felt could be relieved by taking a deep breath but she was unable to do so. She demonstrated this by placing her hand over the heart and taking a deep sighing inspiration. Since the attack she had "gone back to where she was before, after three weeks of feeling better than she has in all her life." She did not dread the test but had been upset emotionally by being taken to class just before the test was done. She did not object to further efforts to inject air. *Subsequent attempts were successful and a good film obtained which showed no evidence of adrenal tumor.*

Hormone assay showed essentially normal findings, which was against the diagnosis of a pituitary or corticoadrenal tumor. The possibility of paraganglioma was still mentioned.

Attack of Pulmonary Edema. After discharge from the hospital she was seen in the out-patient department in a severe attack of pulmonary edema. We had previously doubted whether actual edema occurred when she complained of "attacks of congestion." Now, however, there was no doubt. The face and neck were flushed, she was in great distress, there was palpitation and gallop rhythm, and the lungs were full of moist rales which increased in number and size from the base upwards, leaving only the apices free. Blood pressure during the height of the attack was 210/150 and dropped within a few minutes, as the attack subsided, to 145/105. The attacks recurred in waves. The patient complained of a sweet taste in the mouth as she spat up large quantities of frothy sputum. She stated that the sweet taste was always very pronounced and very distressing; it occurred as soon as she began to cough.

The blood pressure during intervals of freedom from attacks averaged 150–160 systolic and 80–90 diastolic.

LIFE SITUATION

The patient dated all her troubles to her marriage at the age of twenty-nine. She had been brought up in what she considered a cultured and well-to-do family. Although her education was terminated at the eighth grade she spoke of her early life as one of ease and luxury. She was "used to everything" and never worked outside the home. Encouraged by her mother, she studied singing and had always cherished the ambition to become an opera singer.

The mother died of "uremia, stroke and high blood pressure" when the patient was nineteen—a sudden death with no preceding illness. The patient sat up with the mother through the night and felt very guilty for not having been in the house when the attack occurred. The mother was brought to this hospital and died here. The patient had never been able to forgive herself for this fancied defection and stated "my mother is never out of my mind—I think of her all the time."

Marriage

The patient then made her home with her married sister and at the age of twenty-nine married a man "much inferior to her." It was obvious that she approached this marriage in a very immature way. She had had an unsuccessful affair and then married "out of spite" a foreigner for whom she had much contempt. She was shocked when she learned that he could not read or write. She stated that she never intended to "live with him"; hence she continued to make her home with her sister after the marriage. She was always frigid in marriage and finally after a great deal of indecision left her husband only to return to him when he "hounded and threatened her."

Financial Difficulties

Her husband's income was never adequate and he lost his business, including all the money that she could raise. Finally "they went on public relief," which was intolerable to her. It was at this time that her symptoms became exaggerated. As she stated, "Then I really became ill; imagine being on the Welfare when you had been used to everything."

Pregnancy

Finally, after eleven years of married life, she was shocked to find herself pregnant at the age of forty, whereupon began the illness that has been recounted. Now it was necessary for her husband to stay at home to take care of her and her child. The situation reached an impasse. On the one hand she could not tolerate being supported by the Welfare and on the other her illness enforced invalidism which necessitated her husband remaining at home to do the housework, to nurse her, and to care for the child. Her illness had virtually succeeded in emasculating the husband. He complained of the necessity of "being a woman," was very impatient with the child and infuriated the patient when he turned on the child angrily or struck her. She stated, "If it were not for the child I would have committed suicide long ago. I am friends with nobody. You have friends only when you have money." She was intensely bitter against fate, was very irritable and moody, and cried easily.

Social Worker's Report

The social worker reported that the husband was a nice-looking, clean person who, contrary to the opinion expressed above, seemed to enjoy taking care of the house. He kept it spotless during the wife's illness. His desire to find a job seemed questionable. A private family society supplemented relief, even sent a housekeeper so that the husband could look for work, and placed the child in a day nursery. The worker tried to prevail upon the patient to accept her situation and to move to cheaper quarters but she refused to do so.

Repeated Attacks of Pulmonary Edema

When anything happened to remind the patient of any unfortunate circumstance in her life an attack was likely to occur. On one occasion, when the child was singing and dancing "reminding her of happier days, her own ambition; and also 'her inability to live long enough to see her daughter grow up to be a great singer', " an attack occurred.* The husband had just gone out. As she started to read the paper she couldn't see very well, and thought that her kidneys were diseased. She felt a heavy feeling in the heart region and a sensation "like a worm eating her." An attack followed.

On one occasion she visited us with her brother-in-law, who exhibited a great deal of hostility for her husband. It was evident that he held the man in contempt and his feeling was that the patient had been sick since she went back to her husband the second time. Following this visit she had a telephone conversation with the brother-in-law in which she wanted to tell him how humiliated she had been when he had criticized her husband in our presence. Immediately a severe attack with collapse occurred. This was an occasion on which her attending physician, Dr. Morris Kleinbart, thought that coronary occlusion had occurred. At the hospital the electrocardiogram showed progressive myocardial damage; bundle branch block had developed.

---

* It was previously mentioned that the patient herself had always cherished the ambition and was encouraged by her mother to become an opera singer. However, she gave up singing after her mother's death and had never been able to go back to it. Her thoughts about her mother would not permit her to. Apparently it was too mindful of happier days.

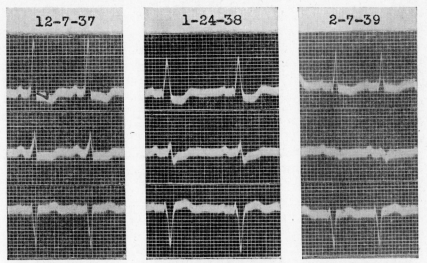

Fig. 6 (Case 10). Electrocardiographic tracing showing progressive myocardial damage. See text for discussion.

Final Hospital Admission

Her dreams concerned churches and religious services and in connection with this it was interesting that as a child she had visited many churches and missions. Just before her final admission to the hospital she had dreamed "that her mother was looking for a place for the patient in the cemetery but couldn't find one. There was no place." She cried in relating this dream and said she wished it was true that they had found a place for her, in other words, that she might die. Her only child, "all I have in the world," was to be put in a boarding school because she could not look after her at home. This was a final blow. Following her discharge from the hospital she did very badly at home, was readmitted into another hospital where she was incapacitated by congestive heart failure. Her final admission to Temple University Hospital was in March, 1939, and death occurred on April 23.

Postmortem Study

Necropsy showed pronounced coronary artery sclerosis and an old area of infarction near the apex. At this point a small aneurysmal pocket contained thrombotic material. The kidneys were sclerotic and showed scars of old infarcts. No abnormalities of the adrenals or ovaries were noted.

SUMMARY

Here was a patient with a very *immature personality*, full of conflicts, who was incapable of expressing hostility in direct action and whose anxiety, readily aroused, seemed to culminate in attacks of pulmonary edema. We had an opportunity to see her during and after many such attacks. It seemed that she had a trigger mechanism which was set off by some emotional circumstance reminding her of her unfortunate position in life. Then apparently a rise in blood pressure would occur and the attack immediately followed. Repeated attacks occurred over a period of years. Progressive myocardial damage and congestive heart failure followed.

Somatic Disease (*Gastrointestinal and Cardiovascular*)
Plus Emotional Factors

CASE 11

The most complicated of all psychosomatic problems are the associations between the gastrointestinal tract and the cardiovascular system. The following case will illustrate some of these problems.

History and Symptoms

H. G., a white man of 50, was first seen in 1929. He complained of pain in the epigastrium. This had made its first appearance about three years before when he noticed a pressure-like sensation. No abnormality was detected in the physical examination except a few bad teeth. These were removed and the patient was advised to stop smoking and his digestion improved. He was not heard from again until 1935 when he complained of fullness after meals. Again no abnormalities were detected except slight elevation of the systolic pressure. At the same time he spoke of being short of breath on exertion but only after breakfast. This again seemed to be a pressure-like sensation rather than dyspnea. However, because of this symptom, special attention was paid to the cardiovascular system but clinical, x-ray and electrocardiographic examination did not reveal any abnormality. When a short time later x-ray of the gastro-intestinal tract showed a typical duodenal ulcer deformity and the possibility of additional esophagitis—on the basis of a rather spastic esophagus with evidence of hyperactive peristalsis—attention was directed away from the cardiovascular system.

LIFE SITUATION

The patient was a very reserved and passive individual with pronounced feelings of inferiority. He had a neurotic and nagging wife, and two daughters, one of whom was hysterical. In addition he had had financial difficulties and it was felt that all these factors entered into his digestive problem. A dream of being in a department store where he could not find his way and nobody could help him led to a discussion of his fear of losing his job and the fact that he was "up against it."

Later History. With superficial psychotherapy and certain general medical measures, such as diet and sedation, he improved somewhat but continued to have the pressure-like, choked-up-feeling, especially in the mornings. Between 1938 and 1941 he was much improved although the symptoms never left completely. In 1941 he returned—the symptom was less pronounced but the blood pressure was elevated and the electrocardiogram showed changes. X-ray showed that the duodenal ulcer had completely healed and there was no further evidence to suggest esophagitis. Attention once more was focused on his cardiovascular system as well as upon his psychological problems.

His daughter's marriage had ended in divorce, his wife was becoming more and more difficult, and for the first time he confessed that he had been "sexually frustrated" for years. In a resigned voice he said "what's the difference" but showed considerable hostility in his feelings.

In 1942 he had a mild attack of congestive heart failure and was sent to the hospital where he made a good recovery. After this he remained at home for several weeks but he was very depressed and complained of headache and nausea. His blood pressure had been steadily rising over the years and he now showed persistent hypertension. His daughter wrote that he was so disconsolate that they did not know what to do with him at home and urged us to give him a "pep talk." On his next visit we talked to him on the necessity for cultivating a fighting spirit. He walked out of the office apparently feeling better and when he got home his family remarked on his improved spirits. That night, after retiring to his room at the usual time, the family heard a thump on the floor and ran up to find that he had collapsed. Apparently he had died instantly. For-tunately for our peace of mind he had not exerted himself after his visit to us. The family assured us that he had done nothing unusual. If he had we would have felt that it was a very misguided "pep talk" indeed.

SUMMARY

A very passive, inhibited man with pronounced feelings of inferiority, complained of indigestion and pressure under the sternum. .He was studied carefully to exclude heart disease. Duodenal ulcer and esophagitis were demonstrated. Emotional factors seemed important. The ulcer healed, but hypertension developed; progressive myocordial changes occurred, and sudden death happened to follow a "pep talk" for depression.

This case once more emphasizes the importance of angina pectoris as a cause of death and, also, the difficulties in diagnosis that are sometimes encountered. Because of the negative cardiovascular findings and the positive gastrointestinal findings it was decided in the early years of his illness that a digestive disturbance, in which emotional factors entered, was wholly responsible for his illness. Later, however, when there was evidence that the ulcer had healed and there was no longer any suspicion of esophagitis and, at the same time, positive evidence of cardiovascular disease appeared, the diagnosis was reversed although we could never be certain that some functional disturbance of the gastrointestinal tract on an emotional basis was not also present. By chance an interview dealing with brief psychotherapy coincided with sudden death from heart disease.

Chapter X

THE CARDIOVASCULAR SYSTEM—ESSENTIAL HYPERTENSION

The most important single process among the cardiovascular diseases is *essential hypertension*. This chapter will embrace a brief reference to the history of this condition, a short discussion of its relationship to arteriosclerosis and kidney disease, a statement regarding the generally accepted clinical concept, and a discussion of pathogenesis. All these are essential because of the interrelationship of psychological and somatic factors in the disorder.

IMPORTANCE OF HYPERTENSION

There is little need to emphasize the importance of hypertension. According to the statistics of the Metropolitan Life Insurance Company every other individual in the United States past the age of fifty years dies of cardiovascular-renal disease. From other sources we have evidence that probably half of these deaths are due to essential hypertension; that is, almost one quarter of all people past the age of fifty years die of the effects of hypertension in one or another of the vital organs. Thus essential hypertension becomes the gravest problem of middle adult life, not even excepting cancer. The hypertension arises from arteriolar vasospasm (whatever its cause may be) and after it has continued for years a compensatory reaction in the arterial system results in a diffuse hyperplastic vascular sclerosis which, in turn, is eventually responsible for failure of such vital organs as heart, brain, and kidney.

Our knowledge of the circulatory disorders has progressed in hundred-year cycles. It was about 1633 that William Harvey reported on the nature of the circulation and about 1733 that Stephen Hales, an English pastor, demonstrated the phenomenon of blood pressure in the horse. In 1833 Richard Bright correctly concluded that an increase in the peripheral resistance caused enlargement of the heart in patients with "chronic granulations of the kidneys," and about 1933 Goldblatt, by his brilliant researches, first produced in the experimental animal a form of hypertension which corresponds to essential hypertension in man.

What have these remarkable observations contributed to the practical management of the individual who has high blood pressure? Not a great deal, we fear, because we are still ignorant as to the cause of hypertension and there is little we can do to eradicate it. In a sense, all that has happened is that the old argument over whether hypertension or systemic arteriosclerosis came first has been narrowed down to the kidney—which comes first, hypertension or arteriosclerosis of the renal vessels? More and more evidence is accumulating to suggest that hypertension precedes arteriosclerosis, but that still leaves us very much in the dark as to what initiates the hypertension.

PATHOGENESIS

Hypertension is a disorder largely confined to occidental civilization. There is a good deal of evidence to support this. Thus studies of African natives, the Chinese, Buddhist priests in Ceylon, and Egyptians of the laboring classes all indicate that hypertension is very rare among those peoples. In this connection it also seems important that the blood pressure of foreigners living in China and in the tropics is lower than when they are living in a temperate zone.

Related to these questions come the important observations of Schulze and Schwab, who found the incidence of hypertension in the American southern Negro two and a half times greater than that of the southern white. They and their associates also showed that the tendency to hypertension, as determined by the Hines and Brown ice-water test, exists to a greater degree in the American southern Negro. This bears on the question of heredity because it is acknowledged that the ancestors of these Negroes could not have had hypertension since the Negroes in Africa do not have it now. Thus it would seem that the American southern Negro in his contact with our civilization over a period of 200 years must have acquired hypertension to an even greater degree than the white American. Kesilman found hypertension three times as common in Negro males in a survey conducted in a northern prison. It is also interesting to know that hypertension runs a more severe course in the Negro (Metropolitan Life Insurance statistics). So that we are presented with this extraordinary fact at the outset of our discussion of constitutional and hereditary factors, as opposed to environmental factors, in the pathogenesis of hypertension.

Relation to the Kidney

Since Goldblatt's investigations attention has been focussed on the possibility that a pressor substance is elaborated by the *ischemic kidney*. This substance, called rennin, presumably interacts with a substrate to produce an effector agent (angiotonin or hypertension), which causes a constriction of the peripheral vascular bed and consequent rise of blood pressure. A great deal of attention has been devoted to the hemodynamics of this situation. The most recent studies of value have to do with the renal circulation. By means of anatomic and physiologic studies based upon the experimental reproduction of the "crush syndrome"

Trueta and his associates have demonstrated a new (medullary) circulation of the kidney, in which the cortex is by-passed. Ischemia of the cortex could thus be brought about and, possibly, pressor substance elaborated. Their work suggests that central nervous system stimuli may be responsible for the vasospasm of renal arteries which initiates this mechanism.

It would seem that here is a clue which may lead to the recognition of the preclinical phase of essential hypertension. Indeed, Trueta and his co-workers state their belief that the primary etiological factors responsible for essential hypertension "will eventually be found in the central nervous system, even in the human mind itself. . . " We doubt that a complete understanding of essential hypertension lies within the province of psychological medicine, but we share with the authors of this remarkable work the enthusiasm for a unique approach to the anatomical and physiological backgrounds of this disorder.

Psyche and Hypertension

It is generally admitted that psychic factors play an important part in essential hypertension. For example, it is always emphasized that we must allow for the emotional element in individual blood pressure readings. Also well known is the large part that rest and reassurance play in the medical management of hypertensive patients, both in relief of symptoms and in reduction of the blood pressure level. The early symptoms of hypertension are often exactly those of a *psychoneurosis*, and the relationship of emotional stress to the onset of hypertension and to the anxiety which is frequently responsible for the aggravation of existing hypertension are well known. Personality study of the hypertensive patient often reveals a deep-seated conflict which stands in close relationship to anxiety. This will be discussed in greater detail in the section on treatment of essential hypertension (p. 313). Therefore, it may be said that in spite of the organic nature of experimental hypertension, the psyche is not absolved as a factor in the etiology of hypertension in man. It is conceivable that a disturbance in the circulatory function of the kidneys could have its origin in impulses of central nervous origin.

The psychic factor thus becomes one of the multiple factors which enter into the pathogenesis of hypertension. An analogy might be drawn to the role of the kidney or the endocrine glands, either of which, in rare instances, may be chiefly responsible for the presence of hypertension but in most instances seems to play a secondary role, depending upon a constitutional or inherent tendency. "The psychologic factor is only one phase, although an important phase, in the composite of the degree and kind of renal, endocrine, and nervous participation" (Corcoran and Page).

Experimental Observations of Renal Blood Flow During Stress

The blood flow in the kidney of the subject with essential hypertension is small in terms of functioning kidney tubular mass, that is to say, the hypertensive kidney is relatively ischemic as compared to the normal. Also, the degree of depression of renal blood flow parallels approximately the duration and severity of the hypertension. The order in which events proceed is indicated by the fact that the glomerular filtration rate in early hypertension is entirely within normal limits, but with advanced hypertension and reduction in the number of functioning glomeruli, the glomerular filtration rate is also gradually depressed. The ratio of renal blood flow to tubular mass is low, indicating a relative ischemia of the hypertensive kidney. As the hypertension advances, the tubular mass decreases but always in such a manner that the renal blood flow is poor in terms of the existing tubular mass. These facts suggest that a defective renal blood flow precedes the onset of faulty excretory function. If kidney ischemia be at all relevant to the occurrence of arterial hypertension, renal blood flow studies in those with widespread vascular reaction to threats become of interest. Before pursuing this topic further, pertinent aspects of the personality of such subjects should be appraised.

Thus Wolff and his associates spoke of their investigation of the renal hemodynamics in subjects with essential hypertension, during a rise in blood pressure initiated by threats in the form of discussion of topics known to have a significant relationship to the personality structure.

In eighteen of thirty-five subjects with hypertension, without evidence of renal disease or abnormality of renal function as indicated by the usual clinical tests, renal blood flow and glomerular filtration rate were ascertained.

Rises in diastolic and systolic blood pressure were induced by discussion of topics of personal significance, usually having to do with family interpersonal relations, without, at the same time, inducing outward evidence of strong emotional reaction. The rise in blood pressure under such circumstances was accompanied by renal vasoconstriction which was either proportional to that of the body as a whole or more intense than necessary to compensate for the rise, reflected by decreases in renal plasma flow of 17 to 25 per cent of control level. The increase of renal vasoconstriction was located principally in efferent glomerular arterioles although both efferent and afferent arteriolar constriction occurred. Fall in blood pressure during induced feelings of security was accompanied by vasodilation of the efferent and afferent arterioles.

"From these and other facts, it may be inferred that the kidney in persons with arterial hypertension exhibits an abnormal vascular pattern, characterized by increased arteriolar tone, and the latter may be further increased by threats or assaults that evoke protective reactions of a pressor nature.

"However, it may not be inferred that the experimentally induced renal vasoconstriction is the cause of the observed hypertension. Thus, preliminary observations have revealed that patients with arterial hypertension exhibit a pressor response during experimentally induced stress both before and after thoracolumbar sympathectomy (T7-L3), although the renal vasoconstriction elicited before is no longer demonstrable after sympathectomy. It is apparent from these observations that the blood pressure may still rise in response to threats, even though the kidney does not participate in the vascular reaction. Secondly, it was possible to demonstrate in those with and without arterial hypertension that the renal blood flow is not increased as the result of renal denervation by sympathectomy, but remains unchanged or may actually be decreased. In one nonhypertensive subject with a unilateral kidney denervation (sympathectomy) equal blood flow in both organs was observed. The meaning of these observations on the relation of adrenergic impulses and kidney blood flow to arterial hypertension in well-established hypertensives is not clear. Certainly, as far as can be demonstrated in the latter, renal vasoconstriction due to sympathetic impulses is not the essential defect in the mechanism of hypertension. Nonetheless, there remains the probability that neurogenic factors are pertinent to the beginnings of the hypertensive syndrome. It is suggested that as part of the protective reaction early in the life of the potential hypertensive, adrenergic impulses induce neurohumoral effects involving the adrenal cortex and the kidney which ultimately result in irreversible kidney ischemia and arterial hypertension.

"Furthermore it is suggested that such renal vasoconstriction may, if prolonged, damage the renal blood vessels and the parenchyma, and lead secondarily to further elevation of blood pressure. The cost of the reaction to the heart and to the vascular apparatus of such organs as the brain and kidney may ultimately be great enough to destroy the organism."

Summary of Pathogenesis

A consideration of the material just presented indicates that hypertension is a constitutional disorder in which both hereditary and environmental (vasospastic) factors are important. Thus it would seem that normal vasomotor activity is superimposed upon intrinsic vascular hypertonus which is maintained independently of the vasomotor nerves. In other words, we may assume that there is an inherent vascular hypertonus fundamentally responsible for increased peripheral resistance in essential hypertension to which may be added vasoconstriction of nervous origin. Nevertheless, it must be acknowledged that the latter may con-

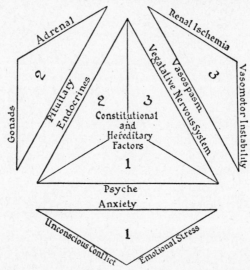

Fig. 7. Diagram to summarize discussion of pathogenesis. The base of the pyramid is made up of constitutional and hereditary factors; the sides consist of interrelated systems which are shown separately as triangles with their sides representing interrelated factors. (From E. Weiss, Psychosomatic Medicine, 1939, Vol. I, p. 183.)

stitute a considerable fraction of the peripheral resistance in persistent hypertension.

In an attempt to assign a proper relationship to the three systems of the body and to the various factors that play a part in the pathogenesis of hypertension a scheme has been constructed as shown in the accompanying diagram. This makes an effort to indicate the relative importance of constitutional and hereditary factors (which make up the base of the pyramid) with regard to the interrelated systems of the body that have to do with hypertension—shown as the sides of the pyramid. These systems are then shown as triangles with the sides of the triangles representing interrelated factors.

It is probable that the constitutional and hereditary factor in essential hypertension is responsible for the inherent vascular hypertonus previously discussed and that environmental influences produce the vasospastic factors which act as precipitating agents. Thus if one were born with a marked predisposition it would probably take little environmental stress to cause hypertension whereas, if the family history were relatively free and one were born with little predisposition then it would probably take a considerable degree of environmental stress to bring about hypertension. In this way we can assume two interacting processes with the environmental stress mediated by way of the vasomotor system.

CLINICAL PICTURE

It is well known that hypertension may exist for a long period without any symptoms whatever. When symptoms finally appear, they frequently arise from the organ or system that is bearing the brunt of the hypertensive-vascular disease process. Thus, the symptoms may be related entirely to the heart, or neurologic symptoms may predominate if the brain is chiefly affected. In terminal stages evidences of renal failure may dominate the clinical picture. However, as previously stated, many of the early symptoms are identical with those that are seen in psychoneurosis. Headache, dizziness, tinnitus, insomnia, and fatigue are prominent symptoms and often are out of proportion to the amount of physical disease that is present.

The Problem in Medical Practice

The problem often met in practice is as follows: An individual of middle age applies for life insurance and high blood pressure and perhaps albuminuria are discovered. Insurance is refused, and, frightened or angry, the applicant seeks the advice of his physician. General physical examination with special attention to the cardiovascular system, particularly in respect to the size of the heart, the condition of the peripheral vessels, including those of the retina, plus tests of kidney function,* will enable one to establish a diagnosis in the majority of instances. The problem resolves itself, with certain very unusual exceptions, into the differentiation of glomerulonephritis from hypertensive-vascular disease. Usually, it will be found that the patient is suffering from essential hypertension and the end result, perhaps five to ten years away, will be cardiac failure in about 50 per cent, intracranial accident (hemorrhage or thrombosis) in about 25 to 35 per cent and renal failure in probably less than 10 per cent. Other accidents and incidental infections account for the remainder of deaths.

If the end result is to be renal failure, the patient, usually over a period of years, will show gradual loss of concentrating power as determined by specific gravity tests of kidney function. The final event, renal failure ending in uremia, will be indicated by the onset of retinitis and progressive nitrogen retention. This change may come about with considerable rapidity; that is, patients who present the usual clinical picture of benign hypertension may quite suddenly complain of severe headaches, show

*Concentration tests, urea clearance and intravenous urography are commonly performed. Unfortunately, there are no simple methods available for testing the circulatory function of the kidneys.

a higher level of blood pressure, especially the diastolic element, increased eye signs (the result of actual retinitis), loss of renal concentrating power, nonprotein nitrogen retention and rapid progression to death. This acceleration of the hypertensive process has been called by Fishberg the malignant phase of essential hypertension.

PSYCHOSOMATIC SYMPTOMS

Ayman and Pratt showed that many of the symptoms of patients with essential hypertension closely resemble those seen in patients with psychoneurosis without hypertension. Closer study of their patients revealed that they really were suffering from psychoneurosis as well as hypertension. In a more recent paper Ayman divided the symptoms of essential hypertension into three groups:

1. Psychoneurotic symptoms
2. Vasospastic symptoms
3. Organic symptoms

Headache and various forms of head discomforts, dizziness and constipation, as well as precordial pain, breathlessness of the sighing respiration variety, and fatigue often cannot be explained directly on the basis of the hypertension. They are out of proportion to the disease. When such patients are studied from a psychosomatic point of view it is often found that there is a great deal of conflict in their makeup and an inability to express their aggression directly, and thus it would seem that tensions which cannot be adequately expressed in words or action seek their way out in the circulatory system. We must repeat that psychologic factors are not the only ones of importance in the clinical picture of hypertension, but they are important because their modification often results in benefit to the patient, regardless of whether the blood pressure figures are lowered or not.

Ayman suggests that generalized arterial constriction may be responsible for symptoms. It would seem to be largely a question of the intensity of the process and the rapidity with which it appears. Ayman points out, and we have frequently seen, patients with very high blood pressure, 250–300 mm. systolic, which may exist for years without symptoms. Yet in other individuals with lower pressures of more sudden onset severe headaches, dizziness, spells of blushing and pallor, temporary pareses and even convulsions seem to appear on the basis of vascular spasm.

When the hypertensive vascular disease advances and vital organs are affected, it is of course true that many symptoms are caused by failure of these organs. Even here, however, it is important that we evaluate the part played by emotional as well as physical factors.

Headache. Janeway observed that headache was the most frequent symptom of which his hypertensive patients complained. He described the typical hypertensive headache which appears on awakening as consisting of sensations ranging from a dull ache to severe pounding distress and as usually being located in the cervico-occipital region. But in addition, he noted that a surprisingly large number of patients had been subject to migraine throughout life. Gardner, Mountain, and Hines found migraine five times as frequently in hypertensive patients as in a control group. Then there is a great variety of head pains, discomforts, and peculiar sensations, such as dullness and fullness with or without vertigo, which occur in hypertensive subjects and are often referred to as headaches. The tendency is to attribute all these "headaches" to the hypertension. Certainly elevation of the blood pressure seems responsible for the so-called typical hypertensive headache. (Even here, however, the anxiety factor enters insofar as it is related to exacerbations of blood pressure.) However, the vast majority of peculiar head sensations and discomforts often designated as headache cannot be correlated with the blood pressure level itself. Here the emotional factor is directly related to the peculiar head sensations.

Recently we studied a patient with severe hypertension and constant headache. She had had a complete physical study. The blood pressure averaged 200/120. The heart seemed within normal limits as to size, as determined by the orthodiagram, and the electrocardiogram indicated only left-axis deviation, other features being within the limits of normal. There was no evidence of impairment of cardiac function. The eye-grounds showed arteriosclerosis of the hypertensive type, grade 1, but no evidence of retinitis. Urinalysis was negative and renal function, as measured by the urea clearance test, was within normal limits. An intravenous urogram was normal. The conclusion was essential hypertension with symptoms out of proportion to disease.

After reviewing the studies, we said to her, "Sometimes tension is related to hypertension." She thought that over for a moment and said, "Well, I can improve on that formula. In my house, it is 'contention-tension-hypertension.' " Then she went on to tell of the role she played as a "buffer" between an irate husband and a lazy son who was in business with his father and of the constant quarrelling between them. The greater part of her sympathy was with the son. She was always trying to shield him. She was a martyr-like person and that kind always pays a penalty, absorbing punches which produce symptoms. This woman's headache was the "body language" means of representing her difficult life situation. It was just as if she would say, "My husband is a headache to me." Indeed he was. He was having an extramarital affair and boasted of it openly. He felt that it was indecent to smoke or drink, but the sexual appetites were normal and were to be indulged and no secret was to be made of the fact. By thus humiliating her in the presence of her friends he added to her problem. Perhaps as a result of the uncritical way this information was received she gained enough confidence to present her husband with an ultimatum and, contrary to her worst expectations, he agreed to end the extramarital affair. It made a great difference in her life. Thereafter, she was well as far as headache was concerned. It is true that this patient still has her hypertension. But the disappearence of the headache was an indication that the symptom was out of proportion to the disease and was related to the anxiety. The anxiety in turn was related to emotional conflict and the conflict could be understood by getting to know the patient as a human being and not just as a medical case.

Migraine presents a more complicated mechanism. It can hardly be assumed, as in the case of anxiety and hypertension, that migraine is so frequent in hypertension because the two are common disorders and therefore must frequently meet. Instead, there seems to be a common denominator, and psychologic study gives a clue. Apparently there is an intimate relationship between the personality structure of the two disorders. Both present evidence of chronically repressed rage. Attacks of migraine occur when situations are met which intensify the rage without providing opportunity for adequate expression.

Constipation. Most patients with hypertension see a connection between headache and bowel function. When they suffer from constipation they are ill, and when the bowel moves freely they are speedily relieved of symptoms. This, of course, is true for many patients who do not have hypertension, but in hypertensive individuals the relationship is especially obvious. Moreover, it is a relationship which is easily exploited and in which the physician becomes a pathogenic agent when he focuses attention on the bowel, as in the days, fortunately not now so common, when colonic irrigations were frequently prescribed for "autointoxication." It is very difficult to overcome a patient's prejudices—and even those of the medical profession—in this regard. But it does seem to be largely a psychologic association, because relief comes too quickly after a bowel movement to be ascribed to physical causes, and, in addition, deeper psychologic study often shows the relationship between ideas of obstruction, "poisoning," and pain in the head.

Vertigo. Patients frequently refer to the symptom of vertigo, which occurs in a great many instances with the head discomforts just described, as dizziness and giddiness. Differentiating syncope, which does not imply a disturbance of equilibrium, and true Ménière's syndrome, one often finds that the symptom of vertigo bears a definite relation to an anxiety state. Frequently in association with ringing in the ears and sometimes with numbness and tingling of the extremities, it is the result of psychic stress.

The early symptoms of anxiety are usually expressed through the cardiovascular, respiratory, gastrointestinal, and genito-urinary systems. It is after the anxiety state has persisted for some time that the symptom of vertigo makes its appearance. When it occurs in association with hypertension the vascular disease often is held to be responsible. However, it is well to bear in mind that, like organ language elsewhere, vertigo (unsteadiness) frequently is the symbolic representation of insecurity, and this is just as true when it occurs in association with hypertension.

Cardiac Neurosis. Pain in the precordium, palpitation, dyspnea and fatigue are a group of symptoms frequently associated with cardiac neurosis. Fatigue may be a prominent part of the clinical picture, in fact, the most prominent symptom, although again and again the patient speaks of pain in the heart region and only after considerable discussion is it brought out that really the most important symptom is fatigue, that it occurred first, and that only later was the pain added. One of the commonest causes of fatigue is emotional conflict, which steals energy that is not then available for useful purposes.

When these symptoms are present with a normal cardiovascular system and the general medical examination otherwise is negative, it is not as a rule difficult to assign them to their proper sphere—the emotions. When hypertension is present, however, it is almost invariably held to be the responsible factor. It is under such circumstances that psychosomatic study will frequently reveal that symptoms are out of proportion to disease, that there is much conflict in the personality makeup, and that it depends on repressed hostility. Moreover, a specific as well as a temporal relationship will be found between the onset of the symptoms and a psychic event.

Thus in regard to symptoms in association with hypertension one must always question their relation to the high blood pressure itself and make an effort to understand them from the viewpoint of behavior.

TREATMENT

Let us take again the example of a middle-aged man refused by a life insurance company because of high blood pressure. His physician rules out glomerulonephritis and decides that the patient is suffering from essential hypertension. Then, all too frequently, attention is concentrated on the effort to "bring the blood pressure down." The patient demands to know the blood pressure figure; on each visit to the physician he waits with anxious concern to hear the latest reading and frequently he has ideas of "stroke," "heart failure" or "Bright's disease" in the back of his mind.

Just what has been done to this poor patient in the effort to "bring his blood pressure down"? Because of an ill-founded idea that protein is responsible for hypertension and kidney disease he is denied meat and eggs, especially red meat, which for some reason is looked upon with particular dread. Then his diet is rendered even more unpalatable by the withdrawal of salt. One would sympathize with this half-starved victim of good intentions except that he probably would not be able to eat anyway, his teeth having been removed on the theory that focal infection has something to do with hypertension. Even before this period he has sacrificed his tonsils and has had his sinuses punctured because of the same theory. In case he actually had been able to eat some solid food, in spite of these previous therapeutic measures, the slight colonic residue was promptly washed out by numerous "colonic irrigations," especially during the period when the theory of autointoxication was enjoying a wave of popularity. To add to his unhappiness he may be told to stop work and exercise, and of course is denied alcohol and tobacco as well as coffee and tea. And now to cap the climax of his difficulties, the unfortunate person with hypertension has been referred to the neurosurgeon, who is prepared to separate him from his sympathetic nervous system.

PSYCHOSOMATIC ASPECTS OF TREATMENT

The knowledge that "every psychic tendency seeks adequate bodily expression" gives a practical hint in dealing with hypertensive patients. An explanation to the effect that inner tension which cannot be released through ordinary channels (action or words) may manifest itself in the circulatory system by adding to the problem of hypertension represents a rational approach insofar as the patient is concerned. This often leads to a discussion of problems which are of considerable interest and importance from the standpoint of illness.

A case, reported in detail later, is interesting from this standpoint. The patient, a young man working for a trucking company in Philadelphia, had rather severe hypertension. His father, who had worked for the same firm, was killed in an accident, and the family was denied compensation. Our patient was "burned up" about it. He wanted to get into union activities where he would have an opportunity to avenge his father. He had been denied this opportunity because it meant "too much work and excitement." We gave him permission. In addition to working eight hours on the job, he had to work six hours for the union. He was an organizer and worked hard, yet he actually improved during the two years he was engaged in union activities. He improved as far as symptoms were concerned and even his blood pressure was lower. Then the union broke up and again he was "burned up." He was "choked with rage," and his blood pressure went up again. As soon as he was denied an outlet for aggression along the lines of avenging his father, up went his blood pressure and symptoms returned. So we think there is something in the personality of a hypertensive patient that suggests a relationship between hostile impulses that cannot find an outlet and elevation of blood pressure. It is not the whole answer—not by any means. We do not maintain that it is the basic cause of hypertension. A patient can be "burned up" all his life and unless he has a predisposition to hypertension, he probably will not get it. Given the predisposition and an aggressive personality with no outlets for aggression, then in all probability hypertension will develop.

Personality Studies

More adequate studies of the emotional lives of patients with hypertension have been published by Alexander, Saul, Dunbar, and Binger.

Dunbar calls attention to the increased tension and sometimes spasm of voluntary or smooth muscles or both that may be alleviated as unconscious conflicts became conscious. She feels that this tension is part of the whole defense mechanism, psychologically and physiologically a general attitude of being on guard. Often its significance is elaborated in terms of accompanying disturbance of tonus in other systems, especially in the gastrointestinal and the genito-urinary tract. Dunbar finds that hostile impulses against which the patient is on guard are as a rule relatively near the surface and accessible to treatment. As these impulses emerge to consciousness there is usually a rise in the blood pressure curve followed by a drop to a lower level as the material is worked through. There are also transitory psychoneurotic manifestations of a phobic or compulsive nature in the course of such treatment. Dunbar has dealt with the subject in detail in her comprehensive book entitled *Emotions and Bodily Changes* in which, among the many studies reported, considerable attention is given to the opinions of Fahrenkamp, whose psychophysical studies on hypertension are noteworthy. Fahrenkamp feels that psychic factors play a decisive role in regard to the blood pressure level in all stages of the disorder and therefore that in all hypertensive patients the major emphasis should be on the treatment of the psychic element. However, it is impressive that this psychologically minded physician does not accept the existence of a functional hypertension of purely psychogenic origin, since he has never seen a patient who completely lost his hypertension. In other words, in his experience the tendency of the circulatory system to pathological reaction remains demonstrable.

Hostility and Aggression

Other investigators, notably Alexander and Saul, find that hypertensive patients show external friendliness and self-control; beneath which there are strong aggressions and anxiety. The anxiety grows out of the danger which these repressed aggressions would create for the security of the individual if they were allowed expression. It is as if the inner psychological tension (force) of the aggression found expression through heightened arterial pressure. We are all familiar with the every-day comment to the person who is about to explode with anger and resentment, "Now, think of your blood pressure!" Of course by discouraging or threatening the person who would relieve his anger by words or action one might be doing just the thing to cause a further rise in the blood pressure.

Latent hostility and repressed aggression are found in every neurosis, but the difference, as noted in hypertension, is explained by Saul who finds the hostility in hypertensive persons to be intense, chronic, inhibited, near to consciousness and perhaps to motility, but not adequately repressed or bound as in an organized neurosis. He finds these people are neither able to satisfy passive, dependent wishes nor to gratify the hostile ones and hence they remain blocked in both directions. Such a psychological structure may develop as follows: With the continuance of the problem of achieving social position, prestige, and a high standard of living, the individual has difficulty in controlling his hostile aggressive feelings. Competitive urges stem from aggression but aggression is often punished and hence fears accompany the aggression. These fears lead to inhibitions which in turn limit an adequate expression of aggressive feelings. This hostile impulse accumulates and increases in intensity, requiring further inhibition in order to keep such impulses from the patient's view or the view of others. The vicious circle goes on and the result is that in some people the emotional energy so generated finds release only through the blood-pressure-controlling physiological mechanisms.

Psychosomatic Observations

In an effort to throw further light on this subject Binger and his associates made detailed psychological and physiological studies of twenty-four patients with hypertension. No effort was made to prove "psychogenesis"; on the contrary, the authors refrained from drawing conclusions regarding the role of psychic factors in the etiology of essential hypertension.

While all of their patients presented evidence of a disorder of the personality which could be classified as "neurotic" the appearance of an organized neurosis with specific symptoms was the exception rather than the rule.

A particular configuration of tendencies was consistently found and an approximate composite picture of the personality and its development described. Regarding this personality they say that "the failure of the integrative functions of personality, the inadequacy of the characteristic defenses against anxiety, the inefficiency of the repressive mechanisms, and the inability to develop an organized neurosis, rather than the nature of the underlying 'instinctive' drives, are what appear to differentiate this disorder from other seemingly similar ones."

Early Insecurity. The outstanding feature of personality study was found to be an early sense of insecurity. In the majority of cases it was possible to discern a critical shock-like reaction wherein the patients felt overwhelmed by danger against which their usual defenses were ineffective. In general the situation which seemed to epitomize the major threat was separation from a parent. The discovery of hypertension or the first appearance of its prodromal symptoms usually occurred in such emotional settings and followed acute emotional disturbances. Study of the childhood of these patients showed that death of the parent or separation occurred in twelve out of twenty-four cases. In twenty-three of the same number of cases the existence of high blood pressure was first observed after the occurrence of an emotional disturbance such as illness or death of a relative; injury, illness, or other trauma to the patient; changes in the patient's life such as separation from parents, marriage, illness of a child, loss of a job, or loss of savings. In thirteen of these twenty-four cases the emotional disturbance seemed to be mainly a reaction to a serious illness or death of a relative. The common factors were loss of security or exposure to the aggressions of the person on whom the patient was dependent.

Personality Disorder. Binger et al. point out that unlike such disorders as asthma and migraine, in which the psychological setting of an attack can easily be studied, it is difficult to show a correlation between psychological situation and physiological response in a disorder like elevated blood pressure, which is not episodic and in which there is not even always a parallel between the level of blood pressure and the existence and severity of symptoms. They review previous observations such as those of Alexander and Saul and agree with the description of the conflict situation in which aggressive impulses are inhibited but not deeply repressed, yet "the assumption that psychic factors causative of the somatic disturbance are of a specific nature, is by no means clear." The authors regard their investigation as a clinical study contributing to the nosology and development of hypertension but not to its etiology. They do not consider the disorder of the personality as the cause of hypertension; rather they prefer to regard the disorder of the personality and the "constitutional vasomotor instability" as different aspects of the same fundamental pathological process.

More study is required in these cases but we trust enough has been said to emphasize the necessity of studying and treating the personality of the patient who has hypertension. These psychoanalytic observations show the necessity for a more adequate approach to their study than "Are you worried about anything?" and a more adequate treatment than "Go home and take it easy." This kind of superficial psychotherapy, if it may be termed that, is in line with the kind of medical management that has been given to the unfortunate sufferer from essential hypertension in the past.

On "Bringing the Blood Pressure Down"

We are referring to the pernicious emphasis on "bringing the blood pressure down" to the exclusion of the much more fundamental understanding of the individual. It is freely admitted that the height of the blood pressure is one of the best indices to the condition and prognosis of the patient with essential hypertension but to put all of our attention on the matter of bringing this blood pressure down is to do the patient an injustice. We say this whether or not psychic factors are fundamental in hypertension.

Redefining Objectives

We must redefine our objectives in the treatment of hypertension. The consideration of pathogenesis must impress us with the necessity for the total evaluation of the patient with hypertension. This will represent a combined physical and psychological study. When we do such a study we will realize that many symptoms occurring in hypertension are of emotional rather than physical origin and that *the incapacity is often out of proportion to the disease.* Hence the importance in a great many patients of reeducation along the lines of "carrying on" rather than urging rest and more rest. Menninger champions this idea on the basis that self-directed aggression may be turned outward by the authority of the physician and that extroversion of the aggression, if not too strenuous, may be of advantage to the patient. We have repeatedly proved this to our own satisfaction in patients who have been invalided by the *knowledge* of blood pressure rather than by the physical effects of the hypertension itself.

Some Practical Points

The knowledge that "every psychic tendency seeks adequate bodily expression" gives a practical hint in dealing with hypertensive patients.

An explanation to the effect that inner tension which cannot be released through ordinary channels may manifest itself in the circulatory system by hypertension, represents a rational approach as far as the patient is concerned; and often leads to a discussion of problems which are of considerable concern and importance from the standpoint of the illness.

To advise the individual involved in mental conflict "not to worry" is valueless, especially when, as is so often the case, no concerted effort is made to find out what is disturbing him. Too often the physician is satisfied that there are no problems disturbing the patient after he has inquired, "Are you worried about anything?" and has received a negative reply. Most of the time the patient really does not know just how much he is disturbed nor does he relate the factors actually responsible for his discontent. He is much more apt to project his worries into questions about his blood pressure, heart, brain, and kidneys. Careful inquiry will bring out that his fears are exaggerated and that the reasons he assigns for them are illogical.

There is only one approach that has any merit, that is, to encourage the patient to talk about himself as a person rather than as a medical case. This will permit some insight into conflict situations and lead often to some relief of anxiety, which is closely related to the high blood pressure. Although this approach does not offer a complete solution of the hypertensive problem and does not even apply to all patients, it is a practical method of dealing with a set of important factors that may be modified, whereas the constitution of the individual cannot be touched. It is an approach heretofore not sufficiently practised. We are too much concerned with physical measurements in hypertension—the blood pressure figures, the percentage of renal function, the size of the heart, the electrocardiographic tracing, the amount of retinal sclerosis—all of which are essential in the study of the hypertensive mechanism but give incomplete information from the standpoint of the total evaluation of the patient. They should represent the beginning and not the end of the study. We are too little concerned with the emotional life, which may hold the key to the satisfactory management of the hypertensive patient.

There is no objection to the effort to lower blood pressure as long as this does not constitute the sole approach to the problem of high blood pressure. This applies to the most recent method of dealing with hypertension by surgical means. In some patients sympathectomy will produce a prolonged drop of the blood pressure. One may say to patients who have hypertension and anxiety (due to the meeting of inner conflicts and external pressures) that our objective in their management is to "take off some of the load." If we can do this by helping them to achieve some insight into their emotional problems, with consequent lowering of tension, well and good; if we can do it by environmental manipulation, fine; but if we have to resort in addition to drug therapy (thiocyanate) or to surgery (sympathectomy) by all means let us use a combination of efforts to help our patients with hypertension. While we believe that essential hypertension cannot be eradicated by any psychotherapeutic process, no matter how intensive or prolonged, we feel also that almost every patient with essential hypertension can be benefited by psychotherapy.

Binger and his associates have the following to say: "The problem is that of treating a severe character neurosis in which anxiety, depression, and suppressed aggression are the cardinal psychopathological features. The method of choice will vary from cheerful neglect to deep psychological exploration. The latter . . . is a matter for the expert. What is to be hoped from it we cannot say. There is as yet no evidence that psychoanalysis or any other psychotherapeutic procedure can reverse the physiological process or change the destiny of this disease—be it benign or malignant. The problem is an open one. It needs further investigation. The ground has now been cleared for such an undertaking."

Another aspect of the problem is referred to by Page and Corcoran who call attention to some of the well known facts regarding the superficial aspects of the relation of the emotions to hypertension and then state: "Such observations, however thoroughly documented, merely establish mental disturbance as coordinate cause; they do not suggest that it can be a primary cause of the whole disease. To establish it as a primary cause, it must be shown (1) that hypertension can arise *de novo* as a sequence of a characteristic mental pattern or (2) that the disease as act and potentiality can be abolished by appropriate psychotherapy."

Conclusions

The organic tradition in medicine has been responsible for a narrow view of the etiology and treatment of essential hypertension. The psychosomatic approach does not neglect the physical problems involved but includes a consideration of the role of the emotions. It does not mean to study the soma less; it only means to study the psyche more. It emphasizes the multiple factors in etiology and pathogenesis and attempts to evaluate the resulting composite clinical picture. Such studies indicate that emotional factors apparently are intimately related to the development of hypertension in some patients, to the production of symptoms in many others, and enter into the question of treament in nearly all patients with essential hypertension.

A common problem seems to be the presence of emotional tension due to chronic repressed hostility. This inhibited aggression (chronic rage) seems to bear a definite relationship to hypertension and if it can be relieved by means of psychotherapy anxiety is diminished and blood pressure is often lowered. Even if the blood pressure is unaffected, the treatment often benefits the patient by making him a healthier and more effective personality. Our objectives in treatment should be readjusted. We must not limit our efforts to "bringing the blood pressure down." There is no reason why we cannot combine physical (medical and surgical) methods with psychotherapy but we must go beyond the physical aspects of hypertension to the personality of the hypertensive individual in order to be successful in the management of such patients.

The following cases have been selected to illustrate various psychosomatic problems in hypertension and their management.

Early Essential Hypertension. Recurrent Attacks of Acute Hypertension with Hypertensive Encephalopathy
Apparently No Harm from Excessive Energy Output When Directed Along Aggressive Channels; Recurrence of Hypertension Corresponded with Period of Throttled Aggression

---

CASE 12

History and Symptoms

A young white man, twenty-nine years old, was first referred to Temple University Hospital on the service of Dr. W. Wayne Babcock, December 12, 1935.

The diagnosis was acute gangrenous appendicitis which was proved at operation. The blood pressure during spinal anesthesia gradually dropped from 140/78 to 86/48. The patient later reported that he had been "scared to death of the operation," that he knew it was a "pus appendix" and that he was fearful that peritonitis would develop. Ten days postoperatively a note on his record stated that he "seemed somewhat hysterical." The blood pressure had been normal and the general physical condition seemed satisfactory so that he was discharged on December 24, 1935.

The same evening he felt dizzy, became delirious and had to be restrained. The following morning he reported that he was "blind in both eyes." He was sent to the psychopathic ward of the Philadelphia General Hospital, where he remained for three weeks. There, according to his later statement, he was treated for "high blood pressure and uremia." From their records it was noted that when he came home from the Temple University Hospital he developed "terrible pain in the suprapubic region which extended into the testicles . . . it made me almost hysterical." He woke up unable to see and became very agitated. At the hospital he had auditory and visual hallucinations in which he saw funny faces and men teasing him. He cried a great deal and was restless and noisy at times. On discharge from the Philadelphia General Hospital, at the end of three weeks, he reported that he was so weak that he was unable to walk. Because of this weakness and nervousness he was readmitted to Temple University Hospital on February 11, 1936.

Physical Examination and Laboratory Studies

Emaciation was pronounced. The skin was warm and moist. The blood pressure during this stay in the hospital varied between 160 and 180 systolic, and 110 and 120 diastolic. There was no evidence of thyroid enlargement. The heart seemed normal in size; the aortic second sound was accentuated. The eyeground examination showed evidence of an acute vasospastic retinitis without organic sclerosis (Dr. Gibson). The nasal retinal arteries were especially constricted. The temporals showed moderate attenuation. There were a few hemorrhages and exudates in the right retina and many in the left. The spinal fluid was clear and no abnormalities were detected.

A psychiatric examination found the patient well oriented and suggested that he had previously suffered from an organic delirium.

The urine examination showed no albumin although there were occasional hyaline casts. Renal function was normal. The blood count showed a moderate degree of secondary anemia. All blood chemical studies, including glucose tolerance, were within normal limits and the basal metabolism was plus 6 per cent.

Additional History

During this stay in the hospital opportunity was afforded for a more satisfactory history. We were told that he had been a healthy child, nursed until one year and then was very difficult to wean; he would not eat and lost much weight. He had diphtheria and scarlet fever in childhood from which he made a good recovery but otherwise had no serious diseases until the present illness. Since about the age of sixteen he would get a "bilious" headache about once a month unless he "warded it off" with a laxative and he reported that his father had suffered from the same kind of headaches.

He completed the eighth grade of school. He married at the age of twenty. His wife had two children, one of whom died in infancy and the other was living and well.

His father suffered from valvular heart disease and his paternal grandfather died of a stroke after the age of sixty. The mother had gallbladder disease and the maternal grandfather died of uremia. The patient was the oldest of a family of six and there was nothing remarkable in the medical history of his brothers and sisters. None of them had hypertension.

After his discharge from the hospital he was carefully followed by his physician who recorded that the blood pressure gradually diminished from 150/110 to 130/88. This last reading was obtained on May 22, 1936, after the patient had returned to his job as truckdriver in a large concern, and had been working for about a month. Meanwhile, his weight had increased from 114 to 127½ pounds and he felt very well.

Hypertensive Encephalopathy

On May 28, 1936, at 4 p. m., he witnessed an automobile accident and although no one was injured the patient became terribly excited over "what might have happened to some children who were playing in the path of the truck." He "knew that he would get sick again," and after a few hours of restless sleep he awakened with abdominal pains, nausea, vomiting, and diarrhea. (Later his physician reported that the first illness, that is, the appendicitis, had begun similarly—"like gastroenteritis with diarrhea.") Nausea and vomiting continued and also the diarrhea. Sleep was restless and fitful and on June 2nd the patient reported blindness on awakening but there was no evidence of this when he was examined by his physician later in the day.

Abdominal examination was negative but the blood pressure was now 160/100. That night he developed *convulsive seizures*. By midnight he was mentally clear but the blood pressure was 190/110. He was readmitted to the Temple University Hospital on the service of Dr. Charles L. Brown on June 3, 1936. On this admission the blood pressure, taken four times daily for a week, remained constantly at 200 to 210 systolic and 140 to 160 diastolic. There were almost no fluctuations. Even during sleep the blood pressure on several occasions was found to be 175/125. Weakness, however, was not so pronounced as before. The temperature on occasions was slightly elevated to 99.4°; the pulse varied from 90 to 120 and the leukocytes ranged from 15,800 to 22,450. Sedimentation time was 10 mm. in one hour and the other laboratory findings were within normal limits. Now the eyeground picture was stated to be acute vasospastic retinitis with arteriosclerosis, grade 1; but the functional (spastic) element was still the predominant feature. There were some retinal scars where previous exudates had been.

Psychologically it was found that the patient had been sleepless and restless ever since witnessing the accident, whereas previously he had always been an excellent sleeper. He kept recalling the accident and thought how "terrible" the consequences might have been. It was obvious that in this patient there was a great deal of unconscious anxiety which, following operation, had resulted in a psychosis, but had then subsided, during which time the patient improved and remained well for more than a month. Then after the accident anxiety broke out again, not quite to the former extent, but with pronounced insomnia and a constant feeling of tension.

Following discharge from the hospital in June, 1936, the patient constantly improved. The weight increased and the blood pressure gradually diminished. During the latter part of June it was reported on several occasions at 140 to 150 systolic over 115 to 120 diastolic. By the latter part of July the blood pressure had dropped to 120/90. The weight had increased to 121-1/2 pounds, and the patient felt perfectly well, eating and sleeping normally, and once more returned to work.

During this period more detailed information bearing on his life situation was obtained.

LIFE SITUATION

According to the mother he was a normal boy, the oldest of six children. Other than difficulty in weaning there were no behavior problems although there were occasional nightmares. He completed the eighth grade at school and began working at the age of seventeen. For some time he was employed as a clerk with a refining company and there he "first developed a fear of operations; a friend had the wrong kidney removed." There he also saw many accidents and deaths and it was largely for that reason that he gave up the position. He was always afraid of hospitals ("a fear of being cut")

He only vaguely recalled any masturbation. He began his heterosexual career at fourteen with an older girl but often suffered from premature ejaculation. After marriage, although his wife was frigid, he indulged in excessive intercourse and asked "whether perhaps that might be responsible for his present difficulties." Occasionally again he would suffer from premature ejaculation. With his illness he lost desire for intercourse. Then when desire returned he could not maintain an erection. Since the illness he developed nocturia. He would awaken with a "water" erection and complained of a pain in the testes.

Marriage

He married at the age of twenty. He became interested in his future wife through a challenge. A friend was attentive to her and expressed himself to the effect that she could not be taken away from him. The patient finally succeeded in winning her away and after a nine month's courtship they were married. During this period he did not have intercourse "because he had too much respect for the girl." His attitude toward his wife was one of extreme jealousy; the following incident is an example: She had been visiting her physician for gynecologic treatments. The patient would go along and wanted to stay in the room while the doctor treated her. "I didn't trust the doctor." His wife did not approve but suffered him to remain. The treatments affected him "in the stomach."

Intercourse was always with condoms which had no effect on his premature ejaculation. While on vacation during the period of rapid convalescence he suffered constantly from premature ejaculation. During the fall of 1936, he carried on extramarital intercourse, still suffering from occasional premature ejaculation.

A child was born a year after marriage but lived only three months. The patient was nervously upset for a time afterwards.

Employment History

For the past eight years he had been employed as a truckdriver for a large concern. On occasions he worked many extra hours; once he worked a hundred hours in one week. Nevertheless, he was always in debt. This was especially so just before his illness. In addition he felt the strain of trying to prevent accidents and stated that although he had a reputation for handling the truck well he, nevertheless, had many accidents and "the more I tried to avoid them the more accidents I had."

Beginning in the fall of 1937, he began to interest himself in *union work*. He stated that his father, who had worked for the same company, had always resented the company's "restrictions" but did nothing, but "my mother is a fighter and I must have inherited it from her." Furthermore, his father was killed by a truck in July, 1937, and the company was fighting compensation. This "makes me more determined than ever to fight the company union." He missed his father very much, because he used to talk to him about union activities. He threw himself into the work with great intensity and after working seven and one-half hours a day on the truck he would then engage in union activities for another five or six hours and in spite of this fact, at the end of six months of such constant pressure of activity, he had gained weight and his blood pressure still averaged 135/90! He stated that when he was under a nervous strain his muscles grew taut and that he perspired freely but that he was able to relax when he left the tense atmosphere. Now and then he felt cramps in the muscles especially of the arms and legs. He became an official of the union and in addition to the long hours of work managed to do a great deal of study. He often worked eighteen out of twenty-four hours and rarely got more than six or six and one-half hours in bed. His activity in the union dated from April, 1937, and in January, 1939, his blood pressure was still 135/90 and he was enjoying excellent health.

Retinal Studies

In October, 1936, Dr. Gibson had found the eyegrounds almost normal. There was very slight attenuation of the nasal arterioles with arteriosclerosis, grade 1, of the hypertensive type, in the periphery of all four arterioles, and residual scars of previous retinitis. All vasospastic features had subsided and a remarkable increase in the caliber of all vessels was noted. In July, 1939, Dr. Gibson found "retinal arteriolar sclerosis, grade 1, of the hypertensive type. There is a very mild attenuation of the arterioles without exaggeration of the reflex stripe. The retinitis has completely subsided. This is a most unusual remission in the retinal picture of hypertension."

Elevation of Blood Pressure

In September, 1939, for the first time since his recovery the blood pressure was definitely elevated (160/105). Union activities "folded up" in the early part of June; he was bitterly disappointed, anxious to do something about it but could not stir up any enthusiasm among his associates. When talking to them he became so "hot under the collar" that he lost the power of speech. He felt very keenly that something should be done but "just couldn't push things through." The injustice was "burning him up" and he felt himself "boiling inside." He had a constant feeling of tension and could not relax.

Coincidentally there had been a recurrence of *premature ejaculation* and a feeling that he could not be satisfied sexually. It seemed very obvious that his throttled aggression manifested itself in the sexual sphere and in his general feeling of not being able to relax, of being irritable and easily angered. We explained that the tension which he used to get rid of in union activities was bottled up and had to find an outlet in bodily symptoms.

SUMMARY

A young white man of twenty-nine with pronounced "mutilation anxiety," first seen in December, 1935, developed high blood pressure and an acute psychosis following an appendectomy, when he became fearful that peritonitis would develop. An acute vasospastic retinitis developed but the heart and kidneys seemed unaffected. The hypertension gradually subsided but in the spring of 1936, following an anxiety-producing episode, hypertension, vasospastic retinitis, and hypertensive encephalopathy again occurred. Once more the blood pressure and eyeground changes subsided as anxiety was reduced and for the next three years the patient remained well, having maintained a normal blood pressure (135/90) since July, 1936.

For almost two years during this period he felt well and the blood pressure remained normal in spite of excessive work. The long hours and intense activity were employed, however, in union activities where he was able to give direct expression to his aggressive impulses. Union activities ceased in the spring of 1939 and in September he was once more suffering from tense feelings, experiencing sexual difficulties, and the blood pressure was once more elevated. It seemed clear that this coincided with the period of "throttled aggression."

Hypertension and Anxiety
Marked Improvement from Superficial Psychotherapy

CASE 13

A white man fifty-five years old first consulted us in May, 1937, complaining of "high blood pressure."

History and Symptoms

At the age of twenty he had rheumatic fever, rested for a year and according to his statement "did not think of his heart again." The tonsils were removed the following year. Although he stated that he was not concerned about his heart he began to have an annual physical examination a few years later. Always he was told that he was normal. Eight years ago he took out a large insurance policy and was told that his blood pressure at that time was 140/90. The following year in his annual physical examination his blood pressure was found to be 150/100 and his physician recommended weight reduction. He dieted, lost weight, and in two week's time his blood pressure was 140/90 and remained at about that level for the following several months.

The next record that he knew about was 1932 when the blood pressure again was 150/100 and about August, 1935, he took another insurance examination and was turned down; he was told that the blood pressure was 180/100. This, he said, was the beginning of his concern about his blood pressure. He was then examined by many physicians and finally was told by a heart specialist, in regard to his hypertension, that he should go home and "take it easy," which he interpreted to mean that he was on his last legs. Then real anxiety attacks began and on his way to another physician he stopped to see a lawyer and have a will made, urging that it be completed immediately because he felt that he had only a few days to live.

Physical Examination and Laboratory Studies

Physical examination showed an obese white man whose blood pressure varied between 190 and 200 systolic, and 110 and 120 diastolic. The heart seemed slightly enlarged to the left and x-ray showed the heart size at the upper limits of normal. The aorta was slightly elongated but not dilated. The electrocardiogram showed slight changes in the T waves in leads 1 and

4 and suggested myocardial degeneration. The urine was normal and renal function, measured by concentration and urea clearance tests, was within normal limits.

The eyeground studies showed arteriosclerosis grade 2 plus, of the hypertensive type. There were innumerable localized areas of narrowing of the retinal arterioles with attenuation of the reflex stripe and generalized narrowing of the arteriolar tree. The impression was of a rather advanced, fairly progressive vascular lesion.

During his study the patient discussed his occasional headaches which extended down into the neck and shoulders and also described a painful penile erection which occurred three or four times at night. The first attack had occurred 8 or 10 years before. He had been informed that this had some relationship to the prostate gland. It was some time later that he recalled that these attacks had occurred a short time after hearing a discussion of cancer of the rectum.

LIFE SITUATION

The patient was of humble origin. He first had limited schooling and then worked at manual labor in an effort to save money to put himself through school. This he accomplished, and finally achieved a position of success in the business world. After jilting a girl whom he had known intimately for many years, he married another who "seemed very kind and considerate" but immediately after their marriage "she changed" and according to his statement "from then on made life miserable for him." They had two healthy children.

Most of his visits now had to do with his marital difficulties. On one occasion his wife suddenly left home but in spite of the fact that he exhibited a great deal of hostility for her he nevertheless urged her to return, which she finally did.

So much of his anxiety seemed to surround the fact that he accused his wife of being psychotic—and it seemed to us without real justification—that we urged that he bring her to the psychiatrist. This he did, with her consent of course, and she remained for several months under the care of the psychiatrist, who reported that she was a maladjusted but not a psychotic person.

Fear of Psychosis

Consequent interviews with our patient persuaded us that these accusations of psychosis regarding his wife were really projections of his own fears for his own condition. It was as though he said, "No, I am not psychotic; you are." In fact, on one occasion he said, "Perhaps I am losing my mind and I ought to see the psychiatrist." He was reassured that no hint of mental disease was present; that it was simply a question of an emotional disturbance.

Improvement

Within a period of a few months he began to improve and by the following year reported that he felt as well as he had ever been. At the same time he stated that his wife was very much better since seeing the psychiatrist. For the first time he began to make some physical efforts such as polishing his car and at our suggestion doing a little gardening, which he very much enjoyed. In fact, he had always enjoyed gardening but during the last few years had been so fearful of straining himself that he had given it up.

His blood pressure was not very different; it varied between 170 and 200 systolic, and 110 and 120 diastolic. All during these months he had troubled dreams but as he improved they diminished and finally disappeared. The night-time penile erections with the pain in the rectum also disappeared. He occasionally had a slight headache which seemed to occur every time he was reminded of high blood pressure, a stroke or heart disease. His visits to us were spaced out. Each time he reported himself well and working to advantage. He had great fun in his gardening and to his great satisfaction his son was also interested and worked along with him.

He was still gun-shy of the blood pressure apparatus but said he was not so afraid of death and was more like his former self.

The eyeground report in 1939 follows: "Retinal arterial sclerosis grade 2, hypertensive type. The right superior nasal retinal artery is spasmed out. There are numerous small retinal scars and areas of pigment proliferation in the retina."

Impression: There has been no increase in the sclerosis since the examination in 1937. There is less attenuation and less spasm. Apparently he has had an acute retinitis which has become absorbed.

Reeducation

Here is another example of great improvement in a hypertensive individual without a real alteration of the blood pressure figures. Nevertheless, by a process of reeducation, removing anxiety over the blood pressure figures themselves, trying to understand the whole personality and the family situation, assisting the patient in achieving the sublimation of which he was capable by gardening and other outdoor activities, we succeeded in obtaining good results. This is an example of the kind of patient in whom a short period of *hospital study* at the beginning was very helpful. It *facilitates a thorough physical study in order to evaluate the cardiovascular-renal situation properly and at the same time furnishes an opportunity to get to know the patient as a human being as well as a medical case.* Also it takes the patient away from his environment in order that reeducation can be promptly instituted. In other words, it is often possible by this abrupt change to bring about some alteration in the patient's attitude toward himself and life. As a great English physician once remarked, "It enables you to make a philosopher of the man before the disease does it for you."

SUMMARY

No far-reaching changes occurred in this man's personality or hypertensive state, yet he became a very different person from what he was in 1937. He carried on his occupation very successfully, was an efficient individual enjoying an ordinary degree of happiness, and his marital situation had been vastly improved. All of this came about with a relatively simple and superficial psychotherapy which consisted in: (1) reeducation regarding his blood pressure disturbance; (2) trying to understand his anxiety which he had focused on his heart and blood pressure; (3) improvement of his domestic situation by getting help for his wife; and (4) encouraging him to obtain satisfaction from a hobby which served as an outlet for some of his aggressive impulses.

Moderately Advanced Hypertensive-Vascular Disease Incapacity Out of Proportion to Disease; Marked Improvement from Superficial Psychotherapy

---

CASE 14

A fifty-year-old white man first consulted us in 1936. He complained of pains around the heart, "high blood pressure," and longstanding digestive disturbance.

History and Symptoms

Trouble began about ten years ago when his boy suffered a head injury and was operated upon, and "surgery killed him." The patient suffered a "nervous breakdown" following this, gave up his business and was told that his blood pressure was high. Ever since that time he had markedly limited his activity, led a very restricted life, and limited his intake of food, expecially salt and protein ("eating very little red meat"). He had also cut down on his smoking.

He had been a healthy child. He had gonorrhea at nineteen but made a good recovery, and typhoid fever at twenty, from which he also made a good recovery.

He had had heart burn and constipation for perhaps twenty years and had taken large quantities of baking soda all during the period.

He married at the age of thirty-four and had two children—the boy who died and a girl of twelve, who was well.

Family History

The mother, age sixty-nine, had had hypertension for ten years. The father was well. There were three brothers and two sisters and one of the sisters, twenty-three years old, also had hypertension.

Physical Examination and Laboratory Studies

Physical examination showed a stocky white man of fifty with blood pressure that averaged about 190 to 200 systolic and 120 diastolic. The heart action was forceful but the size of the heart seemed within normal limits. The sounds were normal. Urinalysis was negative and kidney function good. The eyegrounds showed arteriosclerosis grade 2 of the hypertensive type but no evidence of retinitis.

Continued observation of the patient indicated that *pain in the heart region, headache, and weakness* were his main complaints and that they were precipitated by any circumstance reminding him of the death of his son, death in general, or any topic that had to do with cardiovascular-renal disease and its many complications. He had learned a great deal to his disadvantage from the many physicians whom he had seen.

LIFE SITUATION

Precordial Pain

Pain in his heart region was superficial; he indicated it by rubbing over the apex region. It would appear while we were discussing some subject related to heart disease, and it would disappear as soon as we reassured him that the pain had nothing to do with his heart. *We soon came to the conclusion that the pain in his chest was not of heart origin and, secondly, that his incapacity was out of proportion to his disease.* The treatment from then on was aimed at reeducating him in regard to these two propositions. We soon discovered, and were able to make clear to the patient, that an exaggeration of symptoms always occurred when some emotional circumstance touched upon his conflicts. Gradually over a period of months symptoms diminished and at times disappeared and he was able to work harder and more effectively than before. He enlarged his diet, particulary in regard to meat, which he enjoyed very much, and enlarged the circle of his activities in all directions. The more he accomplished in this regard, of course, the more confidence he had that he was not so disabled as he had thought.

Headaches

Just as pain in the heart region did not seem related to heart disease so did it become apparent that his headaches had nothing to do with hypertension. We could always find some emotional circumstance that antedated the onset of the headache and which, when made clear to the patient, caused the headache to disappear. For example, he was to make a business trip but he was no sooner away from home when he became ill with severe headache, weakness, and pain in the heart region, and he had to return immediately without accomplishing his business. It required considerable discussion to find out that the situation which touched this illness off was the fact that as he got on the train a coffin was removed and this turned his thoughts toward hypertension, a stroke and death. The pain in the heart and the intense headache disappeared when he recognized the connection between the anxiety-producing event and his symptoms.

Symptomatic Improvement

Again and again a cardiac or cerebral accident among his friends or relatives, or even of important persons reported in the newspapers, caused symptoms to recur only to subside one more with reassurance. It also became clear that symptoms recurred on the anniversary of his boy's death without his being aware of the fact that there was such a relationship! It was striking that with the disappearance of symptoms and his increased efficiency blood pressure figures did not change very much. As one so often sees in reports on the *surgical treatment of hypertension,* justifying the procedure, "that although the blood pressure was not modified, symptoms were relieved." This same phenomenon was well demonstrated in this patient as in many others whom we have seen. Such symptomatic improvement does not constitute a justification for a certain therapeutic process because suggestion, reassurance, and enlightenment are enough to accomplish it.

A great deal of the patient's time was given over to a criticism of his wife, toward whom he had a great deal of hostility. He accused her of nagging him, felt that she was acting peculiarly during the menopause and even intimated "that she was going crazy." As with another patient this seemed to be a projection of his concern over his own sanity.

Relation of Headache to Bowel Function

As in so many patients with hypertension he saw a connection between headache, which he correlated with high blood pressure and bowel function. *When he was constipated he was ill; when his bowels moved freely he was speedily relieved of symptoms.* We have seen this repeatedly in hypertensive persons. It seems to us to be largely a psychological association because (a) relief often comes too quickly after a bowel movement to be ascribed to physical causes, and (b) deeper psychological study indicates that there exists in the personality structure of such patients an easily exploited psychological association between the bowel function and head symptoms. Colonic irrigation for "auto-intoxication" is a good example of such exploitation.

Excessive Self-indulgence

An important point in this regard was that with his increased vigor he indulged in extramarital intercourse and even though he did so to excess —previously he had been fearful of a stroke from such excitement and exertion—he always felt better afterwards, apparently with the idea that the emission of semen, like the expulsion of the bowel content, relieved him of some poisonous substance, which made him feel better. Whereas he had previously restricted his intake of protein, particularly "red meat," he now indulged to excess, eating really enormous quantities of meat. He increased his smoking to ten or twelve cigars a day and drank a lot of whiskey, especially at the times of illicit sex relations. In spite of this he remained symptomatically well and we could not detect that the cardiovascular-renal system was adversely affected by these excessive indulgences.

SUMMARY

A typical middle-aged, sthenic, hypertensive man with moderately advanced cardiovascular changes of hypertensive-vascular disease, who had seriously restricted his life and suffered many symptoms, was helped by a psychotherapeutic regimen which emphasized (1) that his symptoms were not due to the hypertension itself and (2) that his incapacity was out of proportion to the disease. By encouraging the outward expression of his aggressive impulses and not forbidding the indulgence of his sexual impulses he was enabled to become a much more efficient and healthy personality. Even against our advice he indulged excessively in all of the things that are so often forbidden to a hypertensive patient—protein food, especially red meat, alcohol, tobacco, and sexual intercourse—and yet this indulgence did not seem to harm the patient from the standpoint of his physical make-up and actually contributed to his feeling of well-being because of his improved confidence in himself. We do not know that the patient is going to live any longer but we are sure that he is living a more effective and happier life. Certainly he is definitely more free of symptoms.

We do not wish to take the responsibility for his excesses—they were his own idea and we did not encourage him—but it is striking that once his confidence was restored he could do to excess all of the things which are usually denied a hypertensive patient, apparently without injury to himself. Again and again we have found patients whose joy of living has been restored by reeducation in regard to their hypertensive disorder, who have to be cautioned not to take advantage of their restored confidence in themselves.

Advanced Hypertensive-Vascular Disease
Marked Amelioration of Symptoms from Superficial Psychotherapy

---

CASE 15

History and Symptoms

A white man, aged fifty-five, first seen in July, 1936, complained of headache, dizziness, and nervousness, and stated that he had been well until four years qefore, at which time a bank in which he was interested failed, and severe headaches and vomiting followed. Prior to that he had known of high blood pressure and had been "warned of a stroke" unless he slowed up in his activities. Then his physician died in December, 1935, and another placed him on an even more severe regimen and according to the patient insisted on nothing but "rest—rest—rest." He lost 8 pounds in weight and in the spring of that year his vision became blurred. He was sent to an ophthalmologist who told him that "his eyes were terrible" and that he had a kidney condition which only medicine would relieve. He became depressed following this consultation and the symptoms mentioned above ensued.

Physical Examination and Laboratory Studies

Physical examination in the hospital showed an obese, middle-aged man with evidences of advanced hypertensive-vascular disease. Blood pressure on admission to the hospital was 228/128 and varied between 190 to 215 systolic and 115 to 130 diastolic during his period of observation of about one week. The electrocardiogram showed changes in the QRS complexes of leads 1 and 2 and occasional premature auricular beats. The eyeground study showed retinal arteriolar sclerosis, grade 2, of the hypertensive type with additional evidence of a vasospastic retinitis, group 3. There were traces of albumin and occasional hyaline casts in the urine but kidney function as measured by the urea clearance test was within normal limits.

It seemed clear that we were dealing with long-standing, advanced hypertensive-vascular disease and that the process had recently become accelerated.

LIFE SITUATION

The patient had entered the hospital for observation without informing his wife "so that she would not be alarmed." The following morning a physician walked into his room in the midst of a scene in which the wife was berating him because he had done this. Shouting, "I have been a devoted wife for thirty years and this is what I get for it," she showed an intensity of affect which seemed out of all proportion to the seriousness of the offense. She paced up and down the room, screaming out vituperation, tearing her glasses from her nose and smashing them upon the floor. When finally things quieted down and she had been removed the patient explained that there had been a long-time religious conflict in his home and that now and always "he had had to swallow everything," otherwise the situation of the moment would fan into flame the old problem of religious conflict. Further details are unnecessary but it was clear that the atmosphere in which he lived had been surcharged with the emotion of this only partially suppressed conflict.

Conflict and Hypertension

It seemed to us that his life situation could not be divorced from his hypertension and that the long-standing tension in the home must have played a part in the hypertensive disorder. Furthermore, we thought that crucial circumstances of recent years (bank failure, physician's death, eye consultation) could well be responsible for the acceleration of his hypertensive process including the eyeground changes which the consultant had said meant "serious kidney disease." We reassured him about his kidneys, informing him that his eye condition had nothing to do with kidney function, and tried to make him see that his hypertensive disorder was in some way related to his whole life situation. This resulted in his saying a few weeks later, "I have an entirely different outlook on things" and "the only complaint that I now have is occasional blurred eyesight." He also stated that he had felt better during the past six weeks than any time during the previous three years. The significance of this is that without altering very much his blood pressure level, and certainly without influencing the vascular changes which had taken place in his organs, symptoms had been almost totally abolished simply by a psychological approach.

Intracranial Vascular Accident

The patient continued to be a useful citizen and died suddenly three years later from an intracranial vascular accident. We have the definite feeling that he lived longer and certainly happier because of the reassurance which followed his hospital study.

Hospital Study

If possible, we always recommend a short period of hospital study in patients of this kind with complicated psychosomatic vascular disorders, because it enables us to study the patient more intensively and thus more quickly get him started on a new outlook toward his illness. By suddenly changing the environment of such a patient from one of protracted tension to one in which he feels secure and at peace, and then adding to his security by the combined psychosomatic study already discussed, we can more readily change his attitudes than in any other way. Frequently such patients will voluntarily submit that their attitude toward long-established patterns of behavior has changed for the better. Then gradual reeducation consolidates the improvement and leads to further degrees of recovery.

SUMMARY

The case is recorded primarily to show that even in advanced hypertensive-vascular disease the psychosomatic approach can be helpful.

Hypertension and Anxiety
The Symptoms Which Precede Hypertension; Relief of Anxiety
Attacks by Psychotherapy

CASE 16

A married white woman of thirty-three years was admitted to Temple University Hospital in October, 1940.

History and Symptoms

Recent History. She complained of palpitation, nervousness, hot flushes, and shortness of breath.

She stated that she had been well until July 7, 1940, when, while at church, she had an attack in which she felt a tingling sensation all over and thought "she was going out of her mind." She had a sensation of heat and flushing of the upper chest, over the face and neck, and had an "all gone feeling inside." Extreme weakness and palpitation of the heart followed. Her physician told her that she had high blood pressure and kidney disease and "that her kidneys were shot," and gave medicine, which, however, did not help her. Instead "nervousness and irritability" increased and, together with palpitation, were especially marked at the time of the menstrual period. She found it necessary to keep herself busy all the time in her household tasks in an effort to allay her nervousness and she developed certain *compulsive tendencies*, such as not being sure that she had accomplished a task satisfactorily and as a consequence doing it over and over again.

Past History. She stated that her previous health had been good but on close questioning admitted that she was not quite up to par just before this illness began in July, 1940. *For about two years she had felt mentally depressed, had restricted her social life, had been increasingly irritable with the children and had been frigid in her sexual life.* The menstrual history had been normal. She had had sighing respirations, which is what she meant when she said that she suffered from "shortness of breath." At times she had band-like headaches and occasionally felt as though her head was "clogged up." She was very sensitive and cried easily. Her weight had not changed.

She was married at the age of nineteen and had two children, eleven and thirteen years old; both were well. Three years ago she had a spontaneous abortion at three months.

Family History. The father and mother were born in Ireland and were well. The patient was one of eight children ranging in age from twenty to thirty-three, all of whom were married and in good health. The mother had hypertension, which was discovered about two years before.

Physical Examination and Laboratory Studies

On admission the blood pressure was 216/140 and there was a pronounced vasomotor flush over the front of the chest mounting up the neck and face. After admission this flushing was less marked and the blood pressure varied between 160 and 200 systolic and 100 to 120 diastolic. Eyeground examination showed rather pronounced angiospasm but no retinitis and this tended to diminish during the hospital stay so that there remained only moderate attenuation of the arterioles. This was interpreted as the preorganic phase of hypertension. The heart was within normal limits as to size; the sounds were normal and the electrocardiogram was normal. The urine was normal and the kidney function (excretory function of the kidney) as measured by concentration and urea clearance tests was normal. Two basal metabolism tests were —2 and —7. Blood count and Wassermann tests were normal. An intravenous urogram showed a normal urinary tract.

The general physical examination disclosed no evidence of disease aside from the vasomotor flush, elevation of blood pressure and the overactive heart; the latter, however, seemed perfectly normal.

We concluded, therefore, that we were dealing with essential hypertension in its pre-organic stages.

LIFE SITUATION

When we first talked with this patient she said that there was nothing wrong, she had no troubles, and her home life was "all right." But after a time by just talking to her casually about herself and her stay in the hospital, the first point of psychological importance was elicited—*that last July was not the real onset of trouble but that for two years "she had not felt like herself."* She had been depressed and had not gone out much socially and had been increasingly irritable with the children and sexually frigid. *Depression of spirits, frigidity, and restriction of the social life are all indications of anxiety.*

Her father, sixty, and mother, sixty-one, were both living. Both came from Ireland. The patient, the oldest of eight children, left the sixth grade of school to work in a large bakery where she held her position a long time and was regarded as a good worker.

Marriage and Family Conflict

She was married at nineteen to a Filipino. The marriage caused great consternation in this Irish family. No daughter in an Irish family had any business marrying a Filipino! As a consequence she was ignored by them. It was two years before her mother spoke to her and five years before her father relented and became friendly again. After her marriage she would enter her mother's home but no one would notice her. She said, "I knew if I just kept going they wou'd finally speak to me but it took two years before my mother did and longer for my father. But now my father is the best one, for he thinks that I have a very good husband." Apparently the family finally came to regard her husband very highly. Once they accepted him they looked upon him as a very good son-in-law.

This period was hard on our patient because she was a very sensitive girl. She had two children and was very fond of them. Nevertheless she had become irritable with them. She had never liked housework very much and it had become more distasteful than ever. She had many times wanted to go back to her former employment and have something to do which would be more stimulating than she had found the care of her home and children to be. Why this prejudice against housework? For the answer to this we have to go back to her early life experiences. Because she was the oldest of eight children she had to do a great deal in caring for the younger ones and was very glad to escape from this responsibility into outside employment. The father and mother did not permit her to go to dances, kept her very closely confined, and did not make home life attractive for her. She had too little fun in her early life to make her eager to perform the poorly rewarded work of wifehood and motherhood.

Inhibited Aggression

Now a few words about the special nature of the sensitivity in this patient. She had great difficulty in talking to people and in expressing herself when she was with them. She was very much afraid she would offend them. She was asked if she ever got angry. She said, "Yes, but I can never do anything about it. I rehearse what I am going to say to the person who makes me mad but when I meet that person I just can't say anything. A lump sticks in my throat. I break down and cry. It is because I feel that I may make a fool of myself. I have become more and more quiet."

For this reason our patient had withdrawn and lived a life very much alone, circulating only among a few neighbors whom she met through the popularity of her son. She was afraid to talk to her husband about home problems. She said, "He might take the wrong attitude or he might not know what I mean." So she avoided even casual conversation with him—this, in spite of the fact that he was judged easy-going and had not shown annoyance with her. An outstanding practical problem was her fear of people and her difficulty in bringing herself to talk to them. She was so afraid that they would regard her as hostile and withdraw their friendship. Thus we could see greatly inhibited aggression in this patient.

Aggression can be regarded in one of two ways. It should be a very real part of any *healthy personality*. We can speak of a person as being aggressive and mean that he gets his job done promptly and well or that he is regarded as a successful person. But we may use the same word to mean something entirely different when we are speaking of another person; we may mean that this person is cruel in his remarks, unpleasant, and destructive rather than constructive in his activities. Both types of aggression, however, arise from the same source, although the constructive kind has more human good will fused with it. This woman was afraid that if she talked to adults her remarks would be regarded as mean and unpleasant. For example, before an election, each woman in the ward was giving her opinion and telling which candidate she considered the best. Our patient had her opinion and she would have liked to speak up and say what she thought. Instead she picked up a magazine and began to read so that she would not even hear what was being said. Just to think of giving her opinion made her so excited inside that she had to stay out of the conversation even as a listener. A fear of hostile expression rendered her more ineffectual and caused her to withdraw farther, just as she had from family and from social life.

Anxiety Attacks

There is no doubt that her attacks since July, 1940, had been anxiety attacks. The sudden onset, palpitation of the heart, sweating, and the fear about throwing herself out of the window—all of these were exaggerated fears that she could not control herself, fears that she had not been able to repel for a long time. She had had social anxiety all her life, an anxiety that made her unable to control herself in such a way as to get on with people and which was finally beginning to show itself in anxiety attacks.

Anxiety and Hypertension

We have said that it has been shown by some investigators in this field that a marked inhibition of aggression has an effect upon the blood pressure. Some of these people who have such great difficulty in releasing their aggression through the usual routes find that their energy is expressing itself in some system of the body, such as the cardiovascular system, and increasing tension results. You know that when you see someone about to get angry and speak his mind it is a common occurrence for those around him to say, "Don't let your blood pressure go up." No one stops to consider where such expressions come from but it is generally known that the emotions do affect the blood pressure.

Apparently in this patient certain emotional tensions were not finding a normal outlet through action or words. Hence it would seem that the feeling was dammed up and was finding its expression through another system in her body. We thought it very important to help this woman to give expression to her feelings by focusing her attention on what was happening to her each day, helping her to know what her thoughts and feelings were, and then giving her encouragement to express them. When we asked her why she couldn't speak her mind about the election she said she didn't know. She had no idea of what lay back of her action. She just knew that she felt uncomfortable and that she had to remain silent. We showed her that it was probable that she was merely afraid that if she said what she thought the other women would hold it against her and think her unpleasant.

TREATMENT

Treatment Approach

First she had to learn what kept her so anxious each day and what made it so difficult for her to relate herself to people in the usual friendly way. We had to teach her that others would accept and tolerate many remarks of a personal nature and that she would be better liked if she got over her timidity. We had to teach her to express her opinions to her husband and family as well. We also told the family how important it was for them to *make it possible* for her to express herself more openly and normally. They were to try to sense when she was angry and urge her to express her mind until she learned to be a more forceful individual and found that after saying what she thought those around her were still her friends. In this way she would feel that she had better control of her thoughts and feelings. As she improved in this sphere she would, accordingly, have a decrease in anxiety. The fear that she would throw herself out of the window was just another way in which she showed a fear of *lack of control*.

In people like this the *fear of lack of control* is usually in two spheres of activity—hostility and sexual expression. We were sure that she had many fears of sexuality. But they would probably not play an important role until the more superficial and everyday anxiety concerning the control of her aggression toward people was dealt with. It was possible that this, in itself, would have a favorable effect upon the illness.

The Earliest Symptoms

The patient, therefore, presented essential hypertension and anxiety neurosis. It is not remarkable that this combination of illnesses should occur in the same person. Essential hypertension, as is well known, is one of the commonest disorders of civilized life and anxiety states are certainly no less common; therefore, simply from the standpoint of their incidence, it is not surprising that the two are frequently present in the same individual. Now the question which must interest us is this—Is there a more specific relationship between the two?

Emotional factors are generally considered to be of importance in essential hypertension. For example, we teach that the patient who presents himself for the first time with essential hypertension is apt to have a higher blood pressure at the first reading than at subsequent readings and this is thought to be due to the tension associated with the first visit to a new doctor. Again we find that very often long periods of emotional stress precede the onset of hypertension, as seemed to be the case in this patient, and that frequently emotional episodes seem to precede aggravation of blood pressure in hypertensive patients. Moreover, again as in this patient, we find that the early symptoms of hypertension are not those which we generally attribute to the high blood pressure itself but rather are exactly the same as occur in psychoneurosis. *In this patient a period of depression, of irritability, of restriction of social life, and sexual frigidity preceded the actual discovery of the hypertension.* And so it is that various forms of head discomforts that cannot be explained directly on the basis of the hypertension, fatigue, palpitation, breathlessness of the sighing respiration variety, gastrointestinal symptoms, constipation, and fatigue out of proportion to disease, are frequently early symptoms of hypertension and not to be accounted for on the basis of the high blood pressure itself.

When hypertensive patients are studied a little more intensively from a psychological standpoint we find that there is often a great deal of conflict in their make-up and an inability to express their aggression directly; thus it would seem that tension which cannot be adequately expressed in word or deed, seeks a way out in the circulatory system. *Please do not understand, however, that we are maintaining that psychological factors are the only ones of importance in hypertension or even that they are fundamentally responsible.* What we are urging, rather, is that they are a set of factors that are important to the patient with hypertension and that their modification often results in benefit to the patient regardless of whether the blood pressure figures are lowered or not.

Personality Study

We are emphatic in saying that emotional factors in hypertension must be studied as well as the physical factors in order that we shall understand not only the high blood pressure, but the person who has the high blood pressure. Then we shall see that anxiety bears some relation to hypertension, which in turn is related to the unconscious conflict in the personality of the hypertensive individual and that this conflict can often be treated, resulting in relief of anxiety. It must be clear that in this patient it was very important to try to analyze and to remedy the anxiety state no matter how it was related to the hypertension, because if this factor was managed, the patient could easily become a more effective and healthy personality. We felt that it would be a great help to her because the anxiety state was very pronounced and the hypertension was in a preorganic phase. *We have no objection to the effort to lower blood pressure so long as this approach does not constitute the sole approach to the high blood pressure problem* because that is what is generally true of medicine today. Both physician and patient put all of their attention on "bringing the blood pressure down." That is the reason for the use of various drugs and various surgical measures to lower the blood pressure. There can be no question that the patient is better off with a lower blood pressure but this in itself constitutes a one-sided, superficial approach. *The whole thing may be summarized by repeating that we have paid too much attention to the physical studies in hypertension and not enough to the emotional factors which may hold the key to the management of the hypertensive patient.*

Follow-up Notes

Upon leaving the hospital, the patient reported every two weeks to the outpatient department. At first her sister was obliged to come with her because she was afraid to travel alone. She reported anxiety attacks which would occur in a setting of emotional tension.

In the beginning she found it difficult to talk to her husband about ordinary affairs of the house, or even concerning the children, without bursting into tears. Every Monday afternoon the women of the family gathered at the house of the mother where they talked over the news of the week. The patient dreaded these gatherings, could not feel herself a part of the group, and often experienced anxiety while there. After about six weeks the patient seemed to gain reassurance and her anxiety attacks decreased greatly. She was able to talk to her husband without crying and also was able to get some enjoyment out of the Monday afternoon gatherings.

Continuation of Anxiety

Her anxiety still showed itself in many ways. She was greatly concerned because the children would not eat breakfast unless forced by her to do so. Even though they ate well at lunch and at dinner she feared that their health would suffer if they did not start the school day with breakfast. As a result of her concern over their health she would scold them severely each morning and then go about the house greatly agitated until their return, fearing that some accident might happen to them. She feared they might get killed and that their last memory would be of an unkind mother. Actually she was afraid that her hostility might magically be the cause of some disaster after they left her presence. We explained to the patient that she did not have to be so anxious about the children's diet. We admitted that it was desirable for the children to eat three times daily. We pointed out, however, that experiments had shown that children did pretty well at selecting their own diet and that if there was plenty of food of an appetizing nature and the children did not feel like eating it, but ate well later in the day, their health would not suffer and she need never reproach herself for being a neglectful mother. We suggested that when the children were at lunch and at dinner and were enjoying these meals she should talk to them about the desirability of eating breakfast and try to win their interest in a friendly setting, instead of leaving the whole matter until morning when they were in a hurry for school. The patient was able to accept these suggestions and this situation improved.

Attacking Problems One by One

One after another, we were able to take up problems which were producing anxiety. The next one was in connection with her son, who was failing in school. The patient felt justified in nagging and scolding him but she could not allow her husband to say anything to him—it upset her too much. We asked if she would allow us to talk to the boy, whereupon she agreed and brought him with her on the next occasion. The boy was a very attractive youngster, well fed, well dressed, and alert. We talked with him about his school work and his outside interests and found him to be quite an average boy. We talked to him about his mother's "nervousness," and he said that he and his sister worried about their mother and often spoke of her and wished she could be in a better frame of mind around the home. We took over the paternal role of being interested in the boy's progress and made some suggestions to the mother and the boy together about helping him with his work. The result of this was gratifying, as the boy passed all his studies that semester with a creditably high grade. He was quite elated and wanted to come at once to tell us about it.

Guilt Over Sexuality

Patients with a great deal of anxiety are often unable to seek reassurance for their anxiety because of guilt over sexuality. They feel that any move toward friendliness and love in some vague way has a sexual connotation. Our patient had a dream of such frightening content that it could, in fact, be regarded as a nightmare, but was also accompanied by some behavior in her waking state which was almost of psychotic nature. She dreamed that a man was breaking into the house and coming to her room. She woke up frightened and with palpitation of the heart, breathlessness, and perspiration. Even though awake she could not get over the impression that her husband, who was lying asleep in the bed next to her, was a strange man. Unable to get over this impression she got up and put on her clothes and lay on top of the bed all night, lest this man should prove to be a stranger to her. This dream created such an impression in the patient's mind that it gave us a good opportunity to discuss her anxiety about the display of affection and the matter of sexual relationship. Improvement then followed in this sphere so that at the end of one year from the time of her hospital admission she was able to report that attacks of anxiety had entirely ceased and that she had been more comfortable physically and more cheerful for a month than at any time during the previous year.

SUMMARY

A young woman developed anxiety attacks after a long period of prodromal symptoms. She had essential hypertension. The blood pressure level was not materially affected but psychotherapy allayed her anxiety and made her a much more effective and contented person.

Hypertension and Anxiety—Hypertensive Encephalopathy

CASE 17

History and Symptoms

A white man of seventy had been aware of hypertension since ten or twelve years ago, at which time he had been refused life insurance. There were no special symptoms, however, and he stated that he had not been much concerned about it until two years ago when he felt a pressure on the top of his head and his physician discovered his blood pressure to be quite high. About one year ago he began to have attacks of unconsciousness. The first one occurred in April, 1938, since which time he had four such attacks at intervals of about four months. All but one had occurred at night and were described as follows: The patient utters a peculiar cry, begins to breathe heavily and then draws up his forearms flexed at the elbow in a spastic manner. There are no clonic convulsive movements, deviation of the eyes or changes of color. The patient has never bitten his tongue. The attack lasts about ten minutes. On each occasion a physician has been called who has administered a hypodermic. Following the attack the patient is exhausted and must lie in bed for from one to three days.

The patient did not complain of headaches, vomiting, or visual disturbances. Sometimes he became dizzy on bending over and complained of occasional fatigue at the end of the day. There had been no impairment of memory or intellect, or any emotional instability. He had never complained of weakness or paresthesias of the limbs.

Past History. The past history was essentially negative. He had been constipated for many years and had always required laxatives or enemas. He smoked moderately and formerly took an occasional drink. When he was forty he married a woman of thirty-five; his wife had never been pregnant. He never had venereal disease.

Family History. His father lived to the age of eighty and died as a result of a "stroke"; his mother died at seventy-seven of "dropsy." The remainder of the family history was negative.

Physical Examination

The patient was a well-preserved, well-nourished, white man, seventy-one years old. The blood pressure varied from 180 to 200 systolic and 96 to 110 diasotlic. The heart seemed normal in size and position. There was a slight systolic murmur at the apex and in the aortic area but no thrill. The abdominal examination was negative and the genitals were normal. The rectum and prostate were normal. The extremities were normal.

Neuropsychiatric Examination*

There was no intellectual impairment, disturbance of memory, or evidence of emotional instability. He appeared to be rather diffident and pleasant in his manner and there seemed to be a very agreeable relationship between him and his wife. Station and gait were normal. There was bilateral arcus senilis. The visual fields were grossly normal; there was no nystagmus, ptosis, or strabismus. The masticatory and facial muscles were normal. Hearing was normal; there was no lateralization on performing the Weber test; the Rinne was negative. There was no palatal drooping or weakness and the tongue was protruded in the midline.

There was no ataxia or cerebellar asynergy. Coarse tremors were present in both outstretched hands. The deep reflexes were hyperactive on both sides, but more so on the right. The cremasteric reflexes were diminished bilaterally and could be elicited only upon reinforcement. A bilateral Babinski sign was present. The right foot was slightly everted; there was no evidence of weakness in any of the limbs. Sensibility was intact in all modalities There was no spinal tenderness or limitation of movements of the spine.

*We are indebted to Dr. Paul Sloane for the neuropsychiatric examination and notes on this patient.

The eyeground examination showed a moderate degree of retinal arteriosclerosis of the hypertensive type; the disc margins were clear and distinct;
there was no evidence of retinitis.

Ordinary urinalysis was normal except for a very faint trace of albumin
and the Addis count was within normal limits.   Renal function, as measured
by the urea clearance test, was normal.   The electrocardiogram was normal
except for an occasional ventricular extrasystole.   X-ray of the skull showed
no evidence of abnormality.   Dr. Sloane suggested that the attacks were "a
subcortical type of convulsive seizure in which the clonic movements of epilepsy are replaced by a spasticity of the limbs.   In view of the hypertension,
the recurrence of the symptoms over a period of a year, without any progressive increase in severity or frequency, and the bilaterality of the py-
ramidal tract signs, we are dealing with a multiplicity of lesions, probably
vascular in nature (hypertensive encephalopathy).   An expanding lesion
can be ruled out fairly definitely."

LIFE SITUATION

The patient had always been a hard worker.   His father was a very
conscientious person and the patient felt that in this respect he resembled
him.   He had been a meticulous person since childhood and had always
been afraid of making a mistake or gaining the disapproval of others.
In his work as a druggist he was always apprehensive and very cautious
lest he make a mistake in filling a prescription.   He devised a method of
checking up on mistakes by having two people go over each prescription.
Despite this fact he frequently left his bed at night to go downstairs and
check up on a prescription that had been filled during the day.   On the
surface he appeared to be reserved and calm, but according to his wife,
"He boils inside of himself."   His ordinary cautiousness had been increased during the last eight years following the death of his partner,
when the entire responsibility of protecting the store devolved upon him.
He had been very careful about protecting the rights of his partner's
widow and seeing that she received an adequate income.   Since the
onset of the present illness the patient had withdrawn from the active
management of the store and had tried to control his usual tendency to
worry

Convulsive Attack

The particular attack which forms the basis of this report occurred in
January, 1939.   He was sitting in a chair reading a newspaper and, according to the patient, he had been reading an item concerning a woman
pharmacist who had made a mistake in filling a prescription, causing the
death of a patient.   The attack which followed was different from the
previous ones in that it was much more violent and the patient became
rigid all over. When he emerged from the original spastic condition he
became "delirious" and kept repeating, "I didn't do it," as if he were

protesting against some accusation. He insisted on sitting up and struggled when the doctor tried to get him to lie down. He did not recall anything until he found himself upstairs in bed, undressed. The attack was so severe that the attending physician thought the patient would die.

SUMMARY

From the psychosomatic point of view this hypertensive patient obviously had an obsessive type of personality and it would seem that reading the news item in the paper so aroused his anxiety as to produce some somatic change which was in the nature of a cerebral vascular spasm. That the attack was accompanied by anxiety was revealed by the subsequent delirium and restlessness in which the patient apparently protested that he had not committed the crime about which he had read.

Hypertension and Anxiety—Spontaneous Subarachnoid Hemorrhage

CASE 18

History and Symptoms

A white woman of thirty-seven years was first seen in the spring of 1937. She stated that hypertension had first been discovered at the age of fourteen. There were no special symptoms, however, until about five years ago when, following financial difficulties, she began to develop anxiety attacks. These would begin with palpitation, extreme agitation, and actual panic so that she felt like jumping out of a window. Because of such an attack she was very thoroughly studied and told that there was nothing wrong with her except hypertension.

The patient had been reared in a small town. The father was a periodic drunkard and the mother a nervous woman whose death was due to "kidney disease and asthma." The patient attributes some of her trouble to the fact that the mother "was suffering from a change of life when I was born." The patient ran away with a much older, married man, and had three children, daughters, one year apart. They were eleven, ten, and nine years of age. When the baby was three months old they separated and she had been supporting herself and the children since.

Physical Examination and Laboratory Studies

Physical examination showed a well-nourished, healthy appearing, white woman. Her weight was 128 pounds and her blood pressure averaged 210 systolic and 140 diastolic. The heart seemed slightly enlarged to the left and there was a systolic murmur at the apex but no thrill. The aortic second sound was accentuated. The remainder of the general physical examination was negative. The urine showed a faint trace of albumin but kidney function as measured by concentration and urea clearance tests was within normal limits. Eyegrounds showed arteriosclerosis, grade 2 of the hypertensive type with no evidence of retinits.

After reassurance about herself the anxiety attacks diminished and she remained in satisfactory health.

LIFE SITUATION

She had three main social-psychiatric problems aside from her physical condition. *First*, she was very ambivalent toward the children, always placing them out to board and then bringing them home again to live with her; *second*, she made a living by keeping a boarding house and was always in financial difficulties. *Last*, she had a lover who, like her first, was married and paid her secret and hurried visits so that she "felt like a prostitute." When any one of these problems became acute, that is, trouble with the children, financial difficulties, or a quarrel with her lover, she became anxious and at the same time the anxiety seemed to reflect itself in an aggravation of the blood pressure level. In spite of her discontent with her present situation and her hostility toward her lover for his bad treatment of her she maintained a kind of loyalty toward him.

In January, 1938, she called a physician at two o'clock one morning to announce that "she had just had a stroke." She stated that she was sitting on the floor and could not move. She was sent to the hospital where the intern reported that "she was just hysterical," and had not had a stroke but that the blood pressure was 250/150. Venesection was done. The following day it was noted that she was drowsy, somewhat confused and disoriented and she remained so for several days. Neurological examination suggested the diagnosis of *subarachnoid hemorrhage*. The patient was somnolent and rather uncooperative. There was marked stiffness of the neck with a positive Brudzinski sign and bilateral Kernig. The left knee jerk, both Achilles and the left biceps reflexes were absent. The remaining deep reflexes were not very active. The spinal fluid was bloody.

Precipitating Factor

After she had become quite clear again mentally she reported that she had been having intercourse that night with another man, that she had been tired after a full day and that she felt "guilty and common' and had been unable to have an orgasm. Suddenly she felt "lifeless' from the waist down. She sat herself on the floor and refused to move and had to be taken to the hospital. She described a pain in her head which felt like a "screw-driver." Later she had a sensation of numbness in the head and still later vomited. There were no new findings as far as the heart was concerned, other than indications of the hypertension; the electrocardiogram was within normal limits. Moreover, the renal function remained good but the eyeground examination now showed, in addition to the arteriosclerosis, very marked vasospasm especially of the nasal branches, and in addition hemorrhages and exudates and some swelling of the disc margins. At first it was thought that the eyegrounds had undergone the changes of malignant hypertension. But this diagnosis was later retracted because the changes subsided and the conclusion was reached that the retinal picture represented a vasospastic exacerbation of the hypertensive changes of severe benign hypertension. In connection with the above episode it was later discovered that on several occasions under exactly the same circumstances attacks of pulmonary edema had occurred.

Recovery from Subarachnoid Hemorrhage

She made a very good recovery and the blood pressure level subsided to 150 or 160 systolic and 110 to 120 diastolic. It remained at this level for several months and then gradually increased and failed to respond to sulfocyanate therapy. Her financial situation became more and more acute and she was again admitted to the hospital in May, 1939, suffering from a slight upper respiratory infection and a state of great anxiety. There were no new findings in the cardiovascular examination except that the eyegrounds no longer showed any evidence of retinitis, and aside from marked attenuation of the nasal vessels there was only arteriosclerosis of the hypertensive type. All evidences of the previous severe vasospastic change had disappeared.

The Necessity for Psychosomatic Study

This case emphasizes one of the points made in the introduction, namely, that diagnosis is not to be made by exclusion only but by a bilateral approach in which psychological and physical factors are given equal weight. When the patient's anxiety began she was told it was due to the hypertension because her physician did not recognize the psychological origin of anxiety and the necessity for the psychological approach in treatment. When she finally developed an intracranial vascular accident her physician, who was too psychologically minded, told her that it was "anxiety hysteria." We repeat that the only safe course will depend upon the proper attention both to physical and psychological factors, which constitutes the true psychosomatic approach. To this end, preparation in psychopathology must be as thorough as instruction in tissue pathology.

SUMMARY

A young white woman with a long history of severe benign hypertension had for several years suffered from anxiety attacks. She had three illegitimate children with a married man who was much older than herself and after his desertion maintained a relationship with another married man. During sexual intercourse, at which time she felt guilty "for her disloyalty" she had an attack which she considered a stroke but which the hospital intern, who was acquainted with her behavior from previous hospital study, considered "an hysterical attack." Neurological studies indicated that she had really suffered a subarachnoid hemorrhage. She made an excellent recovery.

Chapter XI

THE GASTROINTESTINAL SYSTEM

FUNCTIONAL DIGESTIVE DISTURBANCES

The abdomen has aptly been called "the sounding board of the emotions." It is well known that the student before examination may develop anorexia, nausea, or diarrhea. The business man may get indigestion, heartburn, and actual abdominal pain at the time of important conferences or in connection with financial reverses. The worrisome housewife develops indigestion and constipation when there is trouble with the children or housecleaning to be done. Even the child who is not making a happy adjustment with his playmates in the school yard may have an attack of vomiting some morning about school time.

In spite of the fact that this relation beween psyche and soma is well known, it is surprising how little attention is given to this matter in the actual management of gastrointestinal disorders. Rarely is an evaluation made of the personality of the patient or the life situation in which the symptoms occur. The physician may be too busy to try to work this out with the patient. A prescription for a digestive mixture is quicker. Even though he admits that there is a "large nervous element" present he often looks upon this feature as secondary and probably a consequence of the physical disorder. He considers that psychic factors in illness are not on the same scientific level with gastric analysis and x-ray studies, etc., and, therefore, pays scant attention to them. He accepts psychogenesis only abstractly and with vague understanding of the nature of mental mechanisms and the part they play in illness. His formula is:

Cellular disease➤—▸Structural alteration➤—▸Functional disturbance (*i. e.*, Symptom-formation)➤—▸Mechanical investigation➤—▸Evaluation of these measured "facts."

False Sense of Accuracy

The documentation of these measurements gives a false sense of "scientific" accuracy and has led to an even greater neglect of psychogenic factors which, in turn, has been responsible for a lack of insight into the emotional problems and accompanying organ dysfunctions of the sick individual. In other words, it is well understood by many physicians and patients, too, that emotions may be a force that will produce "sick-

351

ness" in various parts of the gastrointestinal tract but beyond paying lip service to this concept very little or practical nature is done about it. Even though the patient understands that he has "nervous indigestion" he still believes that physical measures, diet regulation and medication will provide the answer to his problem. The physician has another reason for trying to find the answer along organic lines—he does not know just exactly what he would do or say if the patient should demand psychotherapy from him.

Organic Treatment

Moreover he knows that if he questions along the line of symptom and circumstance, the patient may prove to be sensitive and conclude that he is being regarded as a weakling who "can't take it" or perhaps actually as a "mental case." The physician, not wishing to arouse ill will or antagonism, just for safety's sake, follows the traditional line of physical and laboratory investigation, diet and medication, and makes no real effort to understand the life situation of the patient.

The matter of *psychotherapy* in gastrointestinal illness has been handled rather superficially in medical articles and textbooks. Advice to avoid worry and strain and to get plenty of rest, and investigation of the work conditions or marital relationship for sources of tension have been the extent of psychotherapeutic investigation. It is hoped that we can carry our readers further into an understanding of the connection between emotional problems and gastrointestinal illness and, by the discussion of cases illustrating various disorders, show the relationship of personality trends to symptoms.

Organ Language

It is understandable that the abdomen should be the sounding board of the emotions since (1) it is so well supplied with autonomic nerve fibers, both of the sympathetic and parasympathetic systems—the lines of communication between brain centers and the viscera—and (2) the behavior patterns of the gastrointestinal tract which have been utilized in infancy are carried to the brain and lodged there in that reservoir of memory, the unconscious mind. Given the proper stimulus, and without awareness on the part of the individual, impulses may be sent out by way of the autonomic nervous system from the unconscious mind recreating that same infantile behavior pattern. The tense business man may bluster about and struggle consciously to be effective while unconsciously there is a strong desire to be a little boy, once again under the protection of his mother and father and depending upon them for his sustenance, rather than trusting, as a mature person would, that a big order from some uncertain source may come his way. Security and sustenance are indissolubly related in the unconscious mind through the very nature of a human being's infantile existence and hence, *if security is threatened* later in iife the organ which regulates sustenance may be disturbed in its normal functioning. The gastrointestinal tract is phylogenetically the oldest system in the body and hence most likely to be used to express an emotion which cannot be dealt with through the regular channels. When urges such as loving or being loved, giving protection or being protected, are not successfully carried out with the mind (emotions) this oldest system of the body will be called into service in a vain attempt to solve the problem in a primitive way. This is what we have referred to as "organ language." Since it is not intended for service of this kind, the gastrointestinal tract is doomed to failure and its misguided effort to be of service for such psychological purposes causes dysfunction and discomfort which results in illness.

Emotional Trends

The most intensive studies of these illnesses have been made by Franz Alexander and his co-workers of Chicago. They have studied the psychological structure and life situations of patients suffering from functional disorders of the gastrointestinal tract as well as of those who have suffered from peptic ulcer and colitis. Their studies led to the conclusion that the gastrointestinal tract, because of its three major functions of taking in, retaining, and eliminating, was especially suitable for the expression of these three elementary emotional tendencies particularly if their normal expression through the voluntary motor system was inhibited. They found some correlation between certain personality trends and different disturbances of the gastrointestinal tract and also a relationship to the part of the tract involved. Thus, the upper end of the tract, according to its normal function, was well suited to express the receptive or taking-in tendencies, whereas the lower end of the tract was more suitable for the expression of the retentive and giving trends.

Gastric Problems

The important personality trends in the gastric neuroses and peptic ulcer cases were intense unconscious receptive and acquisitive wishes which the patient could not admit to himself. It was thought that the stomach symptoms were conditioned by the repressed receptive and aggressive taking-in tendencies which served as chronic psychic stimuli to the stomach function. In other words, many patients who have a strong, unconscious need for affection, a strong desire to be appreciated and taken care of, psychologically translate these trends as a need to be fed. At the same time they cannot admit these impulses to themselves and as a consequence *overcompensate* with a demonstration of great energy and great endeavor. They are afraid to be dependent or in-effectual. Nevertheless, their strong unconscious tendencies to be de-pendent cause reactions in the gastrointestinal tract so that the stomach tries to serve a double function. It tries to serve the function of emotional reception of love as well as acting as the organ of digestion. This is too difficult for the stomach to accomplish because the need to be taken care of (fed emotionally) is acting as an unusual or foreign and constant stimu-lus. This stimulus is responsible for overactivity and excessive secretion beyond the digestive needs. Moreover, this "need to be fed and loved" trend is being opposed by a stronger need to reject the unacceptable idea of dependency and ineffectuality and this conflict may result in stomach symptoms. More will be said on this subject in connection with the discussion of peptic ulcer.

Bowel Problems

The trend of the colitis cases was quite different in that such patients unconsciously felt that they had the right to take and demand for "they always gave sufficiently." They did not feel guilty or inferior because of a desire to receive or take because they were already giving something in return for what they received. This something they gave was the childish substitute of feces for real values—sometimes "given" to express ag-gression. It was pointed out in the chapter in psychopathology that during the period of training in sphincter control the child's first "stock in trade" was his excretions. Up to the time of the beginning of toilet training much had been given to the child and little asked for in return. Then during the bowel training period he learns to attach unusual value to his feces because he is praised so highly for producing them. With his willingness to understand the rules of cleanliness he can give "gifts" of the contents of the bowel or bladder to those who care for him. The emotional value attached to feces may never be sufficiently relinquished to other life values such as work, cooperation, money, or artistic talent. Later in life such people may fail to produce anything worthwhile in these fields and feeling anxiety, guilt, or shame about this, which they cannot admit, they fall back upon the childish pattern of "giving feces." This may sound fantastic to one who has given little thought to such matters or to one who has failed to live closely with the thinking and behavior of children or neurotics. So often we hear it said that the application of more common sense is the answer to these problems, but it takes more than common sense to understand the seemingly irrational behavior of children or the closely related unconscious trends of the neurotic. What it really takes is "uncommon sense" plus a knowledge of psychopathology. It is not to be forgotten that it is during the period of toilet training that a personality trait called *ambivalence* becomes pre-dominant. In other words, the child often develops conflict because of his own desires which are at odds with the wishes or demands of his parent. One part of him loves his parent and wants to *control* the bowel movement as the parent wishes. Another part of his personality defies such wishes and says, 'No, I hate you and do not care about control. I care more for my comfort and pleasure than for your love and I'll spite you by moving my bowels any time I wish." *Underneath a surface attitude of love may rest strong hostile feelings.* Hence a poorly built up control easily breaks down later in life to show an emotion such as hostility by means of a disturbance in bowel function.

Constipation. In patients with constipation the dynamic emotional trends express the idea that since the individual took or received nothing he was under no obligation to give. Alexander and his colleagues assumed that the constipation was a reaction against the obligation to give. Here again we must think of the relationship between mother and child during toilet training and remember that constipation or incontinence may express lack of cooperation on the part of the child. He holds back either to spite the parent or out of a fear that his bowel movements may prove harmful or offensive. He not only believes that his bowel movements offend when deposited in the wrong place but he stretches this belief to cover bowel movements at any time or any place. Most everyone is familiar with the person who cannot urinate or defecate in the presence of others, for example, in a public toilet. It is a short step from this inhibition to the development of constipation even in privacy. Constipation may be a kind of "anal impotence," in some cases growing out of anxiety over offending. In other cases it may mean indifference or stubbornness about producing something for others.

Incidence of Functional Disturbances of the Gastrointestinal Tract

Psychosomatic disturbances of gastrointestinal function occur in healthy people subjected to unusual emotional stress; they are among the commonest manifestations of emotional stress in neurotic people. Of 269 neurotic patients encountered in a medical outpatient department Friess and Nelson found that 41.5 per cent mentioned gastrointestinal symptoms as their chief complaint. The abdomen is, indeed, the sounding board of the emotions.

In a study of 3000 cases from a clinical and roentgenological viewpoint Dwyer and Blackford found that gross lesions in the stomach and duodenum accounted for gastric symptoms in only 15 per cent of the cases. In a consecutive series of 15,000 patients with chronic dyspepsia examined in the Mayo Clinic, 15.5 per cent had deformities which were interpreted as being the result of peptic ulcer. A little more than 2.6 per cent had gastric carcinoma. This made a total of 18 per cent of patients whose digestive disturbances were the result of gross organic diseases of the stomach and duodenum. In commenting upon this material Eusterman stated that these and a few other rare lesions, would account for about 20 per cent of the cases of chronic gastric disturbances. But he added that in private general practice the percentage might not exceed 10. He concluded that gastric disturbances arising reflexly from abdominal viscera other than the stomach are responsible for from 30 to 40 per cent of all cases and that in his opinion the neuroses constitute about 25 per cent of the total. Then from 15 to 20 per cent of gastric disturbances are attributable to disease of organs remote from the stomach, but only on infrequent occasions are such gastric disturbances the sole expression of an extragastric disorder.

Chronic Dyspepsia

Rivers and Ferreira, also from the Mayo Clinic, studied 4223 cases of chronic dyspepsia and divided them into four types: *organic, reflex, systemic,* and *functional.* Under organic causes of dyspepsia they included diseases or anomalies involving the tissues of the stomach or duodenum. Among the reflex causes of dyspepsia they included diseases of the appendix, gallbladder, biliary ducts, pancreas or intestines and renal stone or other conditions which reflexly disturb the chemistry or mechanics of the stomach or duodenum. Among the dyspepsias of systemic origin they included those due to disturbances of metabolism, toxemia, deficiency diseases, or dysfunction of the organs of internal secretion. Functional dyspepsias were assumed to include the disturbances in normal gastro-duodenal activity not resulting from demonstrable disease elsewhere in the body. Of this type they mentioned the various gastric neuroses, constitutional inadequacies and habit dyspepsias and the various dyspeptic manifestations of chronic nervous exhaustion. Their functional cases totaled 25 per cent as shown in the accompanying chart (Chart 2).

Testing Accuracy of Diagnosis. In an effort to test the accuracy of the diagnosis of nervous indigestion, Wilbur and Mills studied the records of 354 patients who after examination at the Mayo Clinic received the diagnosis of functional or nervous indigestion or its equivalent and who were reexamined at the clinic more than seven years later. In 303 cases no evidence of organic disease was found in the follow-up examination. The results suggest a diagnostic accuracy of at least 85.6 per cent for functional dyspepsia in that series. There were thirty-nine cases in which organic disease of the gastrointestinal tract was found at subsequent examination, but in nineteen of the thirty-nine a final diagnosis of duodenal ulcer was made and this represented the most common diagnostic error in the series. We will comment later on whether this represents a serious error in the etiological approach to peptic ulcer.

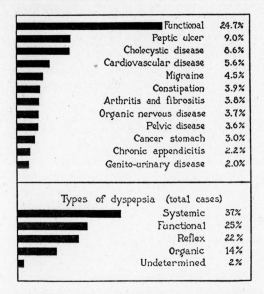

Functional	24.7%
Peptic ulcer	9.0%
Cholecystic disease	8.6%
Cardiovascular disease	5.6%
Migraine	4.5%
Constipation	3.9%
Arthritis and fibrositis	3.8%
Organic nervous disease	3.7%
Pelvic disease	3.6%
Cancer stomach	3.0%
Chronic appendicitis	2.2%
Genito-urinary disease	2.0%

Types of dyspepsia (total cases)

Systemic	37%
Functional	25%
Reflex	22%
Organic	14%
Undetermined	2%

Chart. 2. The twelve most common causes of dyspepsia in order of frequency. (Rivers and Ferreira: J.A.M.A. *110*: 2132, June 25, 1938.)

Diagnosis by Exclusion. Thus when chronic dyspepsia is approached even from a purely organic standpoint the incidence of functional disorders is at least 25 per cent. We have commented previously on the inadequacy of this type of investigation which for the most part represents diagnosis by exclusion. The point that we particularly wish to make is that the diagnosis of functional illness must be established not simply by exclusion of organic disease but on its own characteristics as well. *In other words, neurosis has its own distinctive features to be discovered by personality study.* Only in this way can serious errors in diagnosis and treatment be avoided. If this is true then it must naturally follow that personality studies are just as important in the problems of chronic dyspepsia as laboratory investigations. This applies not only to problems in which evidence of structural disease has been excluded but also to patients who present evidence of physical disease and emotional factors. Just as we cannot limit ourselves simply to the exclusion of organic disease in the so-called purely functional group, so even more importantly is there the necessity for study of the emotional life in patients who present evidence of an organic lesion. The either-or concept in medicine must be displaced by the idea of how much of the problem is psychological and how much of it is physical and what is the relationship between the two. When we come to the question of peptic ulcer this phase of psychopathology will be discussed further.

Psychosomatic Study

Physicians with greater interest in psychological medicine find a much higher percentage of patients with symptoms referable to the gastrointestinal tract in whom emotional factors are chiefly responsible for the illness. Stevenson, in a study of 150 patients presenting themselves to a gastrointestinal clinic, found that there was an important emotional problem in two thirds of the cases and Robinson, in a thoughtful analysis of fifty patients with digestive complaints, found that in two thirds of them no organic lesion or unhygienic habits could be discovered to account for the symptoms. Moreover, the latter author felt that many patients have digestive symptoms as a manifestation of personality disorder before they develop organic disease of the digestive tract and that the latter might be prevented if they were successfully treated. This seemed to be especially true with respect to peptic ulcer. He went on to say that functional nervousness, including fatigue and anxiety, was by far the greatest detectable cause of recurrences of peptic ulcer symptoms, and in many instances it seemed likely that the same etiological factors were initially responsible for the ulcer. He thought, therefore, that the question could legitimately be raised as to how many of these patients might have escaped peptic ulcer if their functional nervousness had been recognized and treated in the first place.

We made a study of 100 consecutive patients encountered in the practice of internal medicine who were considered to be psychosomatic gastrointestinal problems. Forty-four were classified under neurosis with gastrointestinal symptom formation; thirty as somatic disease plus symptoms in part of emotional origin; fourteen as vegetative neuroses.* Seven cases fell in the group of psychoses with gastrointestinal symptoms and five were labeled as hypochondriasis.

Among the neurotic cases with gastrointestinal symptoms twenty-one were listed as anxiety state, sixteen as conversion neurosis, five as compulsive neurosis, and there were two phobias.

Thus, as is well known, every variety of personality from the well adjusted to the psychotic may have psychosomatic disturbances of the gastrointestinal tract. As in other surveys the percentage of somatic disease represented about one third of all cases seen. This leaves, so far as the gastrointestinal field is concerned, about two thirds of the cases in which the gastrointestinal symptoms appear to be chiefly of psychogenic origin.

*A distinction is made between somatic disease with emotional factors, such as structural alterations of the gall tract with stone formation, and the vegetative neuroses. In the latter are included cardiospasm, peptic ulcer and ulcerative colitis.

We are persuaded from our own studies that emotional factors are the *chief* cause of gastrointestinal complaints and many other authors besides those cited could be quoted in support of this viewpoint. Nevertheless, if we took only the organic studies above referred to, in which diagnosis is established by exclusion, we would still have the very considerable number of 25 per cent of all patients with chronic dyspepsia labeled as functional, and to be approached, therefore, from a psychological standpoint.

The Approach to a Digestive Problem

Eusterman believes that when a patient presents digestive symptoms he may be considered in one of the following groups:

1. Unrecognized roentgenologically positive gastric disorders.

2. Roentgenologically negative disorders of the stomach itself.

3. Actual or apparent gastric disturbances resulting from disease of abdominal viscera other than the stomach.

4. Actual or apparent gastric disturbances resulting from disease remote from abdominal organs.

He then discussed these problems somewhat as follows:

1. **Unrecognized Roentgenologically Positive Gastric Disorders.** Peptic ulcer is the commonest intrinsic organic cause of chronic recurrent indigestion. Most such lesions are discovered by means of the x-ray. At least 5 per cent escape such detection. Benign and malignant neoplasm and granulomatous processes also cause appreciable filling defects and rarely escape the detection of the roentgenologist. Gastritis has in recent years assumed greater importance as a cause of digestive disturbance and its various forms have been described as a result of gastroscopy. Diaphragmatic hernias are also easily overlooked on routine x-ray examination and the suspicion of their presence calls for repeated examination with special technic.

2. **Roentgenologically Negative Disorders of the Stomach Itself.** This group is made up principally of the *gastric neuroses*. In a study previously cited by Macy and Allen of the Mayo Clinic in which 235 patients diagnosed as chronic nervous exhaustion were studied again after a period of six and one-half years, the accuracy of the diagnosis was established in 94 per cent of the cases, and of interest in this connection is the fact that the gastrointestinal tract was the point of origin of the major symptoms in the largest number of cases.

Eusterman mentioned certain features common to the gastric neuroses and helpful in their recognition:

1. The disturbances may be of long duration and yet complication or progression may be absent and the patient may be in good nutritional state.

2. Symptoms vary in the region where they appear, are variable in degree and are frequently continuous.

3. There is a lack of sequence so characteristic of the majority of organic lesions.

4. The pain or discomfort, when present, is usually diffuse and is often projected unaccountably.

5. While the patient may complain bitterly of disturbances during waking hours they may be completely absent at night.

6. Intermittent digestive disorders are often coincident with or follow emotional stress.

7. Physical disability is frequently marked and entirely out of proportion to the severity of the complaint.

8. There is usually present the evidence of other indications of a psychoneurotic personality.

3. **Gastric Disturbances Resulting from Disease of Abdominal Viscera Other Than the Stomach Itself.** From one third to two fifths of all chronic gastric disorders have their origin in disease of the gall-bladder, appendix, pancreas, liver, small bowel, colon, or such conditions as epigastric hernia or helminthiasis.

It is well known that *chronic cholecystitis* either with or without stones is the most common cause of the distressing chronic recurring types of dyspepsia affecting adults. At the Mayo Clinic each year 60 per cent more cases of cholecystic disease are seen than of chronic gastric and duodenal ulcer combined. In the study mentioned of Dwyer and Blackford in which 15 per cent of their dyspeptic patients had organic lesions of the stomach and duodenum, 21.3 per cent had disease of the gall-bladder. We believe it is also true that in no part of the gastrointestinal tract are emotional factors more important.

Cholecystographic examination is essential, especially in patients in whom the symptoms are mild and in patients who have not experienced characteristic biliary colic. It is impossible to consider this subject in detail but it may be said that in the absence of a typical train of symptoms and signs, a normal cholecystographic response suggests the necessity for conservative management.

The problem of *chronic appendicitis* will be dealt with separately. In Dwyer and Blackford's compilation of 3000 cases a chronically diseased appendix seemed to be the cause of gastric symptoms in 5.5 per cent.

Diseases of the *liver* and *pancreas* are occasionally responsible for gastric symptoms and the majority of instances of malignant neoplasm of the pancreas without jaundice have symptoms that are purely gastric in nature. The *large bowel*, especially spastic colitis and irritable colon, is responsible for a great deal of so-called "stomach trouble" and rare lesions such as epigastric hernia, Addison's disease, and intestinal parasites are occasionally responsible for gastric symptoms.

4. Gastric Disturbances from Outside the Abdomen. Pathological processes in organs remote fom the abdominal viscera or some systemic disease may be responsible for gastric symptoms. Disease of the circulatory, pulmonary, nervous, or urinary systems deserve first consideration. Next in order of importance are diseases of endocrine organs, deficiency diseases (pernicious anemia, pellagra, and sprue in particular); toxic states induced by noxious gases, heavy metals and drugs; and inordinate use of tobacco and alcohol. These various diseases and intoxications accounted for from 15 to 20 per cent of cases of chronic digestive disorders at the Mayo Clinic. Because of common innervation disease of one organ may reflexly produce spastic and hypersecretory disturbances in the other. It is well known that circulatory failure may produce passive congestion in the stomach, giving rise to impairment of gastric motility and secretion and even degenerative changes in gastric mucous membranes. Rarely are gastric disturbances the only expression of a disorder remote from the stomach. Routine and systematic physical examination, ordinary laboratory studies, and the simultaneous psychosomatic approach will usually disclose the true nature of the underlying cause.

The Clinical Picture of Gastric Dysfunction

According to Eusterman, motor, secretory, and inflammatory changes in the gastric mucous membranes cause symptoms that may be divided into the following syndromes:

1. Vague, mild or nondescript disturbances characterized by "gas," epigastric fulness, mild anorexia, or nausea.

2. Those of the nausea and vomiting type, as seen in the painless form of tabetic gastric crises, in migraine, uremia, and acute hyperthyroidism, and in some cases of cholecystic disease.

3. The catarrhal gastritis complex, in advanced cases the symptoms and signs being strongly suggestive of gastric cancer.

4. Those of the intestinal type, characterized by (a) the "irritable colon" complex or (b) chronic recurrent diarrhea, usually in association with achlorhydria.

5. The hemorrhagic type, in which hematemesis or melena is the predominant or exclusive symptom, as in portal cirrhosis, erosive and ulcerous gastritis, and ulcer in Meckel's diverticulum.

6. Ulcer-simulating, a not uncommon type, and

7. The pain-predominating type, as seen in the painful form of tabetic gastric crisis, in the abdominal form of angina pectoris, in periarteritis nodosa, and in the various sclerotic vascular abdominal conditions.

The cases which follow will illustrate some of these syndromes and call attention to the relationship between personality trends and symptom formation.

Constipation
Related to Social Anxiety; Good Response to Brief Psychotherapy

---

CASE 19

History and Symptoms

M. F., a white girl, aged nineteen, was first seen in the spring of 1942. She complained of constipation of several years duration, headaches, ulcers in the mouth, and fatigue. She had never been seriously ill and there were no other symptoms of importance except that she had had enuresis until she was sixteen. Her father and mother had never been compatible and the patient had always been aware of tension in the household. Finally the parents separated and the four children, of which our patient was the youngest, remained with the mother. At this time the enuresis ceased.

Social Competition

The general physical examination showed no evidence of disease and it quickly became apparent that more important than the symptoms complained of was a high degree of social anxiety in a hysterical person which had interfered with her social development. From a genetic standpoint, insecurity in personal relationships was of course related to the insecurity of childhood and the constipation apparently was a reflection of the tension growing out of social situations. One such situation which seemed to cause the most trouble was an attempt to compete with a pretty cousin. Anticipation of such competition would bring about headache and constipation which were aggravated by erroneous ideas regarding bowel obstruction and toxic poisoning.

Improvement

The origin of the symptoms was made clear and when she was reassured about the insignificance of the constipation and encouraged by the physician, who assumed the role of a friendly parent in trying to give her a little more self-confidence and urging her to cultivate new interests and friends, she improved remarkably and blossomed out into a friendly creature who in turn "found everybody more friendly." Incidentally constipation no longer was a problem.

Recurrence

During a period of a year and a half her progress continued and then suddenly new symptoms appeared. She suffered from vertigo and had pain in the epigastrium. It was not difficult to ascertain that she was forced again to compete with a very attractive young woman in a new circle of boys and girls in which she felt insecure. Once more a single interview succeeded in pointing out the source of anxiety and permitted once again the opportunity for more reassurance and the acquisition of more confidence.

No Mention of Psychotherapy

Here, without mentioning psychotherapy, the physician assumed the parental role, taking the attention of the patient away from the symptom and attaching it to life circumstance. It would be fine for this young woman to have the advantages of psychoanalysis but since that is clearly out of the question we must get along with less. There is no doubt that transference played the important role and was deliberately utilized. Re-education regarding the emotional development was the basis of the brief, and in this case, superficial psychotherapy, although of course psychotherapy is not necessarily superficial just because it is brief. Nor is there any denying that the patient remains dependent on the physician and will have to return from time to time as she encounters new situations. Is it not better, however, to treat a patient with constipation in this manner than to make this young woman dependent upon laxatives or enemas and perhaps start her on a career of gastrointestinal invalidism? So often we find the criticism leveled at the psychotherapist that he does not cure people—they remain dependent upon him. No one expects the diabetic specialist to cure his patient; when he regulates the diet and adjusts a dosage of insulin and carries his patient along successfully everyone is satisfied. Why cannot the psychotherapist be permitted the same privilege of administering reassurance and enlightenment in regulated dosages, knowing full well that in the greatest number of instances he cannot hope to achieve cure but only strive to make the patient a healthier, happier and more efficient individual?

"Nervous Indigestion"
Traumatic Precipitating Event; Relation to Early Life Experiences; Anxiety Attacks; Treatment

---

CASE 20

A white man, age twenty-seven, was first seen in June, 1940. He, himself, stated his complaint as "nervous indigestion."

History and Symptoms

Since the fall of 1934 he had suffered from attacks of "nervous indigestion," and he had been under the care of many physicians. Complete studies had been made which failed to reveal any organic cause. His principal digestive complaint was nausea which came in attacks when there was any variation from his established routine. Further inquiry revealed that the nausea was preceded by loss of appetite, considerable belching, a feeling of tension in the throat, and the fear that he might vomit or have an involuntary bowel movement. Because of these fears he tried to plan his days in such a way that he was never far from a lavatory and it was only after some time that we learned how far his business and social life had been restricted by this necessity. With an attack he had considerable anxiety, the hands and feet became cold, and he perspired freely. The attacks had become more frequent and he had lost a few pounds in weight.

Past History. He had been a sickly child, had had considerable ear trouble and many operations. He felt that he had been much handicapped by his frequent hospital experiences and long illness and that it was only about the time of puberty that he began to develop as a healthy person should. During his teens he considered himself in excellent health.

Family History. The mother had died suddenly of heart disease at the age of fifty-two in 1931. The father died from a gunshot accident at the age of fifty-seven in 1934. More will be said of this shortly. An older sister was in good health. The grandparents had been long lived and there was nothing else of medical importance in the family history.

Physical Examination and Laboratory Studies

The patient was tall and thin and seemed somewhat pale. Temperature, pulse and respirations were within normal limits and the blood pressure was normal. The general physical examination disclosed no evidence of organic disease. Ordinary laboratory studies were within normal limits and a gastro-intestinal x-ray series, including a barium enema, showed no evidence of abnormality. Gastric analysis showed a fairly high acid curve but no other indications of abnormality.

LIFE SITUATION

The patient's family had always been in comfortable circumstances and he had been a pampered child, chiefly because of the many illnesses during his childhood. He had grown up to be a healthy young man, however, and considered himself well adjusted. He took an active interest in his father's business and during the summer months when he was not at school he frequently acted as his father's chauffeur.

Death of Father

In the fall of 1934 he was hunting with his father when a gun was accidentally discharged and his father suffered serious head injuries which shortly proved fatal. In spite of the fact that he was in no way responsible for the accident he continued to blame himself for his father's death and it was at this time that his "nervous indigestion" began. As time wore on and more and more people in whom he had confidence assured him that he was blameless his digestive disturbance improved somewhat but he was never completely free of discomfort.

Dependence on Toilet

Meanwhile he had married and apparently had adjusted well to marriage and had also begun a business career in which he was getting along satisfactorily. His illness, however, had circumscribed his activities severely so that he felt that his opportunities for advancement were limited so long as his illness continued. On close questioning it was revealed that it was not so much nausea which disturbed him as the idea that he might embarrass himself and the people around him by the necessity for vomiting or having an involuntary bowel movement and hence he could never allow himself to be far away from a toilet. His days were planned so that he would always know that he was going to be near a toilet and his appointments were planned with special regard to meal time so that he would be unlikely to vomit. This, in spite of the fact that he never once had vomited. The constant thought in his mind whenever he made any social plans or business appointments was "suppose I take sick—what shall I do?"

TREATMENT

On reviewing his early life history it became clear that he had always suffered from an overstrict conscience and that as a young man he could never forgive himself for any mishaps, actual or fancied. For example, he had done less experimenting with sex than the average young man and yet he could not get rid of his guilt over what were relatively minor transgressions.

The next point of importance which developed was that although he had stated at first that all guilt over his father's death had vanished it became quite clear with detailed conversation that he still held himself responsible and when anything happened which reactivated his guilt an attack of indigestion, which was in reality an anxiety attack, would occur.

Overconscientious Personality

We pointed out that he was the kind of personality that was over-conscientious and overscrupulous and hence burdened with excessive guilty feelings and that he therefore was bound to react as he had to his father's death. He confessed that he always labored under the feeling that he did not deserve to be happy. After this conversation, in which he had an opportunity to air his feelings thoroughly, he felt considerably elated and engaged in some frivolity with his associates at his place of business. He later stated that in the middle of this sudden happiness a thought had flashed through his mind, "something terrible is going to happen." It thus became clear that he did not have the capacity for enjoyment unless at the same time he envisaged the possibility of suffering.

Toilet Training

Conversation with an old family retainer who had acted as his childhood nurse revealed that he had been subjected to very strict toilet training and that during his first year or year and a half he cried a great deal when he was placed on the toilet and finally a physician had said that there was something the matter with the rectum and a minor operation was performed. After that he became very docile but developed some fears, such as fear of the dark, and during the period of his ear infections he frequently became "hysterical when attended by the physician."

On subsequent occasions it was pointed out to him that his fears of vomiting or of having a bowel movement and thus embarrassing himself and other people were probably related to his overstrict training in childhood when he became docile on the surface but probably resentful and spiteful underneath. And now it would seem that his fears of "making a mess" were probably related to unconscious wishes to do just that in order to gain attention. In other words, fears, in reality, are often disguised wishes, and so we can readily understand that as a pampered and spoiled youngster whose attention had been focused unduly on toilet training he may have turned to this means of attracting attention from his caretakers even though it involved censure or punishment. Now as an adult his conscious wish was just the reverse, that is, to be neat, clean, orderly, and overconscientious but still existing within him were certain infantile patterns of behavior which translated themselves into bodily symptoms.

Results of Treatment

For the first month or six weeks he was seen once a week and was given an opportunity to relate the intimate details of the hunting accident which preceded the onset of his illness. It was revealed to him how his overconscientious personality was bound to react to his father's death by his self-accusation of being responsible. By airing this matter on several occasions, combined with the reassurance that we were able to give him, and the conviction that he had taken more responsibility than he should have, his anxiety gradually diminished and his digestive attacks became less intense and occurred at longer intervals. Combined with this was the explanation concerning his early life toilet training and bowel habits and how they in turn were now related to his present difficulty. He became a much happier and more efficient person and was finally able to plan his days so that he no longer thought of the question of being near a toilet. No longer did his "life surround his bowel movements."

SUMMARY

A young man developed "nervous indigestion" following his father's death from an accident for which he felt responsible. Guilt reactivated infantile patterns of behavior of the gastrointestinal tract. After much medical investigation and treatment, satisfactory recovery followed psychotherapy.

An important lesson, which needs constant reemphasis, is the necessity for a balanced viewpoint in the psychosomatic approach to clinical problems. The following case is illustrative.

Syphilis of the Central Nervous System Thought to be "Nervous Indigestion"

CASE 21

A white man of forty-five was first seen in July, 1939. He presented himself with a diagnosis of "nervous indigestion" and said the trouble was due to his business.

History and Symptoms

For about five years he had suffered from loss of appetite, nausea, which was especially marked in the morning, and a gradual loss of weight amounting to about 20 pounds.

He stated that he had never had a serious illness. He had gonorrhea as a young man but made a good recovery and volunteered the information that repeated Wassermann tests since then had been negative. He had been married on two occasions and both wives had been pregnant but apparently had had abortions induced. There were no children.

Family History. Patient was an only child. The parents and grand-parents had been long lived and there was nothing of significance in the family history.

Present Illness. When the trouble first appeared he had had cramps with the bowel movement and occasional vomiting attacks. Then nausea appeared and the cramps subsided. The nausea had been most pronounced in the morning. He confessed that he had been worried about "stomach ulcers." He had always consumed alcohol to excess but since the onset of his stomach trouble he had taken only an occasional drink but he still smoked to excess.

Physical Examination and Laboratory Studies

It was immediately noted in the general physical examination that the pupils were irregular and failed to react to light and that the knee jerks were diminished. The general physical examination otherwise was negative except for a small scar on the foreskin of the penis and on further questioning he then recalled that during the period of the infection with gonorrhea he had also had a small lesion on the penis which, however, promptly healed and he had not shown further concern about it. He was referred to the hospital where a gastrointestinal x-ray series was negative for organic disease but the spinal fluid showed an increase of cells, an increased amount of protein, and a strongly positive Wassermann reaction. Neurological consultation confirmed the diagnosis of *tabes dorsalis.*

LIFE SITUATION

He had always been in the brokerage business and while he had managed to make things go during the early years of the depression he had changed his business connections in 1935 and shortly afterwards noted the onset of his stomach trouble. The circumstances under which he worked were very tense and he felt confident that his trouble was due to the nature of his business and the reversal in his financial circumstances.

SUMMARY

Here was a middle-aged patient who made his own diagnosis of nervous indigestion which he felt was due to the nature of his business and his financial difficulties but in whom studies demonstrated the presence of tabes dorsalis.

A scrutiny of his life history revealed no evidence of previous neurotic symptoms and our admonition will be borne in mind that it is unlikely for a neurotic symptom to appear for the first time at middle age. In other words personality study should reveal some evidence of a neurotic personality to support the diagnosis of neurosis. Moreover, the general physical examination demonstrated evidence of an organic disease which could be responsible for gastrointestinal symptoms.

We have often been impressed by the fact that patients who make their own diagnosis of neurosis or difficulties of emotional origin frequently have organic disease and the reverse is much more frequent, that is, patients who insist "there must be some physical basis" for their symptoms usually have an emotional background for the illness.

NERVOUS VOMITING

In a review of 140 cases of functional vomiting Wilbur and Washburn found that in most cases there were characteristic clinical and diagnostic features. Continued vomiting which is usually without effort, nausea, or significant abdominal symptoms and which occurs within an hour after meals is typically functional. Most patients were women between the ages of twenty and forty years, who, while they were relatively healthy in appearance, presented evidence of instability of the nervous system. In sixty, or 43 per cent of the cases in the series, operation, and particularly appendectomy, had been performed for the vomiting without benefit to the patients.

Many types of treatment had been tried but the keystone of treatment was psychotherapy.

The following case is illustrative:

Nervous Vomiting
Repressed Sexuality; Conflict over Marriage; Favorable Result
from Psychotherapy

CASE 22

History and Symptoms

A young married woman was first seen in February, 1940, complaining of attacks of vomiting, which were usually most pronounced in the morning.

The trouble began about three years before and on two occasions during that period she had hospital observation but no organic cause had been found. The diagnosis on both occasions had been spastic colitis.

Menstruation had been established normally and was always regular but she was often troubled with vomiting at the time of her menstrual period. The patient had been married for a little more than two years but had not been pregnant.

Physical Examination and Laboratory Studies

The patient had lost a few pounds in a recent severe attack of vomiting but still was a well-nourished person without signs of obvious illness. The general examination disclosed no evidence of organic disease. Gynecolological examination was negative.

Routine laboratory studies and basal metabolism were within normal limits. Gastric analysis and gastrointestinal x-ray series disclosed no abnormalities. Biliary drainage and cholecystogram were normal.

LIFE SITUATION

The patient reported that her fear of eating in the presence of others led her to shun people and thus her life was more or less secluded. She became a burden to her husband and parents by restricting their social lives and making increasing demands on their attention.

Her illness began at the age of eleven, shortly after the birth of her youngest sister. At that time, she developed fears for her father's safety whenever he failed to return home promptly. These fears continued for several years. At seventeen she suffered from attacks of nausea whenever she had a date with a young man. On one occasion, when kissed by a man, she suddenly became sick and began to vomit. The vomiting persisted for several days, during which time she was conscious of what she described as a "sexual" odor which had emanated from the man. Shortly thereafter she was courted by another man whom her mother urged her to marry. She resented her mother's interference, but submitted to her wishes, and, as will be seen, characteristically reserved the right to punish her later. On the day of her marriage she felt nauseated and the wedding trip had to be shortened on account of her persistent vomiting. On her return home, she spent a week with her mother until her symptoms subsided. Sexual relations during this period were impossible because of vaginismus. When they did take place later she was, for the most part, frigid.

Dependence on Mother

During the few years of her married life, there had been a number of recurrences of vomiting. The attacks usually occurred when she was angry with her husband or parents. On one occasion, she began to vomit after being advised by a physician to have a child. This, by the way, was his therapeutic advice as a cure for her vomiting. During a period of vomiting, she was troubled by disturbing thoughts concerning the death of relatives. She stated that there seemed to be a "devil" inside her which the vomiting served to get rid of. When well, the patient was a comparatively adequate housewife, but during attacks she became helplessly dependent and spent most of her time with her mother. She had even crept into bed with her mother and cuddled up like a baby and at times had insisted that her mother literally feed her with a spoon. In addition, her vomiting became particularly violent in the presence of her mother, although when alone she could usually control it. She said that she could not give her mother the satisfaction of seeing her comfortable. Once, when her mother remonstrated with her, the patient replied that the mother had no reason for complaining since she, at least, was well; furthermore, she must suffer because the patient was her child. One could readily see the personality of a self-centered individual who had very little consideration for others and tried to dominate them in a passive and dependent way.

Vomiting an Expression of Hostility

Her resentment against her mother at the time of her marriage was based on her belief that her mother was rushing her into marriage in order to get rid of her. This led to a half-conscious desire to punish the mother by her illness, which was actually expressed when she said that her mother deserved to suffer for making her get married when she wasn't ready for it. In her anxiety to obtain affection, however, she had to convince herself that she was in love with her husband lest he leave her. On the other hand, however, she felt that he did not really love her, but had married her because of her money. She suspected that he preferred his own mother to her. This unspoken accusation always came up whenever she quarreled with him; at which times she would feel a surge of intense hatred against him, associated with death wishes. This was tied up with the suspicion that her father did not really love her but preferred her mother, which caused her to be resentful against him. The attacks of vomiting at such times were the result of her unexpressed hostility because her passive nature would not permit her to express her hostility directly.

TREATMENT

As she was permitted little by little to understand some of the forces that were responsible for her vomiting attacks they diminished in number and intensity and for a period of about one year she had enjoyed freedom from vomiting.

SUMMARY

A young white woman, with markedly repressed sexuality, developed frequent vomiting attacks after a marriage to which she had assented because of her mother's urging. Her passive and dependent nature did not allow her to express hostility openly but instead her unconscious mental forces caused her to vomit as though to say, "I cannot stomach this situation." Gradually she was made aware of some of her hostile feelings and hence no longer had to resort to vomiting attacks to express herself. This led to considerable improvement not only in her gastrointestinal function but also in her ability to taste more fully of life in general.

MENTAL DEPRESSION WITH DIGESTIVE SYMPTOMS

Elsewhere we will discuss the clinical importance of recognition of depression as a definite clinical syndrome. One of the characteristic features of this symptom picture is a digestive disorder. The following case is illustrative.

Two Attacks of Mild Depression with Digestive Symptoms; Precipitated by Financial Losses; Prompt Recovery

---

CASE 23

A man of forty years was first seen in 1931. He complained of loss of appetite, sleeplessness, depression of mood, "all-gone" feelings and shakiness.

History and Symptoms

He had always considered himself a healthy person and had never suffered from a serious illness.

Family History. Father and mother were living and well, as were three brothers and two sisters. There was no mental or nervous disease in the family.

Present Illness. He had always been successful in the real estate business until the depression began and then he had lost a great deal of money. He had tried to keep the knowledge from his wife because he didn't want to disturb her but gradually he found himself sleepless and then came loss of appetite and the symptoms related above.

Physical Examination and Laboratory Studies

The patient was a well-nourished, robust, white man with normal blood pressure and normal cardiovascular system. The remainder of the physical examination was negative except for the presence of a few hemorrhoids which he attributed to recent constipation. Routine laboratory studies were negative.

LIFE SITUATION

A review of his life situation indicated how dependent he had been upon his real estate holdings for a feeling of security and now that he had lost considerable of his estate it was pointed out that his "all-gone" feelings and his feelings of shakiness indicated his insecurity. It was obvious that he was in no critical situation from the viewpoint of his financial standing and a discussion of this fact seemed to revive his spirits somewhat. He was placed on 1/4 grain phenobarbital three times a day and in a week reported that he was sleeping slightly better but still felt depressed in mood especially in the morning. His treatment was continued and it was recommended that he once more interest himself in golf, in which he had been active previously but had given up when things were going bad at the office. One month later he reported that he was feeling quite well again. After this the patient was not seen until 1938.

Recurrence of Depression

Once more he complained of "all-gone" feelings in the lower abdomen, loss of strength, no ambition, awakening early in the morning with a feeling of depression, loss of appetite, and a loss of weight.

He himself observed that the same financial circumstances were at work now as had been true on the previous occasion. Not only was business bad but he felt himself under great financial strain. He felt that he had gotten over his previous depression quickly and that he had been well since and he hoped that the same thing might happen once more.

Again physical examination failed to disclose any evidence of organic disease and once more he was reassured when he had an opportunity to discuss his actual financial situation which was in no sense critical. Again it was pointed out to him that he had always been the kind of person who had to accumulate funds and real estate holdings in order to feel secure and that on two occasions in question his losses had been great enough to threaten his security. Hence, he became depressed, symbolized his weakness with his "all-gone" feeling in the lower abdomen, and at the same time lost his appetite as he had lost his zest for living. Once more he was placed on mild sedation and once again he responded although some depression of mood continued for several months.

SUMMARY

A middle-aged white man who presented the clinical picture of mental depression complained chiefly of digestive symptoms. Recovery followed superficial psychotherapy. Recurrence at the end of seven years followed the same precipitating cause. The importance of recognizing the mental depression rests not only upon the psychological approach to the digestive symptoms but on the greater necessity of recognizing a serious disorder of the personality often leading to suicide.

This point is discussed more fully elsewhere (p. 406).

Not all neurotic problems are amenable to treatment. The following case was helped somewhat by superficial explanation and reassurance; he did not seem to be a satisfactory personality for more intensive psychotherapy.

**Gastrointestinal Symptoms; Character Problem
Unsuitable for Psychotherapy**

CASE 24

A fifty-year-old white man was first seen in June, 1938. He complained of fatigue and backache, "slow digestion and accompanying toxemia."

History and Symptoms

He stated that he had never been a very healthy person and that he had always had a poor digestion. In childhood he suffered from vomiting spells and described himself as a sleepy youngster. During his school days he suffered from constipation and a continuation of his digestive trouble. The only times he could remember feeling fairly well were a few summers which he spent on a farm; then he added that he could keep in pretty fair condition if he took outdoor exercise. He admitted that worry and nervous strain affected his stomach but only "because of the weakness existing there."

Present Illness. Trouble had begun about three years ago when fatigue and backache gradually made their appearance. Sometimes he would awaken during the night with a pain in his back and he would be unable to put himself in a comfortable position in order to fall back to sleep. His attending physician thought that chronic appendicitis might be responsible and subsequently the appendix was removed and while he felt he had been benefited to some extent he was still troubled by fatigue, backache and sluggish digestion. He himself suggested that the rest in bed, "thorough cleaning out," and the meager diet were probably responsible for temporary relief. Then he visited a well-known gastroenterologist and was thoroughly studied "without anything of clinical significance being found." Finally he was studied by an orthopedist who suggested that his back discomfort was probably of large bowel origin even though the x-ray study had disclosed no evidence of organic disease.

He felt that his sluggishness was due to a "toxic condition" probably dependent upon his sluggish digestion and poor bowel function. Frequently he would force himself to vomit and he was addicted to the enema habit—both for the purpose of relieving his "autointoxication."

Family History. Father and mother were still living and in fair health. There were two brothers and a sister. All could be described as in fair health, but none was robust.

The patient had been married for twenty-five years and had two grown children both of whom were in good health.

Physical Examination and Laboratory Studies

The patient was a well-nourished, tall, stoop-shouldered person who constantly wore the expression of depression. Blood pressure was normal and the cardiovascular system seemed perfectly normal including electrocardiogram. The examination of the abdomen showed generalized slight tenderness but no rigidity and no organs or masses were made out. The rectum and prostate were normal and the remainder of the physical examination was normal. Routine laboratory studies including sedimentation rate, basal metabolic rate, and Wassermann test were normal. At the patient's own request the gastrointestinal x-ray series was repeated in another laboratory and was found to be perfectly normal and the gastric analysis revealed a normal acid curve.

TREATMENT

We explained to the patient that our examination showed no evidence of organic disease, and then suggested that his symptoms could not be divorced from his life situation. We gave him the further lead that the abdomen is the sounding board of the emotions and that disturbances in the emotional life often cause disturbances in the function of the gastrointestinal tract; hence, spasms of the bowel might occur, gas might accumulate beneath the diaphragm and in that way cause pain in the back. We asked the patient to think back three or four years and see if there was any correlation between a disturbance in his emotional life and the onset of the backache. He then began with a statement that his domestic situation was not too satisfactory, that his wife had lost all interest in sexual intercourse, that he had always practiced withdrawal and that he himself found "that while the biological urge for intercourse was present, the psychological inspiration was lacking." Moreover, during the past year or so he had formed an attachment to another woman "who gave him a degree of companionship that he could not obtain from his wife." He had for some time been considering divorce and was on the point more than once of informing his wife "that he would pack up and get out."

It was obvious from his manner that he lived in a state of hate instead of love and we explained that the aggressive and hostile feelings, being unable to find a normal outlet, expressed themselves in a disturbance of his gastrointestinal tract. We explained to him that we probably were not telling him anything absolutely new; that he probably realized the general background of his trouble but that very often patients didn't quite put two and two together and that this kind of information at least removed any lingering doubt about organic disease and started them in the proper direction. We prescribed a little sedative and antispasmodic, explaining to the patient that it was only for relief of symptoms and not for cure. We did not pretend to give any advice regarding the domestic situation, only urging that he do nothing impulsive as a result of our conversation.

Follow-up. As could have been decided from first contact with the patient (he would be reluctant to acknowledge improvement) he stated that his back was not much better. Then on further questioning he said that perhaps his indigestion was slightly improved and that maybe his sleeping was a little bit better! Apparently he had gone a considerable distance in his arrangement with his girl but had said nothing to his wife nor to his father and mother. He stated that the father was too old and in no condition to be told; that the mother would side with his wife; and the wife, who asked him about a month before whether he had any outside interests, was told "No." "He does not like to hurt anybody's feelings" and yet it was clear that he felt guilty about the situation because otherwise, since he had already made up his mind to leave his wife and the problem was only one of when to do it, there was no longer conflict and therefore no cause for symptoms existed. But it was obvious that he did feel considerable guilt and this was the thing that was causing trouble. He had not had sex experience with the girl—*he* wouldn't want to and he didn't know whether she would or not. He had a cousin who was an intimate friend of his wife and a person for whom he had much respect and for whom he had done many favors. About a month before he told her about the problem and introduced her to his girl—he didn't know just why except "that a woman's viewpoint might be helpful" in deciding how to leave his wife—we thought it was to relieve himself of some guilt and to justify the thing that he was doing. But he chose a prejudiced source.

He was much impressed by the companionship that his girl offered him and it was evident that he derived much emotional satisfaction from the relationship. Since he considered that the decision was made we thought there was no point in trying to show him that his behavior was probably neurotic; it would only incur his displeasure and antagonism. It did not seem to be our duty to try to save the marriage against such odds. If he was indecisive then we might have pointed out that his behavior, just as his symptoms, was neurotic and that he ought to have some expert psychological help before trying to make up his mind. Like so many neurotics he seemed to have a neurotic wife; at any rate, her family background seemed the kind that would promote a neurotic problem.

We explained the simplicity of the prescription since it was not aimed at any fundamental therapy—this apparently appealed to him. The medicine helped him; his digestion, sleeping and the back improved; the ast still bothered him, but did not distrub him so much at night. The lother problem was the same, "he was still looking for advice."

SUMMARY

A middle-aged white man complained of digestive symptoms. Long-standing marital maladjustment seemed to be the background. His was a critical and suspicious personality and we thought it unwise to attempt more than superficial psychotherapy. *Sometimes the neurosis seems to be the best solution of the emotional problem.*

The following is a fairly common clinical problem. Because of the symptom of abdominal pain it will be presented here but the other and more important part of the clinical picture, *fatigue*, will be illustrated by cases to be presented in other chapters.

Pain Right Lower Quadrant; Extreme Fatigue; Low Fever of Obscure Origin

CASE 25

A single white woman, aged thirty years, was admitted to Temple University Hospital in February, 1938.

History and Symptoms

She stated that the present illness had been coming on for a year. She had suffered from increasing fatigue and exhaustion; sweating of hands, feet, and axilla; and insomnia accompanied by palpitation.

Two months before admission acute pain occurred in the right lower quadrant of the abdomen. The pain gradually disappeared, then two weeks before admission a similar attack occurred but the pain was more toward the center of the abdomen. This pain had persisted as a dull ache.

For the year before admission she had had a poor appetite and belching. Since her attack two months before there had been a slight fever (99.2° to 100° F.) in the evening. She had been told by her physician to take the evening temperature.

Past History. A diagnosis of "chronic appendicitis" was made six years ago. She was operated upon but was no different after operation.

A cystic ovary was removed at the same time. The patient had been constipated for a number of years and frequently took laxatives. Menses were normal.

Physical Examination and Laboratory Studies

Examination was negative except for slight fever and slight hypertension, 140 to 160 systolic over 95 to 110 diastolic. Eyegrounds showed vasospasm of terminal divisions of nasal arterioles but no retinitis.

During the first two weeks in the hospital the temperature rose to 99.2 in the evening; during the last week the temperature was normal. The sedimentation rate, repeated on three occasions, was normal.

X-ray studies of the gastrointestinal tract including barium enema were negative. Urine, blood count, blood Wasstermann, blood sugar and urea nitrogen were normal. Basal metabolism was minus 9 per cent.

The patient stated that some doctors called her illness colitis; others had said "nerves," "ulcerous obstruction," or "hidden abscess." She described the attacks as coming on at night like "labor pains" and also said, "it was like a knife being pushed in slowly and drawn out again at regular intervals." She felt as though "food went by the area, like a boil."

LIFE SITUATION

The patient was a stenographer who had worked for twelve years at one job. The father "was always waiting for something to turn up" but had been unsuccessful so that the patient contributed all of her salary to the upkeep of the home. She said that she did not mind this.

Family Problem

The *father*, sixty-nine years old, was described by the patient as being "exactly opposite" to the mother. "My father is weak and quiet. Really, he has a negative personality. When I was little he used to tease me and mock me, but now he doesn't pay much attention to anything. If anyone will listen to him, he talks on and on about politics or some subject like that without showing any interest in the person he is talking to." The patient had never known her father to have a friend. He spent all of his time with his family when not engaged in business activities. He was affectionate but undemonstrative, generous and ambitious but inept and despondent. His family always feared that he would commit suicide. He kept a revolver, which he showed to the patient when she was twelve years old, telling her that he would probably end his life that way. She no longer feared that he would do this because he had become so inattentive, disinterested, and placid in the last few years. He had a very good memory for past events but was inclined to be very absent-minded and forgetful of the present. Since he lost his money in 1929, he had had no employment and had been inactive.

The *mother* was very resentful toward her husband. She was dissatisfied with her own life and that of her children. She resented her husband's financial failure during the depression when he tried to "double his money" in the stock market. So the mother at the age of sixty had given up nearly all of her former friends because she believed that they would not like her since she no longer had money.

The patient described her mother as being very youthful, ambitious, cheerful, but domineering. She had many friends and in spite of her husband's shyness and asocial tendencies, she led an active social life. The patient believed that her mother did not consciously dominate her father but that he always waited for his wife to take the initiative. The mother had always been a capable and energetic person, adhering somewhat compulsively to routine. She had been a strict disciplinarian with her children, not hesitating to employ corporal punishment, but nevertheless she seemed to love, indeed to overprotect them.

The patient had one *brother*. He was thirty-four years of age, married and living in his own home. He was described as being chronically dissatisfied with his relatives, friends, position, school, and possessions. He was irritable, inconsiderate, and quarrelsome.

There was a *sister* two years younger than the patient. The two were constant companions. The patient said of her sister, "She seemed like the older sister; I've always been the baby sister. She is bigger than I am. She was always more active and sociable than I was, and she always took the lead."

Early Life

History of the patient's birth, walking, talking, and dentition was negative. She knew nothing about her toilet training. She was breast fed and weaned when she was nine months old. She was a shy, quiet child, avoiding everyone outside of her immediate family. She believed herself to have been the favorite child of both her parents although no great preference was ever shown. The father favored her, she thought, because she was so much like him. She said the mother could not have helped favoring her somewhat because as a child she followed her mother about continually.

The children were never permitted to leave home to play and other children were not encouraged to visit them. Their companionship was limited almost entirely to several cousins and a favored few children on summer vacations. The patient said, "We were never allowed to play out of mother's sight." The patient said that she was well as a child, but the mother had often said, "You were well as long as you were under my care."

The patient regarded herself as an obedient child and easily controlled, while her brother and sister had to be punished. As she grew older she never argued with her mother as her brother and sister did, but in any conflict she would "walk away and do as she wished."

At night she was often afraid that she heard burglars in the house. She would leave her bed and go to her parents' room where she usually spent the rest of the night sleeping with her mother and father. In her early teens she feared that the world would end. She attended church and tried to act just as her religion required, but she said that she always felt "outside," as if she were "just going through the motions." There was a history of enuresis until the thirteenth year. She felt ashamed of this but since her sister had a similar history the matter did not concern her greatly.

Education

School was delayed until the patient was seven years old because her mother believed children of six to be too young to begin school and be away from home so long. Her progress was normal and her grades were average, but liable to considerable variation if she disliked a subject. She was shy and extremely self-conscious about her personal appearance because she was overweight. She engaged in very little social activity—still depending largely on her sister for companionship. After graduation from high school the patient had no further interest in education. Her mother opposed education for girls and preferred that her daughter take the stenographic position which she had held ever since.

Sexual Life

The patient reached puberty with amazingly little information about sex. Until she was fourteen she believed babies came from department stores and that she herself had been so purchased. She began menstruating at eleven; she had been told the manifestations of menstruation but knew nothing of its significance. She expressed almost no curiosity about sexual matters and seemed completely blind to the whole subject. When she was sixteen friends gave her a pamphlet discussing the anatomy of sexual organs. Even then she supposed that the fetus was normally delivered by cesarean section and not until she was eighteen did she know just how birth was accomplished.

With her "boy friends" she was shy and unresponsive. She said, "I didn't know what to expect nor how to react." She believed that one man whom she had particularly liked left her and married another girl because he found her so cold and unresponsive. At another time she broke an engagement because her fiance became moody about having lost his job. She said, "I didn't care whether he had a job, but he brooded and didn't come to see me; so I sent his ring back." This engagement had been a long one. The patient had put off marrying because a friend of her fiance wished to marry her at the same time and although she had no great affection for him she did not want to "hurt him" by marrying someone else.

For the past eight years a man at her place of employment had been attentive to her but was very unreliable because of his attachment to his mother. The immediate problem which worried her was her unsatisfactory relationship with this man. She felt that they were ideally suited, their interests and personalities being compatible. But he was the only son of a widowed mother who completely enslaved him. The mother had violent temper tantrums if the son had any friendships with women. His dates with the patient had to be kept secret as he feared his mother's outbursts would lead to a stroke. This secrecy was distasteful to the patient and she became very irritable with him, sometimes in a deliberate effort to make him "break away from his mother's apron strings." After one such occasion which led to a break in their relationship another girl in the same office became friendly with the man. The patient stated that "she went around in a daze and couldn't swallow." But she continued to work in the same office under those humiliating circumstances. It was obvious that she was undergoing repeated pain and disillusionment in her everyday contacts and that, as she stated, "she could not find peace or contentment either at home or in the office."

MANAGEMENT

We felt that it would be very difficult to influence this passive and dependent creature but we thought that we did succeed in convincing her that her illness was not of physical origin but rather the result of her continued emotional stress. We tried to show her that her constant pain and disillusionment were responsible for her physical symptoms. In relation to the slight elevation of temperature we suggested that this was only one manifestation of a disturbed constitution and that it had been an error to focus attention on the fever and regard that as the central problem. In reality the fever was one of the less important symptoms and once the patient was thoroughly studied it was dismissed. The *fatigue* was the important symptom because it kept the patient an invalid or semi-invalid. The fatigue, in turn, appeared to be due to the large expenditure of energy on her emotional conflicts. This problem will be discussed in more detail elsewhere (see p. 502). We tried to show her that she must make her own life rather than constantly offer herself up for sacrifice to her friends and relatives.

Follow-up

Two years after her hospital experience we reestablished contact with the patient. She reported that her general health had improved remarkably, that she was more active, energetic, less subject to pain, and consequently more happy. She had not missed any time from work. Nevertheless her problems were not very different, but she was able to handle them without suffering physical distress. Once more the man in question was trying to reestablish his friendship with her but feeling that the situation was hopeless she repulsed him. This we felt was a definite step in the right direction because it was obvious that his friendship could mean nothing to her and that while she was of a marriageable age she must make an effort to establish other friendships.

The problems were no different at home either. The mother was still discontented and the father still more dreamy and unrealistic than ever and there was a great deal of friction between them. She confessed that she was unable to handle this situation and that she and her sister had even considered establishing separate homes, that is, the sister and the mother to live together and she and her father in a separate establishment. It seemed obvious that she must establish her own life if she was going to have any peace and contentment but it was questionable whether she could do so. She had cut herself off from an indecisive man but whether she could do the same thing with regard to her family was doubtful. However, it did seem that she was no longer physically sick. She had at least improved that much.

SUMMARY

A single woman complained of pain in the abdomen, fatigue, and slight fever. She was a passive creature who played a martyr role and expressed her discontent in bodily symptoms. Fatigue was the most important part of the clinical picture and emotional conflict seemed responsible. The slight fever was an insignificant phase of the disordered constitution. Psychotherapy gave some help.

Chapter XII

THE GASTROINTESTINAL SYSTEM (Continued)

CHRONIC APPENDICITIS

Our attention was first called to this important problem many years ago by the following case:

A young woman at the age of nineteen had her first attack of pain in the right lower quadrant. At twenty the appendix was removed. Six months later she had a pelvic operation because of painful menstruation. At twenty-six years she had her third operation for abdominal adhesions. For the next four years she complained more or less constantly and had been in bed for considerable periods because of the pain in the right side. Stricture of the right ureter was suspected but not proved and finally, after a great deal of hospital investigation, a fourth operation was performed in the belief that there was disease of the large bowel, but all organs were found normal.

Here, then, was a patient who had been incapacitated for many years and who during this period of time had been repeatedly subjected to searching physical investigations and many abdominal operations. What the many physicians attending her had not discovered, or did not know the significance of, was that this long illness began shortly after the fourth of her five sisters married and this patient thought that she would in all likelihood remain a spinster and would then endure a life of drudgery and comparative loneliness. Meek and submissive, unattractive and unintelligent, she unconsciously turned to illness when she found it impossible to compete with her sister's superiority. Further personality studies disclosed her very immature emotional development and confirmed the opinion that the sister's marriage had precipitated an invalid reaction in this psychoneurotic individual.

Chronic Invalidism

A great many chronic invalids with multiple surgical scars upon the abdomen have begun their invalid career with the simple removal of a so-called "chronic appendix." Fortunately the problem is not now encountered as frequently as fifteen or twenty years ago. It was then that operations for pain in the right lower quadrant of the abdomen were frequently done for "chronic appendicitis," and the pathologist, we may say, played into the surgeon's hands by reporting *involutional* changes in terms of disease. Please do not understand that we are accusing the surgeon of a deliberate deception—quite the contrary—he was deceived by his organic training into thinking *that he could cut out of the body a pain that had its origin in the emotional life.* We are not going to discuss whether there is such a thing as "chronic appendicitis," but we certainly know that it is not nearly so common as was once believed.

Alvarez, interested in this question, several years ago opened a note book in which he gathered data to help him decide when and when not to recommend an interval appendectomy. Whenever he saw a patient with a scar in the right lower quadrant of the abdomen he asked why the operation was done, what were the symptoms complained of, were there any acute attacks of appendicitis, and what was the result obtained?

Significance of Acute Attack

On studying the histories of 385 patients who, some years before, had submitted to appendectomy, Alvarez found that only two of 225 who had never had an acute attack of appendicitis were cured, while 87 or 67 per cent of the 130 who had had at least one acute attack of abdominal pain, were cured.

He had not accumulated many records before it became apparent what the important point in the patients' histories was. Evidently there was one simple question the answer to which could immediately have told the surgeon whether or not he would be justified in operating for "chronic appendicitis." This question was: Did the patient ever have one or more attacks of abdominal pain around the navel or in the right lower quadrant, pain severe enough to put him to bed, to keep him awake much of the night and to cause the attending physician to diagnose or greatly suspect the presence of acute appendicitis? In most of the cases in which, after one or more such attacks, a young man or woman suffered with indigestion, nausea, loss of appetite, abdominal discomfort, toxic feelings, occasional cramps, and a loss of energy and joy of life, appendectomy worked a decided cure. On the other hand, in almost every case in which there was no history suggesting a previous acute attack of appendicitis, the operation was fruitless.

Alvarez stated that there is still great need for showing the medical profession the almost complete hopelessness of performing appendectomy in cases in which no history can be obtained of acute attacks of abdominal pain and also for showing physicians that appendectomy can no longer be looked to as a cure for neuroses, fatigue states, "mucous colitis," constipation, diarrhea, migraine, duodenal ulcer, cholecystitis, or regurgitation.

In a similar study on a smaller series of patients, Heintzelman and Evans agree with Alvarez but also emphasize that the patients with disturbed digestion on a functional basis (old-fashioned "nervous indigestion") can have—indeed, are more likely than others to have—acute appendicitis. One must be careful not to miss such an attack. Each of their patients with nervous indigestion who had an attack of acute appendicitis obtained relief from the digestive disorders after the appendectomy for periods up to one year. Not one of these patients obtained permanent relief, all reacting exactly as those submitting to operation for chronic appendicitis.

We agree with the conclusions offered by these studies and present the following cases* in some detail in order to illustrate the background of the problem.

"Chronic Appendicitis"
Childhood Neurosis; Neurotic Home Atmosphere; Pains as Protest Against Environment
Appendectomy; Return of Symptoms; Poor Prognosis

CASE 26

A white schoolgirl, fifteen years old, was admitted to Temple University Hospital in March, 1938.

History and Symptoms

She complained of *pain* in the right lower quadrant and stated that she had had vague pains in this region for several years. On December 22, 1937, she was preparing to leave the house when she developed sharp pains, became nauseated and vomited. The pain disappeared and returned February 17, 1938. There was no vomiting with the last attack. The pain radiated around to the back and down the legs and "passed up the spine to the head." She also complained of pain in the mastoid regions.

The pain in the right lower quadrant became progressively worse, was exaggerated by motion and disappeared with rest. On March 16, the pain was so severe that she could not go to school. Her physician found tenderness in the "appendix region" and referred her to the hospital for investigation.

*Additional cases in which the appendix has been removed because of "chronic appendicitis" will be found on pages 395-402.

In the hospital the patient complained of pain in the lower right quadrant, but also in the chest and in the legs. She stated that she had experienced pain in the legs from time to time since she was four years of age, when her mother and father used to take her into bed with them, alternately holding her against their bodies to warm her and relieve the pain. Later they discontinued this practice, left her in her own bed and used a hot water bottle to relieve the pain.

Previous History. The patient had bilateral ear trouble two years before. Otherwise the systemic review and past medical history were negative. The father and mother, each forty, and brother twelve years old were living and well.

Physical Examination

The general physical examination was negative except for general abdominal tenderness which was considerably lessened by distracting the patient's attention during examination. The pelvic organs by rectal examination seemed normal.

X-ray Studies

Gastrointestinal x-ray studies showed a delay in the passage of barium into the cecum. At a point near the terminal ileum there was a well developed sausage-like mass which was probably a Meckel's diverticulum. The barium enema threw no additional light on this finding.

Laboratory and Other Findings

Urine, blood count and blood Wassermann were normal. Sedimentation rate was 4 mm. The temperature, pulse and respirations were normal.

Diagnosis

The surgeon saw her in consultation before x-ray studies were made and suggested the following possibilities:

1. Psychoneurosis
2. Urinary tract infection
3. Parietal neuralgia

The patient impressed us as an intelligent, alert, well-developed and attractive young schoolgirl, who was quite dramatic in the presentation of her various pains. The pain in many areas of the body seemed just as important as in the right lower quadrant of the abdomen.

LIFE SITUATION

Family Background

The patient's father was forty. He was fairly well educated, and until 1931 earned a good salary. Since then his income was unsatisfactory. He was strict with his family, especially with the patient. He seemed reserved to the point of being repressed. He was irritable, the irritability having increased since his financial reverses. He was said to have been extremely interested in the patient ever since her early infancy. The mother said, "Mr. M. didn't have any sisters, and so, of course, she was just the whole world to him ever since she was a baby." The father showed jealousy whenever the possibility of his daughter's having dates with boys arose. He considered the boys in the neighborhood to be undesirable companions for his daughter. He reluctantly allowed her to attend parties, forbidding her the privilege on the slightest pretext. Since she had begun to wear dresses like those of other girls of her age, he had complained that the dresses were unattractive and that they were unsuitable for "a child of her age." He was very insistent that she study in the evenings for a long time, and he usually helped her with the work. Although there had been little difficulty with school work lately, the father seemed to attach an unusual amount of importance to it and spent a great deal of his own time helping the patient.

The mother was about the same age as the father, and her education was comparable with his. She seemed to be a more affectionate person than her husband. She was definitely neurotic, exaggerating her own physical symptoms and those of her children and treating her children as if they were invalids. She was cooperative and pleasant but loquacious and dramatized relatively unimportant details of her life.

Early History

Birth. There was some question as to whether the patient's birth was normal or not. The mother said that labor was induced because she had had scarlet fever some months previous to her pregnancy and her general physical condition was bad. However, the pregnancy continued to term and from her report it seemed that labor began normally. She was ill during the patient's early infancy; she described severe physical illness and extreme "nervousness." She said, "I had anemia of the brain. All the blood left my brain for some time, and when the doctor came he said that if he had come ten minutes later I would have been a dead woman." She described her "nervousness" as follows: "The doctor said that if I had not come to him when I did, I would have lost my mind or gone insane."

Infancy. The baby was bottle fed, and there was some trouble with the feeding during the very early infancy. The mother was unable to remember the details of toilet training but she said that both her children had been completely trained at the age of nine months. She thought that dentition and walking and talking occurred at a slightly less than average age for the patient because friends always considered the baby very "bright."

As a baby, the patient is said to have had an unusually good disposition. But at the age of four and a half, shortly after she left the hospital following a tonsillectomy and pneumonia, she began having tantrums and biting her nails. Her father was very attentive to her, carrying her around with him a good deal and frequently taking her in the car with him.

Childhood. The child was always considered "sickly." Her complaints were numerous. Among them were "sclerosis of the stomach" for which the patient was on a diet for years; "disease of the colon;" mastoiditis; sinusitis; and "weak kidneys!"

Both the father and the mother were overanxious about the child's condition. At one time when the patient had mastoiditis, her mother cared for her constantly for a week without resting—according to her report, she did not even remove her clothes and lie down once.

In 1931 *financial reverses* caused the family to leave home and move to a small apartment in a gift shop which they owned and managed. Although previous to this time the patient is said to have adjusted very well to other children, after the change in residence she was unable to make new friends. She became a timid child, fearing to cross the road, avoiding dark or unoccupied rooms and worrying about possible burglary. Her tantrums increased. Enuresis began at this time, continuing intermittently until her fourteenth year.

School Period. Due to her illness the patient did not begin school until the age of seven. She did very good work in primary and intermediate grades. She skipped the first half of the first, second, third, and fifth grades. There were no behavior problems in this period and she liked her primary grade teachers. She disliked all of her intermediate grade teachers and junior high school teachers, saying that they were "cranky." When she reached high school, her grades became low. She failed in two of her subjects and did poor work in her other subjects.

Sexual Development

Attitude Toward Sex. The patient never at any time asked questions concerning sex. The parents did not think that the fact was unusual. Her mother said that the two children had been reared together and she supposed that was the reason for the patient's showing no curiosity about sex. The mother remembered no incident in the child's life in any way pertaining to sex. She said that she herself was reared without sex instruction and although she did not feel that she was particularly reticent on the subject, she had talked about it very little. She thought that she could not discuss the subject with her daughter because she was like an adult—"you feel that you can't intrude on her privacy."

The patient plainly did not wish to discuss sex. She became very ill at ease, looked away from the examiner, bit her nails, and frowned.

If she was asked a direct question, she answered agreeably but as shortly as possible.

There was no history of masturbation, but the parents were by no means sure whether the patient had shown any tendency to masturbate or not. There was a history of disturbed sleep throughout childhood. Enuresis occurred three to five times a week intermittently during puberty.

Menstruation. Menstruation began when the patient was twelve years old. She knew little about it previously. She had heard girls at school make remarks about "their periods" but she had never asked the meaning of the remarks. When she first menstruated, she was frightened. Her mother told her that the occurrence was "perfectly natural" and the child asked no further questions about the matter.

Attitude Toward Friends and Family

Effect of Parental Restrictions. The patient did not like boys. She stated "They are not dependable. I always have a better time with girls." She admitted shyness in the presence of boys. She mentioned during the interview several older girls whose friendships she valued. She stated a slight preference for her mother, saying that her father was too strict with her and that he did not understand her. The mother believed that the patient preferred her father, but her conclusions seemed to be based on the father's obvious preference for his daughter. The mother said that the patient sometimes kissed her and hugged her until she could not go on with her work. She said, "Of course I feel as if I ought to let her do it because if she doesn't get affection from me, she might get it outside."

Adolescent Adjustments. The patient had been given very little freedom. Her companions had been limited because of the "abominable" neighborhood in which they lived and, due to the child's reticence about sex, the parents were doubtful as to what her attitudes toward boy friends might be. If she was permitted to go to a party, she was required to come home earlier than the other children or she had to take her brother with her to make sure that she would have an escort to accompany her home. She was rarely allowed to entertain her friends at home because the apartment was small and entertaining was inconvenient. She had had dates with boys occasionally, but her father had always objected to the boys because he felt that their English was poor, that their vocational aims were low; in short, that they were not good enough for his daughter.

Effect of Financial Condition. The patient said that she was shy and lonely much of the time. She said that she frequently felt depressed. She was irritable and tried unsuccessfully to control her temper. She said that when their financial distress first began, her feelings were easily hurt, but later she paid no attention to remarks that the girls made about her clothes or her lack of money. She did not seem to attach much significance to the fact that the family suffered financial distress. She said that she tried not to ask for new clothes and other things that she could do without because she knew that is was impossible for her parents to give her these things and that she did not want to worry them She regretted having so few friends and said that her mother's laughing and joking with her relieved her loneliness.

The patient's parents complained that she assumed a "martyred air" and that she behaved as if she was "picked on" by her parents and her teachers. The patient said that her teachers treated her fairly although she disliked some of them. She believed, with some justification, that her younger brother was given more privileges than she received. She felt that her parents were too demanding concerning her homework. She thought that the quality of her school work was improving and that her parents failed to recognize it.

Social Interests. She had almost no *hobbies* or *recreational interests*. She mentioned reading and swimming but did not seem greatly interested in either activity. She was genuinely interested in sewing, especially in making over the clothes given her by more fortunate friends and relatives.

She visited friends and relatives away from home frequently. But even under such circumstances, she did not adjust well to groups of children. She was unsure of her dancing ability and avoided dancing whenever she could. During the past winter while she was a house guest of one of her friends, she was given a birthday dance. The day for the dance arrived and the patient complained of severe pain in the abdomen and of nausea. She told her hostess that she was unable to leave her room during the party, but guests insisted that she come downstairs. The supposed illness prevented her from enjoying the party but cleared up completely the following day.

Morbid Interest in Death. When asked about deaths among friends and relatives, the patient quickly named four persons who had died, none of whom had been very closely connected to her. She was able to tell the exact dates of their deaths and said that she had experienced a great deal of grief on each occasion. On two occasions she said that she had not felt well for a month after hearing of the deaths. A year ago her maternal grandfather was ill. The patient said that she used to lie awake nights worrying for fear that he would die. She was kept close at home because her mother feared that news of the death might come at any time and she wanted the children to be at home.

Significance of the History

The history disclosed *personality changes* as well as symptoms. Her outbursts of temper were frequent and at times violent to the point of throwing objects. She became timid, being afraid to walk into an unoccupied room or to be left alone. She was lonely, wanting her mother to stay with her, talk to her, or play games with her. The quality of school work had dropped below her usual standard. She was failing to make an adequate social adjustment for a girl of her age, due to the fears and prejudices of her parents and the inhibitions they had caused in the girl's behavior.

TREATMENT

Somatic Complaints

We could not be specific as to the mechanism of the pain in this case. We know that as a result of emotion the gastrointestinal tract can undergo spasm in any segment. This may well have produced the symptoms. At any rate there were no objective signs of appendicitis after entry into the hospital.

Meckel's Diverticulum. However, x-ray examination showed another "lesion"—Meckel's diverticulum. Attention had been centered upon this as a possible cause of her trouble, but it must be obvious that this anomaly could not possibly have explained this whole illness. Furthermore, we must realize that without the life story we would have had a very inadequate conception of this girl's illness, in other words, the organic approach alone could not possibly have solved this problem. It required a combined physical and psychological approach.

Neurotic Factors

The Background of Neurosis. Here was a situation in which the sins of the parents were visited upon the child, and we are not speaking of "social diseases." We mean that the atmosphere in which this girl had grown up had resulted in a disturbance in her emotional life which later manifested itself as a physical ailment. In other words, her protest against her environment was to produce aches and pains. The conflicts in her personality sought bodily expression and produced symptoms. How wrong it would have been to operate upon her for "appendicitis" or because of the Meckel's diverticulum. How much more important it was for her to receive proper reeducation and psychotherapeutic guidance. She was young and impressionable and we thought that her personality could be molded. She was not yet fixated upon her neurotic complaints as are so many of the patients that we see. There little may be done; here perhaps something could be accomplished. Thus we felt that we had to help this girl in the emotional growth process of adolescence by education of the parents as well as of herself. We tried to gain greater tolerance on their part for the pleasure, freedom, and prestige to which this attractive girl was entitled. We tried to help her gain a more wholesome contact with the young people in the neighborhood. To reduce anxiety and clear the way for a life of greater interest we thought should help to minimize symptoms in this girl.

Results of Psychiatric Treatment. Upon leaving the hospital it was arranged that this patient should visit the psychiatric clinic. These visits were made once a week. The patient did not seem much interested in these visits but kept her appointments faithfully. Even though she had been assured in the hospital that she had no organic disease she was apprehensive about engaging in ordinary activities. She asked if she could walk home each day, which was a matter of four city blocks. She asked if she needed to undertake the usual gymnastic activities and we urged her to do so. Her mother frequently came with her, as sometimes did her father, and they both made complaints about the patient. They said she was not neat and clean, and felt she did not bathe frequently enough. They were dissatisfied with her choice of friends, especially boy friends. The father characterized them as having "no character and no future." The parents also complained bitterly when the patient's grades were not good and wondered if these grades might not be due to ill health, even though the patient had had such a recent check-up in the hospital.

Continuing Worry over Physical Condition. When the patient was talked to alone she would become unhappy and would cry about the way her parents treated her at home. She said, "They have no confidence in me. They nag me all the time. Nothing I ever do pleases them. I wish I could go live with my aunt. They are so unfriendly to me that I have no desire to please them." The patient went on to say, "They worry too much about me and my friends. I know how to take care of myself with the boys. I have no bad intentions but they won't believe me. They are always afraid I am going to get in some trouble, but I have no wish or desire to do what they think." One day the mother came in excitedly and related a story about her daughter having ridden out in the park with an older man in a Packard car. The mother made it sound like an attempted seduction of a young girl by an older man, but when the truth of the story became known it turned out that a relative of one of the girls in the neighborhood had taken a group of the young people for a ride in a purely friendly way. Nevertheless, the mother and father continued to complain that the local drug store was a den of iniquity and they only wished they could move to a "decent" neighborhood.

Appendectomy

As a result of this tension in the home the patient continued to have symptoms. One day she would complain of a pain in the shoulder, and another day it would be a pain over the eye. On two occasions she had pain occurring again in the lower right quadrant. When these would occur the mother would call excitedly for a physician. Finally, at the time of her third attack it was felt that there was some tenderness at McBurney's point and six months after her original hospital visit for study she entered another hospital and an appendectomy was performed. The recovery from this operation was uneventful and the pathological report was as follows:

"The serosa of the appendix was smooth and the superficial vessels were moderately injected. The wall was normal in thickness. The mucosa was smooth and free of gross ulceration. . . . *Pathological Diagnosis:* Fibrosing appendix with lymphoid hyperplasia."

Whether we should call this a diseased appendix is open to question.

Return of Symptoms

Following the removal of the appendix the mother and father came to the psychiatric clinic to scold the psychiatrist and tell him how irrelevant it had been to concern himself over the girl's emotional state. They contended that the cause of the difficulty had finally been found and now with the removal of the appendix the girl would feel like studying and would have better grades and would no longer be a behavior problem. We said we hoped this would be true. Before six weeks had passed the mother was back in the clinic again with the patient, complaining of her continued poor school work, her lack of interest in her appearance, and the fact that she would pay no attention to her father and mother. On this visit we pointed out to the mother that she seemed unwilling to modify her attitude toward the girl, nagged her too much, instead of trying to create a more friendly family environment in which the girl could mature and have a normal social life. The mother countered by saying it was all the hospital's fault because on the girl's first admission she had had a gynecological examination and the mother feared this had turned the girl's attention toward sex, and she had been worried ever since that she would become a bad girl!

Social Worker's Report

At this point we asked one of the younger social workers of a local social agency to come into the home and occasionally take the girl out for social visits, or to a movie, hoping that this would give the girl a wholesome contact and allay some of the anxiety of the parents. This helped slightly but could not correct the fault-finding in the father and mother. With such continued failure to respond to any suggestion or help, we concluded the parents of this girl were latently psychotic. We tried to arrange to have the girl go and live permanently with an aunt in another state who had shown interest and seemed to be a more understanding person. However, the parents thwarted this move and finally, in February, 1941, the patient came back to the clinic complaining of pains around the heart. These pains came on at any time and were unrelated to physical exertion. She reported on this visit that she had failed in school the previous year but was seeking a doctor's certificate in the hope that she would be allowed to repeat some of the work. The mother was with the patient on this occasion. The resident made a thorough physical examination and except for some dental caries, found no evidence of organic disease. His diagnosis was "a confused, disillusioned young lady who is hard pressed by a domineering, overbearing mother."

Reasons for Failure of Treatment

We regret to report that more progress could not be made in this case, but we present the facts and trust that it indicates that given a bad environmental setting, symptoms may be hard to relieve. Operation may remove a pain at one site, only to have it recur in another.

PROGNOSIS

In view of the course of events since discharge from the hospital, we felt that the prognosis in this case was not good. Since we were unable to get her away from the home environment, it is highly probable that by the time she has reached the age of twenty-one she will be so crippled by the faulty attitude and the fears and prejudices of her parents, and will have acquired so many symptoms that the chances of social and economic success will be limited. As indicated, it has been practically impossible to treat the parents and get them to modify their point of view toward the patient. As explained in previous chapters concerning personality formation, the attitude and beliefs of the parents become incorporated into the child's mind during early development. Sometimes emancipation from the home accomplishes considerable in itself to change a neurotic personality with its symptom formation. However, the process of emancipation has its limits in doing good. The person involved is often unable to do anything once physical emancipation has occurred. He has become so anxious or has developed so much hostility that he cannot relate himself well with anyone since he fears that the bad patterns, which he has been used to, exist in all other people as well as in his parents. We fear that this case fits into that category. In one of the preceding paragraphs, we alluded to the fact that we thought the parents of this girl were latently psychotic. We said this because of what seemed to be a total lack of friendliness and warmth for the child in either parent. Everything done for the child seemed to be done entirely from a sense of duty, rather than from a sense of cooperation with a young human being of their own flesh and blood. Moreover, their fears that there were malicious influences everywhere outside the home, are not far from the feelings of persecution seen in paranoia. Both parents reacted in rather an unusual way to economic insecurity. They did not have the emotional sensibility to make the best of the resources in a poorer community, and they were so extremely anxious with their own sense of failure that they have vented some of the hostility which they have felt against fate toward their children. Extreme sensitivity, emotional rigidity, and so much suspicion related to the environment, made us finally come to think of the parents as psychotic. It is unfortunate that our patient had to be related to two such difficult people during one of the most important phases of her emotional growth.

SUMMARY

Here was a young woman who had been badly conditioned by over-solicitous parents in regard to medical matters. At an age when she should have been oblivious to minor bodily sensations, she dwelled continually upon her bodily discomforts. General examination disclosed no evidence of organic disease and an attempt was made to treat the patient and the parents along the lines of better emotional health. This proved unsuccessful; the appendix eventually was removed, but pains recurred; disability continued and the prognosis, therefore, seemed to be in the direction of chronic invalidism.

Thus by means of an illustrative case we have presented in some detail considerations that must be investigated before one consents to operate upon a patient for "chronic appendicitis."

The end-result of appendectomy for so-called chronic appendicitis is often *polysurgery* and *chronic invalidism*. The following case is illustrative.

> *The Chronic Gastrointestinal Invalid; Sensitive Child; Anxiety Attacks; Polysurgery; "Adhesions"; Chronic Invalidism*

CASE 27

A white woman, age forty-five, was admitted to Temple University Hospital in October, 1940, complaining of sudden attacks of weakness, persistent nausea, vomiting, and loss of weight.

History and Symptoms

The patient stated that nausea and vomiting began in the summer of 1939 and that she had suffered from fatigue, insomnia, and urinary frequency for several years before that. After considerable medical treatment for the nausea and vomiting it was finally suspected that she might have a kidney stone because of a rather sharp pain on the right side of the abdomen. She was then studied in a hospital but no stone was found. The suggestion was made that she might have passed a stone between the time of the pain and the hospital investigation. This was in January, 1940. She then went home, the nausea and vomiting persisted, and she had a good deal of epigastric distress so that she was returned to the hospital in February, 1940, with the diagnosis of probable peptic ulcer. No ulcer was found but it was suggested that she might have adhesions from an operation of twenty years before and that this might be responsible for partial intestinal obstruction. Consequently, she was again operated upon and while recovering from this operation she had an attack of choking, substernal pain, a cold, clammy feeling and, according to the patient, became unconscious and then found herself in an oxygen tent in which she remained for two days. She was told that she had suffered from pulmonary embolism. An electrocardiogram taken three days later showed only changes which were attributed to the effect of digitalis.

She returned to her home on March 23 but still was unable "to digest solid food." Then she developed spells which were described as follows: "The left side of the body would become numb and just before this she would feel cold ascending her legs as though she were sitting with her feet in ice-water. . . She was unable to talk and felt that the power of the left arm and hand were gone. . . The heart would pound, she felt faint and according to observers looked pale. . . The palpitation would last for two or three hours but the left sided weakness did not clear until the following day." This same kind of attack occurred on two or three more occasions but recently the attacks had been chiefly of coldness, palpitation and a feeling of pressure "as though someone were sitting on my chest." There was a great deal of shortness of breath with these attacks and on occasions, some nausea and vomiting. The attacks would come at intervals of a few weeks. Her physician suspected hypothyroidism and treated her with thyroid substance as well as with estrogen, iron and thiamin chloride. Since her operation she had been quite constipated. She had no appetite and as a consequence lost 50 pounds since January, 1940.

Past History. She described herself as a sensitive and nervous child who had the usual childhood diseases and also an attack of chorea. In addition she said that the day before delivery of her first child she developed another attack of chorea but this apparently lasted only one day and consisted of "an inability to hold anything in her hand." The onset of the menses was accompanied by nausea and vomiting and considerable dysmenorrhea. She married at the age of eighteen and at that time the appendix was removed and also the right ovary because of pain in the right side of the abdomen. She was told that the ovary contained cysts. Then she had two pregnancies in quick succession and shortly afterwards the left ovary was removed, also because of cysts. These operations were supposed to have been responsible for the adhesions for which the third operation was done. The patient had not been able to do her housework but had been helped by relatives. The husband was a miner in good health and the children were well.

Family History. The father and mother were well. One brother had a duodenal ulcer and a sister had had an operation for gallstones.

Physical Examination and Laboratory Studies

In spite of the loss of 50 pounds the patient was still well nourished. She seemed quite comfortable in bed. The color was good; the eyes bright; there was no dyspnea or cyanosis and no clubbing. The blood pressure was within normal limits and the temperature, pulse, and respirations were normal. Examination of head and neck was normal except that the teeth were in rather poor shape. The thyroid gland was palpable but not enlarged. The heart seemed normal in size and position and the sounds were normal. Orthodiagram and electrocardiogram were also within normal limits. The lungs were clear and resonant throughout and the abdominal examination showed nothing remarkable. There were the scars of three previous operations and deep palpation in the region of the scar of the right lower quadrant produced some tenderness but this was not considered significant. No organs or masses were palpated. Examination of the extremities was normal. Therefore, we concluded that the general physical examination was negative.

Because of the history that suggested possible urinary stone, we first investigated the urinary tract but could find no evidence of disease. The urine was quite clear; renal function was within normal limits; and the excretory urogram was normal. Next we investigated the gastrointestinal tract by means of gastric analysis and an x-ray series, including a cholecystogram, but could find no evidence of disease of that system. The gynecological examination was negative. The basal metabolism on two occasions showed minus 3 and minus 8. The blood count was good; blood Wassermann negative. Therefore we concluded that in our general physical examination and laboratory investigation no evidence of disease had been discovered.

LIFE SITUATION

Early Life

The father was a street car conductor and both he and his wife seemed very much concerned about the patient. The mother was sixty-three years old. It was interesting, although we did not know how significant, that the mother had had both ovaries removed in her early thirties. In any case the patient was eager to tell this fact when discussing her mother. The parents said that the patient as a child was sensitive and "nervous" and gave the following example of what they meant: each spring by about March or April she seemed "too rundown and nervous" to continue her school attendance and had to be taken out for the rest of the year. When called upon to recite she would become frightened and "too nervous" to do so. She was taken out of school early each year because of this behavior—although it was not called "poor behavior" at that time. It was called "nerves" and she was taken to a physician and medication was given. It is important to recognize that these "nerves" of her early school days were a symptom of anxiety due to social insecurity. Medicines were not indicated at that time. What she really needed was a greater reassurance of friendliness and interest on the part of her parents and greater attention to the school situation rather than to be taken to a physician and dosed with pills and powders. However, the parents felt that they were doing the best thing for her.

Marriage and Pregnancy

When menstruation began she had an exacerbation of vomiting and nervousness over a period of two or three years so that the family felt that a change was necessary. So she left home to live with an uncle in the country where life was quieter. She became interested in Sunday school activities there and met her husband in that religious group, marrying him when she was eighteen. She soon became pregnant and nine months after delivery she found herself pregnant again. Motherhood added to her nervousness, so much so that the mother-in-law took almost complete care of the baby during the first year of its life. The patient continued to get help all through life; her mother, husband, mother-in-law, all came to her aid not only during the interval between births alluded to above, but also since her illness began in 1939. She said she was perfectly well between the births of her children and the summer of 1939, yet when she was questioned closely we found this had not been entirely true. For five years she had been bothered by *fatigue, occasional abdominal pain, and insomnia.* She awakened early in the morning, a symptom which often indicates considerable anxiety. Urinary frequency was another symptom which had been present so that these intervening years had not been so free of distress as she would indicate.

Anxiety Attacks

These attacks of pain, left-sided weakness and distress sounded rather vague when first described. Symptoms limiting themselves to the left side might suggest an intracranial lesion. Yet we found when we studied the symptoms closely that this so-called "weakness" was a numbness and feeling of coldness which ended at a certain point in the arms and legs. It presented the so-called "glove and stocking" type of paresthesia which is found only in conversion hysteria. Symptoms of conversion hysteria may appear in anxiety hysteria just as anxiety attacks may occur occasionally in a case of conversion hysteria. The sensory disturbances referred to were present only in the first two attacks and since that time the attacks had been typical of anxiety attacks with palpitation and dyspnea as the outstanding features, followed, of course, by fatigue.

She had had a few bad *dreams* which were of an anxiety nature. In one dream she and her husband were out on a picnic. There was thunder and lightning. It seemed that she had been struck by lightning and was having difficulty telling her husband that she was not dead. She awoke with palpitation and sweating. It was interesting that in this dream she felt herself half paralyzed by a weakness on one side. The dream was a mental picture showing what was going on in the unconscious mind of the patient but the unconscious material could translate itself equally well into bizarre symptoms during the waking state. The patient had a very vivid imagination. One day in the hospital while lying in bed she happened to look at a patient across the ward. She had a feeling that this patient's face and body were moving nearer and nearer to her until the bed and the patient were almost upon her. At this point the fantasy ended, disappearing without producing anxiety such as that exhibited in the dream.

The Early History of Anxiety

It is important to recognize the anxiety attack as a clinical syndrome with a clinical picture that may be as definite as the rash in measles. Of course, there are all degrees of anxiety attacks. This one was classical. Just as we can often trace physical disease back to childhood, such, for example, as a mitral valvular lesion which had its beginning with an attack of rheumatic fever, so can we often trace anxiety back to childhood. For it is in childhood that anxiety displays itself in its purest form. Accordingly, in dealing with a psychological problem of adult life we must be interested in childhood and the earliest environment to find out whether there was evidence of anxiety displaying itself in behavior or adjustment difficulties then.

Symptoms as Evidences of Poor Behavior

We have discussed the neurotic symptom in terms of anxiety, in terms of conflicts and in terms of persistent infantile trends. We must also speak of neurotic symptoms in terms of poor behavior. Sometimes we meet a child who does not want to go to school so he runs away. Following this he is often called a "bad boy," a truant, and treated accordingly. Why does he behave this way? Because he may not feel at ease with the other children—or because he may be afraid his teachers do not like him. At any rate there is something in the school situation which is making him unhappy and he tries to escape. However, there are people who have not been brought up to think in terms of running away with their feet. Yet they run away just as effectively by vomiting or crying. This patient was frightened about the school situation. It is a frequent reaction of flight or retreat in sensitive people to cry and vomit when they cannot endure a situation. The vomiting is really an inferior kind of adaptation and yet, how often it may be treated as an organic disease! Finding school difficult this patient began to vomit and by this method "ran away" from school very effectively. She was behaving badly and the parents didn't see her reaction in terms of behavior; they thought of it in terms of an illness, a doctor and pills. She consequently did not get rid of her anxiety at that time. It was left untouched, and in adult life, she manifested it in much the same way.

On leaving the hospital this patient was to go home and take care of her family—something very hard for her to do after forty-five years of "running away" through certain symptoms. People had taken very good care of her and she was not going to change that situation. In such a case the attending physician must be prepared to meet hostility when he tries to get the patient to relinquish her symptoms. She is going to be annoyed with anyone who asks her to grow up emotionally and do her job efficiently. Her parents took her to a doctor when she was eight with a condition which remained untreated up to the time of this hospital admission, i. e., anxiety on meeting responsibility. We knew that it would be a difficult if not impossible job at this late date.

Gradual Reeducation

It is not sufficient to tell a patient that the trouble is not organic and that he should go out and do his job. The patient cannot accept the truth so easily. We have to bring about a gradual reeducation of the patient. This means personal help and encouragement in meeting the duties of everyday life. Everyone around the patient must strike a happy balance between giving her friendship and encouragement but at the same time asking her to do something for herself and not to go on believing she has "nerves."

Enlisting Help of the Family. It is sometimes very difficult to enlist the aid of the family, especially that of the husband. How often do we find that the illness somehow fits into his pattern of behavior so that one must be cautious about creating a disturbance in the marital relationship— the illness sometimes suits certain elements in both personalities and to disturb it creates two problems instead of one.

The Patient's Idea of the Illness

In the beginning we must obtain the patient's own idea about her illness. When we asked her what she suspected as the cause of her trouble she said that she had never recovered from the last operation and she suspected that something was not right, in other words, that the operation was not so satisfactory as it should have been. What she believed was that adhesions remained that interfered with the passage of material through the intestinal tract. Thus she had *difficulty in swallowing* solid food and vomited if, for example, she took any meat; but she was able to live on a baby's diet of soft things such as cooked cereals. This corresponded to her idea that solid food could not get past the obstruction but soft food could.

The first thing to try to correct in this woman's thinking was this erroneous notion of what was going on in the intestinal tract. To do that, we felt justified in showing her our gastrointestinal x-ray series in which the barium was well distributed throughout the large bowel. This persuaded her that the intestinal tract was open. It is always important to get the patient's own idea of her illness because in this way you may be able to correct any erroneous idea that is responsible for a great deal of trouble.

The Psychosomatic Approach

But part of the patient's difficulty was due to the fact that the medical approach had been entirely an organic one and that the personality factor had been overlooked. This is an example of the teaching that organic disease must be excluded first and only then the possibility of a psychological disturbance considered. Psychological observations should be made simultaneously with the physical observations and what this patient had to say about herself was just as important as the physical findings that we could elicit. For example, when this patient was first interviewed the intern called attention to the fact that she cried because a patient whom she hardly knew was leaving the ward. At that moment the inquiring physician would want to know why she cried and what ideas came to her mind regarding the incident. In that way we might have thrown some light immediately on the question of anxiety, because it was the heavy burden of anxiety that this woman was carrying that was responsible for the attacks that she had and also for her long-time disability.

Hospital Study. When one deals with such complicated problems as this it is much easier to send the patient into the hospital both for the sake of the studies which are really necessary and for the opportunity to impress the patient with the fact that a thorough investigation has been made. But what we hope is that by using the double approach of psychological observations and physical studies hand in hand, we will, by recognizing these cases earlier, obviate some of the disabilities that result from the long-time purely physical approach. Most problems that the average practitioner sees are not so complicated as this. When they are, we think it is best to urge the patient to be sent to the hospital, at least for the beginning of the study. This again brings up the question of the unfavorable influences which exist for such patients in a general hospital and on that point we will have more to say later.

SUMMARY

A middle-aged woman, the victim of a career of polysurgery, beginning with "chronic appendicitis," presented unmistakable evidence of an anxiety state for which she had been medically investigated and surgically treated from childhood to the time of her last hospital admission. It is the aim of the psychosomatic approach to avoid such tragedies.

GALLBLADDER DISEASE

As previously stated one of the most frequent causes of chronic dyspepsia is gallbladder disease. When a patient has suffered from attacks of gallstone colic and studies demonstrate the presence of gallstones it is universally recognized that operation is essential for cure. Nevertheless, the role of the emotions in the possible development of gall tract disease; in the precipitation of attacks of colic; and in the preparation of the patient for surgery and then recovery from operation, is a matter with which general medicine has not sufficiently concerned itself. We are beginning to realize the importance of emotional factors in the so-called "noncalculous cases" which, in reality, are often simply upper digestive tract reactions to an irritable colon rather than actual gallbladder disease (Tumen). To remove such a gallbladder is very similar to the problem just discussed, that is, the removal of the appendix in so-called chronic appendicitis. All of the evil consequences of *polysurgery*, plus the additional complications furnished by the *difficult anatomy of the gall tract, are apt to follow.

The following cases illustrate some of these points.

Mental Depression
Repeated Hospital Admissions; Cholecystectomy; Poor Prognosis

---

CASE 28

History and Symptoms

A forty-three-year-old white woman was admitted to Temple University Hospital in November, 1938. She complained of crampy pains in the right upper quadrant of the abdomen, referred to the right shoulder region, right pubic region, and in fact, over almost the entire abdomen; frequency of urination during the day, and some burning sensation; loss of appetite; loss of weight; occasional vomiting; irritability. The patient had consulted many physicians and had had many hospital admissions.

Past History. The first hospital experience was in December, 1934, when salpingo-oophorectomy and appendectomy were done. The hospital reported a pathological diagnosis of bilateral pyosalpinx. In March, 1935, the patient was admitted to the same hospital suffering with an abscess of the hand. A good recovery was made. In December, 1935, she was first admitted to the Temple University Hospital for abdominal complaints but did not remain more than twenty-four hours. She refused x-ray studies and signed a release in order "to go home for the holidays." About one year later she was again admitted to the Temple University Hospital, following an attempt at suicide by taking bichloride. She remained in the hospital three weeks. In January, 1937, she was admitted to another hospital where a diagnosis of possible gall-bladder disease was made, because of the same complaint, *i. e.*, abdominal pain. In November, 1937, she was again admitted to the same hospital for four weeks with the same diagnosis. In December, 1937, again she was admitted to the same hospital, diagnosis undetermined. January, 1938, she was admitted to still another hospital where she remained for five days. No diagnosis was made. She returned to the previous hospital, was operated upon for gallbladder trouble and the gallbladder removed. Following cholecystectomy deep jaundice developed. Five days later an end-to-end suture of the cystic duct was performed. The patient remained at home and felt fairly well for about two months but then the same symptoms returned and increased in severity. She continued to come to the surgical outpatient department and finally was admitted to the hospital once more.

Family History

The father was a drunkard and the mother was a highly nervous person. Three brothers were living; one had tuberculosis, one was highly nervous, a third was apparently healthy.

Marital History

The patient was married at the age of seventeen, had two children, and then separated from her husband because "he ran around with other women and contracted a venereal disease." She believed, probably correctly, that this was responsible for her first operation.

She had been married to her second husband for eighteen years and had one child by him. She stated that she loved this husband but was sorry that her ill health had made her a burden to him. He was a textile worker but for the past five years had been irregularly employed.

Systemic Inquiry

There were symptoms in many parts of the body: blurry vision, head-aches, and occasional tinnitus; "a lump in the neck causes nausea"; dyspnea and constipation; frequency of urination; shooting pains and aches in the right leg and weakness of both legs.

Physical Examination

Temperature, pulse, respirations, and blood pressure were normal. Fin-gernails were badly bitten. There was a vasomotor flush over chest and abdomen. The patient was fairly well nourished and appeared quite com-fortable. There was a small nodule in the right lobe of the thyroid gland. It was fairly soft and possible cystic. The remainder of the physical exami-nation revealed nothing unusual. The heart was normal, the lungs were clear. The abdomen was soft and easily paplable without indication of tenderness or rigidity. We were unable to make out any organs or masses. The extremities were normal.

Laboratory Studies

December, 1935, first admission; urine negative, blood count good, serological tests normal. October, 1936, admitted with a diagnosis of mer-curial gastritis following attempt at suicide.

After recovery a gastrointestinal x-ray study, including cholecysto-gram, was negative.

Operation, January, 1938; histological report on gallbladder, "cholester-osis," gross description indicated a normal gallbladder. No stones were found.

Here then, was a woman approaching middle age, who had had ten hospital admissions in the past four years. She insisted that she had had constant abdominal pain for more than that length of time. She had been constantly disturbed by the idea that she might have a cancer. Many doctors had told her that she was "nervous rather than sick" and one even intimated that she was "crazy."

Our complete studies failed to show any evidence of organic dis-ease other than the small nodule in the thyroid gland. There was no question that the first operation was a justifiable one; it is doubtful if the same could be said of the second. It was probably done for the reason that a great many gallbladder operations have been done, that is, because of the patient's complaint of excruciating and intractable pain, and in-sistence upon "something being done" in spite of negative x-ray study. Unquestionably surgeons are becoming more reluctant to operate for supposed gallbladder disease when pain of the type described by this patient is the chief symptom and the findings are negative.

LIFE SITUATION

The patient maintained that she was well until 1934 when she had her operation for pelvic infection. Upon closer questioning, however, we discovered that there was a period of anxiety and depression in 1926, at the time of her mother's death. At that time she also had the same pains and discomfort as on her hospital admission.

Childhood

This patient's childhood was a most unhappy one. She had a father who drank and mistreated the entire family, and who on more than one occasion seduced her sexually. She was always afraid of her father and never felt comfortable in his presence. Her mother seems to have been a passive person who contributed very little to offset the cruelty and lack of affection shown by the father. The patient described herself as always a worrisome person, never happy and never having enjoyed any social life. Her only pleasures were cooking, sewing, ironing. She had never made any close friends nor taken an active interest in anything outside of her home. She was extremely irritable and depressed, and cried a great deal. She was very discouraged about herself and very pessimistic about the future.

Mental Depression

We seemed to be dealing with a woman who had been a chronically depressed person all her life, and at times the depression had reached the degree of psychosis. In 1936 there seems to have been a genuine suicidal attempt.

As in all other severe emotional disturbances there was some conversion of anxiety into somatic symptoms. However, in most cases of psychotic depression somatic symptoms are not in the foreground; instead there is a great deal of guilt and self-condemnation usually over real or imagined sexual advances and over digressions, real or fancied. With what we knew of this patient's childhood there was no doubt that she had a great deal of hostility and guilt over sexual feelings aroused in her at an early age. Many patients, instead of emphasizing self-condemnation, find a solution by punishment through somatic suffering, i. e., somatic symptom formation. We were sure that in this case, the sexual seduction by the father had weighed heavily upon the patient's conscience.

As we observe depressed people we often wonder how it is that they can condemn themselves for so long and suffer so much. We wonder why no one can reassure them. The answer seems to be that the quantity of guilt is so great that a long period of expiation is necessary in order to balance the imaginary sins committed. This patient complained of a terrible feeling of loneliness and sadness which at times was almost unbearable. *From her long list of hospital admissions it would seem that she could endure her feelings only for a certain period of time and then she had to enter the hospital and offer herself up for study and operation in order to relieve her guilt feelings.*

The Unconscious Wish to be Sick

This was the most important question, that is. 'the unconscious will to remain sick." *We could not escape the notion that she achieved a certain satisfaction out of her suffering.* This is a very important consideration in medicine and in this kind of patient is of paramount importance. Because such a patient is really eager to be operated upon and in her very insistence upon the continuous and excruciating nature of the pain from which she suffers one can easily understand how she may prevail on a very sympathetic surgeon to operate. This is particularly true when such patients meet a surgeon who is not loath to operate. Thus, we can say that a willing and even eager patient who derives a certain satisfaction from being hospitalized and operated upon and a surgeon who is ever ready to wield a knife is a very unfortunate combination. A great many patients with numerous scars on the abdomen serve as testimony to this combination.

Sanatorium Care

We felt that following operation this patient should have entered a sanatorium and remained there for a period of at least six weeks where she could have had rest, relaxation, and diversion, and a beginning could have been made in reeducating her emotional life. She needed to become acquainted with her feelings of guilt and hostility, and to realize how much energy she had been using up all these years keeping them repressed. She needed to learn how to enjoy something else besides cooking, sewing, and ironing, and remaining isolated within her own home.

Unfortunately no such sanatorium exists for a patient with a small income. A suitable private institution would cost at least $50 weekly. We felt that unless this patient understood more of her psychic problem, and how it was producing symptoms, then it was highly probable that she would remain just as sick or grow worse.

Threat of Suicide

Furthermore, the danger of another suicidal attempt was always present in a patient as emotionally ill as this one. Any patient who attempts suicide is very sick emotionally, whether neurotic or psychotic. Such persons in one stroke seek to destroy a body they despise and a mind which feels detached from the world.

It was emotional misery which had to be treated in this patient. The husband and two daughters seemed to be of the kind who could give some cooperation. Any relief which could be produced in her emotional state would give a corresponding improvement in symptoms relating to her body. Once the patient had begun to see these connections a beginning would have been made toward a return to health. To be realistic and an entirely symptom-free individual was not to be expected in this woman who has suffered so much over so many years. Probably the best we could hope for was improvement with greater efficiency and less suffering. It is difficult to help a patient who has so few memories of a happy adjustment to everyday life. But even though the therapeutic task was formidable the eventual results would probably be better than symptomatic drugs or surgical treatment could produce.

SUMMARY

A middle-aged woman had repeated hospital admissions because of abdominal pain. On one occasion she attempted suicide. Finally the gallbladder was removed but symptoms returned. Personality study indicated that symptoms of mental depression antedated the hospital admissions and, in reality, constituted the main feature of this clinical problem. Unfortunately we were unable to follow her after she left the hospital.

The following case also shows a recurrence of "gallbladder symptoms" after removal of the gallbladder. A good result followed superficial psychotherapy—listening rather than talking.

Chronic Dyspepsia
Cholecystectomy; Anxiety Attacks; Abdominal Symptoms; Marital Maladjustment; Superficial Psychotherapy

---

CASE 29

A white woman, forty-seven years old, was first seen in March, 1940.

History and Symptoms

She complained of pain in the epigastrium and in the gallbladder region, nausea and heart burn, headache and fatigue. A peculiar feeling in the back "like cold water" extended down to the buttocks. The first attack had occurred twenty-two years ago after the birth of a son. She had been told that the trouble was due to gallbladder disease and the gallbladder was removed. A few years later, however, the same trouble recurred and she had been having attacks which lasted for several weeks at a time ever since. In the summer preceding her present illness an attack had lasted for two weeks and during that time there had been some looseness of bowel as well. There had been no other serious illnesses in the past medical history.

Family History

The father had died of a stomach ulcer twenty-two years before, that is, just before the onset of her illness. The mother had only recently died of heart disease. Three sisters and a brother were living and well.

The patient had been married for twenty-five years and had two children, one twenty-two and the other twenty, both of whom were well. The husband was living and well.

Menses had always been irregular and painful and the menopause had been established at the age of forty-two without untoward incident.

The patient had always been heavy but there had been a gradual increase in weight since her marriage until she weighed 185 pounds. She had always chosen her diet carefully and especially in the last two years because of the digestive disturbance. She felt that cream and milk made her "bilious" and she had cut her diet down in many other respects, eating very little meat, fish, or eggs, so that her protein intake was less than average.

Physical Examination and Laboratory Studies

The patient was an obese woman with normal blood pressure and normal cardiovascular system. There was slight tenderness in the epigastrium but no organs or masses could be made out. Aside from a few varicose veins the examination of the extremities was normal.

Routine laboratory studies, including sedimentation rate and basal metabolism, were within normal limits. Gastric analysis showed normal motility and low acid values. A gastrointestinal x-ray series, including barium enema, was normal. Biliary drainage showed an absence of cholesterin and calcium bilirubin pigment in the centrifuged specimen so that on that basis we felt reasonably sure that gallstones were not present.

LIFE SITUATION

The patient described her life as a happy one. She had been brought up in a comfortably fixed and what she considered a cultured family and had never known serious hardships. At twenty-six years she had married a man who had always been very kind to her, and her children had brought them great pleasure.

In discussing her married life she kept referring to the fact that her husband was very generous and very kind, that he had been successful in business and enjoyed a fine reputation among his business associates and in their social group. The emphasis that she placed on his fine qualities sounded as though she had more to say on the subject, so that while no particular reference was made to the matter upon the first two or three occasions when we saw her, a note was made to reintroduce the subject on a subsequent occasion.

Marriage Problems

Meanwhile with reassurance that there was no evidence of organic disease and the recommendation that she enlarge her diet to include proteins such as meat, fish, and fowl, she reported considerable improvement. On the fourth occasion that she was seen, which was about six weeks after her first visit, she reported that she had been very uncomfortable on that day in spite of the fact that she had eaten very little. She stated that her mouth was dry and that she had an ice-cold sensation in the back which was the same "as her mother complained of just before she died." Conversation was directed along the lines of her day-by-day activities for the two or three days preceding the onset of this difficulty and it became clear that she was disturbed about her *son* who was about to get married and she, like so many mothers, felt that the girl was selfish and not quite suited for him. Although the engagement had been known for some time the marriage date had just been decided upon which brought the acute realization to her that she was about to lose this fine son to what she considered a scheming and designing, selfish girl. When this matter was discussed her behavior revealed that she had a great deal of feeling on the subject. The opportunity was provided to discuss the young lady's qualifications dispassionately and it was pointed out somewhat jokingly "that all mothers felt that way about their sons."

Her Own Marriage. This afforded an opening for discussing her own marriage. With a great deal of reluctance, and with constant apologetic statements that her husband was a very good man, she brought out the fact that her chief problem had been that she considered her husband beneath her from a cultural or class standpoint, that he was a coarse and uncultured fellow while she considered herself a refined and sensitive person. She had never really been happy and had never been free of the thought that she was married to a clod or peasant. The feeling with which she discussed the matter revealed how intensely she felt. It was obvious that beneath these feelings were the physical problems concerning her inability to be demonstrative with him, or for that matter to receive his affections. Consequently she lived a life of fantasy and romance so far as her secret feelings were concerned but felt like a caged animal in regard to her actual life. She had always been frigid with her husband and on many occasions had considered leaving him but had been held back by the thought of her children. But even at this late date she harbored the fantasy that once her children were married she would establish a home of her own. She had a great deal of self-pity and at the same time some apprehension and guilt about discussing for the first time in her life her real feelings about her husband. Still, the matter was received in an uncritical fashion and she seemed to derive a great deal of relief over having unburdened herself at last.

SUMMARY

A middle-aged woman had had her gallbladder removed for epigastric pain but trouble recurred. The remainder of the symptom picture was that of anxiety. Long-standing marital maladjustment, which had been "suffered in silence," stood in the background of the physical complaints. Uncritical listening and reassurance brought relief.

MUCOUS COLITIS ("IRRITABLE COLON")

White, Cobb, and Jones, in a psychosomatic medicine monograph in 1939 and White and Jones in a more recent paper, regard mucous colitis as a bodily reaction rather than a disease entity. They point out that the manifestations are manifold and inconstant and are often overshadowed by other symptoms. They consider that mucous colitis is probably responsible for the removal of more undiseased appendices than any other cause and Tumen believes that more than half of the patients initially labelled as chronic gallbladder disease are eventually identified as having unstable colons. A total of sixty patients were carefully studied by White, Cobb, and Jones over a period of two years. Of these, fifty-seven were studied psychologically with sufficient thoroughness to afford considerable insight into the role of precipitating emotional factors as well as the types of personality encountered in persons with this syndrome.

Clinical Syndrome

In general, patients with mucous colitis suffer from constipation or diarrhea with some form of abdominal pain. In most cases the stools are small and are either mushy or composed of hard pellets. As a rule the symptoms are seen in patients who have a labile autonomic nervous system with associated cardiovascular instability. The lower abdominal pain is generally accompanied by upper abdominal symptoms such as nausea, heart burn, belching, and sour eructations. Cardiovascular symptoms such as palpitation, sweating, faintness, and neurocirculatory asthenia are often encountered. On physical examination the sigmoid colon is often palpable as a firm "rubber hose."

Emotional Factors

Diarrhea as a symptom of nervousness has been recognized for centuries. Moreover, from the very first it has been known that the emotions had something to do with mucous colitis. J. M. DaCosta described the syndrome with accuracy, noted the condition of the rectal mucosa through a speculum and recognized the tense, emotionally unstable nature of the patients. Thus he was responsible for delineating the syndrome to which he gave the name "membranous enteritis." Although infection has been held responsible no one has succeeded in isolating a specific organism. Allergy, of course, has been suspected but repeatedly throughout the literature one meets with the belief that mucous colitis is a secretory and motor neurosis of the intestines.

Severity of Neurosis

Of the sixty cases of mucous colitis fifty-seven were divided into two groups, a more neurotic group, handicapped by neurotic symptoms or personality problems, and a less neurotic group, composed of persons whose personality problems were not incapacitating. With four exceptions all of the twenty-eight less neurotic patients showed a close relation between emotion and aggravation of symptoms. In the more neurotic group there were twenty-nine patients and of these only seventeen showed a close relation between emotion and colonic symptoms. No specific personality type was found and the authors could only conclude that mucous colitis appeared to be a somatic response to a type of nervous tension. Mental states conducive to this response appeared to be anxiety, resentment and guilt. Associated depressive, neurasthenic, and hypochondriacal features were often present and in about half the cases a rigid type of thinking, similar to that seen in the obsessive-compulsive state, was present. Diminution in energy output was also characteristic of the group as a whole. Most of the persons required more than the average amount of sleep. Asthenia was present in the great majority and in some cases was incapacitating. There was a high incidence of sexual difficulties; two-thirds of the women were frigid and libido was diminished in the men.

Thus we have convincing evidence of the *neurotic background for mucous colitis* concerning which Dunbar quotes A. L. Bloomfield as follows:

"No group of patients is more universally misdiagnosed and mistreated and most of the unfortunates who have been told that they have 'colitis' have a neurosis without any real organic disease. Every medical student should read in Axel Munthe's 'Story of San Michele' the amusing but unfortunately true expose of the colitis 'racket.' Others have their symptoms blamed on the shape or the position of their colon, on cecal stasis, or mobile cecum, on the character of the intestinal flora, on a misplaced uterus or a chronic prostatitis, on a 'chronic appendix' or a 'gallbladder' or on what they eat. . . . No attempt should be made to make a final diagnosis without prolonged study of the entire individual from the physical, mental and social standpoints. . . Sooner or later the patient begins to rationalize about his trouble and to blame it on one thing or another—certain articles of food, a past illness or injury, perhaps an operation, or the finding of intestinal parasites. As the years go by he becomes more and more convinced that serious trouble exists and, as a rule, makes the rounds of the 'colon cultists.' Possibly a surgical operation or two has been done to relieve 'dropping of the colon' or to mobilize his cecum. . . In really stubborn cases. . . the cooperation of a good psychiatrist, if one can be found, can be invoked to great advantage."

The following case illustrates some of the points that have been discussed.

Mucous Colitis ("Irritable Colon")
The Conflict of Marriage and Career; Principles of the Psychotherapeutic
Approach

CASE 30

History and Symptoms

A young white woman was first seen in November, 1939. She complained of "colitis," pain in the abdomen, worse after eating, and excessive gas. She also complained of "feeling nervous."

Past History. The past history was negative except that after an attack of scarlet fever in childhood she had trouble with her right ear for a short time. Otherwise, she was a healthy youngster and had remained free of any serious disease. Menses began at the age of eleven, had always been regular and were not painful although for a few days before the period there was some feeling of tension.

Present Illness. The present trouble began while she was at college during the winter of 1937, when she was cramming for examinations. She had an attack of "intestinal grippe" and then the colitis began. Prior to that time she had been constipated on occasions but at the time of which we speak she had five or six bowel movements daily accompanied by considerable amounts of mucus but no blood. She was given bismuth and after about two months the condition subsided. After that she had trouble "only when nervous" but for a few weeks she had been so distressed by the necessity for frequent movements that it was interfering with her work and pleasure. Following her graduation from college she obtained a position in a social agency and in addition took courses in a school of social work.

When her bowels were disturbed she also suffered from poor digestion and had some abdominal pains and bloating. She stated that her appetite was poor and that she "filled up easily after eating." There had been no loss of weight.

In addition to the above complaints she had found herself more nervous and irritable during the month prior to this study.

Family History. The mother and father were living and well except that both were subject to indigestion. There were two brothers and two sisters; one sister had been operated upon for exophthalmic goiter and the remainder of the siblings were well.

Physical Examination and Laboratory Studies

The general physical examination disclosed that she was somewhat overweight and that the blood pressure was slightly elevated (150/100). The hands and feet were cold and moist. Examination of head and neck was negative. The heart rate was rapid but the heart was within normal limits and the sounds were normal. The lungs were clear and resonant throughout. The abdominal examination showed slight tenderness over the descending colon. Urine examination was normal; blood count was good; the examination of the stool showed the presence of mucus but no other abnormalities were detected. The blood sedimentation rate was within normal limits. Basal metabolic rate was plus 5 and the gastrointestinal x-ray series, including a barium enema, showed a normal gastrointestinal tract. Incidentally a small dermoid cyst of the right ovary was apparent in the x-ray film but it was obvious that this had no significance from the standpoint of her illness.

LIFE SITUATION

This young woman immediately revealed herself as a tense, high-strung and unstable person who talked the language of modern psychology and casually considered the idea of intensive psychotherapy for herself. She explained that while she was a junior in college, her mother became nervous and depressed and had to be examined by a psychiatrist, who stated that the mother's condition was due to the menopause. At the same time the patient suffered from sleeplessness and the college physician recommended that she too should consult a psychiatrist. This period corresponded with the former attack of "colitis." She stated that as the mother's condition improved, she, herself, became better.

Already she had determined to major in psychology and to embark upon a career of social service. However, her work in the social agency had not satisfied her and she had become increasingly aware of her limitations so far as advancement in her work was concerned; but at the same time she had been unable to decide between a desire to perfect herself for further progress in her career and an offer of marriage. For about a year a man many years her senior, whom she described as cultured, traveled, and intelligent, had been attentive to her and recently had made a proposal of marriage. She could not choose between marriage and a career but admitted that the thought of marriage and its responsibilities were very disturbing to her.

Conflict over Marriage

The patient was informed that the conflict between marriage and a career probably had some relation to her illness and that it would be helpful to her if she were able definitely to make up her mind. She was seen again a month later and was much improved and announced that she had given up the idea of marriage and had determined upon a period of intensive study to perfect herself for her career.

Once more we see the problem of an immature person finding the hurdle of marriage too difficult and responding by the production of bodily symptoms. Here, obviously, it was the bowel which was expressing fear and insecurity although, of course, there could be other meanings as well. Too often such patients are told that if they will only marry their troubles will disappear. It is unwise to make such recommendations because, as we have said before, marriage should not be recommended for therapeutic reasons. *Marriage is an excellent institution and will no doubt persist but it is not intended as a short cut to the solution of emotional problems*! Neither are we justified in telling a patient not to marry but on the contrary we must allow the patient to make the choice herself, stating frankly that there is a cause and effect relationship between indecision over the marriage situation and the production of symptoms. It is perfectly possible that if such a person can bring herself to marry, sufficient emotional growth may occur so that the illness may be benefited, but it also happens that quite the reverse usually occurs and the marriage situation adds to the emotional problem, causing more symptoms. This is especially true when one immature person selects another immature person as a mate and it is noteworthy that this unfortunate combination occurs with great frequency. The point is, of course, that we must be very cautious about recommendations in regard to such important problems as marriage, divorce and childbearing.

Principles of Management

To get back to the problem of the psychotherapeutic management of such a case as this one we must realize that we are dealing with an emotionally immature and hence weak individual who cannot meet certain life situations in an adequate manner. In the process of treatment they are given an opportunity to release certain tensions and expose psychic weaknesses. The physician who understands and is sympathetic to the idea that it is not reprehensible for patients to have such psychic weakness now has the opportunity to strengthen them psychologically by discussing better ways of adaptation to their specific life situation.

The physician should try to find out by careful history-taking what the bowel function is trying to express, then introduce the formulation to the patient and try to get him thinking of the bowel as misbehaving or as trying to express some attitude he does not recognize or accept consciously. For instance, it can be pointed out that those lacking courage move their bowels under the influence of fear rather than attacking the enemy in the usual fashion. Instead of using the voluntary muscles there is regression to a childish symbolic expression of aggression through the bowel. This reeducational effort helps the patient to meet his situation with the mind rather than by means of "organ language," *i. e.*, diarrhea; and as the individual becomes stronger and able to express his emotions on a more mature level, his bowel, too, should become stronger and better able to "control" its action.

The Organic Approach. P. W. Brown of the Mayo Clinic in a discussion of "Doctoring the Bowels" presents the matter dramatically. We quote his graphic description.

"The following hypothetical history portrays a composite picture of this group which is under consideration: A patient of either sex, but usually a woman between the ages of twenty-five and forty-five years, comes in with the chief complaint of stomach and bowel trouble. During the narrative her memory is frequently refreshed by reference to her notes.

"Her abdominal troubles date back five to twenty or more years, and consist chiefly of distress from gas, bloating, soreness in the right lower abdominal quadrant, and constipation, with occasional attacks of diarrhea which follow catharsis. The stools often contain considerable mucus, and if they are hard, bloody streaks are noticed. The distress has been present more or less all these years, and bears no regular relationship to meals or types of food. The woman never has been strong, although able to attend to usual duties and social demands. Moderate exertion, such as that accompanying a morning of shopping, or having a few guests for dinner is followed by much abdominal distress and fatigue. Dull headaches and a nagging backache are added burdens.

"Further the woman gives the history that because of the distress referable to the abdomen and back, she submitted to an operation, in the hope that appendectomy and straightening of the uterus might help. Prior to operation, a roentgenologic examination had suggested the presence of chronic appendicitis. Relief was obtained for about three months, when the same or even more marked symptoms recurred. Opinions were expressed that perhaps the gallbladder or adhesions might explain the symptoms. In view of the occasional bloody streaks in the stool and anal discomfort, treatment of hemorrhoids was carried out with relief of these local symptoms. Some time later the question of possible focal infection was raised and tonsillectomy was performed. As symptoms persisted, further investigation resulted in a diagnosis of 'chronic colitis.' In consequence, a succession of diets was recommended: no fried or greasy foods, no starches, no meats except fish and breast of chicken, proteins and carbohydrates not to be taken at the same meal, commercial vitamin substances to be included in the diet, only raw fruits and vegetables, only cooked fruits and vegetables, and so on. These diets have resulted in a distaste for food, fear of everything to eat, loss of weight, and actually more or less a state of deficiency. As a logical accompaniment of diet the arch demon, colonic irrigation, was invoked, and the irrigations soon made the mucus and distress worse, in spite of thorough flushing. Other roentgenologic studies resulted in a report of falling of the colon and stomach, for which an abdominal support was prescribed. Almost incidentally, reference is made to peculiar or difficult environmental, social and economic problems, but these are the basis of much, if not all, of the physiologic disturbances. At present the patient eagerly asks, and all in one breath, 'Is the gallbladder diseased and will its removal cure colitis? Will continual abdominal irritation make a cancer? What can be done to restore the normal position of the fallen organs? Just what should my diet be? Are my adhesions causing my trouble?'

"Physical examination reveals an apprehensive, undernourished woman. The abdominal wall is relaxed and all muscles are flabby. A large tonsillar tag is present on the left side. Tenderness is present on palpation of the cecal region. Bimanual examination of the pelvis discloses only retroversion of the uterus.

"The laboratory data are as follows: Roentgenologic examination of the stomach gives evidence of an apparently normal organ. A cholecystogram indicates that the gallbladder is functioning normally. The mucosa of the rectum is normal. No roentgenologic evidence of organic disease of the colon is elicited. The roentgenograms depict the expected influence of the abdominal support on the position of the colon.

"The present condition in this hypothetical case is obvious; it is the end result of *doctoring the bowels*. Interpreted as a group, the diagnosis in such cases is that of functional intestinal disturbance associated with a state of physical and nervous exhaustion. Usually there is a greater or less degree of biologic inferiority, for which the patient is hardly to blame.

It is this, with the characteristic emotional, nervous instability that makes for so much difficulty. We are so constantly harassed by the fear of missing something that we may fail to appreciate how profound are the physiologic disturbances produced by nervous and emotional strain. Although we may need special guidance in some cases, this is not a problem for the psychologist or psychiatrist. It has been suggested that undergraduate training unwittingly stresses organic disease at the expense of a broader and more sympathetic appreciation of emotional and nervous problems. There need be neither thought of curtailing the instruction in organic disease, nor of deprecating correction of organic conditions of nervous patients, but by a fuller understanding of the emotions we may be of greater service."

ULCERATIVE COLITIS

The problem of ulcerative colitis focuses attention on the question of the interrelationship of psychic and organic disease. The general outline of this topic was discussed in the introduction. Here we need only say that we are not interested in trying to prove that psychological factors are directly or solely responsible for ulcerative colitis. Indeed, we do not believe it. In line with our thesis that all illness should be regarded from the standpoint of the whole organism we are interested in psychological factors in ulcerative colitis only as one part of a complicated psychosomatic problem.

Emotional Factors

Unlike mucous colitis, when we come to a consideration of ulcerative colitis, we find general medicine less impressed by psychic factors in the etiology. The opinion is frequently expressed, "Yes, it is easy enough to understand that mucous colitis is a functional disorder but you can't tell me that psychic factors can produce actual ulcers of the bowel." We would be the last to see a direct relationship between psychic factors and ulcer formation. As in many other disorders involving the vegetative nervous system we consider the psychological panel only one phase of this disorder. Some such scheme as that erected for the discussion of the pathogenesis of essential hypertension might apply equally well to ulcerative colitis so far as the part that the psyche plays is concerned (p. 304). However, it is an important phase upon which not a great deal of work has been done. Murray presented some impressive psychological case studies and Sullivan, from the medical standpoint, stressed the importance of psychogenic factors in etiology and considered psychotherapy of the utmost importance in treatment. He felt that when the emotional conflict is solved, the intestinal motility returns to normal, the chief irritative factor is removed from the colon, which can then take care of its bacterial invaders, and the disease may promptly disappear.

Personality Study

Daniels made an intensive psychological study of a case of ulcerative colitis associated with hysterical depression. The patient was a woman of thirty-two years with a history of three previous attacks of ulcerative colitis. Daniels observed her during most of the five years of her fourth attack. Between the third and fourth attacks the patient had two pregnancies. The first pregnancy was terminated by giving birth to the fetus in the toilet, which acted as a great psychic shock, and the second pregnancy was followed by a prolonged attack of tachycardia and a period of partial amnesia.

Psychiatric investigation revealed deep unconscious hostile trends and suicidal drives. The patient was treated by intensive psychotherapy and by this means was able to emancipate herself from her family. Then the social service department assisted her in reestablishing her own home. This was an essential step in treatment. Hay fever and asthma appeared for the first time during this transition and there was an acute flare-up of palpitation and diarrhea when she made the actual step of moving to a new home. Although some frequency of stool persisted and there was an occasional diarrhea brought about by the emotional factors, there was no further clinical evidence of ulcerative colitis. The colon showed chronic changes which suggested that complete recovery was unlikely and the persistence of depressive personality trends further modified the prognosis. The greater severity and duration of the last attack seemed to have been due to an altered life situation with conflict related to a neurotically conditioned marriage reinforced by the childbirth for which she was ill-prepared. Various medical procedures had relatively little effect on the disease process and it seemed fair to assume that psychotherapy had been an important factor in the arrest of the disease and in her social recovery.

Dependency

In another contribution to the subject Daniels states that such persons are apt to be self-centered and dependent. This dependency is shown particularly toward the mother or a mother substitute, frequently an older sister, and is often maintained by an enforced docility on the part of the patient, who says, "My mother would rather have me sick at home than well and away." Dominating in-laws frequently take over this family role.

Furthermore, the ulcerative colitis patients are sexually immature and do not carry responsibility well. They are apt to break in a crisis and have been called the "giver-uppers." In this way they are the opposite of the peptic ulcer patients who as a rule are aggressive and seek responsibility. The males with ulcerative colitis are inclined to be passive, pathologically attached to their mothers, frequently unmarried; the women, who are more frequently married, are apt to be the "fussy" type of housewife.

Relation to Psychosis

Daniels further noted mental depression in association with this disease. He pointed out the importance of recognizing this to be a primary emotional disturbance rather than a secondary reaction to an uncomfortable and disagreeable disease. The depression is usually reactive in nature following some loss or frustration. The psychic structure of ulcerative colitis and manic-depressive psychosis suggests a possible relationship that deserves further study. In regard to precipitating factors it seems that acute upper respiratory infections, emotional upheavals, and possibly pregnancy are the most frequent elements entering into the onset of the disease. The rigid and immature personalities of the majority of these persons make them unable to tolerate reverses or crises well or to undertake the necessary steps in emotional sexual maturity of engagement, marriage, and child-bearing. While many such women get safely through pregnancy, an attack often follows after childbirth. In the men a frequent conflict is that between attachment to the mother and a desire to get married. Sickness or death of a near relative, particularly the mother, seems especially traumatic in these cases. Losses of money or financial worries also act as precipitating factors.

Bereavement As Precipitating Factor

Lindemann, in a study of forty-five patients with ulcerative colitis, noted that various forms of bereavement are the most important precipitating factors. In twenty-six of forty-five patients a close relationship existed between the loss of an important person and the onset of the illness. Dependency became a threat to the patient after bereavement because of a tendency to primitive behavior patterns, colored by fantasies of extreme violence, and asocial behavior marked by aggressiveness and overcritical, demanding, and "spoiled-child" attitudes.

Lindemann cautions against early attempts at exploration with the usual psychiatric technics. He suggests that the contact must be brief, not permitting the development of regressive tendencies, hostile feelings, or affectionate attachment. "The relationship must, rather, be an identifying one, in which the patient copies the behavior patterns of the psychiatrist, and makes use of them in the same manner as he previously did with the patterns of the person who is lost." After such a relationship is established, it is often possible to review the bereavement with the proper emotion of depression and sorrow. The patient may go through a period of "nervousness" and worry, which might, superficially, appear detrimental to visceral functions, but is necessary for readjustment.

Combined Therapy

In discussing therapy Daniels pointed out that the severity of the condition made medical and sometimes surgical treatment necessary. However, in selected cases he regarded psychotherapy as definitely the treatment of choice and actually necessary to get results. Since the patients are usually severely ill physically, frequent contact with the physician over long periods of time is desirable for general medical supervision and to give opportunity for observation, collecting of necessary history and prolonged psychotherapy, either superficial or deep. Some of the cases encountered were largely situational while others had a deep neurotic structure which no one but a psychiatrist experienced in psychosomatic medicine should attempt to treat. He emphasized that it may take weeks or months of observation before relationships between the precipitating elements and the disease become clear. While the problem of a domineering mother or her substitute is one of the most frequent relationships to overcome, the relief of repressed hostility as well as gradual help in bringing the patient to greater emotional maturity is in general the chief aim of the treatment. Psychotherapy can be carried on while the patient is receiving other therapy. The privacy of a room for interviews is important. Daniels also stressed the importance of having other members of the house staff and nursing personnel acquainted with the nature of psychotherapy, and of realizing that following psychotherapeutic interviews the patient might be upset. They should not regard this as a sign that the patient is worse but as a necessary part of recovery through relief of tension. The help of the social service staff is frequently required in making plans for environmental changes and relief from difficult social and family situations.

Physical and Emotional Immaturity

Our own observations support the suggestions that ulcerative colitis is frequently precipitated by emotional factors and that psychotherapy is invaluable in treatment. We have been impressed by the physical and emotional immaturity of patients with this disease. We are not impressed by the argument that this immaturity is dependent upon the disease. As in many other psychosomatic problems we believe that it is the other way around, that is, the immaturity is an index to the kind of personality that is apt to develop a disorder of the vegetative nervous system in which psychic factors play an important part.

In a discussion of Sullivan's paper Jones stated that in easily two-thirds of 100 cases which he and Urmy had followed at the Massachusetts General Hospital psychogenic disturbances seemed responsible for bringing on exacerbations, and that in the whole group acute upper respiratory infections, emotional or nervous upheavals, and possibly pregnancy, were the most obvious elements entering into the onset of the disease. "That there is an infection of the colon is obvious, but that it represents a specific disease due to a single organism is still, I believe, far from obvious." This statement was made in 1935 but we believe that it still holds.

The following case is typical of the kind of personality and psychological background of many cases of ulcerative colitis.

Ulcerative Colitis

CASE 31

A white woman of twenty-five was first seen in 1931. She complained of frequent, bloody bowel movements.

History and Symptoms

Except for an occasional attack of tonsillitis she had always been in good health. The menses had been established at fifteen, and had been regular and normal. She married at twenty-two and had a child one year later. Frequent bowel movements with blood-streaked stools began shortly after the birth of the child. This was in December, 1930. The blood then increased in amount. In March, 1931, the tonsils were removed. Headache, fever, nausea, and vomiting occurred one week later and the bowel trouble, which had partially subsided, returned.

Family History. The father, aged fifty-seven, and the mother, aged fifty-three, were living and well. Three brothers and four sisters were all living and well. There was no history of serious bowel trouble among any blood relatives.

Physical Examination and Laboratory Studies

The patient was a pale, poorly nourished, young white woman with the physical appearance of immaturity and a timid, whining manner. Examination was negative except for slight tenderness on deep pressure over the lower left quadrant of the abdomen. The sigmoidoscopic examination showed a markedly inflamed and ulcerated lower bowel. Barium enema findings were in conformity with the diagnosis of ulcerative colitis affecting principally the descending colon.

Shortly after admission to the hospital the temperature rose to 105° F., then dropped to normal with peaks of lesser magnitude on alternating successive days during the first ten days. Then there was slight irregular fever until discharge from the hospital one month later. She improved during her hospital stay, apparently from topical treatment.

Aside from revealing a marked anemia the laboratory studies were of no importance. No specific organism could be isolated from the stool culture and the blood culture was negative.

LIFE SITUATION

The patient had an insecure girlhood. The parents were incompatible and there was a great deal of contention in the household which the patient seemed to feel more than her brothers or sisters did. They were a hardy lot who openly entered into the family quarrels while the patient, who gave the impression of a refined and lady-like person, suffered the quarreling in silence. She married at the age of twenty-two and a short time before the marriage her fiance, who had been working in Philadelphia, decided to settle in a small town. This was very distasteful to the patient but she did not attempt to express her unwillingness to leave Philadelphia. Then immediately after marriage she became pregnant, although she did not want to, and suffered from severe nausea all through the pregnancy. About six weeks after the baby was born she first noted blood in the bowel movement. Her local physician apparently did not regard it as a serious symptom. However, the bowel movements increased in frequency and the blood increased in amount. She harbored a great deal of ill-feeling for this physician who had made light of the first symptom. She also showed a great deal of resentment in many other aspects of her life. Although she stated that there were no special problems disturbing her, she confessed that she did not get along well with her in-laws who lived in a nearby town and whom her husband insisted upon visiting frequently. She had a child-like *resentment* against them, saying that they held her in little esteem because she did not have a dowry to give their son. Her sexual life during marriage had been unsatisfactory so that she had been resentful of the necessity for permitting intercourse. Her conscious attitude in the hospital ward was one of constant complaining and constant discussion of how long she must remain, insisting that she must get back to her child, and yet it was apparent that she was really satisfied to remain in the hospital as long as we wished her to.

She maintained her improvement after leaving the hospital for a period of about two weeks while she remained in Philadelphia. Then she went home, financial difficulties arose, and the bowel trouble returned. With a second pregnancy the colitis was aggravated and following this incident she never fully recovered. There was constant family dissension, and the patient died of a perforation of the bowel in 1940.

SUMMARY

A young white woman, presenting the emotional and physical aspects of immaturity, developed ulcerative colitis following marriage and the birth of an unwanted child. Her manner was childlike, complaining, and resentful, and it was felt that her personality plus the problems of her life situation had much to do with her illness.

Chapter XIII

THE GASTROINTESTINAL SYSTEM (Concluded)

CARDIOSPASM

Cardiospasm is another disorder of the gastrointestinal tract which touches upon the great borderline problem of the interrelationship of physical and psychological disease. For if evidence were forthcoming in favor of the psychogenic origin of even some cases of cardiospasm it would aid in the establishment of the important concept of the role of psychogenesis in the determination of structural disease, a field of medical investigation that is just beginning to be studied.

Prevailing Ideas of Etiology

Prevailing opinion in regard to psychic factors in the etiology of cardiospasm may be stated as follows: (1) that the disorder is a physical one and psychic factors are considered of no importance or are unnoticed; (2) that it is a disorder of physical origin in which psychic factors are frequently found which are probably secondary to the physical disorder; (3) that it is a physical disorder in which psychic factors are present because these patients are subjects with autonomic imbalance, that is, vagotonics, in whom physical disorders of the vegetative nervous system and psychological difficulties are apt to coexist; (4) that in some way psychic factors, acting through the vegetative nervous system, are specifically responsible for the cardiospasm.

These viewpoints are not so very different from current attitudes in regard to the other numerous functional disorders of the gastrointestinal tract, and indeed, for our purposes, cardiospasm may be said to constitute only one small phase of this larger problem.

Personality Study

In the cases of cardiospasm that we have studied, the disorder seems to have a special meaning in terms of behavior. This meaning can be discovered by a study of the personality in relation to the environment. The cardiospasm often is found to arise coincidently with an emotional conflict, in many instances during puberty, in an individual whose early life gives evidence of personality difficulties. Frequently it is found that at first the disorder seems to manifest itself intermittently; later on, it may become persistently established. Exacerbations occur which often can be correlated with fresh psychic insults touching the particular complex of the individual.

It would seem that the cases correspond to conversion hysteria deeply rooted in the unconscious mental life of the individual. The physical disorder represents symbolically the unconscious conflict—it appears to be a compromise between the gratification of certain forbidden impulses and their rejection by another part of the personality. A superficial but important meaning of the disorder often can be stated in such simple terms as "I can't *swallow* that (situation)." Therefore, this meaning often can be discovered by looking (psychologically) for the situation that the individual "cannot swallow" (Weiss).

The Specific Psychic Situation

This kind of information furnishes a specific background for the cardiospasm and replaces the loose terminology and loose thinking behind such terms as "nervous factors" and "neurogenic background" with a more exact definition of the specific psychic situation. Indeed, to speak of "nervous factors" in the background of the patient with cardiospasm without further defining them seems to us as obsolete as blaming malaria on marsh gas with failure to note the part played by the malarial parasite. In self-criticism, we may say that we have not found the parasite but we do think that we have the mosquito.

Psychosomatic Approach

Whatever one believes regarding the etiological role of these mental forces, it must be apparent that to study patients with cardiospasm simply as physiological mechanisms and treat them by mechanical measures, without making some effort to understand the emotional make-up, is a very one-sided and inadequate attempt to deal with the disorder. The above observations suggest the necessity for a combined physical and psychological study and treatment of the individual patient with cardiospasm. No one can deny the necessity for mechanical treatments in the established case of cardiospasm but is it not possible that this additional psychic approach will help us deal with that group of cases "which tend to recur" or that group "which cannot be cured"? Especially in regard to these groups we must consider the frequent observation that in a patient with a severe neurosis a physical disorder (such as cardiospasm) appears to be that patient's solution of his psychic conflict. The physical disorder, therefore, is necessary to the emotional life and until the psychic conflict is better solved, the particular disorder from which the patient suffers either must be maintained or must be replaced by another illness. Certainly, in an early case of cardiospasm, especially in a young person, psychologic study and treatment seem to us an essential part of the management. Indeed, we venture to suggest that the time is approaching when the physician will consider the neglect of psychological study just as serious an omission, in the total study of the patient with cardiospasm, as the failure to x-ray such a patient or to study him with the esophagoscope.

The following case illustrates the psychological background.

Cardiospasm

CASE 32

History and Symptoms

A fifty-five-year-old white man was referred through the kindness of Dr. C. L. Jackson from the bronchoscopic department of Temple University Hospital, February, 1933, with the diagnosis, established by esophagoscopy and roentgen-ray, of preventriculosis, generally spoken of as cardiospasm. He was receiving treatments in the form of esophageal dilatations.

The patient gave the usual medical history of this condition. He stated that his illness began about eight or ten years before and had been progressive. He had consulted many physicians. Discouraged, he had invested a large sum of money with an osteopath who had promised cure; finally, very sick and without funds, he had come to the hospital. The previous medical history did not seem to bear upon this illness.

LIFE SITUATION

His life situation, however, was interesting. He had been "born into the drug business" and had never known anything except the long hours and tedious work of an underpaid pharmacy clerk. He married young and five children came in rapid succession. It was a great financial struggle to look after them. About 1916 or 1917 while working very hard he had "some kind of a breakdown" during which there were nervous symptoms and he took bromides. In 1922 his oldest and favorite son, then aged twenty, had just obtained an excellent job which paid well. He gave his salary to his mother and the father was overjoyed with the finally achieved prospects of economic freedom. He had always pictured a great career for this able son and had looked forward to his financial aid to help him in his old age.

Marriage of Son

Without warning one morning shortly afterward he learned that this son had just secretly married. He said, "It was the greatest blow I ever received, not only because of the financial part of it but the way he did it" (that is, secretly). The patient went on to say, "I felt like a child crying until his heart would break" and he placed his hand on his epigastrium to show where he felt the blow.

He could not get over this disappointment and even considered having the marriage annulled on the basis that the boy was too young to marry. It was interesting to note, however, that he, himself, had married at the same age. He harbored a great deal of resentment toward the girl's parents who, he felt, had stolen his fine son from him. It was during this period that attacks of *swallowing difficulty* occurred and grew more pronounced and more frequent.

Further Aggravation

A short time later further aggravation occurred. He learned that his brother in England, whom he described as a ne'er-do-well, was cheating his mother of her small legacy. He went to England, brought his mother back and she then made her home with them. It seemed significant that the mother contributed her sole income to the upkeep of him and his family. In other words, while he accused his brother of having "bled his mother" he, himself, had already borrowed money from her and then took her weekly allowance for living expenses. His altruism in rescuing her from his ne'er-do-well brother seemed questionable.

The picture was that of a meek, submissive, and dependent individual who had always worked hard without achieving success. He had strongly identified with his oldest son in whom he hoped to achieve the success denied himself. With his son's secret marriage came a tremendous disappointment from which he could not recover.

Experience with Osteopath

An interesting commentary in line with our thesis was his experience with the osteopath. He consulted him about December, 1931, and was charged $1000, which his sons had to borrow, "for the management of his case." It was interesting to consider why he felt like investing this great sum of money with the osteopath. He said, "The osteopath told me that my trouble was due to a spasm arising from a shock," and the patient went on to say, "he did not know about my son's marriage." He was much impressed by this diagnosis "because it was the first time that any doctor had suggested that shock and worry might be responsible for my trouble." He thereupon placed his entire confidence and all the money that he could raise in the osteopath's hands.

The Meaning of the Illness

In the recital of his story, accompanied by great emotion, this poor druggist made the following significant and perhaps revealing statement, "My son's marriage was a bitter pill that I could not swallow." And who can say that that was not, at least, one meaning of the illness?

SUMMARY

A meek and dependent, middle-aged white man developed cardiospasm apparently in response to a life situation "which he could not swallow."

ANOREXIA NERVOSA

Anorexia nervosa is still another disorder which touches upon the question of the psychogenesis of organic disease. The subject will be more fully developed in the chapter on endocrines and metabolism but a case is cited here only to illustrate that the gastrointestinal symptoms are of psychological origin.

Anorexia Nervosa

CASE 33

History and Symptoms

The patient, a single woman of thirty-two, was admitted to the Temple University Hospital, service of Dr. Brown, September 27, 1938. She complained of weakness, nervousness, and loss of weight. These symptoms had been present for many years but, for the last year, had been so severe that she had spent most of her time in bed.

Past History. The ordinary facts of the medical history follow. She stated that she was a healthy child and recalled only measles among the childhood diseases. No other serious illnesses occurred. She began to menstruate at the age of fourteen and menses were always too frequent. At about seventeen she began to menstruate profusely. At the time she was admitted to another hospital where an *abdominal operation* was done, a bicornate uterus was found; one of the horns was sutured and the appendix was removed at the same time. The operation had no effect on the profuse menstruation. Radium was next tried but neither did this effect a cure. Then she began to lose appetite and weight and suffered from tachycardia, palpitation, and shortness of breath. Her weight decreased from about 110 to 85 pounds and just before her first admission to this hospital in 1931, at the age of twenty-five, the appetite was completely lost, the patient refusing all forms of food except liquid. There was some nausea but no vomiting. She was severely constipated and used enemas as the only effectual means of controlling it. She remained in the hospital for two months; she was considered to have some *endocrine dysfunction*, and was treated by means of *insulin* and managed to gain some weight, which, however, soon was lost after she returned home. The profuse menses continued and one year later she was again admitted to the hospital where a *hysterectomy* was done. The tubes and ovaries were allowed to remain. The patient, however, failed to gain strength and weight and had continued with chronic anorexia ever since, her weight varying between 70 and 90 pounds. During the past year she had become progressively worse, had spent most of her time in bed, and just before admission to the hospital weighed only 70 pounds.

Family History. The mother died in 1929, when the patient was twenty-three, of cancer of the stomach. She had been sick for two years. The father also was dead—the patient thought that he died also of cancer of the stomach, but was not sure. The mother and father had separated when the patient was ten years old. The patient was the youngest of seven children. One of her sisters also died of cancer in 1935. All the rest were healthy. She made her home with the oldest sister, another sister, and a brother.

Physical Examination and Laboratory Studies

Physical examination showed an emaciated young, white woman, but aside from the severe undernutrition, there were no noteworthy physical findings and the routine laboratory studies showed nothing abnormal. Although the breasts were small they were well preserved and axillary and pubic hair were present.

Summary. The illness revolved around two systems particularly, that is, the question of the profuse menstruation eventuating in the removal of a bicornate uterus and the long history of chronic anorexia with considerable undernutrition. Both went back many years, probably to the age of seventeen or eighteen if not before, and resulted in a severe degree of invalidism—that is, an illness necessitating bed care for the past year.

How were we to attempt to work out this problem? When people say they cannot eat one thinks first of the stomach and so here, by means of physical examination, studies of gastric and biliary secretions, and x-ray studies of the gastrointestinal tract, we excluded organic disease not only of the stomach but of the remainder of the gastrointestinal tract and its appendages. Next, of course, we thought of the possible systemic diseases that might be responsible but we found no evidence of heart, lung, or other system disease, including the neurological system, so we then turned our attention to an etiological approach.

Etiological Approach

We discovered no evidence of a chronic infection, "focal" or otherwise; the temperature and pulse were normal; the sedimentation rate was within normal limits; we did not know of any metabolic disorder that could be responsible (aside from the one that we shall mention shortly in another connection); nor were we aware of any allergic process that could give this clinical picture. How about the endocrine system? Certainly this was not myxedema although the basal metabolism was somewhat depressed, minus 14 per cent; nor was there anything to indicate that it was Addison's disease even though the blood pressure was low. But there were certain aspects of this clinical picture that resembled a rare condition that is known as Simmonds's disease or pituitary cachexia. This last, however, presents a profound picture of emaciation with loss of hair from the genital and axillary regions, and wasting of breasts and genitalia, finally resulting in coma and death in a much shorter period than the duration of this illness. This clinical picture might be stated to be a kind of mild copy or imitation of true Simmonds's disease but by no means so profound. Therefore, by means of the bare facts of medical history, physical examination, and laboratory studies, we were unable to say what was responsible for this illness. Let us see what a study of the life situation showed.

LIFE SITUATION

From the psychiatric standpoint we need to know not only from what diseases a patient is suffering but also how the patient is behaving. The taking of food is surely a piece of behavior, as well as a biological necessity, and, as a piece of behavior, it may serve to express something in addition to its normal function of nourishment.

Everybody is familiar with the eating behavior of children, where refusal to eat very openly conveys reaction to disappointment, stubbornness, refusal to cooperate, unwillingness to participate in the environmental routine, or lastly, *a desire to return to an earlier form of feeding or type of food taken.*

In studying this patient we could not reconstruct everything which took place in early childhood. Much was not remembered, and time permitted distortion to creep into what had been remembered. So often in adult patients we must pay close attention to the current behavior and attitudes, and from these reconstruct what has taken place during emotional growth. We have found this to be a safe procedure because early life behavior patterns tend to repeat themselves with but little distortion.

Early Life

When we reviewed the life history of our patient we found that she was the youngest of a large family and that she was always what she called "a picky eater." She was consistently indulged by her mother and the rest of the family, was coaxed to eat more, and became the center of attention in the family group because her appetite was so poor. She stated that her home life was pleasant, although she refused to talk about her father, who separated from the mother when the patient was ten years old, and, as she grudgingly admitted, "drank a great deal but was good to the family."

The patient had a common school education and went to work at the age of eighteen as a weaver, which work, she stated, was too heavy for her and her mother did not want her to continue, but she managed to stay for two years and then had her first admission to the hospital because of profuse menstruation. Afterwards she got a job as a clerk but, following her mother's death in 1929 when the patient was twenty-three, she had what she called a sort of *nervous breakdown*—cried a good deal and had not been able to work since. It was interesting that another sister, who was "wonderful to her, just like mother was," took the patient's position in the clerical job and had continued ever since while the patient remained at home, an invalid, looked after by this oldest, working sister. Another sister, four years older, worked in the same place, and a brother, who was a weaver, had been unemployed for the past four or five years. He, also, made his home with the three sisters. The patient stated that she got anything she wanted—"my sisters see to that."

Her illness, therefore, went back to the mother's death when the patient was twenty-three years of age. At this age we expect normal, well-adjusted people to have a good working ability, a certain recreation program, and to be at least thinking of home formation and community responsibility, if not actually engaged in either of these latter activities.

Immature Attitudes

As we studied this patient's behavior for the past eight years, we saw practically nothing of this more mature attitude toward life. She had done no work at all, she had shown no interest in the opposite sex, home formation, or children, and she had no recreational program. In fact, she became emotionally distressed when she was questioned about her attitude toward the opposite sex or recreation, and stated that she did not feel they were important in any way and certainly had nothing to do with her illness. In spite of the fact that her endeavor in these fields had been so limited the patient tried to give the impression, and actually seemed to believe, that she had been, as she described it, "a very active person." When questioned specifically about the activities she had to admit she never had a date, never danced, never played cards, and that she had never actually participated in any outdoor sport. She maintained that she had many friends, but these friends were those in the neighborhood who came to bring her sympathy and occasional gifts. From these gifts of money, she in turn gave part to those she considered less fortunate than herself. This led her to say that she "is always helping people." She liked to talk of helping people and to listen to her one would get the impression that her activities were of much greater scope than actually turned out to be true upon close questioning.

Emotional Dependency

Emotionally the patient was a very sensitive person. If questioned about the opposite sex she pouted and turned her back upon the examiner. She was unable to think very coherently and was even unwilling to take the responsibility of remembering certain facts out of her past life. One gained the impression that she knew the answer but she said, "I can't remember exactly, you had better ask my sister." She found it difficult to adapt to life in the ward and was eager to return home to her own family. Her eagerness to do this seemed to disregard her expressed desire to get well, to eat better, to gain weight, and to be able to do things. As a result of insulin therapy she had gained several pounds in weight, but seemed to disregard this fact and wanted to hurry home almost as if she wished to lose the added weight and resume her former life of invalidism. During the past year the patient had spent most of her time in bed.

She was fed, and otherwise taken care of by her sisters, like a child of one year, including the regular giving of enemas. Obviously, life at this level was what she wanted but she could not admit it; in fact, she tried very hard to deny it. Her denial took the form of a refusal to discuss why she was not participating in life as a very active individual. This strong, unconscious urge to be dependent, accompanied by a strong conscious need to deny this dependency, has been shown to be a prominent psychological pattern in certain cases of gastric dysfunction. In marked contrast to this pattern we see some people who have no conflict whatever over living at the expense of their family or of friends for an indefinite period. They have an excellent appetite and no conflict whatever over being dependent upon others; in fact, seem to expect it and say they consider anyone unreasonable who tries to change this state of affairs.

Secondary Gain from Illness

Some of the things we have said about this patient and her desire to return home, to be taken care of by her family, might indicate that this was the cause of her illness. It was by no means as simple as that. While it was true that her symptoms permitted her to live in this pleasant, dependent state, she did not consciously seek it and what she obtained in this way is referred to as secondary rather than primary gain. In fact, it was this very denial of her dependency which accounted in no small measure for her inability to eat. By being unable to eat she was refusing to participate even in this simple piece of life activity.

In regard to psychological diagnosis we felt that we were dealing with a person who was emotionally quite ill. She had a very severe neurosis of the conversion hysterical type, but in some ways her regression almost approached psychosis. Unfortunately we were unable to continue treatment after she left the hospital but we were impressed with the unfavorable outlook.

SUMMARY

A young, severely neurotic, white woman presented the clinical picture of anorexia nervosa. Her inability to eat seemed to symbolize her denial of dependency.

PEPTIC ULCER

It was previously stated that in the Mayo Clinic series of 15,000 cases of chronic dyspepsia more than 15 per cent had x-ray evidence pointing to peptic ulcer as the cause. Thus peptic ulcer, especially of the duodenum, is the commonest organic lesion within the gastrointestinal tract itself responsible for chronic dyspepsia. But it is not only because of its frequency that it is easily the most important psychosomatic problem encountered among the disorders of the gastrointestinal tract. The term psychosomatic can be used without hesitation in connection with peptic ulcer because today even the most organically minded physician recognizes the importance of "emotional factors" in ulcer cases.

To be sure, no one doubts the existence of a constitutional factor but, as previously stated, it is impossible in the light of our present knowledge to delimit the role that the constitution plays from the influence of environmental factors. Many instances have been reported of peptic ulcer occurring in infancy and early childhood, certainly at a period when the emotional conflicts, which we shall discuss later, could not possibly enter (Guthrie-Donavan.) This indicates only that the constitutional factor is dominant in these particular cases. But our point of view in regard to etiology is that multiple factors usually are at work: In some instances the constitutional element seems chiefly responsible; in others the environmental influences seem more important, and among these it is now recognized that emotional factors rank first.

Prevailing Views

Cushing, in a noteworthy paper which will be quoted again, observed that all clinicians are familiar with these facts: (1) that highly strung persons are particularly susceptible to nervous indigestion and associated ulcer; (2) that ulcers become symptomatically quiescent or

16

even tend to heal when patients are put mentally and physically at rest; and (3) the symptoms are prone to recur as soon as the victim of the disorder resumes his former tasks and responsibilities. He concluded by suggesting that highly strung (vagotonic) persons subjected to emotional stress, and such other factors as irregular meals and excessive use of tobacco, are prone to have chronic digestive disturbances often leading to ulcer. This was as far as he felt that we could go, with the data at hand, in interpreting the "neurogenic" origin of peptic ulcer and explaining its existing prevalence.

Theories of Etiology

In a splendid review of the etiology of peptic ulcer formation Eusterman discussed the following theories: vascular, chemical or corrosive, gastritic, infectious, traumatic, mechanical, endocrine, vitamin deficiency, allergic, and neurogenic. Although some of these theories had their inception almost a century ago, for example, that ulcer was dependent on vascular disease, and the other theories came along as new developments in their respective fields suggested that this peculiar and baffling disease might be explained on the basis of the newest etiological process, it goes without saying that no one of them adequately explains peptic ulcer.

In appraising the various theories Eusterman stated that all noteworthy contributors agreed that ulcer is not the result of a single agent, but is a product of the interaction of various agents; and that the constitutional or systemic factor is fundamentally essential. He felt that the major facts of the genesis and development of ulcer have been established, and that the causative factor which is operative in the vast majority of cases is the *psyche* mediated through the autonomic nervous system, producing a morbid physiological state conducive to the initiation, extension and chronicity of the lesion. To what extent inheritance or constitution acts in this group he could not say but he was persuaded that conscious and unconscious emotional factors which can be continuously operative are sufficient. Thus Eusterman was apparently most impressed by "neurogenic factors" in the etiology of peptic ulcer. We agree with his critical appraisal and would quarrel with him only concerning the use of the term *neurogenic*. Many authors apparently hesitate to use the term *psychogenic* and therefore all questions dealing with the nervous system, whether they be organic or emotional, are included in the term neurogenic. To this we object because the term psychogenic should be used for emotional factors if we are to respect them as causes of disease and deal with them courageously. Thus even from nonpsychological sources we are confronted with imposing evidence that psychic factors are of the greatest importance as a cause of peptic ulcer and so we have a clear-cut issue of psychosomatic medicine to discuss, namely, on the one hand a definite organic disease—peptic ulcer, which can be demonstrated by means of x-ray and surgery—and on the other hand, emotional factors which seem important from the standpoint of cause and treatment.

That the problem is important from a consideration of timeliness can also be testified to by the fact that peptic ulcer became *a very serious disability problem among the British military forces* in World War II. Here, of course, it is obvious that the matter of psychic stress was important.

In order to replace the loose terminology "neurogenic factors" by Alexander's concept of specific psychogenesis in the etiology of peptic ulcer let us begin by reviewing the work of Cushing, his associates, and others who have been interested in the connection between the central nervous system and peptic ulcers.

Clinical Observations

Cushing cited three instances of perforating lesions of the stomach, duodenum, and esophagus following operations for cerebellar tumor and called attention to further instances of erosions of the gastric mucosa without perforation, after intracranial operations. He reported a case of pathologically verified chronic ulcer in a patient with cerebellar tumor and also cited the case of an individual having a roentgenologically demonstrable peptic ulcer with symptomatic and roentgen-ray evidence of an organic lesion in the region of the third ventricle. He had frequently seen patients recovering from serious intracranial operations in whom during convalescence digestive disturbances strongly suggested incipient ulcer formation.

In an effort to explain these and other similar observations he reviewed the neurogenic aspects of ulcer pathogenesis and called attention to the first observations of that nature by Rokitansky, who believed that the cause of peptic ulcer was "a diseased innervation of the stomach, owing to a morbid condition of the vagus, and to extreme acidification of the gastric juice."

Experimental Observations

From his observations and the investigations of others Cushing undertook experimental studies which showed that intraventricular injections of pilocarpine or pituitrin caused, in man, an increase in gastric motility, hypertonus and hypersecretion leading to retching and vomiting which ultimately contained occult blood. Growing out of Cushing's observations his associates, Light, Bishop, and Kendall regularly produced peptic ulcers in animals with small intraventricular injections of pilocarpine and observed pathologically a local anemia of the stomach mucosa accompanied by surface hemorrhage and necrosis extending to the muscularis mucosae. Beattie showed in animals that direct electrical stimulation of the region of the tuberal centers in the infundibulum not only caused increased gastric peristalsis but also led to small hemorrhagic ulcers of the mucous membrane near the lesser curvature. After section of the vagi these gastric effects were not obtained. In a study primarily undertaken to investigate the heat regulating mechanism of the brain stem in cats, Keller produced bilateral lesions in the expectation of freeing the hypothalamus from its connections with the brain stem. Postmortem studies showed gastric lesions ranging from simple hyperemic areas to erosions extending through all the layers of the gut, and to punched-out perforating ulcers.

From these studies Cushing observed that the reaction of the stomach to intraventricular injections of either pilocarpine or pituitrin in man and to direct stimulation of the tuber or its descending fiber tracts in animals is *hypersecretion, hypermotility,* and *hypertonicity,* especially marked in the pyloric segment. These are the effects commonly associated with chronic peptic ulcer in man. He believed that by the spasmodic contraction of the musculature, possibly supplemented by accompanying local spasms of the terminal blood vessels, small areas of ischemia or hemorrhagic infarction are produced, leaving the overlying stomach mucosa exposed to the digestive effects of its own hyperacid juices. This applies directly to the formation of chronic ulcer in man because Cushing agreed with many others that an erosion of the mucosa must be the primary stage in ulcer formation; "and since there is every reason to believe that acute erosions . . .are of common occurrence, any one of them may well enough be the precursor of a chronic lesion, should the original insult be sufficiently great or should a minor insult be continuous or frequently repeated at the same spot."

Conscious Emotional Factors

For the purposes of the present discussion, it is noteworthy that von Bergmann in Germany and Alvarez in America have insisted upon the importance of nervous and emotional factors in their relation to ulcer formation. Alvarez called our attention to a certain type of individual who is particularly prone to develop peptic ulcer and referred to him as a keen, nervous, active, hard-living individual, upon whom surgeons are reluctant to operate because of the danger of recurrence of ulcer. He felt that arterial spasm may be one of the links between the emotions and ulcer formation and concluded that most ulcers are due basically to emotional factors and nervous tension. Alvarez has gone a definite step beyond the usual medical approach which is considered complete if it enumerates the physical and chemical data concerning the patient.

Wolff and his associates have made significant contributions to this subject. They had an opportunity to make very careful observations of a patient with a gastric fistula and showed that day-to-day life situations which provoked certain patterns of emotional reaction induced hypersecretion in the stomach comparable to that which could be produced experimentally in animals from prolonged absorption of histamine, vagus stimulation and sham feeding. They discovered that:

1. Acid in small amounts was continuously elaborated in the subject under basal conditions.

2. Spontaneous transitory phases of accelerated secretion of acid occurred from time to time, and were accompanied by blushing of the mucous membrane and vigorous contractions of the stomach wall.

3. Emotions such as fear and sadness which involved a feeling of withdrawal were accompanied by pallor of the gastric mucosa, and by inhibition of acid secretion and contractions, a complex encountered infrequently in their subject.

4. Emotional conflict involving anxiety, hostility and resentment was accompanied by accelerated acid secretion, hypermotility, hyperemia, and engorgement of the gastric mucosa resembling "hypertrophic gastritis." (This series of events, much more commonly observed, was associated with gastric complaints of the nature of heartburn and abdominal pain.)

5. Intense sustained anxiety, hostility, and resentment were found to be accompanied by severe and prolonged engorgement, hypermotility, and hypersecretion in the stomach. In this state mucosal erosions and hemorrhages were readily induced by even the most trifling traumas, and frequently bleeding points appeared spontaneously as a result of vigorous contractions of the stomach wall.

6. Contact of acid gastric juice with such a small eroded surface in the mucous membrane resulted in accelerated secretion of acid and further engorgement of the whole mucosa. Prolonged exposure of such a lesion to acid gastric juice resulted in the formation of a chronic ulcer.

7. The lining of the stomach was found to be protected from its secretions by an efficient insulation layer of mucus, enabling most of the small erosions to heal promptly (within a few hours). Lack of such a protective mechanism in the duodenal cap may explain the higher incidence of chronic ulceration in that region.

They conclude that it appears likely that the chain of events which begins with anxiety and conflict and their associated overactivity of the stomach, and ends with hemorrhage or perforation, is that which is involved in the natural history of peptic ulcer in human beings.

Unconscious Mental Forces in the Etiology of Peptic Ulcer

There are many patients with peptic ulcer in whom evidence of continued worry or emotional stress cannot be easily obtained, and clinicians interested in the "neurogenic" aspect of ulcer pathogenesis have been forced to stop at this point in their investigations. Although a distinctive psychosomatic patten of hypersensitivity, hyperirritability, and hyperactivity has been ascribed to peptic ulcer patients these characteristics are often so masked that there are no external manifestations of mental agitation.

The next step, and the one to which we particularly call attention, depends upon the necessity for understanding that forceful influences exist in the unconscious mental life and that these may play a part in causing peptic ulcer.

Draper, long a protagonist of disease as a psychosomatic reaction, pointed the way to a deeper psychologic understanding of personality in relation to peptic ulcer by calling our attention to the unconscious mental life in his studies of patients with ulcer. But it was Alexander who developed the idea that permanent psychic stimuli from unconscious mental sources may be capable of stimulating the subcortical centers similarly to the direct irritations observed by Cushing and others. This constant psychic stimulation of subcortical centers apparently produces local functional disturbances in the upper digestive tract that may be followed by ulcer formation.

Psychological Regression. Alexander informs us that in these patients psychoanalysis reveals a characteristic regression to the early stages of emotional life. In patients whom he has studied a strong desire for dependence on others was evidenced in the unconscious mental life but consciously the patient was dominated by ideas of independence, activity, and success. Thus when unconscious passive-receptive cravings are not satisfied (as they can hardly be in an individual whose conscious life is devoted to activity and independence) they find their expression in this primitive way. The repressed wishes to be loved and taken care of find motor expression in the production of stomach symptoms.

This phenomenon depends upon infantile habit formations which serve as a pattern of behavior later in life. Alexander explains that the first form of being cared for and loved is nursing and the sensations of being loved and being fed become emotionally associated for the rest of life. If the wish to be loved, as one was by the mother, is denied gratification (repressed) the associated tendency for being nourished is energized.

While the personality of the ulcer patient is usually regarded as the efficient, go-getter type, Kapp working with Rosenbaum and Romano in a study of twenty men with peptic ulcer described two additional groups of persons according to their external personality characteristics, in addition to the "classical" ulcer personality type. Although all the patients showed intense, dependent unconscious strivings, in only six was the mechanism one of overcompensation marked by ambition and success.

A second group of five patients reacted by giving in partially to the dependent desires. As a result they appeared passive and shy with marked trends of feminine identification in their overt personalities.

The largest group of their patients, again with deep dependent cravings, utilized socially unacceptable means of dependency, such as chronic alcoholism and delinquency. They had little or no guilt, employed no socially acceptable defenses against selfish, demanding impulses, and were openly parasitic on their parents, wives, or society. They took and grabbed continually and openly. Essentially this is the unweaned suckling type of personality whose oral needs appear to be insatiable.

Thus the majority of their patients with peptic ulcer either were outwardly passive and effeminate or openly acted out their deep oral desires. Ulcer symptoms developed as responses to frustration of these cravings when the various defense mechanisms which they used to handle such conflicts proved inadequate.

Although the conflict situation is similar, the resulting personality facade may vary from exaggerated independence to parasitic dependence.

The Psychic Stimulus. Unconscious forces of such origin may then stimulate subcortical centers exactly like the pathologic and experimentally produced stimulations observed by Cushing; secondary local changes of function in the stomach occur; and ulcer formation may result.

Such studies replace the loose terminology "neurogenic factors," "large nervous element," etc. and the vague thinking behind such terminology, with a more complete and more precise definition of the mental mechanisms that may be concerned in ulcer formation.

The following case illustrates that in some patients, only an understanding of unconscious mental mechanisms will permit an appreciation of the psychic forces that are important in a consideration of peptic ulcer.

Duodenal Ulcer

CASE 34

A white man, thirty-five years old, had indigestion off and on over a period of fifteen years. In August, 1932, there was a large hemorrhage from the stomach and he was rushed to the hospital. Appropriate treatment brought about quick recovery and studies later demonstrated a well marked duodenal ulcer. There were no other medical facts of importance connected with his previous history. When questioned about worry or emotional stress he answered that his only worry was indigestion; he was successful in business and contented at home.

LIFE SITUATION

He was a keen, hard-working, business man; unmarried, living with his family, consisting of father and mother, two sisters, and one brother. The sisters were twenty-nine and twenty-three, the brother twenty-seven, all unmarried. The patient contributed generously to the support of the family.

The mother was an energetic and capable woman who indulged her family and watched over the children unceasingly. Indeed, she still exercised a great influence over the life of the patient. The father was an easy-going, indolent person, apparently little interested· in the family and they took little interest in him.

The mother recalled that as a youngster the patient was "a good boy" and very studious. His grades in school and college were excellent; he took part in many extracurricular activities although he did not enter into athletics. He had some indigestion during his college days at the time of an unsuccessful love affair. It disappeared and returned while he was in a training camp in 1918. Since that time he had been bothered off and on.

Sexual Life

The patient's sexual life was important in this personality study. He asserted that he did not masturbate, and that his first sexual experience was at about the age of twenty-five with an unattractive woman ten years his senior, who made the first advances. This affair continued for a few months and constituted his only sexual indulgence. He gave as his reason for not permitting himself to indulge further that "it was not right," that he had "religious scruples," and that he "feared venereal disease."

Marriage Problem

For the last four years he had been very attentive to an attractive young woman and, although obviously devoted to her, when questioned about marriage he said: he was comfortable at home and didn't want to change; he wanted to be free to pursue his own life as he saw fit; he had seen many unfortunate marriages; he had to contribute to the family support (although his support was not essential to them). More reasons were given which, like the others, could be readily recognized as *rationalizations*. Somewhat casually he remarked that his mother was not in favor of the marriage. Nevertheless, he apparently was deeply impressed by his mother's objection to the girl. Her stated objection was that she did not consider the girl his social equal (although they themselves were of humble origin). During the last several years while at home he had been relatively free from indigestion and almost entirely free during the last year and a half; the hemorrhage came quite suddenly after what he said was a period of hard work and a dietary indiscretion. It was also to be noted, however, that his closest friend, who had experienced marital difficulties and had always advised the patient to stay single, attempted suicide at that time, apparently because of marital reasons.

This period of freedom from indigestion coincided with the attainment of financial success and also with a period in which his mother no longer voiced objections to his companion.

The Nature of the Emotional Conflict

The picture of this man was that of an energetic, hard-working, "successful" person with marked repressions and retarded emotional development, indicated by his strong attachment to his mother, fear to face marriage and compromising the situation by maintaining an engagement for an indefinite period, meanwhile giving a great many reasons, which were obviously not good reasons, for avoiding marriage. Apparently the affair produced a conflict between his attachment to his mother and his desire to establish an independent home and to attain a proper masculine (heterosexual) goal.

His deference to his mother's wishes and his attitude of excessive morality and goodness indicated unconscious strivings of passivity and dependency, while his energetic pursuit of business and indefinite "engagement" to a girl to whom his mother objected indicated his conscious efforts at accomplishment and independence. Such a conflict refuted his denial of any worry or stress apart from indigestion and showed how necessary an understanding of unconscious strivings was to appreciate the forceful psychic influences that were at work in this patient.

SUMMARY

A young man with duodenal ulcer developed a large gastric hemorrhage. No obvious emotional factors were apparent but personality study showed conflict between unconscious strivings of dependency and the conscious struggle for independence and success. This was brought to the surface by indecision over a marriage situation.

A similar problem in another patient permitted a longer period of observation.

Duodenal Ulcer

CASE 35

A young white man of twenty years was first seen in 1932.

History and Symptoms

In the early part of May, 1932, he had fainted while at work, later had a black stool and was admitted to the hospital where a tentative diagnosis of bleeding peptic ulcer was made. This was later confirmed by x-ray which showed a typical ulcer deformity of the duodenum. No food or fluid was permitted by mouth for the first forty-eight hours after his admission to the hospital and then he was placed upon milk and cream feedings according to the Sippy regimen. He made good progress so that at the end of a month he was discharged from the hospital and then gradually returned to activity.

Past History. When first questioned he gave no history of any previous digestive trouble. He had had the usual childhood diseases but had never previously been seriously sick. While in high school some question had been raised concerning his heart because a physician in a routine physical examination thought he had detected a mitral systolic murmur. The patient became somewhat apprehensive and there was considerable concern in the family over the matter of heart disease but further observation proved that the heart was normal and gradually his apprehension had diminished.

On further close questioning regarding gastrointestinal function he stated that his appetite, digestion, and bowel function had always been excellent except that when he was worried about something or had had a quarrel with someone his appetite would leave him. Then he stated that for several months before the onset of his duodenal hemorrhage he had some slight indigestion. He recalled that on many occasions he ate more as a matter of habit than because of any real appetite, and that on some occasions he would have a heavy feeling in the epigastrium after eating.

Family History. The patient was a middle child of a family of five, two brothers and two sisters, all of whom were well. The father and mother were also living and well and there had been no digestive trouble in the family that he knew of.

Physical Examination and Laboratory Studies

On admission to the hospital the physical examination showed a well-nourished young man with no abnormalities to be detected except a moderate degree of pallor. The pulse was rather rapid and the temperature was slightly elevated but both returned to normal within a short period of time. The hemoglobin was 60 per cent and the red blood cells were 3,000,000. X-ray examination was delayed until recovery was proceeding normally and then showed evidence of duodenal ulcer mentioned above. Improvement in blood count accompanied his general improvement and on discharge from the hospital was within normal limits.

LIFE SITUATION

The parents had been in humble circumstances and the patient had worked from an early age and by great effort had managed to put himself through school.

On superficial acquaintance he appeared to have a pleasant and affable disposition and always worked very hard to win the good opinion of his superiors. He had perfected himself as a machinist and held a responsible position.

Conflict over Marriage

In the fall of the year preceding the onset of his trouble, he had met a young woman in whom he became much interested and in a very short time they became secretly engaged and planned elopement. He stated that his reasons for this were that the girl's parents objected because of his limited finances. On further conversation it developed that while it was true that he had paid marked attention to the girl, nevertheless he felt that he had been precipitated into an engagement and as a consequence became sleepless and worried a great deal about the responsibilities that he would have to assume and it was during this period of time that stomach symptoms developed. He had a premonition that he would get sick and, moreover, felt that it would be his stomach "that would go back on him." In spite of his engagement he did not have sexual relations because of moral scruples. To explain his hesitancy about marriage he suggested financial difficulty, the insecurity of his future, and his inability to concentrate upon his work. He recognized that his mind was so occupied that he could not properly concentrate and hence felt that his work was suffering. During this period when he was so worried that he could not concentrate properly on his work he made a serious error which was discovered by his superior who humiliated him by taking certain responsibilities away. He felt the humiliation keenly. Then he became irritable and had a number of mild altercations with other people working in his department. These problems in turn seemed to worry him a great deal and then he would note that his digestion was particularly upset and that loss of appetite would persist until he was on friendly relationship with his associates once more. He had always used cigarettes moderately but during these months smoked to excess, that is 25 to 30 cigarettes daily. He drank only occasionally and then not to excess. He became more and more indecisive about the marriage situation and especially about his financial responsibility and then occurred the digestive accident which resulted in his admission to the hospital.

TREATMENT

Certain medical measures have already been indicated, that is, the withholding of food by mouth for the first forty-eight hours and then the principle of small, frequent feedings. Tobacco, of course, was not permitted and following his return to normal activity periodic rechecks of the duodenum by x-ray were made. The ulcer healed promptly and over a period of the succeeding five years never again showed any evidence of activity.

From the psychological standpoint it was explained to the patient that his conflict over the marriage situation had something to do with the precipitation of his illness and it was felt that so long as this conflict persisted it would be difficult if not impossible to bring about permanent cure. The patient himself readily grasped that this would be the case and hence felt that he must make up his mind either to marry or not to marry. He chose the latter and it would seem without perturbation because it was not long before his affections were engaged elsewhere. We did not believe nor did we persuade the patient that the psychological conflict was wholly responsible for his illness. It seemed rather to be only an activating factor in someone who, for unknown reasons, was predisposed to the development of a duodenal ulcer.

Relation of Emotional Factors to Hemorrhage

The case is cited to illustrate that emotional problems frequently precede the onset of ulcer symptoms and especially sudden hemorrhage. Again and again in our patients with gastrointestinal hemorrhage of ulcer origin we have discovered evidence of a serious psychological conflict related to the particular personality structure of the patient which coincides with the period immediately prior to the onset of symptoms. We of course do not believe that there is a direct connection between psychological disturbance and ulcer formation but rather, as Alexander has stated, that the psychological difficulties may be responsible for changes in muscle tone and secretion which assist in disturbing the ulcer area.

Follow-up

The patient remained free of ulcer symptoms in spite of the fact that within a period of three years he had married another girl. On this occasion, however, he was financially in a much more secure position, had considerably more confidence in himself and, moreover, the engagement was one entirely of his own volition. He still suffered slight loss of appetite when working under stress or particularly when his sensitive nature was disturbed by criticism or altercation but his functioning was close enough to normal so that he was satisfied with himself and we felt that he was likely to remain healthy.

SUMMARY OF CASE MATERIAL

To summarize the discussion to this point it can be said that we have all been perfectly willing to recognize that the obvious emotional disturbances of life may have some effect upon the workings of the gastrointestinal tract but what we have been slow to recognize is that forces within us that are not so obvious have an even more pronounced effect.

Here, for example, were patients who had well-defined ulcers of the duodenum which had been bleeding and therefore constituted a medical emergency. No question was raised about the psychological background of this problem when they were admitted; it was entirely a question of medical measures designed to improve the precarious state. But the question of the future then assumed importance and it therefore seemed that if we could understand them better as persons we would be better able to manage their illness. We need not go beyond that point at the moment. We sketched the life situations and the reactions of these young men as they tried to adjust to them and while there were some peculiarities, chiefly in the direction of exaggerations of normal trends, there was certainly no extraordinary departure from normal. And so it often proves to be in patients like this. The material may be difficult to obtain and the application to the problem of the illness is likewise quite complex.

Conflict over Marriage

Now the point is that these patients had a deep conflict in their personalities which manifested itself in regard to the problem of marriage. They did not recognize this, however; indeed, they refused to recognize it. Their rationalizations for not getting married seemed perfectly satisfactory to them. As Alexander pointed out, a certain drive or urge within them which they could not adequately express in action or words they apparently were trying to express through their stomachs. The stomach apparently was disturbed in its function because they were trying to express certain cravings for love and affection, manifested by "hunger pains," instead of being able to obtain this affection in the usual way. This background has been described as the intimate relationship between the feeding process and the physical satisfaction of infancy. In the study of these adult patients with peptic ulcer and other so-called "functional" disturbances of the gastrointestinal tract we have been impressed that *bed and board in adult life are as indissolubly connected as sustenance and sensuality in infant life.* To put this in another way we can say that men with functional disturbances of the stomach have a very high incidence of marital difficulties. As we have tried to indicate, this is not easily analyzed and so we find many men who are very active, energetic and aggressive in their everyday social and business contacts who, nevertheless, have this infantile pattern deep down in their personality, of craving love and affection and expressing this craving by "hunger pains." Again the symbolism of the body language that we have discussed before will be recognized.

Relation of Psychic Forces to Ulcer Formation

Alexander took pains to point out in the introduction to his studies that he did not consider that the phenomenon of a duodenal ulcer, as an end result of a long series of tissue changes, could be interpreted psychologically. In other words, the ulcer itself has no psychological significance whatever. What can be interpreted as a direct effect of psychological factors are the disturbances in secretion and the change in the motor activity and possibly even the alteration in the blood supply of the stomach. It is not difficult to believe that in the presence of some additional constitutional or acquired factor an ulcer might be brought about.

PRINCIPLES OF PSYCHOTHERAPY IN ULCER PATIENTS

Saul, formerly associated with Alexander, summarizes the psychological management as follows:

"In the first place, we shall concentrate upon the patient himself, and endeavor to discern the major motivations of his life and his relationships to his main feelings, conflicts and tensions. We shall be especially alert to his needs for love, ease, support, and dependence, and to all those desires which can be considered intaking in nature, *i. e.*, of the same direction as the taking in of food. And we shall watch especially for any frustrations of these desires, whether by external circumstances or by the internal attitudes of the patient himself.

"The tempo of the interview is determined predominantly by the patient's personality make-up and by the intensity of his need for help. The physician can rarely force the issue. Rather his effort must be to get the patient to reveal himself. Sometimes, almost all one needs to do is listen. In other cases, the patient not only resists seeing the pertinent emotional forces, but it may even be dangerous to try to force him to do so.

"In the average case it is practicable to begin with a discussion of the physical symptoms. In general, first interviews begin very slowly. As the patient's confidence in the psychiatrist mounts and he feels that there is genuine interest and the possibility of being understood, the pertinent emotional material flows more freely. . . The discussion of the physical condition usually can be led naturally to the emotional setting in which these began, and, once immersed in this discussion, the patient's deeper feelings usually emerge.

"If the patient is too resistant at this point, it is sometimes well to turn to the family background. In the end, one's aim is to elicit the patient's true major motivations and feelings, and how these developed from the emotional pressures of his childhood, on through to their relationship to his present symptoms. While it is impossible to present a list of the questions to ask, one must keep the patient talking, and bring out his feelings in childhood toward those who reared him, and how they shaped his present personality. One estimates the present emotional interplay and organization from his relationships to his family, friends, work, and recreation. One seeks for positive irritants and hardships, as well as for negative factors such as unsatisfied desires. There is no simple method for comprehending the core of the personality, or for estimating the intensity of the feelings and frustrations. This is a matter of psychological sense and psychiatric experience. It is remarkable how much one often learns by merely listening to the patient, while divesting oneself, so far as possible, of one's knowledge and preconceptions.

"Dreams are invaluable in many cases for penetrating rapidly and accurately to the major emotional forces within the person. It is inadvisable for the physician, inexperienced with dreams, to interpret them to the patient, but with a little interest and study he can often glean simply from the topics of the dreams what is central in the patient's mind: hostility, anxiety, desires for ease and escape, the pressure toward work and accomplishment, needs for superiority, etc. What the dreams tell is usually at least a helpful clue, but more often an invaluable aid in clarifying one's understanding of the fundamental emotional forces in the case. This understanding is the indispensable basis of rational treatment. In surgery, the cutting is the least; it is the understanding of the pathological physiology and anatomy, and the utilization of the surgical techniques for accomplishing a rational purpose. The analogy between rational psychiatry and surgery is a sound one. Psychiatric techniques, such as suggestion, reassurance, hypnosis, catharsis, and the like, are significant only when one understands the basic emotional situation and applies them rationally for well-defined purposes. Employed without this understanding, they are little more than a medieval laying-on of hands.

"We have already mentioned some of the therapeutic elements employed in the ordinary interview. The transference, or relationship to the physician, is always present and can be of great value as a means of emotional support. Neurosis is in essence the persistence of childhood desires and patterns. The patient coming to the physician tends unconsciously to adopt toward him the dependent, help-seeking attitude of a child to its parent. This gives the physician tremendous influence. The reaction is of great importance in the ulcer patients, in whom we deal so largely with needs to be fed emotionally. Usually it is not necessary to discuss the transference with the patient, but the physician must be constantly aware of it.

"Insight, properly used, is effective in the vast majority of cases. Like the interview, it must develop slowly and tactfully, at a tempo set by the patient. But where it can be imparted with reasonable completeness it is a powerful instrument, and makes the entire management much easier for the physician; for now the patient himself understands his problem, will himself have ideas for environmental changes, and in the favorable cases will endeavor, with real therapeutic urge, to alter his attitudes. Some patients, who typically are unable to accept anything freely and must be incessantly striving, can be mellowed noticeably in a very few interviews.

"In general, where one cannot relieve the patient through insight, changes in the environment, and relatively simple changes in attitude, one faces major surgery (psychotherapy), and it is necessary to call in the analytically-trained psychiatrist. This specialist is also effective for diagnosis and for brief causal treatment, in which he can often save much time. His contribution is *psychiatric accuracy*."

Chapter XIV

ENDOCRINE SYSTEM AND METABOLISM

There has been considerable discussion in the past decade of the relation between the endocrine glands and the emotions. Books for the public put forth the thesis that personality traits and reactions are largely determined by the action of the endocrine glands. Instead of the food faddists' slogan, "Tell me what you eat and I'll tell you what you are," these popularizers of endocrinology hold that personality types are determined by glandular balances and personality disturbances by glandular dysfunctions. At the same time there are others who are equally convinced that the reverse of this relationship operates, namely, that disturbances in personality may upset the function of the endocrine glands.

Later in this chapter we will call attention to this problem by discussing the relationships of menstruation and personality disturbance. However, it must be confessed that scientific evidence for either of these propositions is meager. Cases of obvious endocrine disease are cited in which psychological disturbances occur; the latter are then attributed to the glandular dysfunction: for example, the emotionalism of exophthalmic goiter. Animal experiments are described in which the behavior of an animal changed following the removal or administration of a certain glandular substance. Here, to an even greater extent than in other fields it is necessary to exercise caution in translating animal experiments into human terms. Even though male rats, after the administration of certain glandular preparations, lose their fighting instincts and assume the emotional aspects of maternity, this does not mean that the human being with his more complex emotional and ideational life will do the same. In an admirable summary of ten years of experimental work on the sexual behavior of animals, Beach concluded that in the course of mammalian evolution several changes in the physiological basis for sexual behavior appear to have taken place. Subcerebral mechanisms, which were capable of mediating sexual responses, have become more dependent upon the higher nervous system, and the development of this increasing dependence on the cerebral cortex has to some degree freed the more primitive sexual mechanisms from strict control by gonadal hormones.

There are many factors in the total problem of thyroid disease and it is not enough to say that the patient with hyperthyroidism is "emotional," or to attribute personality disturbances to overactivity. Some evaluation must be made of the personality make-up before the onset of the thyroid hyperactivity. There is the constitutional factor to be reckoned with, the personality development and evidences of neurotic traits preceding thyroid disease, the activity of the thyroid under so-called normal conditions, and finally the psychological factors which often seem to precipitate the onset of symptoms. Thus we have a series of factors making a complex psychosomatic problem.

THE EMOTIONAL LIFE AND OVARIAN FUNCTION

There are some observers who are so psychologically minded that they ascribe too great an influence to emotional factors in the development of endocrine disorders. In conditions such as disturbed menstruation, amenorrhea, or anorexia nervosa, it may be too readily assumed that only the psychological factor is important when we know very little about the function of particular glands preceding the disturbance. A recent study by Benedek and Rubenstein, truly psychosomatic in its approach, made an effort to determine whether a correlation existed between ovarian activity and psychological processes. Daily studies of vaginal smears and basal body temperatures, and psychoanalytic observation of the emotional life were made independently and the findings then compared. We will quote directly from their study and then discuss some implications of the material.

"During the follicle-ripening phase the psychological material is dominated by heterosexual interest. The libidinous tendencies are concentrated on the male. The heterosexual interest becomes increasingly strong during the ripening phase. With normal sexual adjustment the increasingly strong heterosexual desire finds normal gratification. Without sexual gratification, the heterosexual tension can be dammed up so that increasing hormone production causes an increased tension.

"In neurotic persons we observe that this increasing estrone production activates the psychological conflicts and thus the neurotic symptoms are intensified. The great psychic tension is suddenly relieved (but only for a short time) when ovulation occurs. The libidinous interest is withdrawn from the outer world and centered on herself. She is self-satisfied, wants to be loved and to be taken care of. She is content to be a woman. The period of postovulative relaxation is necessarily of short duration. Hormone production increases rapidly after ovulation. Although both hormones are produced during the luteal phase progesterone now dominates the hormone picture. The psychological material corresponding to this phase of the cycle shows the tendency to be passive and receptive. The tendency to be impregnated, the tendency to be pregnant, the tendency to care for a child and the various reactions to all these are reflected in the psychological material. After this phase of the cycle reaches its peak the corpus luteum starts to regress and with it the production of progesterone diminishes. After regression of the corpus luteum many new follicles begin their development. Ordinarily none of these follicles is destined to mature. However, they do produce estrone in small quantities. This is immediately reflected in the psychological material by the reappearance of heterosexual interest.

"The heterosexual desire of the premenstrual phase is similar to that of the pre-ovulative phase. In the later premenstrual state this heterosexual tension is complicated by the expectation of menstruation. This expectation of the menstruation is in turn reflected in the psychological material."

Scientific Psychosomatic Study

Benedek and Rubenstein showed that following menstruation there is a gradual increase of the estrogenic hormone, and paralleling this, an interest in the opposite sex. Then ovulation occurs and the effects of the estrogenic hormones are masked by the increase of the corpus luteum hormone, progesterone. This is followed by less interest in men and an increased interest in pregnancy and children. In other words, the concern of the organism for pregnancy, stimulated by the hormone of the corpus luteum, is reflected psychologically in the emotional life. Then a few days before the menstrual period, as the progesterone level falls, feelings of frustration and irritability become more prominent in the psychological material. Practitioners will recognize this period as corresponding to what is known clinically as *premenstrual tension.*

Not only do the hormones influence sexual and maternal interest, but the reverse also seems to be true, that is, that the hormonal level is affected by the emotional state. It is common knowledge that emotional disturbances can suppress menstruation. In one of the patients the sexual repression was so great that throughout the study there was no discussion, not even a single dream, dealing with sexuality or pregnancy. This led Benedek to predict an abnormally low hormone level and probably an infantile uterus, both of which were found. It could suggest either that the psychological effect of sexual repression was so severe that it inhibited hormone production and perhaps even affected anatomical development, or that both the physiological and psychological disturbances are parallel manifestations of some basic fault as yet not understood. From our clinical observations, however, it does seem likely that just as hormone production influences the emotional state so may the emotional state influence the hormone production.

The study appeals to us as a scientific effort to discover the relation of the glandular function to psychological processes. First of all, one may say that the glandular function seems to furnish an impetus to the psychological processes, but that there must be a well-integrated psychological structure which can do something intelligent for the emotional needs of the individual who possesses the glands. As the study points out, with the early phase of the menstrual cycle, during the period of increasing estrone production, there is an increase of the heterosexual desires which, if not satisfied, cause tension. With the later phase of the cycle, during the luteal period when progesterone dominates the hormone picture, definite needs and wishes of a passive nature are present, such as the need to be loved and cared for, the wish to be impregnated, and the wish to care for a child. A close correlation between biological functions and psychodynamic processes apparently exists.

However, the woman must have a mind sufficiently *free of conflict* so that she can permit herself to be loved and cared for, to want to be impregnated, and to want to care for a child. If she does not have the opportunity or if she cannot cope with these instinctive needs intelligently and with a minimum of conflict then we have gland activity constantly going on, giving signals each month which go unheeded. Various possibilities of emotional satisfaction are ignored by a woman who may be too prejudiced or too inhibited to want to be loved or to wish to be a mother. Her life is empty of the emotional satisfactions so important to a woman, and when the menopause occurs she becomes neurotic or psychotic because of the lack of emotional sustenance. The obvious conclusion must be that if the psychological needs were not taken care of in a normal manner no amount of injected estrogenic material could remedy the *emotional* defect. Only by this kind of study will we gain insight into the complex problems of correlation of gland function and personality.

Benedek, writing independently, states that more markedly than man's, woman's life is divided into periods which are defined by her reproductive function. During the first period, from infancy to adolescence, the relationship to her mother will determine the development of heterosexual attitudes and the emotional acceptance of the propagative function. The reproductive period is second. Here in cyclic intervals the woman gets ready for conception, failure of which results in the menstrual flow. The sexual cycle evolves from one menstruation to the other corresponding with hormonal stimulation, and during this is repeated the rise and decline of emotional integration of the psychosexual maturation. After a child is born, the mother's psychosexual life is partially externalized; it encompasses the child. The mother repeats with the daughter, more directly than with the son, those emotional attitudes which originally determined her own emotional development.

By living her life with her children again woman is given the chance for final personal integration in mature motherliness. The manifestations of the climacterium and also her emotional life after the menopause will be determined by the accomplishments of the reproductive phase.

THE MENOPAUSAL SYNDROME

One of the most important syndromes met with in relation to ductless gland activity is the menopausal syndrome. It is estimated that at or about the time of the cessation of menstruation, 80 per cent of women experience a variety of unpleasant symptoms. These are *vasomotor disturbances* manifested by "hot flushes" and "cold shivers" accompanied by emotional instability, insomnia, depression of spirits, irritability, anxiety attacks, palpitation, headaches, giddiness, nausea, fatigue, dyspnea, sweating, "tingling" in the skin and extremities, and sometimes obesity. The anxiety and depression of spirits may be of such severity that the patient can no longer carry on her daily tasks, rest comfortably, eat, or control her thoughts and actions. In some instances removal to a mental hospital may be necessary. However, a relatively small percentage of women who have been reported as suffering from menopausal symptoms develop frank psychoses.

The Menopause and the Climacteric

If a woman is "nervous" or presents symptoms of obscure origin she is almost certain to be told that it is the menopause or the "beginning of the menopause." Hardly is she through her twenties before she begins to think in such terms, often, we regret to say, with the assistance of the medical profession. From then on until ten years after the menses cease this shortcut to an involved psychosomatic problem is called upon for an easy explanation, and the injudicious resort to estrogen therapy. It is well to remember that the vasomotor phenomena which are alone characteristic of the climacterium are rarely pronounced in the woman who is still menstruating regularly.

Some observers make a distinction between "menopause" and the "climacteric." They believe that menopause should be used to mean simply cessation of the menses, whereas the term climacteric, which is derived from the Greek and means "rung of the ladder," should be used according to its original meaning to signify a critical epoch of life. These epochs were supposed to occur every nine years, the important ones occurring at eighteen and sixty-three, the latter being called the "grand climacteric."

From a psychosomatic standpoint the epochs of "changes of life" are indeed important. Life is constantly changing and many periods necessitate emotional and ideational adjustment. The menopause is only one such period. Puberty, adolescence, leaving the parental roof, engagements, marriage, parenthood, etc., are all changes which require readjustment. This adjustment process often fails and neuroses and psychoses appear as a result. Hence, we should be careful not to attribute much more importance to either the cessation of the menses or to this particular epoch than to these other epochs. "Nervous symptoms," so-called, occurring at the time of the menopause are frequently treated quite casually by the physician. He says, "Oh, of course. The change of life," or "This was to be expected," and prescribes some glandular preparation. The majority of physicians believe that most of the menopausal symptoms can be controlled by the administration of estrogenic products. The element of suggestion in such treatment is rarely considered.

It is also important to point out that in attributing all symptoms to the menopause equally tragic mistakes are made in overlooking physical diseases. We must emphasize once more that the psychosomatic concept means no less study of the soma than of the psyche. Just as too great an absorption in endocrine matters leads to serious errors in regard to emotional matters so, as shown by Stoddard, many serious physical diseases are overlooked because all symptoms are attributed to endocrine dysfunction.

Estrogenic Treatment

In discussing a paper on estrogenic treatment for the menopausal syndrome, Pratt stated: "It seems increasingly difficult to know what symptoms to attribute to the menopause. A group in Chicago reporting on 1000 women found that 85 per cent had no interruption of daily routine at the time of the menopause and only 15 per cent showed symptoms. If all these symptoms mentioned are due to interruption of ovarian function, it seems strange that the symptoms are so widely different in various individuals and so frequently entirely absent.

"In our own hospital when some physician has made a diagnosis of menopausal symptoms, I ask him to observe the patient carefully and then send her to me for therapy. I will not tell him what therapy is to be employed. I have a preparation of theelin in oil and the same kind of oil without theelin sterilized and ready for injection. Just as much improvement has been noted with the oil without the theelin as there is with the theelin in the oil. I am not the observer, for the physician who refers the patient is the one who makes the notes on the change of symptoms."

Suggestion from Treatment

A healthier attitude and better understanding of sexual matters ought to do something toward the prevention of dysmenorrhea. Swooning, tight corsets, and excessive modesty went out with the "mauve decade" but repression of sexuality is still a part of our culture. If girls can be taught to look upon menstruation as a normal physiological function and as an evidence of "growing up" that makes their parents proud of them, menstruation will be accepted as a part of living rather than a "curse." And it must not be forgotten that a healthy approach to the menstrual life is good insurance against a stormy menopause.

We do not believe that the answer to the treatment of the menopausal syndrome lies in replacement therapy alone. From the above and other similar observations it seems clear that the suggestion value of replacement therapy from the standpoint of *having something injected* has not been granted sufficient importance.

In this connection it is interesting to observe that at the present time psychiatry is going through a phase of "shock therapies." Violent "shocks" are given to the patient by insulin overdosage, metrazol, electrical currents, and even by opening the skull and removing or destroying brain tissue. It would seem that this is rather inconsistent behavior for a speciality which almost unanimously regards personality development as an outgrowth of experience, as a result of the moulding of drives of energy by the impact of persons and experiences upon the developing individual. If this theory of personality development is correct then it seems inconsistent to try to "cure" a poorly constructed personality by brain surgery or the shock of convulsive therapy. We do not deny some of the practical clinical results that have been achieved. We only question the structural approach for psychological problems.

Various theories have been advanced to explain the improvements noted from "shocks" in emotional illness. Chemical, physiological, and metabolic changes of a temporary nature are supposed to be induced. It is well known that major psychological shocks have a profound effect upon the thoughts and the emotional trends of man. The effects of artificially induced shocks upon the psyche need further study. The human body is a complex machine, taking in energy in one form and putting it out in another. Everything which is introduced has an effect upon emotion and ideation as well as upon somatic function. If an injection is given or an electric current is introduced, it affects the feeling and ideas of the person so treated as well as his metabolism. One might say that there is an emotional and ideational metabolism as well as a physical metabolism.

Previous Personality Disturbances

Careful study has shown that patients who develop menopausal neuroses and psychoses have had personality disturbances of long duration. The syndrome occurs especially in people who have lived narrow lives of intolerance and prejudice and who have been worrisome, parsimonious, pedantic, sexually frigid, and poor mixers socially. They have taken little from life and given little. They may have been full of romantic fantasies but lacked the drive to create a life that was romantically satisfying. They have not been able to relax and enjoy life's pleasures but instead have held themselves rigidly to a code of duty.

It is small wonder that when the menstrual bleeding, which is the *symbol* of femininity, motherhood, sexuality, and all the ideas that go with these concepts, is about to disappear, the woman who has led an empty life becomes anxious and panicky. She feels that she is passing into old age without having experienced the things which make life worth living. She is depressed in spirits and irritable at a fate which she believes has cheated her in the past and can promise nothing for the future.

Injections into the body of one so tortured in mind often create the feeling that a deficiency is being supplied—that the force which enables a woman to achieve romance, happiness, love, children, and prestige, is being put back into her. Unfortunately that force has been there within her for a long time and she has not had the personality equipment with which to take advantage of it. The energy of life, as represented by glandular activity, did its best from the age of puberty onward to tell her that she was a woman and that a certain kind of behavior on her part would make her happy. But a bulwark had been erected in her mind built of fear, prudishness, intolerance, and hate, against which the glandular activity was powerless. The secretion of the glands could not coordinate harmoniously with ideas and emotions of loving and being loved, of sexual intercourse with pleasure, or with a desire for pregnancy and motherhood, and as a result the woman has reached the menopause emotionally unfulfilled as well as glandularly deficient.

Need for Further Study

In many cases attempted "replacement therapy" has had no beneficial effect, in fact, has increased the symptoms. But here, as in the cases that have apparently been benefited, both physical and psychological observations are lacking. Perhaps the method advocated by Papanicolaou and Shorr, who recommend control of hormonal therapy by the vaginal smear rather than by subjective symptoms alone, will answer one part of this problem. Then studies similar to those by Benedek and Rubenstein, referred to earlier in this chapter, in which psychological changes in the patient are observed *simultaneously* and *independently,* along with glandular therapy, will help us to understand this complicated psychosomatic problem. In regard to this matter, however, Bennett and TeLinde find that while it is true that most symptomatic menopausal women have vaginal smears suggesting estrogen deficiency and under the influence of implanted estrone, the smears become of the estrogenic type; they also have frequently noted relief from symptoms without any changes in the vaginal smear and are inclined to believe that the dosage necessary to relieve the symptoms in many women is less than that required to alter the vaginal epithelium.

What are the fantasies of the patient concerning the material that is injected into him? To the mind of the average layman a hypodermic injection means that a "strong" drug is being introduced. Moreover, it is introduced in a way that is known to bring quick and often miraculous results. Sometimes it is regarded as a "strengthening" form of therapy. The active principles of the sex glands of both men and women are looked upon as "rejuvenating," "giving new life," and "giving new energy." So in some cases hypodermic injections of such a potent "force" may well stimulate a latent belief within the mind of the patient. Certainly this would seem to be true in those cases in which a neutral solution was injected with such good results. However, the real point is that until more psychosomatic studies have been made simultaneously and independently by the endocrinologist and psychiatrist, neither of them is in a good position to be too positive in his opinion of the causal factor in the menopausal syndrome.

Psychic Factors in the Menopausal Syndrome

CASE 36

History and Symptoms

A woman of forty-four complained of "indigestion" with difficulty in swallowing, distress after meals, belching of gas, constipation, "spells" of nervous agitation with palpitation of the heart, weakness, marked insomnia, hot flushes, and dull headaches. She had been given injections of estrogenic material for three months without effect.

LIFE SITUATION

Her personal history was as follows: She had been the third sibling but the first girl in a family of five children. Her mother was a very strict and rigid woman who made it a point to keep her children as ignorant as possible of the world outside the home. Although they lived on a farm, the patient was not allowed to play freely around the place but was urged to be "in the house" winter and summer. The patient and her sister were taught to regard the farm hands—in fact, any strange man—as "undisciplined cavemen or sex fiends." The patient was given no information on sex matters. She received no instruction regarding menstruation and there was great fright and anxiety when she first discovered the bleeding. During her teens the patient was not allowed to go to dances or parties and any girl who did so was talked about by the mother in a most disparaging way.

Marriage

Finally at the age of twenty-one the patient left home to study music. She met a young man who was very attentive to her and with whom she fell in love. He embraced and kissed her but she felt so stirred emotionally that she refused to see him any more lest her sensual desire lead her to do something wicked, although what this was she did not fully realize at the time. He proposed marriage by letter but the patient did not dare to come in contact with him again. She thought of him "day and night" but steadfastly refused to see him. Finally at twenty-three she was wooed with great persistence by a simple, unimaginative man, untalented and uninspiring. She finally consented to marry him but she "never knew why."

Children

She became the mother of two daughters. For a time after marriage she continued to get satisfaction out of her music but finally she had to give this up because she felt so anxious and uncomfortable when asked to perform. She had enjoyed music and the prestige and praise it brought but now she denied herself this source of satisfaction. Her sexual relations were always without feeling. She curtailed her social relations to a considerable extent because of a fear that she might feel the need to go to the toilet and would be too embarrassed to do this. So this imaginative woman found that because of anxieties placed in her by her mother over ordinary physiological functions she lived a most narrow life devoid of emotional satisfaction. In turn, she disciplined her two daughters in much the same way that she had been disciplined and worried that in spite of her precautions one of them "might do something foolish." Her symptoms were greatly exaggerated when her oldest daughter would have a date with a young man. She would be sleepless, have "anxious spells," and attacks of indigestion.

Psychic Problems

Here were problems of a psychological nature which could not be solved solely by injections of glandular extract. It was necessary to try in a series of psychiatric interviews to show this woman, first, how her way of life had left her dissatisfied and resentful, and second, how to find some substitute satisfactions as well as substitute glandular preparations. She was shown how she had cut herself off from the man she loved, from sexual gratification, from the prestige and satisfaction her music would have afforded and that her lack was more in the emotional than in the glandular sphere. Again we must emphasize that one must be careful to go slowly and to win the patient's good will and acceptance before pointing out the personal failures and subsequent resentment against those responsible for deprivations. If the patient does not have confidence in the physician such efforts will result in the release of more aggression than the patient can handle, anxiety will be increased instead of decreased and often, quite unexpectedly, treatment will be broken off. However, if the patient seems sincere and willing to be taught then she can be shown what has been lacking in her life and she can be encouraged to make such amends as are still possible.

TREATMENT

In the present case we allowed her to express some of her dissatisfaction with her husband and then enabled her to view his foibles with more tolerance and to see that he was not very different from the husbands of her friends. We succeeded in getting her to take up music again after expressing her just resentment against her own early deprivation. She was able to see that her oldest daughter had some rights to a life of her own about which the patient must not be too jealous. As a result of helping her to see things in her life as sources of conflict and hence to attack them as problems to be solved the patient began to take a new interest in life as a wife and mother instead of living as an introspective recluse. Spells of anxiety and "shakiness" diminished and she began to sleep better, eat better, and thus gained strength to resume her social life. This required twelve sessions of one hour each over a period of twelve weeks. A certain innate "love of life" had remained alive in this patient in spite of her impoverished social existence and contributed greatly to so much improvement in so short a time. We do not say that the glandular therapy which she received was of no value but we are trying to show that personality modification must be accorded at least equal standing with replacement therapy.

Waiting Too Long for Help

It is regrettable that so many women wait until the menopause acts as the precipitating factor to make them seriously ill before they seek help along emotional lines. By this time they often are so fixed in their way of life that modification is difficult, if not impossible. Since they have not made satisfactory emotional investments, their personalities become bankrupt. This is especially true if they lack the intelligence and inner resources to permit reeducation and substitute satisfactions. *One of the tragedies of practice is the woman of middle age who has led an impoverished emotional life but has escaped serious neurotic illness (usually by means of repeated pregnancies, often recommended by her physician) and then for the first time at the menopause finally breaks down.* Certainly for some such women it would be better if the breakdown came sooner so that they would seek help when they are in a better position to be helped. To draw an analogy along more physical lines it is often to the advantage of a tuberculous patient if his disease is made known early in life by some dramatic occurrence, such as a pulmonary hemorrhage, which forces him to get proper treatment then, instead of pursuing a subclinical course with slow destruction of pulmonary tissue and discovery of an advanced tuberculous process late in life when little can be done.

Palmer and associates have stressed the matter of "psychological preparation" for the menopause. Slowly American women are learning that the menopause offers no dangers to the body or mind if reasonably healthy physical, mental and emotional life has preceded this period.

THE MALE CLIMACTERIC

With the increased interest of the medical profession in endocrinology and the exploitation of this interest by pharmaceutical houses in marketing endocrine products, a new flood of literature has crossed the physicians' desk on what is termed the male climacteric, or even less aptly the male menopause. This syndrome is said to occur in the middle or late forties and to be characterized by nocturnal urinary frequency, fatigue, indecision, hot flushes, decreased libido, and "impending" impotence. Other symptoms such as vertigo, excessive perspiration, mood changes, headaches, impaired mental concentration, numbness, tingling, tachycardia, palpitation, weakness, lack of endurance, a feeling of inadequacy in undertaking new duties, and a tendency to seclusion are sometimes included as a part of the syndrome.

An Ill-defined Syndrome

Most of these symptoms have been conspicuous in the psychoneuroses, particularly neurasthenia, and were described as far back as 1869 by Beard. Certainly such symptoms often arise from emotional conflict, and can be effectively treated by psychotherapy. We believe that the syndrome spoken of as the male climacteric or male menopause is even less well defined than the menopausal syndrome in the female and consequently that there is less justification for organotherapy, to the exclusion of psychotherapy, in the management of nervous symptoms that appear during this period.

Heller and Meyers, utilizing gonadotropic excretion as well as testicular biopsy specimens in a careful study of thirty-eight cases, tried to find the answer to the following questions:

1. Is there an organic basis to justify the claim that the male climacteric is a true clinical entity?

2. Is it possible to distinguish between the male climacteric and psychoneurosis or psychogenic impotence either clinically, by laboratory methods, or both?

3. If the syndrome exists, what therapy is advisable?

4. Is the male climacteric a normal accompaniment of the aging process or is it a pathologic problem?

Commenting that no objective evidence has been brought forward to prove that the male climacteric is an actual clinical entity or to differentiate it conclusively from psychoneurosis or psychogenic impotence, they say, "Ordinary clinical experience arouses considerable skepticism as to the existence of the male climacteric because of (a) the similarity between symptoms attributed to this syndrome and those referable to psychoneurosis, (b) the retention of fertility by most men well into old age, (c) the absence of regressive changes in secondary sexual characteristics of most elderly men comparable to those which customarily occur in women after menopause. In most elderly women there are unmistakable signs of ovarian failure, namely atrophy of the uterus, vagina, external genitalia and breasts, a deepening of the voice, a tendency toward hirsutism and a loss of feminine bodily contours. In contrast, most elderly men exhibit no physical signs of testicular failure; genitalia and secondary sexual characteristics show no regressive changes; beard and bodily hair remain intact, and bodily contours remain masculine."

The diagnosis of the male climacteric was established in twenty-three cases by the finding of pronounced elevation in gonadotropic hormone excretion, comparable quantitatively to that occurring in castrates. This was corroborated in all of eight cases subjected to biopsy, by histologic evidences of testicular atrophy and degeneration. The diagnosis was further supported in all of twenty cases treated by specific response to a therapeutic test with androgens. A clear-cut differentiation of the male climacteric from psychogenic impotence was made by the urine gonadotropic assays, which were decidedly elevated in the former group and normal in the latter.

Since laboratory procedures which will positively differentiate climacteric from psychoneurotic patients are usually not available for clinical practice, the authors recommend the following therapeutic test: Administer 25 mg. of testosterone propionate by intramuscular injection five days weekly for a period of two weeks. Evaluate the clinical status at that time, noting the effect on symptoms and sexual potency. If at the end of the two weeks trial of therapy the patient has shown no improvement, either of two conclusions may be justifiable: (1) The patient is not experiencing the male climacteric or (2) he will need such an excessively large daily dosage of testosterone that treatment is financially unpractical. If the patient does respond it may be necessary to determine whether the improvement is actually due to specific relief of testicular failure or whether it is merely due to suggestion. Withdrawal of therapy until symptoms return and then reinstitution of therapy with placebos may be required to settle the question.

Heller and Meyers observe that the average male will not experience the climacteric. Their clinical observations and laboratory studies indicate that both the germinal and the hormonal function of the testes is preserved well into senility in the average man. It is true that reduction of function occurs, but there is fairly adequate maintenance in most cases.

So they conclude that *whereas in the female the menopause is an invariable and physiologic accompaniment of the aging process, in the male the climacteric is an infrequent and pathologic accompaniment of that process.*

Need for Psychotherapy

When some method will enable us to say which symptoms are due to gonadal deficiency and which are due to emotional conflict we will be in a better position to combine endocrine therapy and psychotherapy. Meanwhile we emphasize the necessity for scientific psychotherapy rather than empirical organotherapy.

In a case study of the sex hormones and psychic conflict Tauber and Daniels found that the male sex hormone stimulated a special aspect only of sexual functioning. Frequency and strength of erections were increased in the beginning. Priapism or penile response resembling priapism were seen following the *injection of androgenic substances.* These erections were not always accompanied by pleasurable increases of tension or desire for intercourse. In fact with the erection the patient might remain emotionally unmoved. The investigators felt that the sex hormone assists in preparing the individual for sexual activity. Yet the hormone can be utilized to advantage only if, over and above the physiological effect, there is a wish to participate in the sexual relationship.

Although the administration of the male sex hormone temporarily produced a period of sexual rejuvenation, probably capable of repetition, it became evident that the patient's most effective psychic equilibrium was maintained after the discontinuance of hormonal therapy.

A Period of Adjustment

In discussing the menopause in women we pointed out that between the ages of forty and fifty years there were many social and personal adjustments to make. The same is true with men. Many increasing family and business responsibilities are met with. This is a decade fraught with much emotional conflict: Frustrations arouse latent hostilities; the life situation itself, plus a special susceptibility, may well produce irritability, tenseness, mental depression, decreased interest in expressing love genitally, feelings of inadequacy, a tendency to seclusion, headaches and palpitation, without the necessity for a primary defect in glandular function. Whether the psychological factors can, in themselves, give rise to secondary glandular dysfunction is a question that we will reserve for later discussion.

Seeking Quick Cure

There always has been a tendency in medicine to seek a quick cure for mental symptoms—a cure which need not call into consciousness the emotions of the patient or of the physician. Three of the most important magic tools for this effort have been: (1) some appliance through which electricity could be given, (2) manipulation and massage, (3) the hypodermic syringe. The first and second have long been favorites in the treatment of impotence of psychological origin and now the third enters in the cloak of science to "replace the strength of declining manhood." *The lurid literature of certain of the drug firms has been in part responsible for this new method of exploiting neurotics.* We do not mean to say that some form of replacement therapy for gonadal deficiency does not have its place, but just as in the female menopause, we deplore its use as a panacea for the multitude of complaints included under the syndrome of the male climacteric. The psychiatrist rarely sees a patient suffering from neurasthenia who has not been treated over a number of months or even years with tonics, sedatives, glandular injections, and still other methods which have given only temporary relief. The case of mild depression or neurasthenia which will respond to replacement therapy will respond more surely to psychotherapy and stands a better chance of remaining well, because one must not forget that the suggestive effect of glandular injections is short lived.

Psychosomatic Observations

It is always unfortunate for the cause of science when an illness of psychological origin yields to the suggestive effect of another method of treatment. The element of suggestion is not evaluated and a false therapeutic claim is established which provides another hurdle for the cause of psychosomatic medicine. However, better observations are being made. Recently Rosenzweig and Hoskins carefully administered a variety of endocrine preparations to a male homosexual for six months and at the same time studied him psychologically without being able to detect any modification of personality.

The study by Tauber and Daniels, already referred to, combined replacement therapy and psychological observations on a male castrate. In the beginning, treatment with androgenic substance increased sexual desire, but this was followed by a subsequent decline in potency which was influenced only by psychotherapy. Study of the emotional life revealed that there was a homosexual trend, *i. e.*, a wish to play the feminine sexual role. At the same time, there was a conscious rejection of this wish. The patient showed marked hostility toward those people representing father and authority. Castration had actually taken place at the hands of a man (surgeon) and the patient had been made more effeminate. This increased the patient's passive personality trends. Since passivity was a challenge to the patient's security as well as to the cultural tradition of being virile, it naturally produced an aggressive response, in this case directed toward the physicians who treated him. The authors here made the point that inasmuch as castration introduced a greater feminine component into the personality, the patient's sexual conflicts were intensified. Having been made more feminine through castration, he had to struggle emotionally against his passive tendencies. Because of this psychological conflict he was unable to cope adequately with the sexual tension induced by hormones. Thus it became clear that after castration, hormonal therapy might operate to interfere with effective sexuality. Consequently the lesson may be drawn that it is important to study the personality before hormones are administered; otherwise the success of treatment by replacement therapy may be jeopardized.

The Either-Or Problem. Just as we have made the point before, it is not a question of either hormonal replacement therapy or psychotherapy but rather the necessity for a psychosomatic study of the individual to be treated, in order to determine whether one or the other or both will be necessary.

The Male Climacteric?

CASE 37

History and Symptoms

R. K., a white man of 53, was first seen in 1935.

He had an acute respiratory illness from which he made a quick recovery. The illness afforded us the opportunity of getting acquainted with the patient. He had always been a teacher in a small town and had one son, who had referred the patient to us.

We did not hear from him again until 1940, five years later, when he stated that he had been working hard, smoking moderately, and taking an occasional drink. For the last two or three years there had been a gradual diminution in his sex desires — "it had never meant much to him."

Physical Examination

The physical examination was negative except for slight elevation of the blood pressure which had not been noted five years previously. There was slight tremor and on further questioning the patient stated that he had become a little more intolerant to heat and somewhat irritable. Ordinary laboratory studies were negative and basal metabolism was within normal limits.

In a note of that visit we observed the following familiar, differential diagnostic problem with which we were concerned at the time, namely, anxiety neurosis, so-called neurocirculatory asthenia, mild hyperthyroidism and, in relation to the whole problem, the question of the male climacteric.

The son told us that his father had been getting more irritable during the past year and suggested that he was worried about the future. On that basis we began the discussion using the illustration of "body language" — that dizziness and vertigo may be the body's physical expression of insecurity. He said that since the new governor had come into office a bill had been passed forcing the retirement of teachers at the age of 62 and in his case this would provide only a small pension which would be insufficient for him and his wife to live on. He had invested all of his money in his son's education and wondered whether the son would be willing and able to take care of them. As he discussed this problem he became very emotional and it was obvious that this was the point that was disturbing him. We spoke about the son's future and the fact that he wouldn't let his father down and then reassured him as to the absence of organic disease.

17

He remained well for more than three years. Then he began to lose weight, and became worried and fretful. The physical examination showed frequent irregularity in the heart rate, and the electrocardiogram indicated early evidence of myocardial disease. Otherwise the examination was negative and basal metabolism was still within normal limits. The patient was smoking heavily. His wife's illness and the necessity for looking after her himself "had been too much for him." But his son had entered the service and this had reactivated his insecurity.

SUMMARY

Here was an average man reacting to stress and strain by presenting some of the psychic, sexual, and vasomotoi disturbances that are sometimes associated at this period of life and are now often referred to as the male climacteric. Whether they should be is not so much the question except in so far as it bears upon treatment. In general it may be said that too much is apt to be blamed on the menopause and just as in the woman, treatment is apt to be restricted to endocrine products. In this case very simple psychotherapy did a great deal. It was the kind of psychotherapy that any physician should administer and it doesn't have to be called psychotherapy. It is simply a normal part of the physician-patient relationship but it depends upon a knowledge of psychopathology. Here too we see the necessity for equal attention to tissue pathology as we watch this middle aged man developing degenerative heart disease which of course will also enter into the question of his emotional problems to produce indissoluble psychosomatic relationships.

PREADOLESCENT HYPOGONADISM

Concern over the development of small, fat boys is one of the common problems presented to the pediatrician and general practitioner interested in endocrinology. Such boys, who will usually develop in normal fashion if they are given the opportunity, are frequently regarded as instances of dystrophia adiposogenitalis and treated with testosterone. Since the distribution of fat resembles that found in women and adult eunuchs, the physician is inclined to make a diagnosis of obesity due to hypogonadism, particularly since the genitalia appear small. The apparent hypogonadism is due to the fact that the penis is usually embedded in suprapubic fat. When the fat pad is pushed back and the penis and testes are measured, it is evident that the genitalia are within the range of normal when compared with previously established standards. From a study of 1500 males Schonfeld established such standards of development by correlating measurements of penis and testes with the degree of maturation of the secondary sex characteristics. Schonfeld believes that the actual size of the genitalia is of physiologic significance only after pubescence and that "a great deal of therapeutic confusion has been created in the literature by the failure to appreciate the range of normal variation of genital measurements, age of onset of pubescence, and the characteristics of growth of the various types of body configurations (somatotypes). Many of these normal boys have been subjected to prolonged endocrine treatment with the induction of pubescence, and their normal development is fallaciously attributed to endocrine therapy. An accurate evaluation of the existing status and future prognosis is essential for the proper management of the prepubescent and pubescent boy." Schonfeld described a test to prognosticate whether a boy will have spontaneous pubescence. The test is based on the ability of the testes to respond to stimulation by chorionic gonadotropins of human pregnancy urine.

When hypogonadism actually exists the physical and psychological consequences are, of course, disastrous. Boys who in early childhood were active, healthy, husky children suddenly discover at adolescence that they are different from other boys, who make fun of them. Kasanin and Biskind discussed the change in personality that followed specific treatment in seven cases. Their patients had remained adolescent. They showed an abnormal body contour, retained a highpitched voice, and showed no growth of genitalia. Doubt regarding themselves "leads to a great deal of resentment mixed with the feeling of rage and frustration, which is usually repressed, and the only thing evident on the surface is a feeling of bitterness and hostility. . . The most important change effected by successful treatment is a better relationship to the world." All of their patients became more affectionate, less hostile, less jealous, not so bitter, and did not shrink from people any more. They met men and women on an equal basis, and were not afraid to compete.

PUBERTY

Certain emotional phenomena associated with puberty are frequently misunderstood or neglected by the physician. Nightmares, anxiety attacks, and phobias, such as fears of heart disease, lung disease, cancer, or a fear of going insane are commonly encountered. Unfortunately the physician's attitude often is, "He will outgrow it," or "It's only her period. When the menses are regularly established, the trouble will dissppear." We say "unfortunately" because it is true that such symptoms usually do disappear in a matter of months or a year or two, even if neglected. *But they do not disappear out of the personality!* (p. 25). The anxiety which is producing them and the ideas associated with the anxiety are pushed down into the unconscious mind and are carried around for years until some situation arises which produces trouble again. The following case is illustrative:

Masturbation Problem in an Adolescent
Diagnostic Difficulties; Quick Response to Superficial Psychother-
apy; Later Development of Blood Phobia and Inhibition of
Social Adjustment

CASE 38

History and Symptoms

A white girl of sixteen was first seen in 1928. She complained of pains in the abdomen, headaches, and occasional dizziness.

She stated that she had had upper abdominal pains off and on for many years. For the two years past the pain was constant and vomiting occurred. Further discussion revealed that the discomfort in the head was not really a headache but was dizziness, dullness, heaviness, and "inability to think clearly."

Past History. Except for measles and whooping cough and occasional sore throat there had been no serious illnesses. Tonsils had been removed a year before. For about one year she had worn glasses because of the peculiar sensations in the head.

The patient was the youngest of five children, having two brothers and two sisters, all of whom were well. The mother was living and well; the father had died during the influenza epidemic in 1918.

Physical Examination and Laboratory Studies

The patient was a well-nourished and well-developed young white girl. The pulse was rapid but regular and the hands were cold and mottled. The heart was normal in size and position and except for the rapid rate seemed perfectly normal. Otherwise there was no departure from normal physically except that the feet also were cold and mottled. Deep inspiration slowed the heart rate but there was no response to vagus or eyeball pressure.

The temperature was normal and after the patient had spent several days in bed the pulse rate became normal. The basal metabolism was within normal limits. X-ray of the chest was normal both for size of the heart and condition of the lungs. The tuberculin test was normal and the conclusion at the time was that the patient had vasomotor imbalance and a spastic colon.

Subsequent Course

The patient was seen at about monthly intervals and continued to complain. The *menses* were established shortly afterwards. In addition to some discomfort the patient reported that she had *fainted* at the time of the menstrual period on two different occasions.

In 1932 she reported that she was no different than when she had first consulted us. Menses were overdue; there was some *vulvar pruritus* and again she reported that she had fainted. In addition she stated that she was always "shaky and *nervous*." She graduated from high school and then entered business school.

Continuation of Complaints. Because of the continuation of the same complaints and the failure to respond to medication and reassurance as to the absence of organic disease, it was suggested on one occasion that perhaps there were problems that had not been discussed that entered into the illness. The patient did not respond but shortly afterwards we received a letter stating that after a conversation with an older sister concerning this suggestion, she had decided to take this means of informing us of *masturbation* because she was too ashamed to discuss it. She stated that she had masturbated as long as she could remember and that she considered it a degrading and loathesome act for which she could not forgive herself but at the same time she was unable to control the desire.

On her next visit she was *reassured* and *instructed* regarding masturbation. She was told that it was neither a loathesome nor an unnatural act, that it was very common among young people and that, like thumb-sucking in youngsters, it was simply an evidence of emotional immaturity which she had not yet outgrown. It was obvious that her feelings of guilt were immediately relieved and with lightened spirit she left the office.

She returned in a month, to report absence of desire to masturbate since. Any symptoms still present were less intense.

Follow-up

The patient was not seen again until 1941, when she reported that she could not stand the sight of *blood* nor discussions that had to do with sickness or injury. Such discussions would cause her to faint and recently at a motion picture which portrayed an injury she had to leave hurriedly in order not to faint. She also reported that she still had some abdominal discomfort and peculiar head sensations and at long intervals still masturbated though no longer with such feelings of guilt as before.

While she had grown to be quite an attractive young woman she reported that she was ill at ease with men and for that reason had very little contact with them.

Physical Examination

The general physical examination showed a well-developed, young woman whose hands and feet were mottled but not, it was said, so cold or moist as when she was a youngster. There was considerable acne scarring of the face and back. The heart rate was still rapid although the heart seemed perfectly normal.

She had consulted us again chiefly on account of the *blood phobia*, hoping that some magical formula would enable her to get rid of it (probably in much the same way that she was relieved of her guilt over masturbation when she was a child). Since she lived in another city it was impossible for her to come for treatment. The superficial explanation offered to her was that the blood phobia undoubtedly had to do with ideas of injury and bleeding. We felt that this was so because of the sexual fantasies connected with her act of masturbation. These generally had to do with ideas of a man injuring a woman or a child. It will be recalled that at the beginning of her menstrual life she frequently fainted and this in turn seemed to be related to disturbed ideas concerning the sexual act and the birth of a baby.

Chronic Masturbation

The case has been discussed chiefly from the standpoint of the significance of chronic masturbation as an evidence of disturbed psychosexual development. It is true that a great many youngsters, in fact the majority, masturbate during some period of their childhood but this evidence of emotional immaturity is usually outgrown and leaves no permanent marks upon the developing personality. However, in instances of chronic masturbation the act serves as an index to a markedly inhibited sexual development and therefore we may expect that other symptoms and perhaps neurotic illness may develop. In the present case we were pleased with the quick response to reassurance and reeducation concerning masturbation in childhood. But the follow-up experience demonstrated that we were dealing with a severely inhibited personality and that now in adult life a true phobia had appeared as an evidence of the disturbed personality development. Deeper fantasies of injury or harm untouched by simple reassurance had prevented better sexual adaptation and had produced the phobia. The phobia in itself might not prove to be so crippling but it was an index of a disturbed heterosexual relationship which had interfered with her proper social development and would undoubtedly interfere with her ability to marry and make a successful marital adjustment.

Nightmares

Persistent nightmares or anxieties and fears during the day are usually an indication of apprehension over aggressive tendencies or sexual matters. They are indices pointing to important personality difficulties and should not be dismissed by parent or physician any more than a symptom such as hemoptysis should be dismissed. If the anxiety is causing persistent nightmares, the content of the dream may indicate the source of the trouble. The dream can be considered a secretion of the mental apparatus just as the urine is the secretion of the urinary apparatus. To carry the analogy further the one is just as available for analysis as the other and may yield an equal amount of diagnostic information. For example, the girl who dreams that she is always being pursued by men with revolvers or sticks, or by animals with horns, or that a man is breaking into her room or is actually lying upon her and smothering her, indicates fairly clearly in this symbolic way the fear of sexual assault.

Anxiety Develops Early

Evidence already mentioned points to the fact that increase in activity of the sexual glands gives an added impetus to the psychosexual activity. But it would be folly to say that these dreams and and anxiety states and phobias are due to the glandular activity itself. Recent studies show that psychosexual activity does not begin at puberty. As discussed in the chapter on psychopathology, psychosexual development begins at birth. The growing child hears all kinds of statements about sexual functions by those around him. In some children all of this information and misinformation becomes integrated in a well-organized way, the ideas being firmly welded together into a satisfactory whole by a matrix of good will. In other children ideas are poorly understood, poorly integrated, and charged with anxiety rather than being welded into a more stable structure. It is the second kind of child who will develop the nightmares and anxiety attacks. Such signs of insecurity bode ill for the future of that person unless the anxiety state is effectively treated. As illustrated by the case report, if left alone these attacks may subside by further repression into the unconscious, but they tend to return, producing a more serious neurosis in later years. A large percentage of cases of anxiety hysteria of adult life have had anxiety attacks and phobias at the time of puberty. The neurosis develops because during the developing years of adolescence and early maturity the anxious young person never establishes the close emotional relationships with people which tend to strengthen the personality. Fear of exposing sexual or aggressive impulses will keep an adolescent isolated to the point of emotional starvation; an *immature and insecure adult personality* is the result.

Anxiety State of Puberty

CASE 39

History and Symptoms

A boy of thirteen, the healthy son of a farming couple, began to have nightmares in which he would cry out, awake in a panic of fear and state that he had dreamed that he had murdered someone. One of his parents would have to sleep with him the rest of the night. During the day, he would have periods of panic with the same thoughts, *i. e.*, he was afraid that he had murdered a girl and buried her somewhere on the farm. He would insist that his father go with him to the spot to prove that this was or was not true. After being shown that his fear was groundless, he would be reassured for a few hours, sometimes for a day or two, and then the anxiety would appear again.

LIFE SITUATION

When first seen, the boy was too frightened to say anything. After some friendly feeling was established he was told that many young people worry about sex matters and that if this was the case with him he could feel free about discussing his problems and asking any questions. He did not admit anything of the kind in the first two interviews but in the third he told a story of some sex play with the daughter of a neighbor a short time before the onset of his symptoms. He had touched her genitalia and lain on top of her. He had had no information about sexual matters from his parents and had heard only snatches of the sexual talk of older men. He formed the idea that any close proximity to a girl might cause her to become pregnant. He feared censure and disgrace and his mind kept turning to an incident of which he had heard—a man killing a girl whom he had made pregnant and then burying her. This thought became so insistent that it tortured his mind during the day and recurred during his dreams, so that he had to seek constant reassurance that he was not the man involved.

TREATMENT

The physiology of sex relations was explained to him and the necessity for intromission, and the deposit of semen within the vagina before pregnancy could take place was emphasized. He was immensely relieved and that night he had his first restful sleep in several weeks. His anxiety attacks and fears began to subside as his education regarding sexual matters continued. He was frequently reassured with the following statement, "You could not possibly have made this girl pregnant. Since this was not possible you need not worry about having done anything violent." The combination of fear of sexual activity and violence is a frequent source of anxiety. The parents were given some insight into the cause of the symptoms and urged to cultivate a more liberal attitude toward sexual matters. Only a few hours could be spent with this boy and his parents but he was made symptom free. More time could have been spent profitably but at least he received some correct information regarding sexual relations; faulty ideas were corrected so that he could feel that he had not committed any crime; and the good will and a more liberal attitude on the part of his parents had been obtained. It is probable that even this much therapy in each anxiety state of puberty would help prevent many crippling neuroses of later life. In this case, it would have been easy but very inadequate medical advice to repeat the time-worn formula, "Oh, he is thirteen and changing into a man. He'll outgrow it."

Chapter XV

ENDOCRINE SYSTEM AND METABOLISM (*Continued*)

THE RELATION OF DISORDERS OF THE THYROID GLAND TO THE EMOTIONS

It has been known for many years that emotional disturbances often accompany disorders of the thyroid gland. There are the emotional disorders, neurotic and psychotic, which occur as a part of the clinical picture of hyperthyroidism; the autonomic imbalance and psychic shocks which often seem to precede hyperthyroidism; and lastly the anxiety states associated with thyroid enlargements without hyperthyroidism. The *emotionalism* of hyperthyroidism is well known and is not our special concern. It is equally well known that this emotionalism diminishes when recovery from the disease occurs. What we are especially interested in is whether personality disturbances of long standing may lead to an alteration of thyroid function, or to put it another way, whether hyperthyroidism may represent a characteristic response of a special personality type to a specific psychic insult.

Preceding Emotional Disturbances

Many observations have been made on the emotional disturbances that precede hyperthyroidism. In 1925, Nolan D. C. Lewis reviewed the literature and concluded that there was no generally accepted theory of the pathogenesis of exophthalmic goiter. That is still true today. Nevertheless, increasing attention has been paid to the incidence of emotional difficulties in the histories of patients with hyperthyroidism. Moschcowitz, Bram, and Hyman and Kessel, are among the clinicians who have been impressed by such factors. Hyman and Kessel, who studied the problem of the relation of autonomic imbalance and hyperthyroidism, reported that "our patients almost without exception gave a history of psychic trauma preceding or associated with the development of the symptoms of exophthalmic goiter." But hints from life situations in series of cases compiled by clinicians and flashes of intuition by psychiatrists who have studied occasional cases, are not enough to establish the importance of psychopathology in the etiology of hyperthyroidism. Felix Deutsch approached the problem psychoanalytically and postulated that a constitutional degenerative "Anlage" could be lighted up into exophthalmic goiter by nervous influences such as might arise in hysteria.

473

B. Mittleman, in a recent discussion on the psychogenic factors in hyperthyroidism, felt that no work existed which used full modern psychopathological knowledge in its dynamic and descriptive aspects covering a large series of cases. Therese Benedek in the study and treatment of two cases, thought that the increased activity of the gland helped to *release* the emotions of *anxiety* and *aggression* which in turn often gave rise to the clinical picture of mental depression. In a study of considerable importance 166 women and 34 men with hyperthyroidism were observed from a psychiatric standpoint by Conrad.

Psychosomatic Observations

Conrad began her examination with a careful check of the exact time and sequence of the appearance of symptoms of hyperthyroidism. This was followed by a review of the family situation. Particular attention was given to any alteration in any situation showing a time relation to exacerbation of symptoms and a constant watch was kept for signs of unexplained emotion. In this connection she called attention to a *flushing* of the neck and lower face which showed a high degree of specificity in leading one to the conflict over which the patient had "decompensated." If the patient was interviewed in a good light, this was frequently noted in mild form. The degree of severity showed some correlation with the elevation of the B.M.R. and also with the violence of the trauma recalled. The blushing extended from the upper chest to the middle of the cheeks and occasionally to the forehead, with the neck veins standing out and pulsations in the neck increasing in violence, so that in extreme cases the thyroid gland itself appeared to increase in size. This flushing was noted when specific sensitiveness of the individual to an emotional experience had been "touched off." In mild form, such a blush repeatedly established points leading to the patient's major unconscious conflict. Conrad remarked that once noted it was a signal for as much caution as the appearance of pain in palpating an acute abdomen. She was also impressed by the appearance of confusion when the patient was questioned about dates and a sequence of events focusing upon a traumatic situation.

It was increasingly evident that instead of long periods of worry and deprivation there was usually an *emotional conflict* at the time of onset of the first typical symptom of the disease. Many times a patient repeated a story of shock as the cause of illness and this later proved to have come after typical symptoms had been present for some time. Thus she emphasized the necessity for an exact study of the onset of the very first symptom and of the personal life situation at that time.

Disturbance in Mother-Child Relationship. Many hyperthyroid patients showed endocrine imbalance in their development and family history. The body form was often that of hypogonadal development. So far as the psychic situation was concerned some abnormality in the mother-child relation was usually obvious. Examination of the female patient often revealed anxiety at the time of onset of acute symptoms, which followed in the main two patterns: (1) a fear of loss of shelter and affection, often apparently equivalent to deprivation of the mother or loss of the mother's approval, and (2) a fear of the dangers of the mother role. Many of the patients had been subjected to a strain with a resulting sense of inadequacy in the "mother's care of child" relation which seemed to be badly tolerated by them. This kind of strain appeared to precipitate the syndrome or to bring about an exacerbation. A large number of patients had been deprived of their mothers at an early age and often the death was due to child bearing. These persons appeared to make desperate and life-long struggles to win the mother's approval and to achieve likeness to her at the same time that they feared the responsibilities which she had. Worry over the mother's lot, however, was not limited to the dangers of pregnancy. It was often noted that the patient had been selected by the mother to share her anxiety and burdens even when there were older and stronger siblings. Even the male patients showed in a number of instances a disturbance in the mother-child relationship. Often there was conflict over partial identification with the mother. It was also noted that there was a tendency in a rather high percentage of cases to be dependent on the wife as a mother.

Previous Emotional Trends. Usually there was one or more previous episodes of nervousness or breakdown before the overt onset of the actual illness. Several cases who "never felt the same after the mother died," then showed a typical sudden onset following another traumatic experience. Hysteria, anxiety, and paranoid and manic-depressive tendencies were often observed in these patients prior to the onset of their hyperthyroidism.

Anxiety Takes the Visceral Path. Therefore, Conrad suggested that the emotional pattern of these personalities may be explained by hypothesizing a pathological development, often a frustration, in the normal attempt to establish independence of the mother. She remarked that the classical neurotic symbolizes his conflict without somatic pathology—he suffers at a cortical level. In other words, instead of showing physical symptoms he presents disturbances in thinking and attitudes. But when conflicts in the personal life discharge energy into autonomic channels, pathological tension, congestion, and imbalance of secretion may occur and may increase susceptibility to physical disease, precipitate it or cause an exacerbation of disease that is already present. As Deutsch suggested, Conrad also believed that this occurs in individuals with more or less hereditary weakness or acquired pathology. For anxiety to take the visceral path, there must also be an instability of integration for one's role in life, originating in the early formation of the personality, probably in the process of establishing independence of the mother. This pattern may be linked with a typical neurosis or occur without it. In the latter case the patient's relation with other people appears undisturbed while his attitude toward himself shows pathological insecurity.

Psychic Trauma. So far as etiology of hyperthyroidism was concerned she obtained a history of psychic trauma in 94 per cent of cases by a method of examination which stressed (1) the investigation of new developments in the life situation and personal relations at the time of onset of hyperthyroid symptoms; and (2) the evaluation of unconscious conflicts which were indicated by the appearance of a specific sign of emotion during history-taking.

Treatment Suggestions. In regard to treatment she suggested the necessity (1) for increasing the stability of autonomic function as, for example, by partial thyroidectomy or x-ray treatments and (2) for psychotherapy aimed to increase the independence of the personality. To the extent that this is impossible of realization, the maximum of physical and emotional shelter becomes imperative. Insight into the specific threat to which each patient was sensitive aided in the establishment of security from within or from without.

Psychological Invalidism in Thyroidectomized Patients

Ruesch and his associates explored the problems of personality structure in relation to the onset of symptoms and recovery in forty-three patients who had been subjected to subtotal thyroidectomy. There were thirty-five women and eight men in the series; thirty-two had toxic and eleven nontoxic goiters.

The study indicated that patients afflicted with thyroid disease fall into two distinct entities as far as their sociopsychological aspects are concerned: the normal, or almost normal girl (one third of the total) and the hysterical or anxious type (more than one half of the total). In the case of men it was a question of dependent personalities. Although surgical procedures were tolerated well by the normal girls, delayed recovery was pretty much the rule for anxious types and hysterical characters.

Ruesch noted that the conformist attitude in these patients was outstanding. There was a great need for recognition and for dependence. Self-love and inability to express anger were the outstanding character problems; overconformance to accepted ideals was the principal defense. In about half the cases a necessity to adjust to environmental changes was found at the time of onset of the disease. Because of their childhood pattern, the patients were poorly equipped to face these environmental changes; broken homes, for example, burdened them with premature responsibilities, producing feelings of insecurity. Ruesch recommends psychotherapy before and after this operation. His comprehensive article contains an appendix summarizing the sociopsychological aspects of patients with hyperthyroidism.

The following case represents a characteristic background of a typical case of hyperthyroidism.

Hyperthyroidism

CASE 40

A white woman of forty-four was first seen in the summer of 1938 complaining of nervousness and loss of weight. She said that she had always been nervous but that it had been worse in the last few months and that there had been a loss of about 10 pounds in weight in the last two months. Except for heart consciousness there were no other symptoms.

Past History

She had been married for fifteen years and had a son, aged ten, who was living and well. Prior to the birth of her child she had suffered from dysmenorrhea but that was no longer present. Nevertheless, she had had a long period of invalidism after the birth of the child—this she referred to as "a nervous breakdown."

Family History. The father had been a dreamy, incompetent creature who died suddenly from heart disease at the age of fifty and the mother, an accomplished and domineering woman, had been forced to earn a living for the family. The family consisted of three brothers and a sister. One brother, somewhat younger than the patient, suffered from manic-depressive psychosis and had been an inmate of institutions on numerous occasions. Still another brother was brilliant but erratic. Whereas the sister had enjoyed a college education and had married successfully, the patient had been saddled with responsibilities at home and denied educational opportunities.

Present Illness. At first the patient was unable to find any emotional circumstance that coincided with the onset of her illness but after some discussion admitted that once more the family was torn with conflict over the question of the disposition of the manic-depressive brother. It always fell to the patient's lot to be responsible for him at such times as he was not in an institution. Just prior to the onset of this illness she had been faced with numerous responsibilities and suddenly was presented with the necessity of once more taking this brother into her home. She said, "I didn't know whether to mother him or smother him." Thus her conflict of maternal devotion and hostility was symbolized by this casual expression. Nevertheless, she took her brother, hardly recovered from a manic attack, into her home, felt great tension, smoked and drank to excess, and kept herself busy in order "not to have time to think."

Thus it was that increased "nervousness" and loss of weight became evident to her family and friends even before she herself noted it. Finally she was persuaded to seek medical attention and the classical picture of hyperthyroidism was found.

TREATMENT

The background out of which the hyperthyroidism seemed to arise was made clear to her and it was explained that the immediate problem could be met by surgery or x-ray but that the emotional tensions of the past had to be dealt with differently in order for her to achieve permanent cure. She chose to be operated upon. The surgical removal of the major part of the gland was successful and she made a speedy recovery. Then with the help of medical advice she adopted a more realistic attitude toward her brother's illness, insisting that other members of the family assist in his care, and placed him permanently in an institution so that he would not prove to be so disruptive a force in the family situation.

The following cases represent various problems associated with or related to thyroid disease.

Nodular Goiter with Anxiety Symptoms; Suspected Hyper-thyroidism
Psychological Preparation for Surgery; Thyroidectomy; Excellent Recovery

---

CASE 41

A young, married white woman was admitted to the hospital on October 7, 1940. She complained of a lump in the neck and nervousness.

History and Symptoms

She considered herself in fairly good health until about one year before, at which time she developed attacks of nervousness, especially in the morning, which were accompanied by a feeling of "a lump in the throat," tremors, and nausea. They occurred frequently and especially about the time of the menstrual period. The attacks might last an hour or might last all day. She felt that they were often precipitated by emotional disturbance. She had had frequent nightmares so that she awakened with a start, was very frightened, and perspired freely. Following such attacks she was apt to have diarrhea. When she was nervous she had deep sighing respirations.

Past History. She was a premature baby and was considered a frail child, but had no serious illness. About four years ago in school it was noted that the thyroid gland was large. One year ago her father was operated upon for goiter after having had medical treatment without help for a long time. Following his operation he did very well, gained weight, and regained his health. It was about this time that the mother called the patient's attention to the fact that she also had a goiter.

Menstruation. Menses, established at the age of eleven, had always been painful and sometimes were accompanied by nausea. As stated above, the choking feeling in the throat was worse during the menstrual period.

Family History. Her family history other than the note mentioned regarding her father did not seem to have any bearing on this illness.

Physical Examination and Laboratory Studies

Examination showed a small, thin girl with nodular enlargement of the left lobe of the thyroid gland. Other than this finding the physical examination was essentially negative. There were no objective evidences of hyperthyroidism. The urine examination was negative and the Wassermann was negative but the blood count showed leukocytes varying from 10,000 to 17,000 and the temperature chart showed that her temperature averaged about 99° or 99.2° F. with one elevation to 99.4° F. Pulse and respirations were not increased.

Basal metabolism tests had been plus 8, plus 14, and after a few days in the hospital plus 1 without any medication. The sedimentation rate was within normal limits. The gynecological examination was negative.

The patient was sent into the hospital first, to determine whether she had hyperthyroidism and secondly, to decide, even if she did not, whether to operate upon this enlarged gland. On the basis of the observations up to this point we concluded that there was no evidence of hyperthyroidism. The second question we will reserve for later discussion.

LIFE SITUATION

Unfortunately, terms for describing personality changes are not so precise as those for describing pulse or basal metabolic rates. But we have to do the best we can with close observation and description to make clear the pathological disturbance in the temperament of our patients and thus realize that this factor may be just as important as a very high basal metabolic rate.

Childhood

The mother died when the patient was born and she lived in an orphanage for three years, whereupon her father married again and she was taken home. Certainly three years in an orphan asylum was not the most auspicious way to begin life, even though this orphanage may have been an unusually good institution. A child placed in an orphanage is not likely to get the individual personal interest and love that a child obtains with his own parents. Even after she came to live with the family in her father's home she says she never knew until the age of fifteen that her stepmother was not her real mother. She had two older brothers but evidently the siblings weren't close enough to discuss such matters. When she found this out at fifteen she felt she understood why she had been neglected and why there had been a lack of personal warmth for her in the home. Of course it is common for children to feel neglected in *any* home but it may well have been that the stepmother was not able to feel the same interest in the patient as in her own child.

Shyness

The patient was unusually sensitive. An illustration of her sensitiveness follows: During her teens she was given a surprise party by a friend which affected her adversely because when she was with people she was inwardly very uncomfortable. At this party she could not "pull herself together" for about an hour and when she finally did she was still shaky, felt dizzy, and could not sleep that night. This was the first of many such attacks occurring under similar circumstances.

She went to school to the twelfth grade and did well. She had few close friends and never felt at ease in the company of strangers.

Work

After leaving school she went to work, first as a waitress, then in a women's clothing business, where she had been working up to the time of admission to the hospital. She got on well at work but she paid in emotional tension for the calm she exhibited externally. She took a certain pride in telling us that no one knew how she felt inside. It "took a great deal out of her" to hide any feelings of depression.

Marriage

She was married nine months before admission, to a man she had known for some time and liked very much. She had been very happy. At the same time anticipation of sexual relations disturbed her and during the first week of her marriage the idea of sexual intercourse was so distressing that her husband was not able to approach her. It took some time for her to become adjusted to the sexual relationship. Later, according to her statement, intercourse became quite satisfactory. We have learned that we cannot accept such a statement at face value in the beginning of psychotherapy. In fact we must not dwell too much upon the subject of sexual functioning. Later the importance of any disturbance in this field can be more easily discussed and understood.

Anxiety Attacks and Anxiety Dreams

In the past year and a half she had had what will be recognized as anxiety attacks, usually occurring at night, preceded by a dream in which something unpleasant was happening. Sometimes she was being pursued by animals or men. Sometimes in the dream she was falling from the roofs of houses and then would awaken in the anxiety state. Recently, she dreamed that a dog was biting her hand and she could not get away. She awoke crying, felt cold all over, and had palpitation. She had also dreams in which actual violence, such as a murder, had taken place.

On coming home one day she found the mother of her fiancé dead. Again this caused her to "break down." For several days all she could see was the dead face of her fiancé's mother in front of her and she was many weeks getting over this fright.

Up to the time of the present illness this girl had done well in meeting her tasks as far as the casual observer could see. But fear and anxiety existed within and as a result of it she had begun to display symptoms and her efficiency had begun to fail.

She had difficulty in adapting herself to the hospital environment. On one occasion we saw her about an hour after visitors had left. She was asked about the effect of the visitors upon her, as well as the effect produced by her interviews with the physicians. She said that all of these situations were an ordeal, producing cardiac palpitation, sweating, tightness in her throat and stomach, and a sense of uneasiness.

Many patients with *social anxiety* do not develop anxiety attacks until much later in life than was the case with this patient. Fortunately, she had not developed a belief that she had a heart condition and was willing to listen to advice that could help her to understand her illness. She apparently was willing to believe that she did not have thyroid disease, although this had been suggested as the cause of her distress and she had been much impressed by the facts of her father's illness.

Relation of Shock to Hyperthyroidism

It has been noted that there is a tendency to develop increased thyroid activity after a severe shock or fright. Sometimes a patient who has seen a murder or an accident ending in injury and death develops hyperthyroidism within a few days. The German expression *Schreckbasedow*, meaning "Basedow's disease of fright origin," has been used to describe this phenomenon. Whether the event which our patient witnessed—the death of her fiancé's mother—was especially significant and had any effect in aggravating the anxiety in this girl we could not be sure. But she claimed that this was the most serious shock in her life.

TREATMENT

From a psychiatric standpoint we felt that it was very important to treat the *existing neurosis* at this early stage. This patient had marked anxiety which was being condensed into anxiety attacks and these had been advancing very rapidly in the last nine months. If this aspect of her illness was not treated she could soon become incapacitated.

We felt that the *prognosis* was fairly good, the chief reason being that the anxiety state was in its early stages and the patient was in the frame of mind to accept help. She had not yet come to the point where she wanted to lay the blame for her attacks upon some obscure organic disease. She seemed to have the capacity for reeducation and emotional growth. For some time this patient had been weak because anxiety had prevented emotional development from taking place. Thus there occurred a frequent personality disturbance—an inordinate wish to be strong; she wanted to deny that she was frightened; she wanted to do her work and conceal from her husband and from us that she was inwardly so sensitive. Most neurotic people react in this way. We must help them to expose their weaknesses and then help them to grow stronger through reeducation.

In the past year the patient had not been getting any emotional satisfaction at home or at work. She was so frightened about coming to the hospital that she derived no satisfaction from her stay here. Her inability to relax, and a complaint which she referred to as "this emptiness inside" (an indication of her great insecurity) suggested the possibility that this patient could develop a psychosis if any marked degree of thyroid overactivity should occur. We concluded that the patient needed psychiatric help at regular intervals, probably once a week for several months. The family as well as the patient had to be made to understand that the proper medicine for this patient was an understanding of anxiety and how to combat it.

The Question of Psychological Preparation for Surgery

The first question to be decided was whether this patient had hyperthyroidism and we came to the conclusion that she did not but that she did have a *simple goiter*. Then the question arose as to whether she should be operated upon anyhow and here a number of considerations entered. She was a young woman and the lump in the neck might be removed for cosmetic reasons if for no other. In addition there was always the possibility of further growth, of hyperthyroidism, and of the development of a cancer. Besides all that, and very important in this case, the patient had the knowledge of her father being treated for goiter for a long time without help and then the quick recovery following surgery. Then came the question of psychological preparation for surgery, which we consider one of the major questions in medicine. Surgeons are always so careful to prepare their patients physically for surgery; they would never think of performing a major operation without knowing that the cardiovascular-renal system had been surveyed but they almost never give any consideration to the kind of personality that exists in the individual who is about to be operated upon, how much anxiety is there, and what the effects of a surgical traumatic experience may be as far as the personality structure is concerned. We recently had in the hospital ward an old woman who had a huge enlargement of the thyroid gland which was removed because it was pressing upon the trachea. She had some discomfort but not severe dyspnea. The anatomical problem loomed large in the clinical picture but the patient was very apprehensive prior to operation and after operation became completely psychotic. As it turned out we wonder whether perhaps she was not better off with the lump in her neck. Similar instances of how badly some patients react to surgery are dealt with elsewhere.

Line of Inquiry to be Followed

Therefore, the matter of preparation for operation especially interested us in this patient. We allowed about six weeks for seeing the patient once a week and getting acquainted with her problems. Here were some of the things we wanted to find out: Had many people noticed or commented upon the lump in her throat? How much would she like to have it removed? We tried to estimate from what she said just how important this lump was to her. Sometimes people are very sensitive in many other fields and yet the enlargement does not distress them or at least disturbs them very little. In that case one would not think of operating for cosmetic reasons alone. We tried to find out how much she feared an operation and how much of a shock she thought it would be to her. We put the question something like this, "How many people who have had operations do you know? Have they suffered from pain or distress during or after an operation? What did she fear? Was it pain or the effects of the anesthesia or the scar or discomfort connected with the scar?" Each time we talked to her about these things we tried to estimate what her reaction to operation would be.

Listening Instead of Talking. We felt that in a month or six weeks the patient should get an increasing amount of confidence and should receive definite and precise information in place of her hazy and ill-formed fears.

We spoke of getting acquainted with the patient. Inexperienced physicians often have a great urge to interpret things to the patient, to talk a lot to the patient about mental mechanisms. We advise that it is better to listen than to talk. In the beginning one should be satisfied simply to get acquainted with the patient. The visits should mean an opportunity for questions and discussions of the patient's feeling about life in general and, of course, the particular problem that is disturbing the patient. Also in a case like this it was important to know whether or not the patient was going to remain in our care both before and after the operation. If some change was made and she came into the hands of another physician there might be enough difference in opinion to cause worry and conflict in a patient as sensitive as this one. For the next few years it would be important for this girl to be in the care of one physician or one group of physicians until she was properly educated and stabilized. There must be a consistency in her life if one would try to stabilize her thinking.

Therapy in Outpatient Department

The patient reported to the psychiatric outpatient department one week after her discharge from the hospital. On this visit she was again informed that as a result of her study in the hospital, no cause of an organic nature had been found for her fatigue and her weakness. Her personality needs were put before her again and it was explained how important it would be for her to recognize these needs and so relate herself to people as to get some satisfaction for these needs. On this visit a maternal aunt had accompanied the patient. She seemed a kind and understanding person and so we explained to her in the patient's presence something of the latter's problem. This is a safe procedure when we are sure that the relative is really kind and understanding. In some cases a relative or friend may use such information to ridicule or harass the patient rather than to be helpful. But in this case we felt the aunt was sincerely interested in our patient and understood her problem. The result of this was to make the patient feel that she was not carrying the burden of her emotional problem entirely alone.

Inferiority Feelings. The patient was seen every two weeks in the clinic and as time went on she began to understand why she had developed such a sense of inferiority. The stepmother had always browbeaten the patient and scolded her with such statements as "You are a stupid girl. Why do you have to be so dumb all the time?" Apparently the stepmother could not tolerate the idea that the children should cherish any thoughts or feelings toward the real mother. Hence our patient grew up without having any older woman as a close friend. The result of this was that she was always trying to make a good impression upon other people and would not allow them to do anything for her. For instance, while she was in the hospital the stepmother visited the patient every day. The latter did not feel that the stepmother did this out of any real interest in her but only out of a sense of duty for which she expected something in return. Therefore the patient, on leaving the hospital, purchased a smoking stand for the stepmother's home. In relating this the patient said, "My stepmother always says she does not want anything in return for what she does for me, but I know differently. When my father makes such a statement I know he means it but not so with my stepmother. Had I not bought this smoking stand, I know she would have felt unrepaid for her attention to me while I was ill."

Anxiety Continues. At the end of the first month the patient reported that her anxiety attacks were decreasing but might still occur in the presence of people when some incident of emotional significance occurred. For instance, on her return to work her fellow employees had made a collection and given her a purse of thirty dollars in order to help her pay her hospital bill. When this was presented to her she became anxious, her heart beat rapidly, she perspired, and was not able to utter a single word of appreciation. It took her several days to get over the feeling of what a fool she had been on that occasion when she could not say a word in response to their kindness.

We explained to her that her desire for evidence of love and friendship was very great—so great in fact, that she was afraid to admit it lest she lose complete control of herself. We reassured her that to want friendship is normal and mature and that she must be more understanding in this regard when she was with her family, her fellow workers, and her friends. People who pretend to need or want nothing can be baffling and unsatisfying to the average person who wants some chance to be of value to others. Although she was at first skeptical, this discussion of human nature interested her and she said she would like to learn more about herself and other people.

In the next two weeks the patient reported that she was feeling still better and had had only one mild period of anxiety. This occurred when a new situation presented itself. She had her first altercation with one of the employees who tried to impose additional work upon her. On previous occasions our patient had always given in although there was inner rebellion. On this occasion she spoke up in defense of herself and declined to accept the additional work. The patient felt rather good about this in spite of her mild anxiety.

Readiness for Operation. We inquired about the lump in her neck and she reported that the swelling seemed more pronounced and caused a sense of pressure. She also felt that for cosmetic reasons she would like to have it removed. Her friends remarked about the lump and it embarrassed her to have attention called to it. As she was so extremely neat in her appearance it was understandable that this asymmetry of the neck would be a psychological problem for her. We discussed the matter of operation. We asked her how she would feel about the resulting scar upon the neck and her reply was that she thought she could endure the scar much better than the present lump. We warned her that an operation might not remove the sense of pressure of which she complained, at least not more than temporarily, since a sense of pressure in the neck was often of nervous origin and not due to pressure of a small growth such as she had. The patient felt that she would be willing to take this chance. At the end of two months the patient reported that her anxiety attacks had entirely disappeared. She was not busy at her place of work and therefore wanted to have the operation performed then. We felt that since her desire for operation had been consistent ever since leaving the hospital and that since her anxiety attacks had subsided and she was making a better social adjustment, she was in a satisfactory emotional condition to meet the operation.

Operation

The operation was successful and the patient was then sent to a convalescent home to recuperate. A small stitch abscess developed which she tolerated without a return of anxiety. This healed without producing a disfiguring scar and the patient felt well satisfied with the result. Her social adjustment has not been as satisfactory as we would like to see but there has been no return of anxiety attacks and it seems likely that further improvement will occur.

The next somewhat similar problem did not yield so happy a result.

Nodular Goiter; Thyroidectomy; Neurasthenia; Dependent Person with Strong Unconscious Desire to Remain Sick; Bad Prognosis

---

CASE 42

A single white woman of forty-seven was first seen in the medical outpatient department in September, 1939. She complained of epigastric distress and a pulling sensation in the neck, sometimes extending up into the face to the ears.

History and Symptoms

She stated that she had been a healthy young person but that when she was eighteen a goiter appeared and soon afterwards she became nervous and had rapid heart action. Nevertheless, she continued to work until about the age of thirty but since that time (*i. e.*, for the last seventeen years) she had led a life of *invalidism*, remaining at home and being looked after by the mother. She stated that she was not operated upon sooner because the family doctor was not enthusiastic about the chances for cure and the mother consequently had forbidden operation. A sister-in-law stated, however, that the mother was not so decided against operation but said, "If I do have her operated upon she will find something else to complain about!" How prophetic the mother's words were we shall soon see.

The *mother died* in February, 1938, and immediately the patient began to complain of epigastric distress and the sensation of a lump in the throat. A short time later, in June, 1938, she was studied in another hospital and *thyroidectomy* was done. She is stated to have had a large, nodular goiter. Almost immediately after operation the epigastric distress became more marked and was accompanied by a pulling or clutching or *choking sensation* in the throat. When this was severe it extended up into the face. She received much medical care and many studies were done but according to the patient no diagnosis was established. She had been told that she was anemic and was being treated for this condition.

Family History

The father died of tuberculosis at the age of forty-two when the patient was seven. He was sick at home for six or seven weeks. The mother died of diabetes at the age of seventy in February, 1938. She had been sick for about two years with diabetes, high blood pressure, arteriosclerosis and gangrene, and finally became psychotic. She was always a nervous person. One brother was living and well, age forty-nine, married and had two children.

Physical Examination and Laboratory Studies

After her first interview in the outpatient department she was referred into the hospital for complete study. There we observed that the patient was a fairly well-nourished white woman who was very cooperative and was looked upon as a "good patient" by the nurses. The general physical examination was negative except for slight tenderness in the epigastrium. It should be mentioned that the patient was edentulous, her teeth having been removed with the idea that "focal infection" might have been responsible for the illness. We felt that it was necessary to study the gastrointestinal tract carefully and also to pay some attention to the basal metabolism and the question of parathyroid insufficiency following operation. Gastric analysis showed low free acid but the gastrointestinal x-ray, including cholecystogram, was entirely normal. The urinalysis, complete blood count, and blood Wassermann were all normal. The basal metabolism was minus 6 and the blood calcium and blood phosphorus and also phosphatase were all within normal limits. This was also true of the cholesterol figure. During a week's observation the temperature, pulse, and respiration were normal and blood pressure was within normal limits. We felt that we had excluded any evidence of organic disease.

LIFE SITUATION

We will discuss this case in the following order: *First*, the life situation; *second*, the personality trends brought out by the life situation; *third*, the diagnosis; *fourth*, the meaning of symptoms, and *fifth*, treatment orientation and management.

This patient continued at school until the eighth grade and then engaged in factory work for a few years. About the age of thirty, however, she was forced to give up her work and then continued to live with the mother who supported her and took care of her. She insisted that the mother would not permit her to be operated upon but just where to place the responsibility for her failure to have proper treatment was a question that we could not be sure about.

Dependency

Patients often place responsibility for such action, or rather inaction, on the shoulders of others when it properly belongs upon their own. During these years she did not live a useful kind of existence. It might be said that she utilized her goiter for the purpose of escaping real responsibilities in life. For example, when we asked her whether she regretted not having married, she answered in the affirmative but did not give the reason that one would naturally expect, that is, of not having a home and not having children, etc., but rather said, "Now that I am sick it would be nice if I had someone to look after me." This was a strong indication of her passive and dependent make-up. After the mother died she went to live with her brother. Already she had pronounced stomach symptoms and was urged to do something definite about herself. It was then that she was operated upon but the symptoms became more severe and this made her more of an invalid than she had been. These symptoms did not seem to have an organic basis. They could be explained on the basis of dependency which was innate in this person and in turn was fostered by the people with whom she lived.

Gastric Symptoms

We said that there is a definite relationship between the dependent role and disturbed gastrointestinal function. Dependency indicates a need for love and affection and this in infancy is closely tied up with the function of eating. Getting food and getting affection go hand in hand. Later in life when these people are denied the affection which they so strongly need the gastrointestinal function becomes disturbed through undue stimulation by unconscious love hunger which has the same physiologic effect as food hunger. It was striking in this patient that as soon as her mother died the gastric symptoms began.

Diagnosis and Treatment

Because she lived so useless an existence in so passive and dependent a fashion, with emphasis on fatigue and gastrointestinal symptoms, and because she exhibited so much concern about herself and the harm that she might do herself through activity, we concluded that this illness was *neurasthenia*. In her brother's home she was called upon to do very little and rarely volunteered to do anything. She had given up all social contacts and according to the sister-in-law would do nothing but sit around and mope all day. When we considered treatment in this woman we faced a very difficult problem. She was a very passive and dependent person and if we urged her to be more active, to attempt to accomplish something in the world, she would become very irritated with us. And yet this was a responsibility that we could not shirk. So long as her dependency was encouraged she would remain an invalid. Only by coming in closer personal contact with life and trying to do something for herself would she overcome her symptoms and really become a useful citizen again. This, of course, we recognized as a very difficult task in a person who had neglected life so long, and we were prepared to meet and deal with hostile feelings in such a patient as one of our responsibilities. Physicians must be aware that hostility and dissatisfaction with life are present in every neurosis and cannot remain hidden if the patient is to be made well.

We felt that we must let the patient, and the family also, see and know the source of her bitterness and dissatisfaction in order to try to remedy it. As unconscious emotional needs are forced out, by encouraging a patient to act more like a normal person, some means of gratification must be found. It is true that this may tax the resourcefulness, or even call for sacrifices, of patients or relatives and they must realize it. While we felt that the prognosis was not too good in this case we thought that at least we could remove the aura of illness which surrounded the patient and set her apart from her family, even if we could not make her an entirely happy, well-adjusted person. That would be worth the effort of a psychiatric-sociological approach.

Unconscious Wish to Remain Sick

We considered this a very important case because there are many such patients in the world and they are often badly treated by physicians who do not appreciate the unconscious tendency to remain sick. Here, for example, was a patient studied by an excellent physician, who, because of his organic training to the exclusion of psychological training, sought an organic explanation for this illness. All that he could find was a mild anemia for which he was treating the patient. This, of course, played right into her unconscious wish to remain sick. If she was anemic then she was weak and if she was weak then she could not work! Our efforts had to be exactly the opposite. We had to encourage such a patient, by assuring her that she had no organic disease, that she was capable of doing something and then insisting that something be done. Of course we were not very hopeful because anyone who had demonstrated such dependency and passivity is certainly not good material to work with from a psychological standpoint. Regardless of who was responsible for her failure to have been operated upon sooner we must realize that here was a patient who had lived with a disfiguring and disabling goiter up to the age of forty-six before she finally decided to have it operated upon.

We did not say anything about a little horny, epithelial *growth* that this patient had on her nose and which we removed while she was in the hospital. It played very little part in her illness but helped to indicate the kind of person we were dealing with. In other words, just as she tolerated a disfiguring goiter for all of her adult life, so for the past four or five years she had permitted this horny excrescence on her nose and we doubt whether she would have done anything about it except for our urging while she had been here in the hospital. Certainly no ordinary woman would allow herself to be so disfigured in this day and age.

The "Good" Patient

A word also about the "good" hospital patient. Patients like this often accommodate themselves very well to the hospital routine. They feel secure, taken care of, and all of their dependent wishes are gratified. Hence, they are pleasant and cooperative. *We must be suspicious of patients who accommodate themselves too well to hospital routine.*

Cancerophobia

This patient was convinced that she had a *cancer*. This was not unique because a great many patients think they have cancer and indeed most women who consult physicians will at some time have the idea in their heads. They do not always express it, in fact, they rarely directly express their cancer fears. They often disguise it by a complaint about a lump, a swelling, or a curious sensation in the abdomen or breast, and when they are assured at the end of a complete physical examination that they are free from organic disease they heave a sigh of relief and say, "Oh, I am so glad because I thought I might have a cancer." With all of the *propaganda* for the early detection of cancer these fears are exaggerated and we presume it is the price that we must pay for instructing people about cancer. We are not, of course, advising against such instruction; it is only that we must realize that we add to the apprehension of many patients by our emphasis upon the early detection of cancer.

Reconversion of Symptoms

We have often spoken about the conversion of mental conflict into physical symptoms. Now we must realize that in the treatment of such a patient as this one it happens that when we make an effort to abolish symptoms there is a "reconversion" of physical into mental symptoms, manifested by dissatisfaction and depression. It is because of this inevitable "reconversion" that we speak of being prepared to deal with *negative feelings* in our patients. Such negative feelings may impel them to break off treatment. Such a situation must be guarded against by preparing the family for such an attitude and enlisting their cooperation beforehand. However, there is always one strong factor in our favor: the neurotic patient needs a friend badly and this the physician can be at the same time that he is an educator. They need someone to be interested in them and hence when the family or their conscience does not permit them to avoid life through symptom formation they are most likely to seek the physician's help.

Follow-up

The patient returned to the outpatient department on several occasions during which an effort was made to follow up the principles of treatment just outlined but she was incapable of accepting any insight, insisted on receiving medicine, and finally broke her appointments and failed to return.

The next patient was at first treated as thyroid disease and later, for no better reason, as pituitary disease.

---

*Early Schizophrenia (?); Anxiety Attacks
Differential Diagnosis from Endocrine Disease*

CASE 43

A single white woman, age twenty-two, was first admitted to the Temple University Hospital, February 21, 1939. She complained of a burning sensation in the stomach which extended "like a wave all the way to the genitals"; attacks of palpitation, sweating and faintness.

History and Symptoms

She had been well until one evening in August, 1938, when, in a motion picture theater, she had a feeling of oppression on the chest, palpitation, and sweating which caused her to leave the theater. On the street she felt faint, was taken to a nearby drug store and later to the office of a private physician. There the diagnosis of a *heart attack* was made. She was later treated for *thyroid disease* until November, 1938, when her physician sent her to another hospital for laboratory studies. Following this study she was admitted to the Temple University Hospital for further investigation. The history at this time indicated that she had been short of breath since her "collapse" in August but that this had no relation to exertion. Palpitation occurred whenever she became nervous or excited and she said that it was in December, 1938, that she observed that the hair of her arms was getting longer, blacker and coarser and that there was an abnormal growth of hair on her lip and chin and also upon the abdomen. About the same time she began to complain of a loss of appetite, a sensation of heat or a hot flash arising in the epigastrium and lasting several seconds to hours. This would extend like a wave down to the genitals. Since the beginning of the illness she had also complained of "fainty spells with a dizzy sensation." She became very weak and exhausted on walking and had to lie down.

Past Medical History. She had measles and whooping cough as a child and at the age of nine an incision and drainage of a thyroid abscess with a resulting sinus and fistula which took four years to heal. There had been no other illnesses. The menses had been regular up to the time of admission; they were profuse and the last two periods were associated with dysmenorrhea. Her best weight had been 165 pounds at the age of sixteen and on admission she weighed 130. She had been constipated for many years and used a laxative nightly.

Family History. The family consisted of a father, fifty-four, and mother, fifty-five, who were living and well. There were two brothers and three sisters all of whom were well. A grandfather died of carcinoma of the stomach.

Physical Examination and Laboratory Studies

On admission the temperature, pulse, and respirations were normal. The blood pressure was 120/85. The skin of the face was rather coarse and oily and there was some excess hair on the upper lip and the chin. There was a moderate amount of acne on the back. There was a small scar just at the right of the midline over the thyroid region but the thyroid seemed normal on palpation. The cardiovascular system seemed normal and the lungs were clear and resonant. The abdominal examination showed some striae atrophicae over the lower abdomen and hips, and there was some extension of pubic hair toward the umbilicus.

The urine and blood count were normal; a glucose tolerance test was slightly altered in the direction of diminished tolerance; the blood Wassermann was negative and basal metabolism was minus 3. Eyegrounds were normal and visual fields were normal. An x-ray of the skull was normal. The electrocardiogram was within normal limits. In spite of these negative findings it had been assumed that the patient had *pituitary basophilism* and she had been treated with irradiation to the pituitary gland. About the only change noted was that she missed a menstrual period. The same symptoms continued, and she was then treated elsewhere with some kind of injections of glandular substance, and returned to the Temple University Hospital in October, 1939, for further studies.

Second Hospital Admission

The complaints were the same but on several occasions the blood pressure had been slightly elevated. Studies were repeated. This time the glucose tolerance test was normal and two basal metabolism tests were minus 5 and minus 6. Neurological examination was negative and the eyegrounds and fields were normal. Gynecological examination was negative. The general physical examination showed nothing different from before. The patient was normal in appearance except for the slight hair increase that we had already noted. She felt well when she was lying down but complained that after she was up and about she became very fatigued and had to lie down. Electrocardiograph studies in the recumbent and upright positions showed very slight evidence of postural circulatory changes. Slight flattening of the T wave occurred in the upright position. Pulse and blood pressure were practically unaffected.

LIFE SITUATION

Early Life and Family Background

We have seen that regardless of what organisms invade the tissues, or what anatomical deviations may be present, the physician interested in psychosomatic medicine is curious to know how the patient has lived. In fact, even in the presence of tumors or broken bones we are interested to know in what kind of personality the tumor growth or broken bone is found. The symptoms just described were present in an individual who had lived an unusual kind of existence. She had lived a very secluded life, entirely within her own family. As a child she was not allowed to play with the neighborhood children because the parents felt that she was superior to the others. They seemed to feel that she would learn something unpleasant or be contaminated in some vague way by the children of other families. This same attitude persisted throughout adolescence when she was not allowed to associate with the other young people of her town because they were not "the right kind." As a result this girl enjoyed no hobbies and no sports. She never learned to dance or to play cards. She had no special interest of any kind. She had never done a single day's work! On one occasion she started to work in a factory, but after being on the job for a few hours she began to feel tired and weak and had to go home. Therefore we found her at the age of twenty-two having made no contribution, either to her own welfare or to the welfare of society.

Her father was a Catholic and her mother a Protestant. About the age of eleven this girl became interested in the Catholic church (according to her statement because of a girl friend who became a Catholic) and she joined the church but had not kept up her interest. She did not seem much concerned about this and stated that the family was not concerned and it may be that this was true. Nevertheless, as we have discussed elsewhere, such a situation is often associated with conflict during adolescence.

Failure to Develop a Normal Personality

A normal personality has been defined as one which is *free of symptoms, unhampered by mental conflict, has a satisfactory working capacity, and can love someone other than himself.* This girl deviated markedly from this definition. She had many symptoms. It is true that she displayed little obvious evidence of mental conflict, but she had no working capacity and was unable to love anyone but herself. The mental conflict was latent within this person, and was absorbed, so to speak, by the symptoms. Mental conflict would have been produced if she had been forced to live a normal existence. Never having learned to associate with other people, or to make friends, she would have had great anxiety if forced to take up these activities. Fatigue, one of her chief complaints, was due to the energy which she had to expend to maintain even her poor contact with reality. In the hospital she made friends with a few of the patients and said that she was happier here than she had ever been at any time of her life, and that she had made more friends than ever before. But even these few contacts proved too much for her, so that she remained fatigued most of the time.

Secondary Gain from Neurotic Illness

The patient saw nothing particularly unusual in the way she had lived, and excused her lack of productive activity by the fact that she had not been feeling well. She believed herself to be seriously sick and to have the rare and unusual disease of an adenoma of the pituitary gland. Naturally any such diagnosis was eagerly seized upon by this girl who had been so poorly trained to meet life, and the diagnosis was used as an excuse for her invalidism. This case illustrated especially well the secondary gain of neurotic symptoms. We often see rather active, energetic people who have neurotic symptoms but the symptoms are only a handicap to them, not totally incapacitating. They do not give in completely to their symptoms, they continue to work, and continue to live a fairly normal existence. This girl never had any such ambition and through her symptoms she gained many of the things she was looking for, namely, the interest and attention of her family, especially the solicitude of her mother, the kind and thoughtful attention of nurses and doctors, and in the hospital she gained the opportunity of making some friends for the first time in her life. All these things were important, and in this case had been an obstacle to cure. However, a point which should be stressed is that *this secondary gain is by no means the cause of the illness.* We have heard it said in the past that neurotics have symptoms in order to gain attention and to seek refuge from life's difficulties. This is only part of the story because there must have been certain personality trends which brought on the symptoms in the first place. Then the symptoms, once under way, bring a secondary gain of variable importance to the patient, but this should in no sense be regarded as the cause of the illness itself.

The Nature of the Illness and the Diagnosis

The difficulty in this patient was due to great *anxiety* at the slightest undertaking. Every effort toward work or social intercourse brought a fear of disapproval by some authority, a fear of rejection or a fear to compare herself with others. Her longing to be fed or taken care of was expressing itself through the gastrointestinal tract by means of a disturbance in function, rather than being recognized consciously in her psyche. From the standpoint of *differential diagnosis* what had to be recognized here was the social anxiety and social prejudice, the extreme childlike dependency, the great poverty of ideation and affect about what her place in life should be at the age of twenty-two, and finally the rather unshakable conviction that she was seriously organically ill. All this added together would indicate that this girl was an unusually severe case of *neurasthenia*, or possibly in the hypochondriacal stage of *schizophrenia*. It is true that the clinical picture was not that of a well-developed psychosis. However, it must be remembered that schizophrenia is a disease which develops gradually, and that patients with this disorder who finally reach a psychiatric hospital have usually been seen during the developmental stage by the family physician or have spent some time in general hospital wards. From the standpoint of therapy it was encouraging that while this girl had led such a seclusive, unsocial life up to the time of admission to the hospital, she still had some capacity while in the hospital to make friends and be interested in other people. We hoped that this hospital visit would clarify finally for her and her family the true nature of the symptoms which were disabling her. We tried to make clear to her and her relatives that she was physically well and able to work and live a normal social life. We felt that she must be urged to do this and thus have it proved to her that she was physically able to carry on, and that a more gregarious life was neither immoral nor beneath her dignity.

Notes of Student Clerk. In looking over the notes of the student clerk we observed that he was very much impressed with the idea of endocrine disease and made a great many suggestions for the investigation of the patient from that standpoint but no place in his notes was there any indication that he was concerned about the life situation of the patient! As has been stated elsewhere the organic tradition in medicine is so firmly rooted in many of our medical students that, unless a patient is labeled as suffering from a functional illness, such a diagnosis can be considered only after the exclusion of all organic processes. Meanwhile, the life situation of the patient, which may hold the key to the solution of an obscure illness, is not investigated.

Prognosis

Unlike patients we have seen who have been chronic invalids and led seclusive lives until middle age, we were more hopeful that this young woman could be rescued from invalidism by encouraging her to turn her attention *out* upon life instead of *in* upon her organs.

Follow-up

A year later the patient reported that most of her symptoms had completely disappeared but that on occasions she had slight attacks of dizziness, nausea, and a burning sensation in the epigastrium. After the attack she felt a depressing weariness. However, she reported long periods of well-being between attacks, during which time she was able to work and to attend movies, parties, and dances. She had gained 26 pounds in weight and altogether reported herself and her family as much pleased with her recovery.

SUMMARY

Here was a young woman who, aside from a slight excess of hair on the lip and chin, seemed quite normal on physical examination but who had been incapacitated for more than a year. The chief feature of the illness had been attacks of rapid beating of the heart, sweating and faintness with marked fatigue, and a sensation of heat in the abdomen. The laboratory studies showed nothing remarkable and yet this patient had been considered to have a disturbance of the endocrine system, probably pituitary basophilism, and had been treated with irradiation of the pituitary and injections of glandular extracts on that basis. We must not forget that she was at first considered to have heart disease and some of that thought still lingered with her.

The next case illustrates a problem which was thought to be one of hypothyroidism.

Neurotic Invalidism—Neurasthenia Following Childbirth
Differential Diagnosis from Endocrine Disease—Hypothyroidism

CASE 44

A white woman of forty-two was admitted to the Temple University Hospital in October, 1940. First we present the history and physical findings just as they were described by the intern. Then a few additional comments are made.

History and Symptoms

Chief Complaint. (1) Profound weakness (bedridden one year). (2) Attacks of faintness. (3) Sensation of pressure under lower sternum. (4) Attacks of palpitation and pains in left arm. (5) Soreness of the abdomen. (6) Gaseous eructation and distention. (7) Sensation in left leg of "blood trying to get past clot" following phlebitis one year ago. (8) Inflammation and swelling of left clavicle several months ago. (9) Repeated attacks of phlebitis in legs.

Present Illness. The patient was well until thirteen years ago when she had phlebitis of both legs complicating her first and only pregnancy. She was in bed for six weeks following the birth of the child because of this. Afterwards, although she was out of bed, she "lost her strength" and had never regained it. Two years later she injured her right leg and developed an open lesion which did not heal for fourteen weeks. Then she was fairly well although weak until two years later when the left ankle "broke open" and began to drain. She was in bed for ten weeks before this healed. One year before admission both legs (ankles) broke open (same sites as previously) and drained. About the same time she had a "fungus infection" of the skin of the neck, chest, and back manifested by a rash. With this she was sick one week. She felt that the present marked weakness dated from this affair. Shortly after this (October, 1939) she went to bed in order that her legs might heal and had been in bed ever since (one year). A few days after going to bed she suffered a "complete collapse" which apparently was severe weakness—she was "so weak that she could hardly talk or eat." Since then she had lost about thirty pounds in weight and she reported that she had been unable to sleep.

The attacks of *faintness* mentioned in the chief complaint appeared about two years before admission and had become more severe. Since the spring of 1940 she had several of these attacks in which she thought she lost consciousness for several minutes.

Attacks of pain in the chest had occurred for over a year, originally without radiation to the arm. They were apparently sensations of pressure as if tight bands were around the chest. They were made worse by exertion and sometimes occurred while lying down. Recently there was radiation of pain down the left arm.

There had been soreness of the abdomen and anorexia for four to five weeks although she had had some tenderness when she went to bed one year before. Previously she ate fairly well. Ordinarily she was constipated but for the few days before admission she had diarrhea.

Several months before she had swelling which she said was in the left clavicle region and which she thought was due to the thyroid. It subsided gradually.

In the year before admission here she had been in hospitals five times for study of the general problem without any definite diagnosis or improvement. She said that the basal metabolisms had been subnormal and hence that *she had taken thyroid extract daily for six months.*

Past Medical History. Usual childhood diseases, diphtheria, pertussis in adolescence. Otherwise nothing of significance prior to thirteen years ago.

System Review. Head—Frequent headaches regularly. Eyes—Wears glasses—no other complaints. Nose and Throat—Negative. No sore throats. Mouth—Negative. Upper teeth removed. Cardiorespiratory—No significant cough recently. Did have difficulty breathing, usually precipitated by excitement. Occasionally waked up in sleep by dyspnea. No hemoptysis. Gastrointestinal—Anorexia recently. Recently also had much gas and belching after eating. No vomiting. No melena and no clay-colored stools. General—Always felt cold. Could stand heat more comfortably than other people. The patient's highest weight was 243 pounds in 1932. The weight was 172 when she went to bed one year ago. On admission it was 142.

Physical Examination

A middle-aged white female, not acutely ill, with anxious expression, showed evidence of marked weight loss. Collection of fatty tissues under arms, long pendulous breasts, large apron of abdominal fat and configuration of hips showed that at one time she must have been very obese.

Skin—Warm, moist, not jaundiced.

Eyes—Pupils regular and reacted to light and accommodation. Fields of vision grossly normal.

Head—Negative. Mouth: Oral hygiene, fair. Tongue, moist, moderately coated, no glossitis. Tonsils: Atrophic.

Neck—No masses nor nodes palpable. Thyroid not felt. No pulsation nor tracheal tug.

Chest—Expansion fair and equal.

Lungs—Resonant throughout. Breath sounds normal. No rales.

Heart—Normal in size. No thrill. Sinus rhythm. Sounds of good intensity. No murmurs. B.P. 124/72.

Breasts—Flabby, pendulous; no significant masses.

Abdomen—Large apron of fat, flabby musculature. Generalized tenderness most marked in right upper quadrant. Spleen not felt, liver questionable. Slight tenderness in epigastrium but no mass made out. Ascending and descending colon palpable and tender. Peristalsis hyperactive throughout.

Extremities—Large pigmented scarred area medial surface right ankle (2 × 4 cm.); two smaller similar areas same location left ankle. Reflexes generally brisk. No pathologic reflexes. No edema.

Pelvic and rectal examinations negative.

Comment

The outstanding points in history and physical examination were the marked weakness, obvious weight loss, chest pain, poor tolerance to cold, gaseous eructation, and indigestion. Many of the complaints, especially the chest pain in the left arm, were rather vaguely stated and it was difficult to pin her down to a clear description. She seemed quite proud that she had confounded various hospital staffs and all physicians who had seen her. *"It seemed as if there was a large functional element present, yet there must be organic disease, probably of metabolic nature."* Myxedema seemed quite likely yet did not explain everything.

In going over this history with the patient the most remarkable fact was the *disproportion* between the complaint of such profound weakness that necessitated bed rest for a year and the paucity of physical findings. The only additional points to be noted were first of all, that *sleeplessness* had been quite a problem with her especially during the last year. When questioned about how she had occupied herself while in bed, she said that she was unable to concentrate on reading or the radio, which frequently was disturbing to her, that noises bothered her and that she had been very irritable. About the only occupation had been seeing friends and even this was very fatiguing to her.

Laboratory Studies

Routine laboratory studies did not show any abnormality. The urine and blood count were normal, blood Wassermann was negative, blood chemical figures including blood sugar, blood urea nitrogen, CO_2 combining power and blood cholesterol were all within normal limits and gastrointestinal x-ray studies were normal. Just as the cardiovascular examination was normal physically so did the orthodiagram and electrocardiogram fall within normal limits. Repeated basal metabolism readings varied so widely that the reports were held up for one week while readings were repeated almost daily. They varied from minus 9 to plus 51 and no adequate explanation could be given. Technical error did not seem responsible. The variability will be discussed later but at the time we felt that there was no serious organic disease present and also felt that even if a certain degree of hypothyroidism was present it did not seem sufficient to account for the amount of disability.

LIFE SITUATION

Family History

The patient's father died in 1939 of apoplexy and the mother died of cancer of the uterus, complicated by kidney and heart disease. The mother underwent "change of life" at forty-two and from that time on she did not feel well. Our patient was the fifth of nine children, eight of whom were living. Most of them were working and doing well. However, it was noteworthy that one of the sisters, younger than our patient, was said to have a thyroid condition accompanied by fainting spells.

Our patient said of this sister, "She's got the same thing I have, only she hasn't given up yet." A younger brother had suffered from a pain in the neck for some time. In spite of medical study no cause could be found.

Before continuing let us say a word about large families. Sometimes the desire to have more children ceases, yet there is no knowledge of the use of contraceptives and the parents continue having children with little or no interest in their emotional needs. They may do a fair job at first but by the time four or five children have come along the parents find that their energy has run out and in these cases it is the young siblings who suffer. We noted that our patient was one of the younger children in her large family.

Marriage and Childbirth

Our patient finished one year of high school and then went to work in a clothing factory. She married at twenty-two. Her husband was a machinist. She had one child, who was thirteen years of age at the time of her admission. *Our patient says she was well until this child was born and that she had not been well since.* It would seem that this was not entirely true as she occasionally had fainting spells before the child was born.

We have already emphasized the fact that there are women who are never the same after a child is born. Some women do not wish to fulfill their destiny of being mothers. They hate childbearing and fear motherhood, although these emotions may be unconscious. Consciously they say and believe that they want children. When you come to know these people well you find out what they really think. They feel that the child "feeds off them" and "saps their strength" to such a degree that, as we see in this patient, they are "never the same" afterwards. Another idea that they may harbor is that they are "torn to pieces at childbirth and that they never get put together again." They do not expect to get about in the same way after they have gone through the "terrific ordeal." They feel that a child is a great sacrifice—a great gift which they give to the world. Having given it they feel that they should be entitled to rest for the remainder of their days. These are a few of the ideas buried in the minds of these women who become so ill after childbirth. We cannot be sure which of these ideas existed in our patient. She was unable to say these things to herself or to anyone else at that time. She was not even aware of them.

Loss of Strength. The statement is often made by physicians and nurses to pregnant women—and we see no reason why it shouldn't be made, for it is true to a certain extent—"The child has to feed off you during his life in the uterus." This should have no frightening effect because it is a very normal process and should be so regarded by the mother and by those around her during pregnancy. However, some mothers seem to feel that a child being fed from their blood stream in this manner saps their strength—*takes something away which is never replaced*. This patient told us, "I feel that everything has left me. My strength was sapped by that pregnancy; it took everything out of me." Those expressions mean that from that point onward this woman had too little interest in going on with her job as a mother and a wife.

Loss of Interest. At the end of our conversation with her she was asked if she had lost interest in life because of having been sick for thirteen years. She exclaimed, "Oh, no! I have been no mother at all—indeed, I want to get well and work again." Consciously she had to say that. But in helping this woman get well and getting her to talk about her pregnancy and its effect upon her we observed that unconsciously she had just the opposite ideas. She wanted to rest and be cared for herself like a baby.

Anxiety Symptoms

The patient and her husband moved to Philadelphia and lived here until she was well along in her pregnancy. At that time her husband's family lived in a small town and they wanted her to come there in order that she might have her child with them. She wanted to remain in this city. Her husband and his family finally persuaded her and reluctantly she gave in and left the city she liked so well. The child was born in this small town but the business depression followed and they had been forced to remain there ever since. While the patient was in this city she was interested in going to the movies and various entertainments. These things were her pleasure and her greatest interest in life. When she became pregnant and moved to a little country town all of these pleasures stopped and she had not enjoyed life nearly so much since. The patient said her trouble had come since childbirth but when one examined the rest of her symptoms—the fainting spells, the attacks of weakness, palpitation, fatigue, dyspnea—we have the typical picture of *anxiety attacks*. Every few days she had a feeling of shortness of breath and palpitation which came on suddenly and which was the effect of a quantity of anxiety being set free through the autonomic nervous system. After the birth of her child when it came time for her to get about again she said she felt she "just couldn't . . my strength was all used up."

Fatigue

Her husband had sensed that she felt a lack of the things which formerly interested her and he had taken her to movies and even to night clubs. But regretfully she had to leave. No longer was this sufficiently entertaining to occupy her attention and make her have any feeling of well-being. When questioned about what symptom she would most like to have removed she answered fatigue and indeed that was the most significant and important part of her illness.

Significance of Fatigue. In dealing with fatigue orthodox medicine looks for an organic condition such as tuberculosis or anemia, or other physical disease, yet a great deal of the fatigue commonly found in people comes from the fact that they have too little interest in doing their work or that it is too difficult—there are too many conflicts which induce anxiety. They are working overtime as it were. Through having lived each action over many times in fantasy, they are tired out before they start to do anything. Such was this woman's difficulty and that is what had to be treated in order to rid her of fatigue and of exhaustion spells. This patient had become discouraged after thirteen years of this condition and no doubt the family had become discouraged too. This woman would have profited most by being sent to a sanatorium where she could have had a pleasant routine among strangers, occupational therapy, and psychotherapy. It was difficult to ask this woman to pick herself up from her bed and walk immediately and alone. She would be weak and frightened. A sanatorium where there would be regularity in her sleeping hours and meals and where she would gradually find pleasant work with her hands, such as going to the occupational therapy department to learn some new hobby, would help to keep her from dwelling upon the sensations of her body and be a helpful transition step between a hospital ward and normal activity.

TREATMENT

Then we felt that this woman's thinking would have to be changed so that when she went home she could take charge of her household and live her life in a small town. We began this task by reminding her that studies showed that her body was functioning well and that what she needed was to look to human beings for help rather than to physicians for medicine and to get from people a sense of security through being like them and one of them. If we could help this woman to forget about her physical condition and show her that her body would function and that it was mainly a matter of fear which prevented it she would probably be able to do more and more. She had some very concrete beliefs about certain disease processes. From this standpoint she needed a great deal of education so that she could believe that she was well enough to work. We had to assure her repeatedly that since neither her child nor the phlebitis that followed childbirth harmed her body, there was no physical reason why she could not live an active useful life as well as a happy one. What she had passed through was not enough to bring her to this weakened condition. In emphasizing the emotional side of her illness and asking her to do better in spite of her fears we, of course, brought out her doubts and hostility. But we were patient and insisted that she try each day to function better and thus she would learn that her illness was only part of a faulty reaction to life itself.

Diagnosis of Functional Illness

The first comment that we must make is that even on our first contact with this patient it seemed obvious that her disability was out of proportion to any disease that might have been present. She had been studied on numerous occasions in many hospitals and by many doctors and yet no one had the knowledge to tell her that the illness was of emotional origin or nobody had the courage to do so. Her frequent hospital studies resulted only in the diagnosis of hypothyroidism with the statement that perhaps something else was present in addition but "they weren't able to put their finger on it." We have stated before that doubt arising from this kind of indecision is the factor often responsible for continuing neurotic illness. Her own physician insisted that "there must be some glandular disturbance" that was responsible. We were unable to establish a diagnosis of hypothyroidism or other glandular disorder. Some variability in results is often seen in repeated basal metabolic readings but never, in our experience, to the degree noted in this patient. We can draw no conclusion except to express the necessity for further caution in trying to evaluate the basal metabolism test in psychoneurotic patients.

Exclusion of Organic Disease. Much of the difficulty of making a diagnosis of functional illness comes because of our determination, founded on the organic tradition, to establish such a diagnosis only after the exclusion of physical disease. The result is that we continue to study our patients indefinitely because "something will show up if we are only thorough enough." What we say is contrary to much of orthodox medical teaching, but we think that *one of the great mistakes in medicine is to relegate the diagnosis of a functional disorder to the background, to be considered only after physical diseases have been excluded.* To a certain extent it represents an effort on the part of medicine to say, "It is reprehensible to have an illness of emotional origin and therefore, we can make the diagnosis only if all physical diseases have been excluded." But more especially it represents the fear of missing something organic and thus being held responsible for a serious error in diagnosis. Now we are trying to teach that physical or functional illness must be regarded in the same way—the patient is no more to blame for one than for the other—and the possibility of functional illness of emotional origin must be entertained from the beginning.

Personality Observations. In other words, we must recognize that because functional illness is so common and has such definite earmarks of its own, we must be prepared to entertain the suspicion that it is present from our very first contact with the patient and that just as we immediately try to establish certain indications of a physical disorder so we ought in our very first contact with the patient to observe him from a personality standpoint so that we may establish positive evidence that will aid us in making a psychological diagnosis. If such ideas had been entertained in the present case and had the physicians who attended this patient been as well educated in psychopathology as in tissue pathology, we feel sure that this long invalidism would not have been permitted. Even if the patient had two or three different diagnoses—let us say neurosis, hypothyroidism, and a skin disorder—we must realize that the neurosis was just as capable of being treated and indeed was the first consideration in treatment because it was contributing most to the degree of disability. It was necessary for this patient to realize that the fatigue was her most important symptom and that the cause of the fatigue was emotional conflict. Moreover, the *sleeplessness* of this patient should immediately have aroused the suspicion of neurosis because in the absence of pain or grave organic disease, either general or neurologic (and we distinguish between neurologic and psychologic), sleeplessness is always a neurotic symptom, and we must always inquire about it.

Neurasthenia

A few words regarding the term neurasthenia. This is a greatly misused term in general medicine because it is used as a catch basket into which to throw all functional problems that are not well understood. We will not make great progress in this field of psychosomatic medicine until we are able to make the same precise diagnoses and apply the same terms with precision as we do in regard to disorders of other organs and systems. This was true, for example, in cardiac diagnosis where real progress was not made until we applied a satisfactory nomenclature. It is also true in kidney disease. So often in dealing with patients the doctor will say, "Oh, she is a neurasthenic" and thus indicate the derision or contempt in which he holds such a patient and also the lack of knowledge regarding the meaning of the term. But neurasthenia is really a very definite diagnosis and has a characteristic personality structure and clinical picture. Hence, we should use the term in the limited sense in which it is intended. Therefore, when medical training is as thorough in psychopathology as in tissue pathology, we will be able to make a precise diagnosis of neurasthenia and to know something about the approach so far as psychotherapy is concerned because knowing the personality structure of such a disorder, we will know how to deal with it.

Follow-up

Because this patient lived in a small community a considerable distance from Philadelphia it was not possible for her to return for treatment. We were unable to do more during her short hospital stay than reassure her regarding the absence of organic disease and indicate the general emotional background of the illness.

Yet a year later she reported that she was much improved and was able to do light housework. Her social adjustment was far from satisfactory but at least the complete invalidism had been broken up and she was once more of some use to herself and her family.

ADDISON'S DISEASE AND THE ADRENAL SYNDROME

In 1855 Thomas Addison described the syndrome of adrenal cortex insufficiency. It is characterized by insidious onset, progressive development of fatigue, and asthenia to the point of exhaustion, associated with varying degrees of anorexia, nausea, and vomiting. Sometimes abdominal pain or diarrhea is present.

Pigmentation and arterial hypotension are the physical signs usually exhibited by patients with adrenal cortex insufficiency. The pigmentation is brownish and may be either diffuse or blotchy in distribution. It is most typically observed in the mucous membranes of the buccal cavity. However, there are patients in whom no pigmentation develops. Hypotension is almost invariably present. During crises it falls to strikingly low levels, and the patient presents a picture of dehydration and shock.

"Low Blood Pressure"

Although a definite and serious condition, Addison's disease is relatively rare. However, numerous patients who present fatigue and asthenia as their outstanding complaints are said to suffer from lesser degrees of adrenal insufficiency and are treated with adrenal extracts. Or they are told that they suffer from "low blood pressure and anemia" and efforts are made to raise the blood pressure and correct the anemia usually, nowadays, by means of vitamins and the administration of iron by mouth or injection. Seldom is any effort made to study the life situation of such patients in spite of the fact that anyone familiar with the symptom picture of neurasthenia will be struck by the similarity of the complaints. Neurasthenia likewise is slow and insidious in onset, is marked by fatigue, asthenia and gastrointestinal disturbance, and some degree of hypotension is the rule.

In other words, there are many physicians who when confronted with the much more frequent condition of neurasthenia insist upon thinking in terms of adrenal insufficiency as a cause of this symptom picture. Neurasthenia is due to disturbances in the emotional and ideational life of the patient and the treatment, therefore, must be psychotherapy.

Chronic Fatigue

In an effort to study this common problem, Allan compiled data on 300 consecutive cases from the Lahey Clinic in which weakness, fatigue, or weak spells were the chief complaint. In only one case was vitamin deficiency held responsible for weakness. Anemia was found in only five cases. "Certain conditions, such as vitamin deficiency and glandular disorders, considered widespread causes of weakness by both the laity and the medical profession, were actually found to be rare, and not a single case of weakness due to liver trouble, poor elimination, or low blood pressure was encountered." Thus no evidence was found to support the theory that vitamin deficiency seriously affects the health of a large percentage of the population or that low blood pressure is related to weakness.

The origin of the complaint was found to be physical disorder in only 2 per cent. In the remainder it was the result of a nervous state.

The following case is cited to illustrate the diagnostic problem that we have been discussing. The treatment problems of neurasthenia will be discussed elsewhere.

Neurasthenia with Somatic Disease

CASE 45

A forty-eight-year-old Russian Jewess was admitted to Temple University Hospital in October, 1938, complaining of weakness, burning pain in the epigastrium, loss of appetite, and loss of weight.

History and Symptoms

This woman had been ill for a number of years—it was almost impossible to date the illness exactly but she had been worse for the past two or three years and very sick, according to her statement, since July, 1938. It was very difficult to obtain an accurate history and the emphasis on the complaints varied from time to time. Usually, however, she paid most attention to the gastrointestinal tract. Her mood was one of depression and in addition she appeared anxious and apprehensive.

The past medical history was uneventful. She had never had a serious ailment. She had been married for twenty-six years and had two sons, aged twenty-five and twenty-three. In 1923 an abscess had been opened in the left axilla and the tonsils had been removed some time later. No other operations had been done. Her menses had ceased two years before and other than burning on urination there had been no complaints referred to the genito-urinary tract.

The family history did not seem important from a medical viewpoint.

Physical Examination and Laboratory Studies

Examination showed a slight, undernourished, apprehensive, middle-aged woman with no definite abnormalities in the general physical examination. Gnyecological examination indicated old inflammatory pelvic disease for which the gynecologist recommended radical surgery, that is, hysterectomy.

Routing laboratory studies were within normal limits including normal sedimentation rate. The question arose whether we should carry out the recommendation of the gynecologist for radical surgery.

Because the complaints were so numerous and seemingly not referred to the areas where we found evidence of organic disease we asked for an analysis of the life situation.

LIFE SITUATION

The patient was born in Russia. The paternal grandfather was once a man of means but his property had been confiscated so that the patient had known only poverty since an early age. She started working as a domestic at the age of ten. The father died when the patient was fifteen. The patient came to the United States at the age of eighteen, began to work in a factory and attempted to go to night school for a time but could not continue. She found the work a drudgery and married without romance to get away from the factory. The marriage was entirely one of expediency. According to her description her husband had always been an anxious and worrisome man. When she went to live with his parents they emphasized that "life is a struggle" and she was told always "that she must not look up—she must always look down and must struggle."

She had two sons, one of whom entered the army three years before and the second left also to enter the army six months before, and it was significant that there had been an exacerbation of all of her symptoms coinciding with these two episodes. Moreover, she told us that her illness really dated back to her first childbirth. She admitted that marriage was an attempt to escape from the drudgery of factory work but it developed that this was no solution, for marriage had also become a drudgery and a duty for her. Her husband, who was first on salary, managed later to obtain his own shop but had never been able to succeed.

During her illness the patient consulted many physicians and was told that she had low blood pressure, that she was anemic, run down and nervous, and told to "fight her 'nervousness,'" but she did not understand what it was that she had to fight. She had received all kinds of medication including injections of glandular substance.

From this information it was evident that although the patient had a physical disease this did not account for her symptoms which appeared to be chiefly neurasthenic in origin.

Neurasthenia

In neurasthenia there are three outstanding symptoms: *first*, fatigue or weakness; *second*, poorly defined gastrointestinal symptoms; *third*, irritability and depression of spirits. The neurasthenic syndrome, however, is rarely limited to these three symptoms. There is expansion in the number of complaints and involvement of almost all parts of the body. Sufferers from neurasthenia are usually chronically depressed, anxious people who have few life interests. They want success and contentment but have little available energy to achieve success or little ability to enjoy life because of the amount of anxiety and guilt which they constantly carry with them. These people have passed through a difficult childhood with little love or interest from their parents. There has been failure of proper psychosexual development. They remain "fixated," as we say, to early stages of psychological development and tend to emphasize the sensations and attitudes associated with the function of the gastrointestinal tract in childhood. They are sensitive and feel themselves unloved and thwarted. Their psychosexual development has usually become retarded so that they never reach a stage where they may have acute conflict over genital sexual expression, as we see in hysteria.

Hostility. With such a life history these patients naturally have a great deal of repressed hostility which is a very important part of the psychological structure. All of the hostility is not repressed; some of it emerges as the symptom of irritability. Much of that which is repressed is responsible for both the depression of spirits and somatic symptom formation. The patient feels that it is understandable that he is irritable because he does not feel well, and it is one of the tasks of therapy to get him to see that something more nearly the reverse is true, *i. e.*, that he does not feel well because he is so full of hostility and anxiety.

Anxiety. Our patient had always been worried about financial matters, and even though at times there apparently had been real cause for anxiety it is important to note that when conditions were good the amount of anxiety and worry was unchanged. As the patient put it, "When we had no money I was, of course, worried, but when we had money I seemed just as worried about when it might give out. I have always worried that something might happen." One of her most outstanding fears had been that she and her husband would starve to death. Actually the husband was making a living, their home was in a good neighborhood where they were respected by their friends and neighbors, and both her sons were gainfully employed, yet she continued to be apprehensive that some tragedy was impending.

TREATMENT

The first question in the management of this case concerned what treatment was to be given to the pelvic disorder. After an explanation of the serious degree of emotional disturbance in this patient one would have to consider very seriously the necessity for the operation suggested. If bad results were sure to follow without operation then, of course, it would have to be done, but neither the patient, the gynecologist nor ourselves should be led to believe that this would favorably affect the illness as a whole. In such a case as this the most conservative surgical treatment is usually the best. Operations only tend to fix the patient's invalidism because in the first place treatment of a limited area produces little improvement in a patient who feels so uncomfortable all over. In the second place they are disappointed that anything so important as an operation has failed to bring the desired relief, and lastly, operative measures tend to focus the patient's attention upon the organic rather than the psychological side of the illness. We felt that the important therapy here was to treat this individual as an unhappy personality, to consider the family and social problems, and to try to bring something of happiness and reassurance into her life. Some discussion should be had with the other members of the family as to the cause and meaning of neurotic illness, and their help should be enlisted.

Emphasizing Security

Cases have been cited of patients who were very complacent and satisfied with invalidism and we stressed the need of putting some pressure upon such patients and upon the family to increase activity and in this way bring out anxiety which could then be dealt with. In this woman it seemed important to do just the opposite, for a time at least. It seemed better here to lessen the idea of "struggle" in her mind and emphasize the available security. This did not mean that we should overindulge her for a long period without explaining why these efforts were made. This woman had actually struggled and we should try to teach her and those around her that she deserved some appreciation and some reward for her struggle. We had to help her to see that life from day to day was not so dangerous and burdensome, and educate her to get more enjoyment out of life in the neighborhood where she lived. All this could not be done in a few days or a week, but had to be done through continued contact with the patient and the family.

Precision in Diagnosis

A whining woman like this one would promptly be dubbed neurasthenic even on a cursory examination because neurasthenia is a term carelessly used to cover all neurotic problems. If we are to make headway with such illnesses we must be more precise in our diagnosis because the psychological structure differs and hence diagnosis and treatment and prognosis differ. The situation is much the same as it was in regard to heart disease a quarter of a century ago when everything was likely to be called myocarditis. Now we have a much more scientific approach to heart disease and hence a more satisfactory treatment and better understanding of prognosis. We must pass through the same stages in regard to psychological ailments, realizing that psychopathology is just as necessary for their scientific understanding as histopathology is for an understanding of physical disease.

Chapter XVI

ENDOCRINE SYSTEM AND METABOLISM (*Concluded*)

ANOREXIA NERVOSA

One of the clinical syndromes perhaps most responsible for bringing the medical profession to believe that there may be a psychological background for certain physical diseases has been the condition called anorexia nervosa. Within the last few years a number of excellent papers in which the psychological background is emphasized have appeared on this subject. Prior to this time the diagnosis of *Simmonds' disease* was almost invariably made whenever the syndrome of anorexia, emaciation, and amenorrhea was encountered.

In 1874, Sir William Gull observed a disorder of young persons characterized by the following symptoms: emaciation, scaphoid abdomen, amenorrhea, and the appearance of age. He noted the slow pulse and subnormal temperature, the equivalent of the depressed basal metabolism so frequently mentioned in case reports labeled Simmonds' disease. He made shrewd observations as to the psychic behavior of his patients. In particular, he noted their sense of well-being and their excessive activity in spite of extreme emaciation. He pointed out that this degree of activity would be impossible if the inanition were due to constitutional disease. After discussing hysteria, he chose the term anorexia nervosa as a name for the disease. He pointed out that all of the symptoms could be explained on the basis of the undernutrition which, in turn, was due to a "morbid mental state." This was a time when the function of the pituitary gland was unknown. It is remarkable that in spite of this clear description so much confusion still exists in regard to this disorder.

Simmonds' Disease

At about this period of medical history many morbid states, which had been considered to be of psychological origin, came under the influence of the new cellular pathology with its structural orientation and from then on were considered of physical origin. Moreover, the recent interest and activity in the field of endocrinology has been a further reason for including this syndrome among the endocrine disorders. Simmonds in 1914 described the destruction of the anterior lobe of the pituitary gland which he observed at autopsy in certain cases of cachexia and reconstructed from the history the clinical picture of the disease that now bears his name. The syndrome is a chronic, progressive disorder characterized by loss of weight, asthenia, atrophy of the genital organs with decreased sexual function (in women, amenorrhea—in men, impotence), loss of the axillary and pubic hairs, changes in the skin, and decreased basal metabolic rate. Hypotonia, hypothermia, bradycardia, hypoglycemia, gastrointestinal disorders, anemia, and achlorhydria may also appear. Cachexia is a late phase of the disease. The pathologic changes besides those already mentioned are atrophy of the pituitary, skin, sexual glands, thyroid, parathyroids, and adrenals. In advanced cases the internal organs are atrophied.

Differential Features

While the clinical picture of anorexia nervosa may reproduce all the symptoms of true Simmonds' disease the changes usually are not nearly so marked as in the true pituitary cachexia and autopsy observations prove that the pituitary is structurally intact. Recently McCullough and Tuffer demonstrated an increased gonadotropic hormone excretion in some cases of anorexia nervosa, a finding inconsistent with severe pituitary failure.

Functional Pituitary Depression

From a psychological standpoint it has been said that "just as these patients are physically starved so are they emotionally starved." We would put that the other way around, because we must be very careful in the consideration of psychosomatic disorders not to put the cart before the horse. In other words, this condition differs from true pituitary disease because it is the psychological conflict which brings about the loss of appetite and undernutrition and, very likely, this in turn affects the pituitary function which is closely tied up with the cessation of menstruation and lowered basal metabolism. It seems that this is a true interference with the function of the anterior pituitary but the latter occurs as a result and not as a cause of the disorder. One piece of evidence to suggest that this is a functional depression is that, when the patients improve as a result of psychological management, their menses begin again and even pregnancies occur.

Psychic Traits

In all cases of this condition studied psychologically there have been serious neurotic traits and sometimes even psychotic manifestations. Most patients showed a noteworthy reticence in discussing themselves and particularly in discussing sexual topics. Masturbation was minimal or absent. In other words, there was a strong repudiation of sexuality and if sexual relations occurred they often had a marked traumatic effect upon the psyche. In fact, starvation, emaciation, and the resulting unattractive appearance in many instances made an excellent defense against establishing healthy social contacts with the opposite sex. Sometimes this state of undernutrition led to the breaking of a marriage engagement. Eating sometimes symbolized impregnation to these people and obesity represented pregnancy. Some of the other personality characteristics encountered were perfectionism, overconscientiousness, neatness, seclusiveness, shyness, and dependence upon others. Such patients had difficulty in making friends and of necessity had a poor relation to parents. In many cases the parent had shown preoccupation with gastrointestinal functions and the patient as a child had been a "feeding problem."

A detailed study by Waller, Kaufman, and Deutsch showed the symbolism of "eating as impregnation" in two patients whose personality structure was of the compulsive type. The whole syndrome represented an elaboration and acting out in the somatic sphere of a specific type of pregnancy fantasy. Secondary gain allowed the patients to obtain affection, to be the center of the family, to work out hostilities, and to provoke the environment to certain acts of punishment which would alleviate guilt.

Lorand likewise found that there was great immaturity in the personality development, which interfered with normal psychosexual development. In his patient, refusal of food also arose from fantasies of oral impregnation.

Clinical Findings

The clinical findings in addition to emaciation may be dry scaly skin, cold extremities, low temperature, slow pulse, and amenorrhea. In some cases amenorrhea may precede the loss in weight, but return of menstrual flow usually follows improvement in nutrition without hormonal therapy. In fact, treatment with anterior pituitary lobe growth hormone or estrogenic hormone has not seemed to bring any permanent benefit to the cases of anorexia nervosa. Basal metabolism is usually low but this is due to inanition rather than to thyroid deficiency and attempted replacement therapy may be injurious instead of helpful. Insulin treatment may or may not add some weight but even if it does, such weight gain usually is only temporary and the persistence of the psychological conflict causes the added pounds to melt away again.

Principles of Treatment

Treatment, then, consists in making the patient aware of the nature of the mental conflicts underlying the condition, and at the same time trying to reeducate the patient to express himself in a more adult fashion than *by the rejection of food.*

While the fully-developed syndrome of anorexia nervosa is a rare disorder, lesser degrees of poor appetite and inanition based upon the same psychological principles are exceedingly common. As we have pointed out before, the taking of food is the chief activity during the first year of life and continues for some time to be connected in an important way with the child's entire relation to life. If he is restless or tense he is fed and comforted by the mother. A mother who cannot understand the child's need for physical and emotional closeness to her may offer only food to the child. Parents often reward a child with something good to eat when some other reward would be more desirable psychologically. Thus it is that our relation to life starts through the feeding mechanism and may be continued almost exclusively through this channel. Appetite for food therefore becomes a substitute for and symbolic of an appetite for life activities. In all cases of anorexia nervosa we find the relation to life, usually expressed by enthusiasm for work, hobbies, and friends, to be as inadequate as the appetite for food. Thus we see that anorexia nervosa is a complex psychosomatic illness involving the whole personality, and that the treatment can never be limited to the administration of tonics or endocrine products.

The following case illustrates many of the points that have been mentioned. (See also Case 33 p. 428.)

Anorexia Nervosa

CASE 46

A white girl, aged nineteen, was admitted to the hospital in October, 1938.

History and Symptoms

The patient complained of loss of appetite and loss of weight, cessation of menstruation, and increasing irritability.

Present Illness

The patient first consulted a physician in the fall of 1936 because of a slight eruption on the face which was diagnosed as acne. She was advised to cut down on sugars and starches, which she did, and she blamed loss of weight upon this fact. The loss of weight began about November, 1937, at which time she weighed 105 pounds. Her menstrual periods ceased in March, 1938, and for this she received "gland injections" from her attending physician. For a few months before admission she noted an increasing irritability and this she attributed to the fact that the family tried "to force her to eat." Her weight was finally reduced to about 74 pounds and due to the persuasion of her family and her physician she entered the hospital for study. It was not because she felt bad. As she stated, she was just as active as the rest of the girls in her group and would not have sought hospital care if her family had not insisted upon it.

Past History

The systemic review did not reveal any additional information of importance and the past history was not significant except for an illness which was diagnosed as rheumatism shortly after she started school. Her mother stated that this was not rheumatic fever and that she was told that there was no evidence of heart involvement. She was a thin but healthy child.

The patient was the third in a family of four children. The mother and father were well and the other children were well and none had ever suffered from any serious physical disease.

She graduated from high school and had been employed as a secretary from January, 1938, until August when she lost her position, but not because of illness.

Physical Examination and Laboratory Studies

Physical examination showed a small, thin girl who appeared alert and intelligent and seemed entirely comfortable and at ease in the ward. She had a few marks on her face of the previous acne eruption but they were entirely healed and not very noticeable. The body and limbs were very thin although the breasts were pretty well preserved. There was considerable hairy development on the arms and legs. The heart and lungs seemed entirely normal; the abdomen was scaphoid but otherwise there were no special findings. The temperature on admission was 97.5°F. the pulse 52 and regular, the respirations 14 and the blood pressure 94/56.

Routine laboratory studies—urine, blood count and serological tests— were all normal. Because the general physical examination and ordinary laboratory studies were normal we turned to the life situation of the patient before considering the question of differential diagnosis.

LIFE SITUATION

Family History

The father of this patient was the owner of a store. He was described as a friendly person who had always been on good terms with the patient. The mother was also said to be a friendly person, interested in her children. The patient was the third in a family of four, the oldest a married sister who had no children. The brother, twenty years old, a college student, had been close to the patient and they discussed some of their life problems together. If we had accepted a superficial description of her she would have seemed to be what is called an extroverted person. She danced a great deal, went to movies and the theater, had many friends, and was socially popular. It is to be remembered, however, that there are no true extroverts or true introverts. Some apparently extroverted people are very sensitive, and due to this sensitivity avoid many things which go to make up a well-rounded personality.

Adolescence

It would appear that some external change in personality took place in this girl about the time of puberty. Previously affectionate, she became, as she termed it, "selfish and a snob." She became very interested in her appearance and in her clothes. She had a great desire to be liked and to associate with people whose appearance was very neat and striking in some way. She said, "I cannot endure people who are sloppy."

Attitude Toward Marriage

She had never been able to tolerate any love-making of any kind. She was aware that many of her friends of both sexes indulged but she could not endure coming in too close contact with anyone. Not only was she unable to endure the idea of body intimacy but the idea of marrying and becoming a mother was unattractive to her. She felt that pregnancy and the nursing experience would spoil her appearance and be both painful and "messy." She thought that having children would spoil her figure, which in itself was a remarkable statement for one who presented the appearance of a scare-crow! When she pictured marriage at all it was only the social side—entertaining, travel, and luxuries— which a man of means could provide. If she had children she would want to adopt them, obviously to avoid the responsibility, and what to her would be the unpleasant duty, of nursing and toilet training. She had no desire to prepare meals or take care of a house. She said, "I might if I loved someone." But she had never permitted herself to love anyone but herself. On two occasions she had felt emotionally and somewhat physically drawn to young men. This feeling seemed to disturb her, however, and she found a reason to break off these friendships. It was as if she sensed that to foster such a feeling would bring a sense of responsibility toward someone and hence change her position to that of being self-sacrificing and perhaps maternal instead of being able to enjoy the position of being the loved one herself.

Summary of Findings

So here was a girl who was unable to give much to life but only wanted to receive. She realized that she was selfish and possibly had some desire to change, but so far she had found it difficult to do. At the age of nineteen she should have been able to take some responsibility in relation to other people. She had not been emotionally educated to do so; instead she had been allowed to overemphasize appearance until this was her only source of satisfaction. And now she was becoming too thin, even in this age of slimness, to gain satisfaction.

It usually is true that people who have too much interest in themselves and too little for other people only end up by cheating themselves. Such was the case here. This girl's loss of weight, which was rightly regarded by her relatives as serious, was only an incident in the life of a person poorly adjusted to reality. She not only had starved herself physically but she first had starved herself emotionally. She had recently occasionally found herself crying without reason. This symptom plus irritability must be regarded as indications that this girl was unhappy and that her way of gaining satisfaction through overattention to appearances was failing her. She sensed that something was lacking and that something was the satisfaction which comes from being able to have a warmer interest in others and to be able to express this interest.

Differential Diagnosis

There was really only one clinical condition with which this illness could be confused. Was this a primary endocrine problem such as pituitary cachexia or was it anorexia nervosa?

Further studies showed that the basal metabolism was reduced just as the temperature, pulse, and respirations were, but there were none of the profound changes that are associated with true Simmonds' disease. The latter is a disease which occurs usually in the child-bearing age after some destruction of the pituitary body has occurred. As a result there are profound changes leading to wasting which involves the breasts as well as the genitalia, loss of axillary and pubic hair and the process eventuates in coma and death. The clinical picture presented by this patient was like a mild form of this disease. All of the changes were present but they were not nearly so marked as in the true pituitary cachexia. Thus from a physical viewpoint the evidence was against Simmonds' disease and from a psychological viewpoint we were impressed with the fact "that just as this girl was physically starved so was she emotionally starved." In other words, this differed from true pituitary disease because it was the psychological conflict which brought about the loss of appetite and this resulted in the undernutrition. This in turn affected the pituitary function which was closely tied up with the cessation of menstruation and the lowered basal metabolism. It seems likely that this is a true interference with the function of the anterior pituitary but occurs as a result and is not the cause of this disorder. The best evidence for this that we have is that as these patients improve as a result of psychological management their menses begin again.

Therefore we had *negative* evidence from a physical standpoint and *positive* evidence from a psychological standpoint to say that we were dealing with anorexia nervosa.

These are difficult problems and often the psychological background is anything but obvious. It is certainly not the kind of situation which will yield information to the inquiry, "Are you worried about anything?" Unfortunately we cannot tell a neurotic by looking at him and it is only by calmly sitting down and permitting the patient to talk about himself as a human being rather than as a physical mechanism that we will come to understand his other "troubles" and when we do we will then come to a closer understanding of the reason for which he consulted the physician.

The Marriage Problem

This girl had difficulty in regard to marriage. Her attitude was not quite what we would expect in a girl of her age. *So often physicians recommend marriage and child-bearing as a short cut toward the solution of emotional problems.* Unfortunately people who are so immature as to find marriage an emotional hurdle which they cannot negotiate are the very kind of people who find difficulty in meeting the responsibilities of marriage. And then marriage serves not as a cure for but as a cause of the onset of many of their nervous symptoms. So that if such persons have not been brought up properly prepared for marriage it is much better for them to have a psychological preparation rather than to be forced or to force themselves into a marriage situation which may prove to be the cause rather than the cure for an illness. The same may be said for child-bearing. To the person who is emotionally immature having a child may increase rather than alleviate troubles. It is true that such persons are often very much better during the period of pregnancy (although this is by no means the rule) but it is after the child is born that trouble starts. Anxious mothers often make anxious children and thus we have an endless repetition of the neurotic problem.

In the question of *treatment* we must emphasize that simply adding a few pounds to this patient by means of forced feeding with perhaps the use of insulin would really be only a temporary measure because as soon as she went home and met another emotional situation difficult to handle she would once more reject food just as she tried to reject life, and the added pounds would melt away. In other words, the only intelligent approach to this problem was to make an effort to reeducate this young woman in a new approach to life.

Prognosis

It appeared that this patient was fortunate in at least one respect. She was only nineteen, her illness had not lasted very long, and a correct diagnosis had been made and treatment started in the proper direction. Unlike patients who have reached mature years, who in other words have already lived their lives and for whom little can be done, and unlike patients who are so fixated in their invalidism that probably nothing can shake them loose from it, this patient was considered much more amenable to treatment because she was young and her psychological structure could perhaps be modified. In other words, it is much like the problem of tuberculosis. When the patients are far advanced in that disease there is little that we can do to restore them to normal but when they come in because they have had a dramatic episode (*e. g.*, pulmonary hemorrhage) as the very first manifestation of the disease and we find on physical examination that there is only a small lesion in the lung, we are very hopeful that a cure can be brought about. This patient from a psychological standpoint seemed to be in the latter position.

TREATMENT

Treatment, therefore, consisted of attention to the personality. We tried to show her that no one can be complete in herself, that her interest in being admired was too great and would bring her increasing disappointment as she grew older. We tried to help her to be more tolerant toward people generally, and to see that virtues may exist in people who did not put so much emphasis on neatness as she did. Her marked antipathy to lack of neatness had come from an overscrupulous regimen during the period of *toilet training* as discussed in the chapter on psychopathology. Her training had been accomplished by the inculcation of an excessive disdain for anything which was not neat and clean. When such an attitude is taken in order to help accomplish toilet training and neatness the emotions spread away from excretions to include other things such as food, dress, environment, and even thinking itself.

On first entering the hospital the patient was unable to eat food from the regular house trays. When she was later put on a special diet, and extra care was given to the neatness of her trays in the diet kitchen, she was able to eat more. The food was the same but because it was more neatly served she found it more attractive and acceptable.

Discussion of a Plan for Living

In treatment sessions with this patient a discussion of a woman's appearance during pregnancy, her feelings over nursing, and the responsibility of toilet training were discussed with her. We tried to enable her to see that while these things had their unpleasant side they bring compensations which should far outweigh feelings of antipathy. We tried to show her that if she continued to avoid these necessary contacts with everyday life she would be missing emotional experiences that make life of value to most people. If it should actually turn out that this girl would want to renounce marriage completely, with its necessary intimate contacts with a man, then more emphasis would have to be put on some other kind of life work. She had vaguely thought of taking a course in accounting but as yet nothing had been done about it. She was drifting and hoped that some solution to her emotional needs would come without any definite plan. But we tried to show her that a girl must plan her life along one of the acceptable channels which will bring satisfaction. We tried to make her see the necessity of choosing either marriage or office work and of making a more definite preparation for one or the other. In some families an emotional preparation for family life takes place imperceptibly but thoroughly from childhood onward. In other families this is not the case and special attention has to be given to it later.

Tasting Life and Tasting Food

We thought that as this patient learned to get into closer contact with people instead of remaining aloof and waiting to be admired she would lose her irritability and depression, and her desire to starve herself. An ability to taste life would probably mean that she could begin to taste food and her zest for life and zest for food would increase together. Superficially, anorexia had meant a wish to avoid any imperfections in appearance. It had meant avoiding food which did not seem entirely neat and clean, and it had meant avoiding responsibility. Finally it had meant something still deeper from the psychological standpoint and that was the rejection of people as well as food. To be in love or to like someone means a taking in of that person into one's thought and feeling. This is regarded unconsciously as a process which takes place by way of the gastrointestinal tract. The expression "my thoughts are full of you" means that the individual making this remark has taken something of the loved person inside himself. This girl had scrupulously avoided falling in love or emotionally taking anyone inside of herself. This attitude and her rejection of food definitely had something in common. To correct the rejection of food one must correct the attitude of rejecting love and its responsibilities. In other words, she must not be overscrupulous in regard to neatness and orderliness and even cleanliness, because to put it frankly there is a certain amount of dirt in the world that we have to learn to accept. Modern pediatricians are not afraid to allow children to come in contact with a little honest dirt and adults too must learn to accept reality. In other words, this immature young woman had to be helped to grow up emotionally. She had to be taught to behave different-ly toward people and although this might stir up a little anxiety the phy·

sician must then occupy a position of confidence and authority so that he can allay this anxiety and thus permit a little more emotional growth.

Follow-up

Treatment sessions were broken off after several visits to the psychiatrist but she continued under the care of her family physician who had a good understanding of the psychological background of the illness. No improvement was noted for many months but finally, for reasons that were not very apparent, she began to eat and gain weight, improved in her social relationships, got herself a job and at the end of a year was working steadily and again "tasting of life just as she was tasting of food."

DIABETES MELLITUS

Primitive man had to have a mechanism of homeostasis (Cannon) which would enable his endocrine-sympathetic nervous system quickly to prepare his body for fight or flight when his physical safety was threatened. In civilized man the same mechanism exists and apparently is called into action when man faces threats not necessarily to his physical self but to his security and prestige. One of the central factors of this homeostasis is a mobilization of the sugar in the blood leading to a hyperglycemia. It is strange that this mechanism has not been alluded to more frequently as a possible background for diabetes mellitus. It is true that emotional glycosuria and hyperglycemia, due to conscious fears or threats, are recognized but it would also seem that fears and threats of which the patient is not wholly aware could, by the very nature of their unconscious energy, act as a chronic stimulus to the insulin-producing mechanism and hence might have something to do with the development of true diabetes.

Flanders Dunbar, in her book on "Emotions and Bodily Changes," summarized the studies of emotional glycosuria and hyperglycemia. She referred to the classical experiments of Cannon which demonstrated that cats, if excited or enraged, developed glycosuria. Sugar was found in the urine of football players after an exciting game and in students after a hard examination, and hyperglycemia occurred in aviators and in soldiers exposed to danger. The anxiety in some patients before operation has induced hyperglycemia. Suggestion under hypnosis has altered the blood sugar level.

Although recent evidence (Mirsky) throws doubt on hyperglycemia as the responsible factor for the glycosuria which occurs with emotional stress and suggests that it must be attributed to a decrease in absorption of glucose from the kidney tubules, the clinical fact that emotional stress can produce a rapid rise in blood sugar concentration in diabetics, thus causing an exacerbation of the disorder, is generally recognized

History

Haagensen and Lloyd tell us that the beginning of our modern under standing of diabetes dates back to the opening year of the American Revolution, when Matthew Dobson, physician to the Liverpool Infirmary, discovered that the urine, which is passed in too great an abundance in this disease, contains sugar. This discovery led the way to attempts to control the disease by limiting the amount of sugar in the diet, a method which was not very successful. And so the matter stood for another hundred years, until in 1889 the experimental attack on diabetes was begun by a Russian physician, Oskar Minkowski, then a young assistant to Professor Naunyn at the University of Strasbourg. Minkowski removed the entire pancreas in a dog and discovered that severe diabetes at once developed which persisted until the animal succumbed a few weeks later; he also found the sugar content of the blood elevated. The next step was made in 1900 by Eugene L. Opie, at that time a young instructor in pathology at Johns Hopkins. Studying the microscopic sections of the pancreas of a little girl who had died of diabetes, Opie saw that the islands of Langerhans were so degenerated that they could not be identified. His observation led the English physiologist Sir Edward Schafer in 1916 to postulate the theory that these special pancreatic cells produced some form of internal secretion which controlled the metabolism of sugar. Shortly afterwards came the epochal observations of Banting culminating in the discovery of insulin.

We believe that psychological medicine also has important contributions to make to the subject of diabetes but, aside from some excellent studies to which we shall refer, no concerted efforts have as yet been made to study the emotional component of this disease.

Emotional Factors

There are very few references to emotional factors in the disease from the field of internal medicine but several have appeared in the last few years from the field of psychological medicine. Of these, Daniels contributed a most authoritative and comprehensive review. The following material is taken from his study.

In going over the literature on diabetes Daniels was impressed by the fact that from January, 1934, through March, 1939, of 3333 articles on diabetes listed in the Quarterly Cumulative Index Medicus, there were only twenty-three with titles which called attention to emotional factors in diabetes; and on going over the rest of the literature, little or no reference to psychic factors was found. Even the subject of fluctuation in the disease due to emotional factors—of which almost every physician is aware—was neglected in the medical literature.

Daniels felt that the chief case against the importance of emotional factors in diabetes as reflected in the literature could be enumerated under the following heads: (1) recent studies showing heredity to be the determining factor; (2) the experience of World War I, in which the evidence seemed to indicate that military life did not predispose to the development of diabetes; (3) the impression that nervous strain or shock does not lead to more diabetes or to any appreciable increase in hyperglycemia or glycosuria in those already having diabetes; (4) confusion between organic neurological changes and emotional tension which uses the autonomic system for discharge.

Experimental Studies

In his summary Daniels stated that he gave a considerable amount of space to the experimental field because at the time it appeared to hold out the best prospect of ultimately furnishing the key to the psychosomatic problem presented. Impetus was furnished to all branches of research in metabolism by the discovery of Houssay and Biasotti in 1930 that diabetes of depancreatized animals could be attenuated and their lives prolonged by extirpation of the anterior pituitary gland.

Houssay's work and its consequences have revolutionized theories of the mechanism of diabetes and have led to the relinquishment of the simpler insulinogenic concept. This has broadened the base for the understanding of the influence of emotional factors.

Numerous extracts of the anterior pituitary affecting metabolism have been described. One of the most important extracts is made from crude gland which has a diabetogenic effect on the normal animal. Young, by a series of brilliant experiments, has shown that repeated injections of such extracts result in a permanent diabetic condition after treatment is discontinued.

Many modifications of the original Houssay experiment have been tried to test the diabetogenic influence of other participants. Long believes that the adrenal cortex is essential. A modification of the diabetic condition similar to that produced by Houssay and Biasotti has been obtained by bilateral injury to the hypothalamus. Other evidence of implication of the hypothalamus in disturbed sugar metabolism, its importance as a center for the involuntary nervous system, and its participation in automatic emotional discharge make it a focal point in attempts to understand degrees of emotional participation in diabetes.

Personality Studies

Studies of the hereditary factor in diabetes show quite conclusively the importance of a diabetic anlage and there is some evidence that this may be passed on as a recessive Mendelian trait. In evaluating the emotional factor in the etiology of the disease the constitutional predisposition should be taken into account. It seems unwarranted, however, to dismiss the importance of the psychic factor either on account of hereditary predisposition or on the evidence of the first World War that "shell-shock" is not an important etiological factor because recent psychiatric contributions to the subject, though scattered, show an awakened interest with a new approach afforded by psychoanalytic insight. Emphasis is away from settling the whole question of psychogenesis in diabetes on the frequency of traumatic diabetes but is laid rather on the presence of anxiety, concealed or overt, which is unable to discharge through the conscious voluntary system and is forced through regressive changes to discharge at more primitive autonomic levels. It is well established that emotional changes can affect the blood sugar level. Up to the present time it has not been definitely proved whether or not it is possible to precipitate diabetes by such influences. Cases in which emotional disturbances seemed of importance in the causation of diabetes were cited by Daniels, including the first report of a case of diabetes to be psychoanalytically investigated.

The importance of attention to personality factors in the uncooperative case, as well as in those cases which react to emotional conflict with increased sugar, was stressed.

From the Psychiatric Field. That neurotic manifestations occur frequently in association with diabetes, is becoming increasingly clear as cases are studied systematically by observers trained in psychiatric methods. W. C. Menninger in two articles reviewed previous literature, reported on thirty cases of mental disorder associated with diabetes, and analyzed this material along with that of ninety-three cases of uncomplicated diabetes and 400 uncomplicated cases of mental disorder. Daniels, and Dunbar and associates, reported studies on successive diabetic admissions to a large general hospital which allowed them to contact cases that ordinarily would not be seen by the psychiatrist. Dunbar contrasted the diabetics studied with a parallel series of fracture and cardiovascular patients.

Menninger called attention to the present viewpoint of psychiatry that some of the most severe emotional conflicts are entirely unconscious to the patient, but with the exception of three authors there was no recognition of unconscious emotional conflicts. He listed nine of a series of thirty cases studied by him as psychoneurotic. Five of his cases seemed to be the result of a psychological disturbance, appearing either with a mental disorder or during its course. These cases conformed to the following arbitrary requirements of such relationship: (1) Obvious psychopathology was evident prior to the development of the diabetic state.

(2) The mental picture was quite different from the toxic state occasionally seen in either hyperglycemia or hypoglycemia. (3) The course of improvement of the mental picture was paralleled by the glycemic and glycosuric levels, with fluctuations in these as emotional upsets occurred in the psychic life. (4) The metabolic disorder was indicated by a persistent glycosuria (without dietary control or insulin), retarded glucose utilization curves of the blood sugar, and a response to dietary, and in some cases, insulin therapy. (5) With mental recovery, the diabetic condition cleared, requiring neither insulin nor dietary treatment. Menninger considered this the only such group described in the literature and gave abstracts of the cases in both of his articles. He stated that none of the cases lent themselves to psychoanalytic investigation so that the unconscious forces could not be determined. Actual psychotherapy was mentioned in only one case.

One of the questions which repeatedly occurs is whether or not there is any characteristic mental picture in diabetes. This has various aspects. The first is the question of toxic psychoses attributable to diabetes. Menninger reviewed the literature and came to the conclusion that "such a group of toxic cases represents a small percentage of the number of cases in which diabetes and mental disease are associated." He cited three such cases in his own series.

Depression is among the most frequent of the mental symptoms described, according to Menninger's summary of the literature. Daniels found depression to be an important complication in ten cases of the twenty-three diabetic admissions studied, either from the history or while under observation. In five cases the depression was reactive to the loss of a love object prior to the onset of diabetes. When possible it is useful, in the case of depression, to make the distinction between a depression of a primary nature which might or might not be related to the diabetes, and a depression secondary to the diabetes. The knowledge by the individual that he is suffering from an incurable disease which, on account of the care necessary in treatment, sets him apart from the rest of his fellows, in many cases explains the reaction. Much of the hypochondriacal self-observation which often accompanies such depressions can be explained in the same way. Because it is so natural, however, to conclude that such a patient is upset over his condition, it is possible to miss more fundamental neurotic reactions which may play a primary role. Cases of manic-depressive psychosis, appearing coincidentally or alternating with the diabetic picture, have been described.

Anxiety. Daniels stressed the factor of anxiety in his cases and thought the anxiety may have expressed itself through disturbed metabolism. He felt that since diabetics frequently have severe neurosis an opportunity is afforded to study the interaction of the two conditions.

The fact that the diabetes might not be cured along with the neurotic symptoms does not prove that the neurosis may not have set the diabetes in action. We know too little about the problem of reversibility in organic disease and the point at which this is no longer possible because of structural changes. Daniels analyzed a case of diabetes and anxiety neurosis. Although the diabetes was not cured some interesting observations were made concerning the resemblance of the anxiety attacks and hyperinsulinism and the relation of hyperglycemia and glycosuria to emotional conflict.

Fatigue and Deprivation. Menninger found psychic trauma important in the precipitation of two of his ninety-three cases of uncomplicated diabetes. Dunbar found that such emotional traumata preceding diabetes occurred less frequently than in the cardiac and fracture patients, and that a long period of stress and strain was a more frequent occurrence. She pointed out, however, that such a period of stress and strain or definite emotional trauma immediately prior to illness is a frequent finding in numerous disease pictures and needs further evaluation. However, Dunbar felt that *a frequent pattern in diabetics was a steady grind of fatigue and deprivation with an increase in passive personality tendencies*. Resentment is called into play by daily life situations in contradistinction to the repressed unconscious hostility of hypertensive patients.

Type of Conflict. The essential feature would not seem to be the trauma, although this may play an important part, but the type of conflict measured in terms of tension and anxiety. Another important condition to have in mind is that it is not conscious emotional conflict, which has greater opportunity to discharge through the voluntary nervous system, that is most important but emotional tension that remains unconscious. This explains much of the seeming contradiction in the effect of transitory emotional upsets on the sugar level which has so confused diabetic specialists and led them to rule out the whole phenomenon as of little importance.

Psychic Conditioning. Daniels has pointed out that trauma which precipitates a neurosis has its effect because it impinges in many cases on an infantile neurosis which it reactivates, thus releasing more primitive anxiety patterns. Dunbar and associates in discussing diabetes stated that "from the psychosomatic point of view there is no more fundamental determinant of the organism's equilibrium together with its capacity to make adjustments than anxiety." In the diabetic and cardiovascular groups they found anxiety a prominent factor. In these groups the somatic and psychic conditioning and expression of anxiety presented a contrast with the fracture group. From the patients' subjective viewpoint there was a significant contrast because in the diabetic and cardiovascular groups the danger, as well as the handicap, was more diffuse and threatened from within, whereas in the fracture group the danger, as well as the damage produced, was concrete and seemed to come from without.

The Refractory Patient. An interesting note concerning a refractory patient, as well as a hint on the usefulness of relaxation therapy in diabetes, was furnished by Dunbar. The patient was an Austrian Jewish seamstress of forty-three years who had been treated for diabetes for seven years.

"In addition to her diabetes, she had suffered from pain around the heart, shivers and pain in the left shoulder and arm (which had been considered diabetic neuritis), numbness of the tongue, the left hand and of her leg, attacks of dizziness and headaches. These symptoms had come on suddenly twenty-one years previously when she received news of her father's death in the war. In general they had become progressively worse but with marked exacerbation at the time of certain events in her life. This patient was rather uncommunicative, and showed a high degree of muscle tension. When put on the examining table and asked to relax, she burst out crying and showed extreme anxiety. Later she said: 'I feel safer when I am stiff. My aggravations don't bother me so much. That's why I go to sleep stiff like that, only when I wake up in the mornings sometimes I can hardly get out of bed.' After this the patient became communicative; this point is stressed because of the well-known role of muscle tension in connection with the attitude of being on guard, resistance, and repression.

"The patient had been originally referred because she was refractory in following her diet. She explained to the psychiatrist that she knew that diet had little to do with the amount of sugar because she had made an experiment by eating all sorts of foods that were supposed to increase the sugar, had a test made at a drug store, and only a faint trace of sugar was found. On the other hand, another day when she had a lot of 'aggravations—so many aggravations that they made me feel as if I must have sugar,' she went to the drug store and found a four plus sugar. This made her decide not to bother with her diet. She explained that, 'of course, the doctors would not understand this.' " Dunbar stated that this patient's life followed very much the same pattern to which attention previously had been called in connection with diabetes, namely, a "steady grind of fatigue and deprivations with an increase in passive personality tendencies. Her resentment was constantly called into play by life situations, not deeply repressed and unconscious as is usual with the hypertensive patient." The major aggravations (as she called them) in her life situation were summarized and discussed in relation to treatment. "In the course of treatment the patient developed conversion symptoms not peculiarly associated with diabetes, such as inability to walk, and now and then aphonia. The original hysterical symptoms cleared up with relatively superficial psychotherapy and she began to lose weight, the polyuria disappeared, and the diabetes began to improve."

Psychologic Problems in Children

A long-term study by Fischer and Dolger of forty-three patients whose diabetes began in childhood called attention to the fact that diabetes is similar to other chronic illnesses in its effect on the psyche. Just as a hunchback or a cripple is always aware of his deformity, so the diabetic child is always conscious of his condition. He cannot escape the daily injection and is constantly reminded of his affliction by the discomfort produced by the needle as well as by the restriction in diet. Further-more, there is always the fear of a possible hypoglycemic reaction. Good adjustment is possible, however, if there is understanding, harmony, and security in the home.

Bruch and Hewlett also reported on a psychologic investigation of a group of twenty-one diabetic children. In a third of the cases diabetes developed at the time of a disturbance in family relationship such as boarding out with relatives, divorce, deaths in the family, and so forth. Infection preceded the onset in less than a third of the cases. The first reaction of the families to the diagnosis was often one of great emotional disturbance and bewilderment. Frequently the mothers were responsible for dietary cheating because they could not bear to see the child deprived. Many children became adept at manipulating the diet and insulin so that before the next visit to the clinic a "clean" specimen could be produced. In emotionally disturbed families poor cooperation became the center of existing conflicts and was frequently associated with poor regulation. The authors shrewdly observed, however, that cooperation does not necessarily mean absence of neurotic conflicts. On the contrary, it may express a repressive, perfectionistic attitude toward the child so that a more lenient medical regimen would sometimes help such families to accept diabetes with less guilt and anxiety, and this offer the child a better opportunity for normal personality development.

Illustrative of the influence of adaptive stresses on the course of diabetes is a case reported by Mirsky of a 17 year old boy whose mother died when he was two and who never had the security of a stable home, living either with relatives, his alcoholic father, or in institutions. His diabetes was discovered at the age of 13 while he was living in a school for delinquent boys and where he was most unhappy. In the four years following the onset of diabetes he was hospitalized on 19 occasions because of the severity of the acidosis that he developed in spite of an insulin dosage of 110 units per day. Although the urgency of adhering to a specific diet was emphasized by his physician, the patient frequently ate excessively between the prescribed meals. For an interval of nine months he was removed from his unhappy environment and put into a more permissive one where he was allowed to eat whatever he wished, where he was encouraged in his expressed desires to go to school but not forced to do so, and where his pseudomasculine strivings to be a "big-shot" were accepted. During that interval he developed no symptoms whatsoever, nor did he have a need to eat between meals. Twenty-four hours after he was precipitously evicted and returned to his former environment, the patient again developed acidosis and had to be admitted to a hospital.

Psychotherapy

Psychoanalysis. In addition to the patient analyzed by Daniels, a psychoanalytic study of two well-controlled cases of diabetes was reported by Meyer, Bollmeier and Alexander. Their method of observation was to correlate the psychoanalytic material with fluctuations of sugar output as determined by four to six daily quantitative urine examinations.

The first patient, a highly intelligent young man of twenty-nine, developed severe diabetes following an infection but during the course of serious psychologic conflict. He had been gravely ill as a young child and starved under a strict diet for almost a whole year because of a severe gastrointestinal disturbance. Apparently as a result he retained much of his infantile dependent and demanding attitude and was never able to accept the responsibilities of adult existence. He always felt frustrated and responded with hostilities because no one could gratify his demands for attention and love. These hostilities revived the old anxiety that he might lose love and security just as he was deprived of foods during the severe illness in early childhood. Emotional maturity was blocked by this anxiety and the patient never reached the psychosexual attitude of adult age. Diabetes developed at the height of emotional frustration which arose in relation to a sexual problem. A diagrammatic representation of sugar output showed that when his wishes to receive love and security were frustrated sugar levels were high but when he escaped the conflict by turning to a neurotic solution characterized by depression and a withdrawal into self-pity lower sugar levels occurred.

Followed for six years after the completion of a successful analysis, he was well adjusted in his marital life, successful in his profession, and much attached to his child born a year after his marriage. He was in good physical health and the urine was free of sugar.

A second patient, a young woman, also developed diabetes under the strain of an emotional conflict of a striking similarity. The patient retained an infantile dependent and demanding attitude, and felt frustrated because her demands for attention and love were out of proportion to the reality situation of an adult and consequently were never adequately satisfied. To this frustration she reacted with hostility. Diabetes developed when these infantile wishes conflicted with the demands that were frustrated, and the sugar output decreased when her demanding attitude was temporarily renounced. Just as in the first case the sugar output was increased under the strain of this conflict, and decreased when the patient indulged in self-pity and passivity.

Brief Psychotherapy. Although psychoanalytic study gives the most thorough understanding of the personality structure and life situation of the diabetic patient brief psychotherapy, based upon psychoanalytic understanding, is more available to the majority of diabetic patients. Commenting that diabetes is associated with almost every type of psychiatric disorder, with correspondingly varied personality structures, Daniels in a more recent paper suggested that these personalities are frequently under "forced draft" from endogenous or exogenous chemical substances associated with the disease or its treatment, so that repressed aspects of the personality or neurosis become highlighted. This emotionally, as well as chemically charged atmosphere, makes brief psychotherapy as important for regulation in some patients as diet or additional insulin.

In the majority of patients help was asked by the medical service because of a tendency of the patient to shock easily or because of confusion in distinguishing between true insulin shock and a clinical picture which resembles shock with normal or even high blood sugar. (page 535).

Reporting on eight young patients, Daniels found that conflict between parental dominance and repressed hostility was present in all cases, and a direct relationship between this and sexual conflict was most marked in the females.

In passing, Daniels commented that one important therapeutic element which should not be ignored is the effect of group classes on diabetics, now employed in many clinics while patients are learning the necessary dietary and other regimens. These frequently act as a form of group therapy by showing the patients that they are not the only ones afflicted with the disease, giving them the opportunity to exchange experiences, and furnishing the encouragement and support of the doctors and dietitians. This established class instruction should furnish a valuable guide for further development of group therapy.

Discussing a test based upon the urine sugar output, which was used to differentiate between emotional glycosuria and stabilized diabetes mellitus, Bollmeier and Meyer felt that psychotherapy has great therapeutic possibilities in the first group of patients—indeed, that it may prevent some from becoming true diabetics.

Mirsky insists that the physician should treat the urine less and the patient more. "He should be concerned with the amount of calories the patient retains rather than the amount that the patient eats or excretes. The proper use of insulin permits this on a normal diet. Even with the free diet the physician cannot shirk his responsibility since giving a patient freedom insofar as choice of food is concerned is of little avail unless, at the same time, the patient is handled sympathetically. Given an opportunity to mature emotionally, the diabetic patient will confront his wishes and his frustrations and make such compromises as are more consistent with both his chronologic age and social milieu. Then, he will act and eat as a normal individual and neither harm himself nor his environment."

The following case is an illustration of one of many that we have studied indicating the kind of life situation that frequently is found in diabetic patients. It lends point to Dunbar's observations regarding the *steady grind of fatigue and deprivation with an increase in passive personality tendencies as the psychological background of many cases of diabetes.* However, we are not concerned to try to prove that emotional factors are responsible for diabetes. What we are interested in is to show that the emotional part of the problem of diabetes has been neglected and that it is an important phase of the problem with which we must concern ourselves.

Diabetes Mellitus
Passive Personality; Fatigue and Deprivation

CASE 47

The patient was a young white man, studied at the Jefferson Hospital on the service of Dr. Thomas McCrae, in June, 1932. He had five admissions to the hospital. The first admission was in March, 1930, and the last in June, 1932.

History and Symptoms

The diabetes was discovered following loss of weight which was noticed by friends. On his second admission an observation was made by one of the physicians that excitement caused a rise in his blood sugar. His diabetic condition always responded well to treatment, but he was very careless about insulin after he left the hospital. His fourth admission to the hospital was for *coma* which came on during the night. Recovery was prompt and thereafter he promised to take better care of himself.

LIFE SITUATION

The *mother*, to whom the patient was greatly attached and whom he described as "sweet and altruistic," died in 1924 at the age of fifty-five when the patient was twenty. She had been sick about a year with carcinoma of the stomach and had been invalided for several months. During the latter part of the illness the patient took care of his mother at night.

The *father*, whom the patient always hated and whom he described as "selfish and mean," died at the age of seventy-two, in June, 1930, of pneumonia after being sick only a few days. He had previously always been well. The patient was at his father's bedside after an absence of ten or twelve years. During that night he sat in a nearby room and "searched his memory for traces of love for his father" but he could find none.

The *patient*, twenty-eight years old, was the youngest of a family of six children, two brothers and three sisters. The oldest sister was operated upon three years before for tumor of the stomach and had been well since.

Childhood

The patient was a fairly healthy youngster always deeply attached to his mother. As long as he could remember he knew that his father was mean to his mother. The father would frequently leave home and about three or four years before the mother's death definitely separated from her. The father contributed very little to the support of the family so that his mother from the earliest days of the patient's childhood was forced to work (domestic service). It was necessary, therefore, for the oldest sister to help take care of the patient during his infancy and childhood. One of the patient's earliest memories was of being thrown out of the house by his father on the occasion of the birth of his sister's baby.

He attended high school for two years and then quit to go to work at the age of fifteen. For a time while working he went to a preparatory school in the evening thinking that he would later study pharmacy. About the age of eighteen, he worked for his brother for two years in the paper business, which he did not like (the father was once in that business).

Mother's Death

The mother, by hard work and great saving, had managed to purchase a small home. It was placed in the name of the brother. During her last illness she said in the presence of the brother and the patient that she expected the brother (six years older than the patient) to look after the patient. The patient looked upon this as a "verbal will" and considered that he would share one half of the estate. He looked after his mother very tenderly during her final illness. "The brother was also very good to the mother but not so demonstrative in his affection."

The patient took the mother's death very hard. He was unconsolable, despondent, seclusive, and tortured with suicide thoughts. According to their religious custom they continued to live in the house for thirty days and then he and his brother went to his sister's home. The first night away from his old home he woke up with a choking sensation and this happened again a day or two later. A physician treated him and referred to it as a nervous affection of the throat. A month later he left town to visit the oldest sister. He stayed for six months, had a job, and because he felt that "nothing mattered" he had an affair with a married woman ten or twelve years older than himself. This was his only sexual experience. His explanation of this episode was that he "just didn't care what happened."

Quarrels with Brother

He returned to Philadelphia in order to dedicate a stone for his mother's grave and then he, with his brother, continued to live with a married sister. During these two years the mother's house was rented and the patient took it for granted that eventually he would get his share. At the end of two years the estate came up for settlement and the brother broke "the verbal will" and refused to give the patient his share. A terrible scene followed in which he felt like killing the brother. Thereafter for about three or four years there was constant tension and much quarreling with the brother about his share of the estate. Each time that he saw him a quarrel would follow in which the patient would always come off second best because he would get so angry and excited that he was unable to express himself. Furthermore, he would deliberately "hold himself back" so as not to prolong the quarrel. At the end of about two years the brother married and found further justification for keeping the estate. He brought his wife to live in the same house with the sister and after about six months the patient left to live with a younger sister to avoid so much quarreling. He lived there about two years and then took a room by himself because he desired to be "independent" and a month later he was admitted to Jefferson Hospital, his diabetes having been discovered.

The interviews with the patient would leave him nervous and excited and interfere with his sleep. After the last interview his hands were cold and damp and he complained that the left hand, that is, all of the fingers and the thumb, felt numb and it was observed by the physician that the middle and ring fingers of the left hand were paler than those on the right. The patient called this condition "neuritis" and said that he had had it ever since his coma attack. Apparently, however, it was of *vasospastic* origin.

SUMMARY

A soft, effeminate, passive young man with marked attachments to mother and hatred of father, transferred the hatred to a brother when the latter took from the mother something which belonged to the patient. Constant quarreling with the brother for a period of three or four years preceded the discovery of diabetes. Between hospital admissions he received only indifferent attention to his diabetes and occasionally let up on dieting and insulin.

After the attack of coma he promised to do better but frequently expressed the wish that he had not recovered. The patient himself was of the opinion that constant quarreling may have had something to do with his illness. His passive personality was long subjected to the steady grind of fatigue and deprivation.

SPONTANEOUS HYPOGLYCEMIA (HYPERINSULINISM)

Still another aspect of carbohydrate metabolism which has not been sufficiently dwelt upon is the confusion which exists between the clinical condition known as functional hyperinsulinism—a form of spontaneous hypoglycemia—and the anxiety state. This same confusion occurs in diabetics when it is suspected that an overdose of insulin has been given. Both occurrences are frequent. Repeatedly patients with anxiety neurosis and anxiety attacks are said to be suffering from hyperinsulinism and the diagnosis is thought to be confirmed if the blood sugar, taken at the time of the attack, is found to be low. Even if the blood sugar is not low, so great is the confusion in regard to this subject that the term *dysinsulinism* is frequently applied simply because organic medicine will adopt almost any subterfuge rather than use the term anxiety neurosis. We do not deny that there is such a clinical state as spontaneous hypoglycemia due to hyperinsulinism. Indeed a number of cases have been proved to be due to pancreatic adenomata and after their removal the patient has recovered. But a great many patients labeled *functional hyperinsulinism* are suffering from *anxiety neurosis* and the differential diagnosis is not difficult if one will just take time to make fasting blood sugar tests as well as a study of the personality and life situation of the patient before jumping to a hasty conclusion. So-called functional hyperinsulinism is not associated with low levels of the fasting blood sugar, and the depression by provocative tests is no greater than that produced in the normal individual (Conn).

Another clinical point utilized in supporting the diagnosis of spontaneous hypoglycemia is the tendency for patients who suffer from weakness and feelings of anxiety to carry candy or to eat some other food when they feel an anxiety attack coming on. It is presumed that the body chemistry is calling for carbohydrate. This presumption does not, however, take account of the psychological needs of the organism which can also be satisfied by swallowing. Referring to our discussion of the association between gastrointestinal function and anxiety (page 25) we will recall that the anxious and irritable infant is soothed by swallowing milk and the pattern is established so that the anxious and irritable adult unconsciously seeks to comfort himself in the same way. The implications for obesity will be discussed later (page 544).

Psychic Manifestations

The psychic manifestations of spontaneous and induced hypoglycemia are well known, the latter particularly because of the wide use of insulin. In general, these symptoms consist of anxiety, irritability, excitement, confusion, and finally complete loss of consciousness (hypoglycemic coma).

Diabetes with Anxiety Attacks, Thought to be Hypoglycemic

CASE 48

History and Symptoms

A patient, a young white man with a neuropathic background, was first seen because of indigestion which was proved to be of functional origin. Prompt recovery followed. In spite of his obvious neurotic tendencies he was an efficient and capable business man and shortly after he came under our observation was elevated to an important position in the concern for which he worked. On his next visit to us, at which time he again complained of indigestion and buzzing in the ear, which we also thought was functional, he reported that his responsibilities were great and "that the person who had previously occupied his position had died of overwork."

Blood Sugar Normal

The pressure of meeting these responsibilities seemed to weigh heavily upon him and within the following six months he developed glycosuria which at first was transient and later became permanent with an elevated blood sugar. Control of diet and insulin was begun and he got along satisfactorily for the next few years. Then he developed acute appendicitis and during his hospital stay, while recovering from the operation, he was very apprehensive about "complications," and frequently showed anxiety symptoms that he felt were due to overdosage of insulin but on each occasion it was found that his blood sugar was normal or beyond the normal. Again and again it was necessary to prove to him that these so-called hypoglycemia attacks were in reality anxiety attacks.

Functional Hypoglycemia

CASE 49

A white man of thirty-four was first seen in the fall of 1942. He complained of fatigue and exhaustion, abdominal discomfort, a sense of pressure in the head, and occasional sharp pains in the head followed by palpitation and sweating.

History and Symptoms

At first he stated that his trouble had begun in the previous spring when he began to feel fatigued in the early afternoon. Then came an exhausted feeling in his legs. The exhaustion became more general and more pronounced and was followed by poor digestion and loose bowel movements. In spite of frequent eating he had lost about 10 pounds in the last year.

The sharp pains in the head occurred only rarely and were associated with dizziness, palpitation, and sweating.

On close questioning he stated that he really had not been well since the age of nineteen. At that time he had begun to have pains in the back and in the legs and later suffered from indigestion. He had been under the care of many physicians, and while at times he felt fairly well, he was quite sure that he had not enjoyed good health since 1927.

Following a glucose tolerance test the patient was told that he had spontaneous hypoglycemia and was encouraged to eat frequently.

Family History. The father had died suddenly in his sleep at the age of seventy-three in 1937. Previous to this he had suffered from a mental depression, and the patient felt that he resembled his father. Otherwise, the family history did not seem important.

Physical Examination and Laboratory Studies

The patient was an alert and intelligent young man, who was obviously quite apprehensive about himself. He was fairly well nourished, in spite of the loss of about 10 pounds during the previous year, and the general physical examination disclosed no evidence of organic disease. He was then referred to the hospital for special study.

A glucose tolerance test was done with the following results: Fasting sugar 82 mg. followed by a curve of 100, 62, 60, and 55. This was repeated with a slightly better response: fasting sugar 80 mg. followed by a curve of 131, 133, 90, and 57. The temperature in the hospital fluctuated between 97 and 98.6, in other words, there was a tendency toward hypothermia. Basal metabolism was found within normal limits and a salt deprivation test for adrenal function showed a normal response, indicating that there was no evidence of adrenal dysfunction. Sedimentation rate was within normal limits and other ordinary laboratory studies were normal.

LIFE SITUATION

The patient was born and brought up in a small community in the Middle West. He described his father as a successful and important member of the community who was very religious, strongly opinionated, and a strict disciplinarian in the rearing of his children. In spite of his devotion to the church the patient had never felt that the father had any real warmth of affection for him. The patient felt that perfection was demanded of him and he was fired with ambition to get ahead. He tried very hard to excel both in regard to studies and athletic endeavors. Although not gifted intellectually and small for his age, he exerted himself to compete in scholarship and in athletics and made fair success at considerable effort. He had his heart set on a professional career but the father lost considerable money in 1929 and thereafter became depressed, and the patient was advised by his mother to take a position with his uncle (the mother's brother) who was a storekeeper in another town. After he had formed this connection at the age of nineteen he became ill and, as before stated, he had never felt right since.

Shortly after moving to the new community he married and his wife had three children in rapid succession. All during the years he worked faithfully but received no advancement and, as a consequence, had a difficult time getting along on the small salary of a clerk and "was never out of debt." He felt very strongly that his work was not appreciated and during the last spring he had made some ineffectual efforts to find another position after concluding that the work was monotonous, that he was in a rut, and that he could never "find his way out."

Explanation of Illness

After giving this picture of driving energy and throttled ambition the patient was told that all studies were negative for evidence of organic disease and that the low blood sugar was probably of functional origin, in other words, very likely due to the excessive production of insulin— functional hyperinsulinism. It was also suggested that perhaps throttled energy, which could not find an outlet along normal aggressive channels, might have something to do with the excessive secretion of insulin—that his pancreas was being driven to too much activity. He became very excited at this suggestion that energy for driving ahead had been dammed up in him and was seeking a way out by disturbing the function of his organs. He insisted that he had always known that he could never get well so long as he was in his uncle's store and that in order to recover, he must get out and be "on his own." It seemed very reasonable to him that his dammed-up energy was trying to find a way out by means of excessive pancreatic function. We suggested that perhaps the satisfaction which he craved was the cause of his abdominal discomfort—that here was a displacement of his craving for recognition, forming a void which he was trying to fill by frequent eating.

We discussed this problem of his eating between meals and suggested that perhaps he really was not so hungry but that it was just an attempt to satisfy this craving which represented something else, that is, in early life the need for recognition that he had been so eager to achieve in the eyes of his father and, later, the need for recognition of his real worth by the uncle.

It occurred to him that the pressure in his head might also be due to throttled energy—"like steam under pressure trying to find a way out." The patient was cautioned not to make any impetuous decisions until he had had time soberly to review his feelings.

On a subsequent occasion he informed us that he had had a talk with his wife about the material that we had discussed and then had a talk with his uncle, whom he found "surprisingly understanding." He had served notice on his uncle rather indirectly that he might have to leave the business in order to get well and the uncle assured him that this was not necessary, that he would receive some immediate recognition, and that his future was assured—that when his uncle retired he would become the manager of the business.

Follow-up

The patient improved immediately, and within a period of about two months he had lost most of his symptoms, and "for the first time, was really enjoying life."

SUMMARY

A young white man presented symptoms of exhaustion and anxiety which were attributed to spontaneous hypoglycemia. It was true that he had a hypoglycemic reaction to the glucose tolerance test but it was felt that this was functional and secondary to his anxiety state. The life situation showed evidence of long-time frustration and when it was suggested that this dammed-up energy was finding a way out by means of excessive secretion of insulin, the patient seized upon the suggestion with a great deal of avidity, unburdened himself of some of his anxiety and aggression, and made an excellent recovery.

To have called the illness spontaneous hypoglycemia or hyperinsulinism, to have encouraged frequent eating, and not to have made an effort to find out the nature of the anxiety which stood behind his functional hyperinsulinism, would not have helped this patient.

OBESITY

One does not have to be a physician to hear a great deal about the matter of weight. Next to the state of the weather, there is hardly a topic of conversation mentioned as frequently as weight loss or gain. This applies not only to women but to men as well, particularly in the last two decades when the obesity problem has been stressed from a health standpoint as well as for appearance's sake. It is recognized that the latter factor is not confined to women.

Excessive weight brings people into conflict for several reasons. First, overweight makes people look older and less attractive from the standpoint of our national ideal of good looks. Secondly, many people are aware that obesity may have something to do with the development of such disease as diabetes, hypertension and heart disease. Then, of course, conflict occurs when they attempt to do something about it for they would like to maintain an attractive figure without foregoing the pleasure of eating. To avoid the unpleasantness of dieting, patients often resort to harmful drugs or injure themselves by overexercise. When they are finally forced to restrict foods, the choice of diet is often injudicious, based chiefly upon the desire to prevent "hollow hunger."

Intake of Food

Exercise and the functioning of the ductless glands have something to do with the problem of weight gain but the most important factor is food *intake*. As stated in the chapter on psychopathology there is a great deal of sensual pleasure associated with the function of the mouth area of the body. The lips and tongue are well supplied with nerve end organs highly sensitive to food and drink. The greatest pleasure to the human being during the first year of life comes through this mouth area in the acts of nursing, eating and drinking. As the months go by other pleasure stimuli should enter his range of vision or feeling and should be incorporated in his developing personality.

Emphasis on Eating. However, whether or not this is so depends largely upon the family background of the child. Some families are quite "oral" in their orientation to life. The parents pride themselves upon having good food. The mother says, "Whether we have enough of other things or not we'll have good things to eat." A treat for such a family will be a good meal rather than creative work or play. They talk about food and the various ways it should be cooked and other interests in life suffer proportionately. If a child grows up in such a family he is almost certain to place an overvaluation on food and eating. When the child goes to school or camp the mother voices her fear that he may not have enough to eat. The impression is gained that if he does not eat well something dangerous will happen to him. Everything about the offering and receiving of food is endowed with a high emotional value.

Food Instead of Emotional Sustenance. This excessive interest in feeding is an unconscious effort of the mother to treat her children well and to strengthen them for life's battles through food because of her weak emotional relationship to them. She is unable to give them the strength of her love. It is as if the desire to satisfy the child with abundant nourishment has been exaggerated by the mother's reluctance to give something of herself. She fails to make them independent and self-reliant through emotional strength and wisdom but tries to make them grow strong through size alone. They are not taught to derive pleasure through learning, play, competition, and social contacts but are kept overprotected and overindulged. The result is often a lack of ambition, poor social adaptation, unhappiness and *obesity*.

Endocrine Glands. It may well be that the endocrines play a part but that part may be a secondary functional disturbance as a result of the psychological situation. For example, when menstrual irregularities occur in obesity, they appear to be secondary because the menstrual cycle can often be restored simply by getting rid of the fat. At any rate it should be obvious that the interrelation of personality, social situation, and glandular function is a highly complex one.

Richardson reported that obesity which is demonstrably of endocrine origin is rare even in an endocrine clinic, whereas fat people constitute a large section of the general population. Moreover, in ordinary obesity he found little evidence of endocrine disturbance; the obese woman has normal skeletal and sexual characteristics. "It often happens, of course, that an obese patient receives an endocrine preparation of some sort and loses weight. But this is no evidence that the preparation has any biological action on the fat apart from its psychotherapeutic effects. When the emotions are involved, as they usually are in any deviation from good health, it is enough that the patient should believe in the remedy to produce a psychological effect on the disease. If endocrine preparations were not available for the treatment of obesity the patient would probably be equally benefited by some other form of medication."

We do not deny the importance of the endocrine glands in the problem of obesity; we only urge psychosomatic consideration in every instance of this disorder.

Personality Studies

Some of the above observations were made by Bruch in an important study of 140 obese children and their parents. Marked delay in ability and willingness to take care of themselves was noted in three fourths of the group. A concurrent evidence of *immaturity* in emotional development was shown by the symptom of *enuresis* which occurred in 40 per cent of those studied.

Physical Inaction. Entrance into school marked the first opportunity for social contact in these children. About two thirds of the group were considered physically inactive. Few of them made use of the opportunities for muscular exercise provided by the school playground. They remained isolated and without playmates. Even in recreational activities involving other than muscular exercise there was little indication of creative self-expression. The majority of them sought the "made" entertainment of movies and radio. Only a small number of parents had encouraged activity or initiative in other ways. In fact, their overprotection of the child was extreme, sometimes to the point of wanting to accompany the child to school and even to the classroom door to help him remove his outer clothing. It is small wonder that these children expected that everything would be done for them. Slow and awkward movements were thought to be due to lack of training games and other activities rather than to any abnormality in the mechanism of transformation of energy.

Family Setting. Although obesity apparently often "runs in families" this fact does not exclude more than one mechanism. Richardson emphasized that transmission can take place in one of two ways, or both of them at once: by genetic inheritance, or through the medium of the family life and its social and cultural setting.

In a study with Grace Touraine in relation to the family setting from which obese children come Bruch observed that in such families the amount of money spent for food was disproportionately large. The obesity was rarely a matter of concern to the parents although concern over minor physical ailments was excessive. Many of the fathers were weak, unaggressive people with little drive or ambition. The mothers had suffered from poverty and insecurity in their own childhood. In only a few families was there marital happiness. At times there was open fighting and frequently contempt was expressed for the father by a domineering mother. The families were usually small in size. Seventy per cent of the children studied were either an only child or the youngest child. One half of the children were admittedly unwanted. Sometimes hostility was openly expressed by cruel punishment or shown through unreasonable and severe discipline. But the most conspicuous feature in the attitude to the obese children was *inconsistency*. Most prominent was an open display of protectiveness. But this seeming manifestation of devotion and affection was frequently like a thin veneer that barely covered the underlying insecurity in relation to the child. *The fundamental rejection was compensated for by overprotection and excessive feeding.* These contradictions were more frequently observed in mothers than in fathers.

Psychic Conditioning. Muscular activity had been associated with the idea of danger in these fat children. Hence the lack of muscular activity and excessive intake of food were both factors in obesity, to which social and emotional adjustment were intimately related. Of course, all obesity does not have its beginning in childhood. It may come on at any age. What that age will be is determined in many cases by the same factors that cause the onset of any neurotic symptom. When insecurity or need for affection and attention become more pronounced than the maturity of the personality can cope with, anxiety appears. If the pattern of that personality has been set up so that oral gratification through eating allays anxiety then obesity is likely to result. If this conditioning to excessive eating is great enough, obesity may occur in childhood. If the conditioning is only latent in the framework of the personality, indulgence in overeating may not occur until some stress makes itself felt later in life. For example, an adolescent moves to new neighborhood or enters a new school. He or she fails to get off to a good start in making friends and entering into social activities. Denied such pleasures he regresses to oral gratification, eats excessively, withdraws to himself, further limits his muscular activities, and as a consequence gets fat. More than likely the obesity will be blamed on "glands."

A married woman of about forty-two, a large, soft, dependent and passive creature, took care of her husband and his business as a mother would and had little of the pleasures, satisfactions, and responsibilities of a wife. After several visits to us she volunteered the information that some six or eight years ago she discovered that her husband was having an extra-marital affair and that thereafter "she had let herself go." That is, she had given up trying to dress attractively and had eaten as she pleased. As a consequence she gained a great deal of weight. It was obvious that when she was denied certain satisfactions in life she regressed to oral satisfaction and as a result she became very heavy and, of course, even less attractive to her husband. It was not too difficult to point this out and to hold out as the incentive for a strict reduction diet, the possibility of regaining her interests in life and regaining her husband's interest in her.

Psychological Aspects of the Treatment of Obesity

Therefore, whether the endocrine factor is large, small, or nonexistent, it is necessary in approaching the obesity problem to study the emotional life. We should elicit a history concerning the parents and siblings which will show the influence of the family situation in the development of the patient's personality. Was the mother herself a deprived and insecure person? Bruch and Touraine noted that common factors in the background of mothers of obese children could be found not only in the actual events of their lives, but that even more important aspects were reflected in their responses to them, in their self-pitying attitude towards the past. Resentful submissions, incessant preoccupation with their misfortunes, and condemnation of others for their frustration manifested itself in their words as well as their behavior.

Mother's Attitude. What was the mother's attitude toward the patient during his gestation and at birth and in his developmental years? What was her attitude toward food in general and toward the feeding of the patient in particular? Did she encourage play and exercise, stimulate initiative and imagination? Was she overprotective in her attitude and strict in her discipline or was she friendly and tolerant? Were her mother and father compatible, and what was the father's role in discipline and in the inspiration of the patient? Were food, drinks, and candy used as rewards for good behavior or were rewards less related to oral gratification?

Attitude Toward Reduction. Had the patient resorted to food and especially sweets to assuage anxiety or disappointment? We would have to ask him to watch himself very carefully to see if he was nibbling at candy and taking food snacks to a greater extent than he was consciously aware. A patient can consciously desire to reduce and unconsciously cheat on his resolve. To make a reduced caloric intake effective the patient may make a great deal of effort to focus his attention upon the problem at hand. Every psychiatrist frequently observes the paradoxical situation of the patient who comes for treatment of a symptom and yet in his treatment sessions or in the intervals between will not focus his mind upon his symptom or the probable causes for it. The man being treated for impotency may stubbornly refuse to think or talk about sex or women. The man being treated for alcoholism will refuse to discuss his drinking experiences. The reason for this is fear of something unpleasant in connection with the symptom. The patient who wishes to reduce may consciously want to limit his food intake but another part of his personality fears deprivation. It is quite common for such patients to feel that disease may attack a thin body. In fact, when we get into more deeply unconscious ideas we find that some are even more bizarre. For instance, the very woman who consciously wants to diet to lose weight and become more attractive has at the same time a marked anxiety about becoming more attractive. She is afraid she will fall into sexual temptation or if she is single she is afraid some man will really ask her to marry him and she will be drawn into responsibilities which she is afraid to face. Obesity in some women has the unconscious significance of pregnancy because of the primitive belief that impregnation occurs through eating.

Obesity as a Manifestation of Neurosis. Richardson reported in detail a case of obesity in a woman which began before the age of ten. The central psychological features were deprivation by the parents in childhood, for which she blamed chiefly her mother, and an atmosphere of severe sexual repression. She early relinquished the expectation of affectionate care and understanding from the mother and regarded herself as a waif. She longed for a family and children but was strongly inhibited and rejected men. To a large extent eating took the place of affection but she also invested it with the symbolic meaning of impregnation following the childish idea of gastrointestinal pregnancy and parturition.

"Examples could be multiplied to show neurotic symptoms in the obese: the destructive effects of the obesity; anxiety, guilt, self-depreciation, depression, and a compulsive type of eating analogous to alcoholism or a drug addiction. That the neurosis affords a psychological gain is indicated partly by the fear of losing weight. Fat is used as a barrier against men and marriage and against other affectionate relationships of adult life."

Nervous Hunger. Patients do not present themselves for psychological study because of obesity. But treatment of patients for other conditions has revealed valuable information regarding the matter of overweight. Either sex may use the *eating* process to *allay anxiety* or to gratify pleasure cravings which should be satisfied in other ways, as for instance through a better sexual and social adjustment. A nagging, intolerable sensation in the epigastrium often referred to as "nervous hunger" is symbolic of the emptiness of the emotional life. The effort to fill this void with food instead of emotional sustenance is a frequent cause of obesity. A woman who had been married twelve years, childless, and twenty pounds overweight, reported that whenever she felt unhappy or depressed she felt that she must have a good meal. She would describe the meal in great detail, how good the food was, and how kind and friendly the waitresses were. Psychological study showed that she had a strong need to be loved but an even stronger need to hate, to criticize, and to be unreasonable and disagreeable. After she was permitted to express a great deal of her hostility she was finally able to be friendly and tolerant. Then she made up her mind to reduce. She said, "I guess I felt so mean I didn't care whether anyone liked me or not." A deeper study of her unconscious mental processes showed that her fat abdomen symbolized a pregnancy. When she was able consciously to bear the idea of a child the normal way she wanted to get rid of her fat. Naturally all of this material was not disclosed at one time. She would get discouraged occasionally and then eat too much. But as treatment continued, dieting became easier. She said, "I didn't realize how much I nibbled all day long. I didn't know I was eating much when really I was eating most of the time. It was like having company to eat a little something. Now I'm on a diet and I feel I have enough. It's really easy when you have a definite purpose and nothing pulling you the other way."

Psychotherapy Versus Calculated Diet. The effect of psychotherapy without the use of calculated diets was studied by Nicholson. Ninety-three patients were divided into the following four groups:

1. Thirty-eight patients were treated by superficial psychotherapy without calculated diets and without medication; the patients were offered a simple explanation of energy exchange and the caloric value of foods.

2. Thirty-five patients were given a calculated diet of 800 calories. An experienced dietitian explained the diet and, when desired, further instructions were given on return visits. There was no medication, nor was any effort at psychotherapy attempted.

3. Ten patients were given 5 mg. of amphetamine sulfate three times a day. No psychotherapy was attempted and no calculated diet was offered.

4. Ten patients were handled as in Group 3 except that thyroid substance was administered instead of amphetamine.

All obese patients studied were found to have some type of psychoneurosis in varying degrees. Psychotherapy resulted in a higher percentage of successful results than was obtained from the other methods of attempted reduction. Nicholson concluded that both psychotherapy and the reestablishment of proper dietary habits are essential for permanent weight reduction.

Obesity and Reduction Problem
Unilateral Kidney Disease (Kidney Stone)

CASE 50

A married white woman of thirty-three was admitted to Temple University Hospital in November, 1939.

History and Symptoms

She complained of a sharp pain in the left flank; intermittent pains low in the right side of the back and abdomen; loss of appetite and nervousness.

The pain on the right side began about January, 1939. She described it as a sensation of a hot coal in the lumbar area with a "drawing effect" on the right side. The pain also extended up toward the umbilicus and down toward the genitals. Her first idea was that this had "something to do with adhesions," possibly from a former appendectomy; then a slight change in the character of the menses occurred and after consultation with a gynecologist there was some question as to whether an operation should be done to free "the adhesions." Following a vacation during the summer when she began to feel better and considered the question of returning to work, she again had an attack of pain on the right side of the abdomen associated with vomiting and diarrhea which was diagnosed as "intestinal flu." It was after this that she came to the Temple University Hospital outpatient department where she was studied for a short time but on November 1 she awoke with intense pain on the left side of the abdomen which came through from the back and extended toward the genitals. There were no urinary symptoms but she said that the urine was bloody and her physician reported that he found blood in the urine. She had to receive morphine to get relief and it was because of this attack of very severe pain that she was sent into the hospital.

Past History. She considered herself a healthy person but had always been overweight, even from childhood, and during adolescence her weight increased a great deal. She stated that she had an enormous appetite and a great craving for sweets and her parents indulged that craving. They placed no limit on the amount that she could eat.

At the age of eighteen, she had discomfort in the right lower quadrant of the abdomen associated with nausea and thought that she might have appendicitis. A physician agreed with her and the appendix was removed. A perfectly clean "chronic appendix" was found. A short time later while at work she had a sudden peculiar attack in which the left side of the body, including the left side of the face, became limp and numb—this she referred to as a "slight stroke." She was incapacitated for about three months; she told us that the left arm hung limply against the body but that the left leg was not affected. We were at a loss to understand this particular episode but will refer to it later in the discussion.

Fluctuation in Weight. She married at the age of nineteen and her weight steadily increased until she reached 235 pounds. At this point, for reasons to be discussed, she went on a reduction diet and managed to lose 70 pounds within a year. Shortly, however, "her craving for sweets was so great and her appetite so enormous" that she gave up the diet and steadily increased her weight again until about six years ago when she was back at the same level of 235 pounds. Now she sought medical attention and a physician prescribed a pill containing "thyroid, pituitary, and ovarian substance" and informed her that with this pill she would lose weight without paying much attention to her diet. However, she found that this was not so and once more by means of dieting, together with the pill, she brought her weight down gradually over a period of three or four years until she weighed about 135 pounds. In other words she lost 100 pounds! She then managed to hold her weight at this level but it was only a short time before pain began in the right lower quadrant of the abdomen.

Family History. The patient was an only child. The father died at the age of fifty-six of high blood pressure and a "stroke." According to her statement he had never been well. She described him as a quiet, ailing man, interested in music but never successful in life.

Physical Examination and Laboratory Studies

The general physical examination disclosed very little of significance. The patient seemed perfectly comfortable. The temperature, pulse, and respirations were normal. The blood pressure was normal and the cardiovascular system seemed perfectly normal. Examination of the head and neck showed nothing significant; the chest was clear; the breasts small but showed no abnormality. The abdomen was flat and soft and while there seemed to be some tenderness on the left side on admission, it soon disappeared There were no organs or masses palpable. The gynecological examination was normal, although the uterus was rather small. The rectal examination was normal. The extremities were normal.

Examination of the urine showed a faint trace of albumin and a few red blood cells and gave a positive occult blood reaction. Other laboratory tests showed nothing remarkable. Renal function was within normal limits; the blood Wassermann was negative and the blood count good. The Addis count of the urinary sediment showed four and a half million red blood cells and six and a half million white blood cells thus indicating a slight increase beyond the normal limits.

An intravenous urogram was done which suggested impaired filling on the left side with a statement that there might be a lesion of some kind in the left kidney pelvis but a retrograde pyelogram later showed normal filling. At the same time urine was collected from the left kidney which was perfectly normal microscopically and bacteriologically. Apparently, therefore, this patient may have passed a stone and the residual irritation interfered with function of the left kidney as demonstrated by the intravenous urogram. This seemed the only likely explanation.

LIFE SITUATION

Family History

There were some very interesting facts in the life history of this patient. Her father was a musician, a quiet, retiring man, a dreamer rather than a doer, who, according to the patient's statement, "never had a well day in all his life." The patient gave us the impression that the father was a frustrated dreamer who found the realities of life too much for him.

The mother, on the other hand, was described as a vigorous, healthy, and loquacious person who was forty-one years of age when the patient, an only child, was born. The patient felt in her father's quietness and taciturnity, a kindness and understanding which the mother did not possess.

Early Life. The patient graduated from high school and then went to business school. Following this she did office secretarial work up until the last few years when she started to do dental laboratory work. In all she had worked very steadily up until six months before admission to the hospital.

One of the first symptoms in which we were interested was the paralysis which occurred at the age of eighteen. A paralysis of the arm and face, on one side, is a rather unusual occurrence at this age. It was said to have cleared up promptly in three months and to have left no residual changes. Although it is a little unusual for the face to have been involved as well as an upper extremity there is a strong suggestion that this illness was an hysterical attack.

Death of Father. While the patient was convalescing from appendectomy, word came to her that her father had died. Her physician broke the news to her very gently and remained near expecting an outburst of emotion. The patient stated that she did not feel anything, did not say anything, did not cry nor carry on in any way. Instead of an emotional outburst she said, "My grief all went down there," pointing to the right lower quadrant of her abdomen. On the same day her fever went up and an intra-abdominal abscess developed which required re-operation and drainage and the patient was incapacitated for several weeks.

The reaction to her father's death did not seem to end here, however, for she went on to say that for the following two years there was "something inside of me that was not right." She was unable to express any feeling over her father's death but retained this general discomfort until one day when visiting her father's grave she cried for two hours, and then went away feeling entirely differently from that time onward. She said, "I could not believe that he was dead until I had a good cry." From this history we could surmise that this patient was one in whom emotional relationships were not easily handled, that tension piled up with consequent bodily discomfort, and emotional release took place with difficulty.

Personal History

Marriage. She married at the age of nineteen a man who proved to be an *alcohol addict*. Their married life had been marked by several separations and returns. The husband had experienced many vicissitudes in his early life. The patient stated that she was at first easy on him because she felt he had gone through a great deal and therefore had reason to be emotionally unstable. Finally, however, she made up her mind she could put up with the drinking no longer, and told him forcibly that if he did not give up drinking she would have nothing to do with him. He accepted this ultimatum and had not used alcohol since. We can understand how she could deliver such an ultimatum and stick to it. It was because she herself could endure a great deal of self-denial and did not see why others could not do likewise. We know that this is unusual, however, because experience proves that the wives of alcoholic men are not usually able to come to such a definite decision and stick to it.

The Reduction Regimen. The matter of the patient's diet made a very interesting story. At one time she weighed 235 pounds. One day a friend of her husband visited them and made the remark, "You are falling away to a ton." Although many remarks had been made about her weight before that time, she was particularly nettled by this remark and resolved then and there that she would lose weight. She promptly went on a severe diet, cutting out all sugars and carbohydrates, and restricting fluids as well. Within a year she had reduced her weight from 235 pounds to 165 pounds. This took a great deal of will power on the part of the patient because "I loved to eat, especially sweets" and "I used to eat one meal a day which began when I got up in the morning and lasted until I went to bed at night." Her feelings as she discussed this dieting episode left no room for doubt that she had obtained a great deal of gratification from eating and required great will power to make this weight reduction. Having denied herself the gratification of eating over this length of time, and done it successfully, she was able to insist upon the same oral deprivation on the part of her husband regarding his drinking.

Medical Assistance. After all her work, however, it was not long before the craving for food overcame her good resolutions and she began to eat greater quantities again, and in a short time her weight was back up to 235 pounds. Once more uncomplimentary remarks began to come her way and this time she thought she would like to have the help of a physician in the matter of reducing. She was told that with the use of a pill she would not need to pay any attention to food intake. However, it turned out that the use of the pill itself effected no weight reduction; on the contrary she began to gain still more. So she again had to use her will power and cut down on the amount of food. This time she did not attempt to lose weight so rapidly but combining a careful selection of food and reducing her intake, with the continued use of the pill she was able finally to reduce her weight to 135 pounds. The patient felt that the pill was definitely helpful and that she did not have to reduce the food intake so drastically as on the first occasion. In the spring of 1939 the patient began to feel pains about the site of the appendectomy, complained of fatigue, and for the first time in her life lost her desire for food. It was then that she was examined by a gynecologist and it was thought some operation for adhesions might be necessary. She stopped her work, however, made two short vacation trips out of the city during the summer, and came back in September feeling quite well. She was reexamined by the gynecologist, who felt that in view of her good health no operation would be necessary and she was advised to return to work. But a few days later she developed the severe gastrointestinal disturbance previously mentioned and following this fatigue, anorexia, and occasional abdominal pains had troubled her ever since.

Sexual Life

Gynecological examination revealed that the hymen admitted only one finger, but in spite of this observation the patient, when questioned about her marital life, told us that sexual relations had been regular and thoroughly satisfactory up until recently. The sexual act "had never meant much" to the patient, but on the other hand was not actually distasteful. She was desirous of being a good wife and inasmuch as the husband was considerate and gave her no actual discomfort she made no complaints about this aspect of her married life.

Psychological Significance of Reduction

From a study of this patient's past life and the emotional make-up which she revealed to us it would seem that her excessive appetite was an attempt to gain through eating the love that she had been denied by her mother, and by the world in general, ever since her childhood. When she came to a certain point where her weight was too excessive she found she was losing her prestige and people were disapproving of her. It was at this point that she could make up her mind to discipline herself very severely and achieve a figure more in conformity with the popular ideal. She was able to accomplish this partly because her will power was apparently well developed, but of course she was aided by a mental picture of the approval which people would give when she had reached a more desirable weight. It would seem, however, that the gratification she obtained when she had reached a weight of 165 pounds did not compensate sufficiently for the pleasure she had in taking food and as a result she gradually gained weight again. On the second occasion the goal did not seem worth quite so much effort and she sought the aid of glandular therapy and dieted much more slowly. Finally after a second reduction she still had not found the attention and prestige she was looking for, and a feeling of depression, fatigue, and gastrointestinal symptoms began to appear as a result of her internal conflict. As the patient herself expressed it, "Life lost its zest during the past six months."

Narrow Interests

A review of this woman's history showed that she had too few interests in her life. She was brought up as an only child, emotionally more attached to her father, but not particularly inspired by either parent. She had no special interests beyond her work. She studied the piano and violin as a child and adolescent, but never touched either after the "paralysis" of her arm at eighteen. She had never cultivated any hobbies, she had never wanted any children, she took no pleasure from social life, she had an alcoholic husband whom she had kept in control with difficulty, and while she had tried to make herself agreeable she had never been close to and enjoyed the companionship of people in any deep way.

Summary of Psychic Aspects of Illness

So here was a patient whose emotions played a considerable role in the matter of her obesity and weight reduction, as well as in some of her more recent symptoms. The patient's inordinate appetite throughout her life had been symbolic of a desire for love and affection which she could not gain through the ordinary means but sought through food, just as the need for love and food are so closely associated in the life of the infant. Our patient was not able to gain this love and affection from her mother and her father and consequently did not learn how to gain it from others. Hence as she grew older, she resorted to food instead, just as some other people resort to alcohol.

Significance of Neurotic Symptoms. A very pertinent question might be as follows: If the patient used this method successfully for a long time why was it not still successful? The answer lies in the fact that a neurotic symptom does not serve a useful purpose indefinitely. A normal individual has his plans well laid for what he would like to accomplish in life, and he works to achieve these ends. A neurotic person also hopes to achieve but he does not have his ideas clearly formulated and hence struggles more blindly toward an uncertain goal. This woman had no special goal during the past ten years but used her energies in thinking of producing a change in her body configuration and had her mind on little else. As a result she found herself at thirty-one doing nothing which she enjoyed particularly and having accomplished nothing of which she could be proud.

Chapter XVII

THE GENITO-URINARY SYSTEM AND THE SEXUAL FUNCTION

The derivation of the word *hysteria* from the Greek word for uterus emphasizes the long-recognized kinship between disorders of the genital tract in women and psychological disturbances. More and more gynecologists are recognizing that probably a half of all patients who present themselves for treatment have no gross disease in the pelvic organs. The mechanistic view of the origin of symptoms in gynecology is being replaced by new developments in physiology, endocrinology, and psychology. A great many of the operations which were so common fifteen or twenty years ago, such as suspension of the uterus, are now much less frequent. It was discovered that operations alone did not relieve the symptoms in this area, and as more knowledge has been gained about the varied manifestations of neuroses, an operation is no longer regarded as the magical influence needed for cure. Gynecologists have learned that they must be constantly on the watch for a background of emotional disturbance which may be producing the disordered function and the distress in the pelvic region.

Karl Menninger has pointed out that surgery is often sought by the patient who fears something else more than she fears surgery, and cites the case of a young woman who postponed her marriage date five times because of a right-sided abdominal pain. Finally the patient begged for an operation and it was performed. Her attacks of pain in the lower right quadrant were relieved, however, only until the approach of the postponed wedding date. Then they returned and she insisted upon returning to the hospital. Such a case illustrates that the demand for surgery was only the lesser of two evils—the greater evil being a heterosexual relationship which she was emotionally too immature to face.

INSTINCTUAL FORCES

As stated in the chapter on psychopathology, there are two main instinctual drives which are always asserting themselves in the individual who is trying to make an adaptation in a busy and none too friendly world. These are the aggressive drive, leading toward a mastery of the environment, and a sexual drive, leading toward reproduction. Through the first, man seeks to gain sustenance, comfort, possessions, and prestige.

He must learn to control the aggressive force skillfully lest it show harmful and destructive tendencies which will either bring punishment upon him and alienate him from those who could help him or will turn back upon him in the form of disease or accident. Through the sexual impulse—broadly speaking, an instinctual drive for sensual gratification—man seeks to give and receive pleasure in close physical contacts. Through the contact of the genital organs, man reproduces himself. Through gratification of the senses, through food, warmth, kind words, sweets, etc., children learn to feel love for those who treat them well, and become willing and able to feel the same for others—their playmates, friends, sweethearts, marital partners, and finally their own children.

GENITAL FUNCTIONING

This process seems a natural and harmless one, and yet it must be admitted that there is a great deal of social condemnation of genital functioning as a whole without consideration of the fact that there is a right time and place for this kind of behavior. Rarely is there any intelligent consideration on the part of parents and teachers of the purpose and importance of genital function. As a result the genital tract as a body system falls most directly in the path of a deluge of human emotions of a most unfortunate character.

The genital organs have their own physiological functions to perform as well as being the most important organs of love-making and the *only* organs of procreation. As a result they fall heir to many taboos, feelings of disgust, shame, fear, anxiety, and even hate. *None* of these feelings *should* be associated with the reproductive organs. It has been definitely shown that with intelligent information and the development of love and good will associated with sexual functioning, human beings will conduct themselves in a highly satisfactory fashion; but that fears, taboos, and prejudices on the other hand, may lead to crippling of the behavior.

EDUCATION IN SEXUALITY

In this chapter considerable material will be presented concerning the sexual function and the emotional problems concerned with satisfactory sexual relations. The relation of the sexual function to health has not been adequately dealt with in medical teaching. The study of medicine is to a certain degree a sublimation of the desire to know more about the human body and its functions, of which the sexual function is by no means the least important. Medical students are eager to know more of this subject, and rightly so, for they feel that the more they know of this vital factor the better they will understand human behavior in general and therefore the better physicians they will become.

Furthermore in recent years college students, engaged couples, and many young groups have asked to know more about sexual function in order to prepare themselves for a happy marriage. Physicians are expected to know much about sexuality and often imagine that they do, but when questioned by their patients or by a group of curious young people they often find themselves not only inarticulate but lacking in knowledge. Accordingly there are many good reasons for a physician to be aware of the role of sexuality in physical and emotional health.

FRIGIDITY AND IMPOTENCE

The inability to function normally with the genital organs either for procreative purposes or for pleasure is fairly common. This condition, called *frigidity* in the woman, is much more common that its counterpart, *impotence* in the male. The proportion of adult women who are unable to achieve complete sexual satisfaction is more than 50 per cent. There is a large number of women who never achieve orgasm at any time in their lives. Others have sexual satisfaction for a period of from one to five years after marriage and then the capacity for achieving satisfaction is gradually lost. Others do not begin to have orgasm until six months or a year have elapsed after marriage. Then they enjoy sexual pleasure for a time and once again lose the capacity for satisfactory sexual relations. Some women enjoy love-making before marriage, have an active erotic fantasy life and imagine that they have considerable sexual feeling, but in the marriage relationship are disturbed to find that actual sexual relations mean very little to them. Many women will enjoy sexual relations when on a holiday or vacation away from home but with the responsibilities of everyday life they derive little romance or pleasure from the sexual act.

Thwarted Sexual Development

It is not surprising that capacity for sexual feeling is poorly developed in the female. Too often in the past, and even quite commonly now, a great deal of pressure has been exerted upon the female which tends to thwart psychosexual development. She is usually kept in ignorance ot sexuality as long as possible, and when grudgingly permitted to know anything about sex she is often told that the sexual relation for the woman is "not nice, degrading, wicked, dirty, disgusting, impure, shameful, dangerous." She is told that no nice woman has sexual desires, and that such desires lead to impulsive, uncontrollable sexual behavior resulting in disease, pregnancy, and social ostracism.

Marriage and the Sexual Function

The reader already knows that when a human being has been taught to hate or fear some idea or act long enough and intensely enough it is with great difficulty that he can change his point of view. When this point of view is acted out by an organ of the body, that organ can be stubbornly obedient to the old prohibition long after a need for change has taken place. Marriage does not change points of view regarding sexual behavior. Marriage gives only legal and religious sanctions. The capacity to make full and wholesome use of these sanctions must be present in the personality through sensible and friendly education. A girl cannot be taught to hate and fear sexual relations for twenty years and then overnight accept them as correct, dignified, and pleasurable. Hence it is important for the growing girl to have *enlightenment as she asks for it* concerning the functions of the genital organs and the sensations associated with them. It has long ago been proved that information about sexuality does not lead to vicious and immoral behavior. When children are given credit for common sense and restraint in their sexual lives they will behave better than if it is assumed that they have no intelligence or average consideration or will power. At the same time they will develop the feelings in the sexual organs so necessary to a happy, well-regulated sex life in marriage. As Menninger reminds us, sexual feeling does not arise in the prostate gland or the uterus, even though these organs are often indicted in impotence and frigidity and treated by manipulation and surgery.

The capacity for sexual feeling is present in every healthy man and woman. But whether those feelings are permitted to be felt in the sexual organs depends upon whether the right ideas and emotions concerning sexual functioning have been allowed to develop during the growth of the personality, or whether these ideas and feelings have been smothered by fear, guilt, shame, disgust, and hatred for anything and everything sexual.

Psychosomatic Background of Impotence and Frigidity

We recognize that not all cases of impotence and frigidity are psychological in origin. In rare instances certain organic diseases of the nervous system such as multiple sclerosis, transverse myelitis, tabes dorsalis, anterior poliomyelitis, and others, may cause this condition. We recognize also that acute financial problems, grief, overwork, and other circumstances that induce emotional stress may temporarily reduce or abolish sexual desire. But we do wish to emphasize that the physically and emotionally healthy man and woman should have a capacity in the marital relationship for sexual function *with pleasure* if the ideas and emotions in relation to this function are rational and well integrated.

Even though many husbands pay too little attention to achievement of orgasm in the female (often referred to as "having a climax") the common saying, "There is no such thing as a frigid woman—it is only the man who is clumsy" is not true. Women too must share the responsibility for inadequate sexual expression. The man or even the woman herself often concludes that she is "probably cold by nature" or that "women weren't meant to feel the same way in sexual relations as men." On the contrary it is quite important that the woman share equally in the pleasure of intercourse. Just as the husband wants his wife to share his vacation pleasures or sit at the same table and enjoy his food with him, or share the beauty and sensual pleasure of a painting or sunset, so he should want her even more to share this most meaningful experience of all. There is no human relationship in which so much can be shared, so much of emotional and spiritual value given to each other as in the sexual relationship, if the attitude toward each other as man and wife is normal.

Orgastic Pleasure

There is considerable variation in the time taken in coitus for both parties to achieve orgasm. It is a well-accepted fact that the female, because of her nature and training in these matters, is slower to come to the point of sexual excitement and orgasm than the man. It is important that before coitus is undertaken the man should attempt to bring the woman to a state of sexual excitement by kisses, caresses and fondling of the breasts and genitals. Preliminary sex play of this kind should last for a number of minutes in order that the woman become interested for actual coitus to begin. The period of time during which the genitals are united may vary from two or three to fifteen or twenty minutes. It is not easy for many women to achieve orgasm in less than two minutes of genital union and coital movements. Ejaculation in the male occurring before this time is likely to result in disappointment in the female and chagrin in the male, particularly if the latter has any feeling whatever for his partner's pleasure.

RELATIVE DEGREES OF SEVERITY OF IMPOTENCE AND FRIGIDITY

Male	*Female*	
1. Potent but coitus lacks pleasure	1. Occasional failure to obtain orgasm	
2. Potent but has coitus under protest	2. Only occasional orgasm	
3. Interested in coitus but cannot always have erection when desired	3. Mild pleasure in coitus *but* without orgasm	Usually accompanied by some lack of vaginal secretion
4. Inadequate or partial erection	4. Vaginal anesthesia with no special aversion to coitus	
5. Premature ejaculation		
6. Impotence complete but interest retained in coitus	5. Vaginal anesthesia with aversion to coitus	
7. Impotence complete with no interest in coitus	6. Dyspareunia and vaginismus	

MALES

Potent But Coitus Lacks Pleasure. There is a group of men who are able to achieve erection when desired and are interested in the sexual act but for whom, when it actually takes place, there is always something lacking in the achievement of the anticipated pleasure. Some of these men seem to take more pleasure in boasting of the number of their sexual conquests than they take in the sexual act itself. Their pleasure is not so much in the company of women as in discussing their sexual feats with other men. One cannot actually say that they achieve no pleasure at the height of orgasm; rather the pleasure is not what is anticipated. When such a sexual difficulty occurs in the marriage relationship it discourages them from frequent attempts at intercourse.

Potent But Has Coitus Under Protest. There are some men who have little difficulty in achieving erection and having intercourse. However, they believe that intercourse is harmful and saps the energy and strength from a man, leaving him tired, exhausted, and unfit for his work the following day. In marriage such a man has intercourse infrequently, or if the wife's sexual desire causes him to have coitus more frequently than he desires, he acquiesces under protest.

Interested in Coitus But Cannot Always Have Erection When Desired. In this group of men coitus has considerable attraction at all times, but when the opportunity for intercourse arises the capacity for erection disappears.

Inadequate or Partial Erection. Some men who are interested in coitus and are consciously eager to satisfy the woman sexually are unable to obtain a vigorous erection. Only a partial erection is achieved so that it is difficult to enter the vagina, or if the vagina is entered, the man is unable to be sufficiently forceful or vigorous in his movements to bring satisfaction to the woman.

Premature Ejaculation. This is the most frequent disturbance of sexual functioning in men, causing them frequent humiliation and feelings of inferiority, and producing a lack of sexual gratification in the female. In some cases ejaculation of semen takes place before the male has actually inserted the penis within the vagina. In other cases ejaculation takes place almost simultaneously with entrance into the vagina or a few seconds later, entirely too soon for the woman to have received any stimulation from the penis which would aid her in achieving orgasm. In some married couples premature ejaculation is the cause for an inability in the female to achieve orgasm. In some men this symptom is looked upon as a personal peculiarity rather than a symptom, and hence they do not consult a physician. Often neither party regards this condition as anything unusual since neither has obtained information which makes comparison with others possible.

Defect in Emotional Development. In many cases of premature ejaculation the male is too embarrassed to consult a physician for his difficulty, and the woman has too much consideration for him to force him to do anything about it, and a long-standing sexual disharmony results. Sometimes, unfortunately, when the patient has consulted a physician who knows little about the subject, the condition is treated casually or even jokingly and he comes away worse than before. The patient should at least be informed that he suffers from a defect in his emotional development which has interfered with his ability to exercise control over ejaculation and that such a condition is amenable to psychotherapy, rather than being made to feel that he suffers from some organic defect or glandular deficiency which has to be treated by injections, manipulations, or surgery.

Impotence Complete but Interest is Retained in Coitus. There are cases in which the ability to achieve erection is lost and yet emotionally the man is interested in women and interested in functioning sexually with them. Inasmuch as a capacity for erection depends so much upon psychological factors, it is of some importance to distinguish this group from the next group of those having *complete impotence with no interest in coitus.* The man who is impotent and has no interest in coitus is likely to have many more inhibitions and a more severe neurosis underlying his symptoms. Other things being equal, it would take a longer period of treatment in such a case because those factors which were interfering with his interest in sexual functioning would have to be dealt with before getting at the factors which were merely interfering with erection itself.

FEMALES

Occasional Failure to Achieve Orgasm. Women have many fantasies of which they are not aware regarding sexual functioning, and are more sensitive in matters of love and sexuality than men, so that it is not unusual for them to have an occasional failure in achieving orgasm during intercourse. However, it is important to pay some attention to these occasional failures lest they gradually become more than occasional and mark the beginning of a definite problem of frigidity. If the husband neglects or is unable to be ardent in his love-making before intercourse is begun, or if the woman is under special stress (for example, unusual concern with the children) enough psychic energy may be lacking to result in a failure to achieve orgasm. If this happens too frequently, however, it should not be looked upon as something natural but as a defect in the woman's capacity to function normally in the sexual sphere.

Only Occasional Orgasm. In taking the histories of many women patients we are told that their sexual life is "normal." If we inquire a little further and ask if they achieve orgasm or "reach a climax" they reply "of course." As we come to know them better and they in turn learn to speak more freely we find that their capacity for orgasm occurs very occasionally indeed, and that most of the time sex relations occur without orgasm and with a limited amount of pleasure.

Mild Pleasure in Intercourse but No Orgasm. Many women say that they enjoy intercourse, but by this they mean only that in sexual relations there is some mild pleasure as a result of coitus. They achieve little if any increase in sexual pleasure to correspond to the increase in pleasure of the male, and never reach the height of pleasure which ends in orgasm. Most of these women do not know what orgasm really is, not knowing that women are supposed to have a pleasure corresponding with that of the man.

Vaginal Anesthesia with No Special Aversion to Coitus. In this group of cases are the many women who have never allowed themselves to have much sexual feeling. They say that they never became sexually excited during their adolescent years, and either not at all or very mildly excited during their engagement period, or as a result of love-making prior to marriage. Following marriage, they accept intercourse as a responsibility of married life in which they take no pleasure, believing that any pleasure the man derives from intercourse is just one of the many advantages of being a male. In these women, intercourse causes no special discomfort since they feel nothing. They are not aware of dissatisfaction since they have no conscious sexual desire. They are willing to cooperate dutifully in the sexual act in much the same spirit as in keeping the house clean and getting the meals. The husband may protest at the lack of interest shown by such a woman in regard to coitus or he may care little as long as he has an opportunity for sexual expression. Such women are very prone to have neurotic symptoms or to suffer from premenstrual tension, or to have an unusually difficult time during the menopause, because of the fact that the psychosexual needs have never had conscious expression.

Vaginal Anesthesia with Aversion to Coitus. Women in this group derive no pleasure from sexual intercourse and in addition resent it. They feel that they are being exploited, imposed upon, degraded, and made to suffer unnecessarily. They often utilize the fear of pregnancy in order to avoid intercourse. Sometimes they pretend to be menstruating in order to escape participation in the sexual act and they may either distrust contraceptives or deliberately say they do in order to avoid intercourse. In discussing contraception (p. 581) we shall have something to say regarding women who learn the method but fail to continue to use it. Many such women belong to this group.

Dyspareunia and Vaginismus. In some women intercourse is always painful. The pain may be so pronounced as to prevent the insertion of the penis. If the penis can be inserted, pain may be felt only at the beginning or sometimes during the entire act. As one might suppose, abundant and pronounced early life fantasies of the sex act as a horrible, painful, and harmful experience are to be found in the psychological study of these women.

As noted in the chart on page 581, any interference with a free flow of psychic energy into the sexual act may cut down the secretion of the mucous glands of the vagina which is intended to facilitate the act of coitus. In other words, the woman may consciously permit intercourse but unconsciously try to deny entrance to the penis by failing to provide secretion.

CAUSES OF FRIGIDITY AND IMPOTENCE

1. *Fear of disapproval or punishment*
   - (a) Fear of criticism or ridicule.
   - (b) Fear of bodily injury from some disapproving person other than the partner.
   - (c) Fear of pregnancy.

2. *Hostility toward the partner*
   - (a) A general resentment toward the opposite sex with desire to do them harm.
   - (b) The woman resents what she considers domination by the man.
   - (c) The man is envious of the woman and her role in life and refuses to give her pleasure because of this envy.
   - (d) A fear of one of the partners of injuring the genital organs of the other.

3. *Conflicting loves* (usually unconscious)
   - (a) Man loves some other woman and is unconscious of it (mother, sister); or woman loves some other man (father, brother) and cannot accept husband sexually.
   - (b) Latent homosexuality; i. e., persons of the same sex are loved rather than persons of the opposite sex.
   - (c) *Too much self-love.* Love of another person is an overflow from self-love. In these cases there is no love left for the sexual partner.

Fear of Disapproval or Punishment. It has already been pointed out that criticism and ridicule regarding matters pertaining to sex are too often exerted upon the child and adolescent. Masturbation is the first genital sexual act which is indulged in, and this is often severely criticized or ridiculed. Later the same child may be criticized or ridiculed for his attempts to come in contact with the opposite sex in normally acceptable social relations. Through such unfortunate attitudes he comes to associate so much that is shameful or harmful with sexual behavior or with advances toward the opposite sex that it is very difficult to overcome these attitudes after marriage has taken place. The married person still feels that disapproval, criticism, or ridicule are bound to come from some source because of a normal interest in sexual pleasure, and this may prove to be an important factor in determining the onset of impotence or frigidity. Some people never get over a long-standing threat that they will be punished for sexual activities.

Young married couples who have to live in the same home with the parents of one partner may be greatly inhibited in sexual relations, fearing they will be overheard, or fearing that the act of intercourse will be assumed and they will meet with disapproval the following day. In more than one instance we have seen the inability to achieve orgasm cured merely by the young people moving out of the parents' home and taking an apartment of their own. The sense of freedom obtained in this manner was sufficient to remove an inhibiting fear of censure. Sometimes the fantasies in the minds of these young married couples are poorly understood by persons uninstructed in the evils attached to such unfortunate early attitudes as we have just discussed. We have known many a newly married man living in the home of the father or father-in-law who has had the feeling that each morning when he came downstairs he would be soundly thrashed for having had intercourse with his own wife. In the same way the newly married woman meets her parents the next day with the fear that she will be scolded and put out of the house for having had intercourse with her husband.

Fear of Pregnancy. This is one of the most common inhibitors of free sexual expression. It is for this reason that contraceptive advice is so helpful in removing some of the anxiety and hence some of the inhibiting influences connected with sexual intercourse. It goes without saying that this is only one of the more superficial rationalizations of inability to perform normal intercourse and therefore contraceptive advice cannot cure deep-seated inhibitions. On the other hand, there is still a belief common among many women that if they do not become sexually excited and do not have orgasm they will not become pregnant. While there may be a very remote relationship between the orgasm of a woman and the possibility of becoming pregnant it is an everyday occurrence for completely frigid women to become pregnant. In other words, for practical clinical purposes there is no relationship between frigidity and the ability to conceive.

The "Clumsy Male"

Speaking as a gynecologist, Furst mentioned the harmful effects of initiating intercourse in a clumsy manner. He says, "The first cohabitation performed in a rough manner may render every following cohabitation unpleasant, a reaction that may persist for the rest of a woman's life. I use the term 'unpleasant' advisedly, because from the medical standpoint these cases are so slight that they seldom reach the doctor. One discovers them as a kind of side-line problem when women report other complaints. Most of these women have been married for many years and have borne children, yet they complain they have never experienced an orgasm, that they submit to intercourse as a matter of duty, or because they desire to have children. When the physician attempts to ascertain the reason for their lack of response, one invariably elicits the reply, 'It is painful.' By psychotherapy we can successfully treat this very common condition. In such cases it is correct to tell the patient that because of her fear complex she is always inclined to contract her muscles before and during cohabitation, which causes her to suffer pain; but that by 'pressing down' her vagina, as in going to stool, her vagina would open, the muscles would then relax and she would feel no pain. Following this explanation one should demonstrate on an examining table with a gynecological speculum how easy it is to introduce this large speculum into the vagina, when the patient cooperates by pressing down.

"These patients are very grateful for this help and in many cases report later that they have experienced orgasm *for the first time*. These cases are characterized by some gynecologists as 'light' cases. That is a matter of opinion; for many husbands, particularly those who are sexually experienced, do not understand why their wives are so unresponsive to the marital embrace. As a result of this disappointment they may break up their homes, causing misery and misfortune to their families."

Hostility Toward the Partner

Unconscious hostility is one of the common causes of frigidity and impotence. Many men have suffered so much at the hands of their mothers that they never overcome an intense hostility toward women in general. A man so affected may see many desirable qualities in his wife and wish to treat her kindly, but the accumulated unconscious hatred does not permit him to do so. He may have a strong unconscious desire to hurt, punish, or soil her with his penis—a desire so strong that the result is a reaction in quite the opposite direction and he becomes completely impotent. In the same way there is the woman whose relations with her father and brothers have been of such an unfriendly nature that she finds it very difficult to love another man or make him happy with her body. She will not give him the gift of an orgasm nor allow him to make *her* happy. In some cases the woman will actually taunt the man for being unable to arouse her and condemn him for a weakness which is really her own. Some women have grown up so deprived in their own lives and yet seen the advantages accorded to their brothers, that they learn to hate the male genital organ, which seemed to them to be the one reason why brothers had been granted so many privileges which had been denied them. As a result they have no pride in their own sexual organs, feel inferior, and in their envy of the male role are unable to have sexual pleasure.

Attitude of Men. Just as some women are envious of the prerogatives of men there are men who have the same feeling about women. Some men envy women the opportunity to stay at home, to wear pretty clothes, to bear children, and their role of passivity in the sexual act. They resent the attention which women receive. These men are reluctant to give the woman sexual pleasure or to give them a child. They resent having to take care of the woman and child, and unconsciously wish to be taken care of as children themselves. When these passive trends are strong impotence may be the result.

Sadistic Concepts. Some individuals have been brought up with a sadistic concept of sexual relations, fearing that sexual intercourse will result in some harm to themselves or to their partner. Many women have the idea that to participate in sexual relations means to be hurt by the man's sexual organ. Some carry into adulthood a childish fear that the penis is so much larger than the vagina that they will be torn and injured. One patient said, "I know it's foolish but each time I am faced with sex relations I feel I am going to be pierced with a sword." Even if the woman does not have definite fantasies of injury it is likely she may feel that the sexual act is humiliating and degrading and is an act which no man with any kindness and consideration would perpetrate upon a woman. In the same way that women fear injury by the male organ, men fear injury at the hands of the woman. Many stories are told among boys and young men of how the vagina may contract and constrict the penis so that in some cases an operation on the penis has been necessary in order to bring about separation of the couple. While many boys and young men hear these stories and pay little attention to them others take them quite seriously and *never* lose the fear that such an occurrence *could* take place. Of course no such possibility has any basis in fact, but the idea that the vagina is a mysterious organ with possibilities of harm latent within it may have sufficient force to inhibit erection. Further, the fear that the woman may have a venereal disease which will cause the man much pain and incapacity is quite common, and it is well known that this belief is often based on warnings uttered by the parents, intended to keep young people continent, in place of giving a well-rounded, wholesome sexual education.

Just as the partners may fear harm coming from the other, so may they also fear *doing* harm. The fear of injuring the partner in the sexual act may be just as strong and just as inhibiting to satisfactory relations as the fear of being harmed one's self. Of course, just as with many irrational fears, underlying the fear of doing harm to the partner, there is implied some degree of a wish to do this very thing.

Conflicting Loves (Usually Unconscious)

Anyone who has been at all observant knows of cases in which a man has such a strong attachment to his mother that he has very little interest in any other women. Of course, such an attachment with a sister could also take place, or even with some more remote relative who had played an important role in the man's life. Should he become interested in marrying, his early emotional attachment may be so strong as to prevent him from functioning sexually with his wife. Such men will often say, "My wife is a wonderful woman, very capable and very important to me, but I just can't seem to love her in an intimate sexual way." The same conflict in sexual love can take place in the woman who has an overstrong attachment to some man with whom she has been closely related during her developing years. This is most often the father but may be a brother or an uncle. She has never realized the sexual component of this emotional bond and feels that she is in love with her husband until the sex relationship demonstrates the emotional barrier between them. Such women will say, "My marriage seems like that of all my women friends until my husband wants to make love with me physically—then I feel he is an alien, an outsider, as if he were someone I never could know well enough for that."

Latent Homosexuality. There are some individuals who have never developed enough emotionally to be able to love intimately a person of the opposite sex. Their interests and emotional satisfactions lie with those of the same sex, and sexual relationships with those of the opposite sex seem meaningless. The latently homosexual woman remains frigid and the latently homosexual man is likely to be completely or partially impotent.

Bearing on this question are the important studies by Kinsey, who finds "that something between a quarter and a half of all males have demonstrated their capacity to respond to homosexual stimuli; that the picture is one of endless intergradation between every combination of homosexuality and heterosexuality; that it is impossible to distinguish so-called acquired, latent, and congenital types; and that there is every gradation between so-called 'actives' and 'passives' in a homosexual relation."

Taking issue with theories of homosexuality based on urinary hormone findings Kinsey asserts "any hormonal or other explanation of the homosexual must allow for the fact that both homosexual and heterosexual activites may occur coincidentally in a single period in the life of an individual; and that exclusive activities of any one type may be exchanged, in the brief span of a few days or a few weeks, for an exclusive pattern of the other type, or into a combination pattern which embraces the two types.

"Any explanation of the homosexual must recognize that a large portion of the younger adolescents demonstrate the capacity to react to both homosexual and heterosexual stimuli; that there is a fair number of adults who show this same capacity; and that there is only a gradual development of the exclusively homosexual or exclusively heterosexual patterns which predominate among older adults."

Self-Love. Again there are some individuals with such great self-love that they have little emotion free with which to love other people. They have difficulty in sharing even time and effort with anyone else, let alone having that amount of energy directed toward others which is necessary for sexual relationship. Such a state of affairs is frequently seen in the severely neurotic and the latently psychotic. They are entirely absorbed in concern with their aches and pains or their bizarre ideas about themselves or the outside world, and they have no thought or interest in sexual functioning. However, as we leave this extremely pathological group we come to some people in the ordinary walks of life who may be doing a fairly good piece of work, all of whose available energy is channeled into this activity. For instance, a man may have a work project which means a great deal to him. He works and dreams of the success and acclaim which will be his, and is so preoccupied with his work and his dreams that he has no interest or energy for sexual functioning with a woman. Certain artistic temperaments fall into this group.

There are women who may be doing good work but the interest they center upon themselves in relation to their work and the prestige obtained through it, or their interest in clothes, jewelry, and the appearance they make or the social success they can achieve, occupy them to such an extent that they have no emotion left over for loving a man in a sexual way and giving him anything so personal and intimate of themselves as sexual feelings. Some women can extend their feelings of self-love to cover their children and take great pride in the children and their appearance and the children's success as though the children were part of themselves. To these women a sex relationship with a man is only a means to an end, and it does not enter their thinking to share with him a feeling of pleasure during the sexual act.

Effect on Spouse. These people who try to be so complete within themselves and will not permit themselves to be dependent upon their marital partners for the emotional satisfaction which sexual relation affords are often very baffling to their spouses, who feel left out, excluded, and eventually inferior. Such self-absorption on the part of a woman often drives the man to a house of prostitution or to a mistress who gives him something which the wife never does, namely something of herself emotionally. When the husband is of this self-loving and self-contained type the wife is usually in a somewhat more difficult position. It is not so easy for women to seek extramarital relationships, and they often suffer in silence, become hostile, and develop neurotic symptoms.

Psychosomatic Problems of Frigidity

It is easily understandable that the effect of frigidity on the woman is different from that of impotence on the man. Whereas an impotent man is incapacitated in regard to the act of intercourse, a frigid woman submits to the wishes of her husband and the lack of enjoyment leads to indifference, resentment, or even disgust. Growing out of these reactions are various physical problems. Ruesch and his associates, in a monograph devoted to a study of chronic disease and psychological invalidism, discussed some of these problems.

The life histories of the frigid women in their series resembled each other closely. They were characterized by a high rate of marriages, marriages at an early age, greater than average divorce rate, and a large number of medical experiences and operations. There was a great lack of love and security in their childhood. Marriage often served the purpose of breaking away from home at an early age, looking for security and love, and to prove that they were grown-up people.

The Abuse of Surgery

One of the most frequent syndromes encountered in Ruesch's patients was that of the patient with a history of many abdominal operations. The case is cited of the girl who marries early and soon afterwards develops abdominal pain, which is followed by appendectomy. At short intervals other abdominal operations follow; finally ovaries, tubes, and uterus are removed. The castration effect of the loss of the uterus is often a great blow from which a woman may find it impossible to recover.

Unfortunately attention to the emotional life usually comes only after irreparable damage has been done. (p. 407)

One or more major operations occurred in more than 65 per cent of frigid women contrasted with about 40 per cent in nonfrigid women. Ruesch commented as follows regarding the abuse of surgery:

"In surgery, as in all other disciplines of medicine, there exist fashion trends. In case of doubt the choice between conservative treatment or operative treatment will be decided by the personality of the patient, the personality of the surgeon, and the fashion trend. A large percentage of our women, for instance, had a small ovarian cyst removed at the time of their appendectomy. According to competent gynecological opinion there is no factual indication for such procedure. While this large-scale castration of women is in part due to old-fashioned medical concepts, it is in part also a function of the personality of these "operators." They start with intention of removing the cyst, underestimate the difficulty, and have to proceed with an ovarectomy. While these men would seriously consider and hesitate in removing a testis, they castrate women by the hundred. This practice reflects the mutual satisfaction of the needs of both patient and operator. The surgeon with his aggressive personality castrates the woman, and she in turn seeks this aggressive action in order to gratify her masochistic tendencies." (pp. 383, 483)

Many patients who avoid surgery nevertheless abuse medicines, diet, and rest, (page 313). Not only vitamins but sleeping tablets and cathartics are among the worst offenders.

Related problems are illustrated by a recent experience: A plumber's wife complained of pain in the back, nervousness, and fatigue (a familiar triad in gynecologic practice) and, as so often happens in such cases, the gynecologist found a reason to operate and the patient gladly assented. (Anything is welcomed to escape the environment and enjoy a rest in the hospital, being waited upon by nurses, and so forth.) For a time after the operation the patient seemed better but then began to complain of headache, nervousness, and even greater fatigue. By this time her plumber husband had been presented with a sizable bill. He visited the gynecologist to complain that his wife was no better; in fact she was worse. The gynecologist insisted that the new trouble was unrelated to the old—that it was "mental." "Listen," he said, in defense, "if someone gives you a job to fix the pipes in the cellar and then the roof starts to leak, that isn't your fault, is it?"

EMOTIONS AND MENSTRUATION

We might well begin by examining some of the prevalent attitudes toward the normal function of menstruation. An excellent monograph on the "Psychological Effects of Menstruation" by Chadwick should be read by every practitioner of medicine. It treats of the many emotional attitudes toward menstruation held by both ancient and modern cultural groups as well as by the individual. All races have shown guilt over menstruation and according to their folklore they have needed some impersonal or plausible way to explain its occurrence. To account for the onset of menstruation at puberty there was an early belief that some snake or wild animal had injured the girl, or that the spirit of an ancestor had had intercourse with her. The idea grew that the monthly flow of blood in the woman was accompanied by cruel and hostile wishes within her, and as a result, women were dangerous at this period and needed special taboos erected against them, and some degree of seclusion from others, lest harm arise from contact with them.

Menstrual Taboos

It is important to consider these old beliefs and superstitions because, as we know, such beliefs die out slowly in mankind. Many centuries of education and enlightenment are necessary for the individual to be entirely rid of their influence. We must admit that the girl of today, while not told exactly the same things as her sister of a thousand years ago, is nevertheless placed under certain restrictions and taboos just the same, and many superstitions are established for her concerning the menstrual function. In our society it is common for a man to regard a menstruating woman as dirty and disgusting, and so she often regards herself, and this may be in part responsible for this fear or anxiety on the part of one or the other, or both. Some groups of people have menstrual taboos which are intended to protect the man against the dangers of the menstruating woman. In these groups the menstruating woman, her bed, and her clothes are dangerous to the man and should not be touched until eight days after the cessation of the menstrual period, and until after the woman has completely immersed herself in water. (See p. 669).

Anxiety and Superstition

Women, likewise, have anxieties, suspicions, and superstitions relating to menstruation. They often refer to themselves as "being ill" during the time of the menstrual period. They often do not dare to bathe during this time and only wash themselves to the waist. Many women prefer to remain in bed for a day or two because they were taught to do so by their mothers or some other woman, lest the bleeding become too profuse or stop completely if they go about their work in the usual manner. Among certain people menstruating women are forbidden to sew, to knead bread, to handle cut flowers, to preserve fruit, or to water young plants. While menstruating, a woman's touch is considered capable of blighting crops, withering gardens, bringing fruit from trees, killing saplings, turning wine to vinegar, or causing mares to miscarry. If we ask why the menstruating woman is regarded as so dangerous to growing things, the following answer has been suggested: In primitive tribes menstruation was regarded as a sign of sexual excitement. As culture changed, the sexually excitable woman was regarded as a danger to the stability of the home, and to the legitimacy of the heir. This original connection of sexual excitement and menstruation has been lost and remaining we have the taboo against menstruation itself. Nevertheless, many civilized women still exhibit considerably increased sexual excitement around the time of the menstrual period.

Childhood Fantasies

Many people of both sexes regard menstruation as unpleasant or dirty because they associate the menstrual flow with urine or with feces, in short, an unpleasant excretion which cannot be controlled. They feel that a discharge from that portion of the body must be regarded as dirty or contaminated. In both sexes, menstruation arouses some anxiety because the bleeding stirs up some childhood fantasy that an injury has been done to the female and this *same* injury could occur to the male. Some women regard menstruation as a repeated confirmation *each* month of a belief that they have injured themselves through masturbation.

Effect on Children

Chadwick thinks it is important that the child is subject, year after year, to the effect of a periodically recurring indisposition of the mother at the time of the menstrual period. At these times she may be irritable, self-centered, often depressed, and may remain in bed a day or two. At the same time, children, because of their curiosity or because of the carelessness of the mother, become aware that bleeding is taking place. Rarely is any explanation given and the child is left to draw its own conclusions, which are often bizarre but fairly certain to include the idea of injury and pain. Menstrual bleeding stirs up anxiety and fear of *genital mutilation* in the minds of both the little girl and the little boy. At the onset of menstruation the girl is often treated unkindly and unsympathetically, is not enlightened by the mother, and hence concludes that she has some unspeakable condition for which she feels unpopular and cast out. The girl realizes that she is experiencing something about which people just cannot express themselves. She feels the hostility of everyone for being in this state. She regards herself as unclean and unwanted by her parents, her brothers and sisters, and society in general. At this time activities and pleasures have to be curtailed, or at least she is too often told that this should be the case. With all of this taking place in the mind of the child at puberty, not to mention what takes place afterward, it is small wonder that women grow morose and irritable as this phenomenon recurs each month.

Hostility

In the female child who may have been envious of the privileges of masculinity and who still had the hope of some day growing into a boy, these hopes are blasted when menstruation begins at puberty. The bleeding is a very definite evidence of the need to accept the feminine role, and if the advantages of the latter have not been portrayed to her, this realization may have a very saddening effect. Furthermore, many girls approach puberty and menstruation with some hope that when menstruation begins they will be accepted by the mother and the sisters and other women into a greater intimacy and friendship. They often find that this does not take place since the whole subject is one with which women generally associate little dignity or prestige. Hence the girl finds that she has all the discomforts of menstruation and none of the advantages of her growing maturity. Thus we see this phenomenon of menstruation as one which, each time it occurs, stirs up fantasies of hostility toward both sexes—toward women because the mother let her be born that way, and toward men because of envy of the freedom to which their organs seem to entitle them.

DYSMENORRHEA

Dysmenorrhea is a symptom rather than a disease. It occurs with great frequency. In a study of a large group of student nurses dysmenorrhea occurred in 52 per cent. It may be due to pelvic disease but usually occurs in the absence of any recognizable cause and is then spoken of as functional dysmenorrhea. Montgomery suggests that even when pelvic lesions exist caution must be exercised in attributing menstrual pain to the disease process, such for example as displacement of the uterus or a simple cyst of the ovary, which may have little effect in the production of dysmenorrhea. The mere existence of some abnormality in the pelvis is not positive proof that it is the cause of menstrual pain. That is the reason why careful study, prolonged observation, and the psychosomatic approach are important before surgical measures are tried.

Clinical Aspects

In addition to pain various other symptoms are frequently encountered such as general lassitude, headache, gastrointestinal disturbances, mental depression, and emotional instability. The explanations that are usually advanced for menstrual pain are mechanical obstruction of the cervical canal, hypoplasia of the pelvic organs, congestion, and other vascular disturbances, constitutional defects such as structural or physiological inadequacies, endocrine disturbances, allergy and psychogenic factors. It is usually stated that no one theory adequately explains all cases and, like many other psychosomatic problems that we have discussed, in the majority of instances there is probably more than one cause. It is probable that a structural or physiological problem plus a psychological factor may be in the background of a large number of cases.

A General Problem

Therefore, so-called *functional dysmenorrhea* presents a general more than simply a pelvic problem, and a general survey rather than just a pelvic examination is essential before treatment can be instituted. A general physical examination not only may reveal organic disease but gives information concerning general nutrition, constitutional defects, endocrine abnormalities and neurological disturbances. Examination of the pelvis may reveal evidence of genital hypoplasia, such as poorly developed external genitalia, short interior vaginal wall, shallow posterior fornix, infantile-like cervix and acute pathologic anteflexion of the uterus. Psychological study often reveals emotional instability and a background of psychoneurotic tendencies such as we shall discuss shortly. In the majority of instances of functional dysmenorrhea we deal with young unmarried women and emphasis upon mild anatomic or developmental anomalies of pelvic organs, persistent and ill-advised local or surgical treatment, or a long series of injections of questionable value, may give temporary benefit but in the long run are distinctly harmful. In this connection let us refer once more to the statement made by Clifford Allbutt in 1884 regarding a neuralgic woman (p. 7). Dysmenorrhea may occur, like many other neurotic symptoms, in women who do not "appear" nervous. The fact that a patient appears calm and poised does not exclude a psychogenic cause for this symptom.

Psychological Study

In personality studies on patients with dysmenorrhea Wittkower and Wilson found that many patients suffering from dysmenorrhea had been either unusually aggressive and boisterous tomboys resenting their feminine role or ailing, complaining children unwilling or unable to give up their childish dependence on their parents and possessing strong needs or cravings for sympathy and protection. As adults the dysmenorrhea patients were deeply resentful of their feminine role or obviously immature physically and either shy and shut-in or chronically anxious and complaining.

Nature of Sexual Fantasies

Others have noted the physical masculine attributes—voice, hair, bones—that coexist with distinct masculine attitudes and aversions against the female role. This is by no means the rule, however, and often an absolutely female habitus exists along with the same emotional conflicts. Karen Horney noted that dysmenorrhea usually starts, if not at puberty, at the time when the patient comes in contact with adult sex problems. In patients suffering from this condition there are unconscious fantasies of the sex act as something cruel, bloody, and painful. One of her patients felt sexually aroused whenever she heard or read of cruelty. (See illustrative case, p. 468.) She described the pain which she had at the time of menstruation "as if her insides were being torn out." As a child she had the idea that in intercourse the man tore something out from the body of the woman. In her dysmenorrhea she emotionally acted out these fantasies.

While the subject is far from solved there is enough evidence to suggest that the psychosomatic approach is essential in the study of functional dysmenorrhea and certainly should precede any attempts to cure the condition by surgical means.

PREMENSTRUAL TENSION

It is well known to every physician and to many husbands that women are prone to undergo certain emotional changes for a varying period preceding menstruation, sometimes terminating when the menstrual flow begins, and sometimes continuing until the menstrual flow has ceased. The term *premenstrual tension* has been applied to this syndrome. Important symptoms are a varying degree of depression of spirits and irritability, headache, insomnia, outbursts of crying, physical unrest, a sensation of the entire body described as "being jittery" or a feeling that "they would like to jump out of their skin." This syndrome is usually attributed to menstruation by the patient and is often explained by the physician on the basis of dysfunction of the endocrine glands. Many glandular preparations have been used in its treatment. Medical writers, in discussing this syndrome, often refer to the 40 or more per cent of *normal women* who suffer from this condition. There are others, however, who disagree with the point of view that these are normal women. They regard these symptoms as being evidences of an underlying neurosis and hence due to the expression of unconscious fantasies. They believe that if endocrine imbalances or deficiencies exist, they are either secondary to the underlying psychological disturbance, or just another phase of the disturbed psychosomatic make-up. Hence, it would be understandable that endocrine therapy might produce temporary alleviation of symptoms, either by substitution or through the effect of suggestion, but in neither case would the deeper cause of the condition be eradicated.

Premenstrual Tension;
Relief from Superficial Psychotherapy

CASE 51

A white woman of thirty-nine complained that for a year or more she had been tense and "jittery," demanding and quarrelsome, and suffered crying spells for several days before the menstrual period. She expressed herself as worried that she could no longer "cope with things."

History and Symptoms

There had been no serious previous illnesses. The menses had begun at fifteen; there was always some irregularity and dysmenorrhea. The patient had been married for fifteen years and had two children, both of whom were well. The husband, who was the same age as the patient, suffered from neuralgic pains which the patient thinks "have something to do with her."

She came from a large family, the members of which she described as emotionally well adjusted and of whom she stated, "They all got along together nicely."

Physical Examination

The general physical examination disclosed no evidence of organic disease and routine laboratory studies were within normal limits. Pelvic examination revealed a low-grade endocervicitis which had been cauterized successfully.

LIFE SITUATION

The patient stated that she thought her trouble was due to "change of life" and hoped that the slight pelvic operation together with hormone injections would help her. She was reluctant to talk about her family, insisting that all was well and that no blame could be attached to her emotional life. She did admit, however, that she had become "a little more irritable" with her husband and owing to the fact that "he had also changed" there had been a good deal of quarreling between them.

Husband's Illness. Some four years previously the husband had begun to suffer from neuralgic pains and after receiving a great deal of treatment finally found his way into the hands of a physician who placed the responsibility on his relation to his work and his attitude toward his family. As a result the husband's pains seemed to diminish but at the same time "his attitude changed" so that he was no longer so subservient to his boss as he had formerly been and acted differently toward his wife, and she was "not so sure she liked it."

Husband's Family. After the above discussion the patient had less trouble talking about herself. She spoke of the manner in which her husband had been "taken advantage of" by his family and how she, of course, also had to bear the brunt of this responsibility. She complained, moreover, that she had devoted herself to her husband when he was ill and now she is "taken for granted."

Subsequent Course

The following month the patient reluctantly admitted that she felt better but expressed the belief that she had "talked too much" on her previous visits and "felt silly" about returning. She had no objection to visiting the gynecologist for a checkup but thought it unnecessary to talk about herself further. She did confess, however, that she was worried about the emotional upbringing of her children. She did not want them to have the difficulties that she and her husband had experienced. On this basis she was encouraged to talk further about her family, which she did with essentially the same trend as before.

SUMMARY

A woman approaching the menopausal age suffered from typical premenstrual tension. Pelvic surgery and hormonal injections failed to help her but superficial psychotherapy, which gave reassurance that she was not "changing life" and at the same time permitted her to vent some hostile feelings, accomplished satisfactory relief of symptoms.

Encouragement to talk about her feelings raised certain resistances, but these were expressed in a satisfactory manner with the result that the patient was able to benefit from the treatment and at the same time maintain a good relationship with her physician.

Follow-up a year later showed that she had remained free from symptoms.

AMENORRHEA

Few studies have been done on this subject by those working in psychosomatic medicine. One reason has been that amenorrhea, to an even greater extent than the conditions just discussed, has been assumed to be caused by a defect in the endocrine system and endocrine therapy has been prescribed. The second reason is that amenorrhea is not a particularly distressing or incapacitating symptom, and hence study has not been so urgently demanded. Nevertheless, Dunbar in her book on "Emotions and Bodily Changes" gives a number of references to observations which European observers have made on this subject. They felt that a large number of cases of amenorrhea seen during the war were due more to the lack of men than lack of nourishment. The condition was found in well-nourished women as well as in the undernourished, and often disappeared as soon as opportunities for sexual relations with men were restored, even though coitus did not actually take place.

Some very interesting observations on the subject of amenorrhea were made in an internment camp in the Philippines during World War II. Among 1042 women of menstrual age (American or British) Whitacre and Barrera found 125 patients with amenorrhea which had developed since the outbreak of the war. Of sixty nurses who had been through the campaigns of Bataan or Corregidor, 50 per cent exhibited menstrual disturbances; amenorrhea was present in 23 per cent. In many of these patients the menses stopped abruptly after the first bombing of Manila, or soon after internment and before a food deficiency could have had any effect. The physiologic amenorrhea of pregnancy, or the fear of it, was ruled out as a cause, and patients with chronic diseases were omitted. It seemed clear that emotional shock was responsible. In spite of the difficulties under which they worked an effort was made to study ovarian and anterior-pituitary-like gonadotropic excretion. In two selected patients estrogen was absent from the urine while gonadotropin was present, probably in increased amount. The investigators felt that worry and fear, acting through the autonomic nervous system, had caused a complete suppression of ovarian function. Most of the women overcame the difficulty within a few months and the good results were probably due to psychological influences.

Cases of amenorrhea cured by hypnosis have been reported. In fact, through hypnosis it has been possible to regulate menstruation so as to have it occur on the same day of the month, regardless of the number of days in the month preceding.

Unconscious Influences

It is well known that the wish to be pregnant may result in amenorrhea and distention of the abdomen. On the other hand, fear of an unwanted pregnancy may cause cessation of the menstrual flow for a month or longer. That is to say, the menstrual flow, while linked up with ovarian function and tending to follow a definite cycle, nevertheless seems to be under the control of the emotions in the same way, if not to the same extent, as the secretion of tears, saliva, and perspiration. Emotions quite profoundly regulate the discharge or retention of secretions, and in the case of the menstrual flow, may have as powerful an effect as the endocrine regulatory mechanism itself.

LEUKORRHEA

Here again, as in the subject of amenorrhea, the majority of studies along psychological lines have been made by Europeans. Dunbar has collected the observations of the outstanding authorities. E. Graefenberg stated that the psychogenic component of leukorrhea is little disputed. Psychogenic leukorrhea is particularly resistant to the customary gynecological treatment, and for this reason patients often go from physician to physician until the psychological background of the condition has been recognized. One case was reported by Bunneman in which the patient's leukorrhea had stubbornly persisted for twelve years in spite of all gynecologic procedures. It was cured by hypnosis. After a year's time the leukorrhea began again following sexual excitement. It again disappeared in response to hypnotic suggestion and remained absent for six months. In order to convince himself that the cessation of the symptom could not possibly have been an accidental coincidence Bunneman brought it back again by suggestion.

Naussauer termed leukorrhea the "headache" of the lower abdomen, thus indicating that it develops without disease of the genital organs. Mayer felt that unconscious sexual ideas led to hyperemia and hypersecretion in the genital region with a decrease in tonus of the smooth musculature.

Psychological Factors

Two cases of leukorrhea in which psychological factors seemed important have been observed by one of us. In the first the symptom was precipitated by constant sexual excitement from much erotic fantasy occuring each day. Treatment was not sought for this symptom alone, even though it was rather annoying at times. Inquiry revealed that following marriage and satisfactory sexual adjustment and the living out of the sexual fantasies and erotic desires, the leukorrhea disappeared.

Another case was observed in a quite different type of personality. This patient was single, twenty-one years of age, and came from a very happy home. As a result of large quantities of repressed hostility she had frequent cramps and diarrhea which would last for days at a time. She had been treated as a case of colitis. After months of intensive psychiatric treatment and readjustment of the personality the colitis was cured. In the course of treatment, however, it was observed that when diarrhea was controlled there was a leukorrheal discharge. Both of these symptoms cleared up simultaneously and it seemed that the leukorrhea, like the diarrhea, was a production from the body of something unpleasant, one purpose of which was to vent repressed ill-feelings upon the environment.

From the accumulating evidence it surely is a physician's duty in a case of leukorrhea in which disease or infection does not seem responsible, to inquire of the patient what ideas are associated with the discharge, and to acquaint the patient with the existing knowledge of what such a discharge may mean from the standpoint of behavior.

FUNCTIONAL URINARY DISTURBANCES

It is quite well recognized in medicine that functional disturbances of urination may depend upon emotional factors. Nocturia in a medical history does not necessarily mean kidney or prostatic disease but may indicate a functional disorder. The bladder, like the stomach, may register emotional disturbances. The difficulty has been, as with so many problems in psychosomatic medicine, in having some practical approach which the patient could understand and which could be of actual value to him in the control of his symptoms.

A Substitute for Sexual Activity

The function of urination from the physiological standpoint is periodically to relieve the discomfort of accumulated urine within the bladder. However, this function may serve different psychological ends. It has a pleasurable erotic component in children as urination is the first excitement and source of gratification associated with the genital organs. It is the fore-runner, so to speak, of later orgastic pleasure in coitus. Bed-wetting is succeeded by masturbation and nocturnal emissions and the prohibitions of the toilet are succeeded by the prohibitions of society against sexuality. Hence just as various sexual acts may be resorted to surreptitiously for sources of gratification so urinary symptoms may represent at a more unconscious level a substitute for sexual activity. It is quite common for women to have frequency of urination when thrown in company with the opposite sex. Children and adolescents will often have an erotic dream and awaken to find that they have urinated in bed. Adults will often dream of urination accompanied by highly pleasurable sensations and men may awaken to find that there has been a seminal emission.

Aggressive Component

The *aggressive component in urination* is well shown in our coarser vituperative language since expressions referring to urinating or defecating upon the victim or the hated person are so common. Such ideas date back to early childhood when the child discovers that the contents of the body can be used to express hostility. Children and adults often urinate with marked frequency, the idea expressed to those in authority being, "Since you want me to behave properly and not wet myself *or anyone else* you must let me go to the toilet any time I like." This may be a very time-consuming and wasteful gesture in a group of workers. They capitalize in an aggressive way upon a necessity which cannot be refused. Finally, frequency of urination may be used to punish one's self in that it leads to great inconvenience and the necessity of curtailing social life. A reduction of usefulness takes place just as in phobic behavior or in the compulsion neuroses.

Lack of Emotional Control

In short, a persisting defect in sphincter control means a lack in emotional control either in the erotic or aggressive parts of the personality or both. If these secret childish erotic desires or aggressive impulses can be discovered by the physician and explained to the patient the urinary frequency can be cured as the patient learns to express himself more maturely.

A woman of twenty-five years who was subject to attacks of mild anxiety and irritability with the people in her environment had urinary frequency. No physical cause could be discovered. As a child she remembered telling her younger brother that if he did not stop teasing her she would urinate on his bed and on his clean clothes. We told her, "Obviously you were saying with your bladder what you could not adequately express with your tongue. Try to be more realistic in your contacts with people." After a few weeks her behavior at home and at work became more mature and her urinary frequency ceased.

A married woman of twenty-three years was troubled with the desire to urinate whenever she became sexually aroused. This sexual excitement might come about through dancing with a man or even sitting beside him, or by stories which pictured sexual situations. In spite of this easily aroused eroticism in a social situation she was *frigid* in sexual relations with her husband. She had received no sexual information as a girl and did not realize what a woman should experience in the sexual relation.

We explained that both the clitoris and vaginal wall should be sensitive to pleasure and said, "The first pleasurable erotic sensations in the human being occur in connection with urination. But you are no longer a child and what you feel should be transferred from the urethra to the vagina proper." This state of affairs was explained to the husband who was an understanding and considerate person. The patient expressed vaguely formed beliefs that women who felt pleasure in intercourse were not virtuous. She was assured that this was not the case and that urinary urgency was no more virtuous than vaginal excitement. She also felt that to feel too much pleasure in her vagina might lead to infidelity on her part. We told her we believed she was well able to control this.

Reeducation in thinking and feeling about sexual activity resulted in removal of the frigidity and coincidental disappearance of the urinary urgency in eight treatment sessions. In other words, the urinary frequency was a childish substitute for a normal sexual feeling which she should have experienced. In helping her to advance to the normal sexual adjustment the need for perverted pleasure in the urethral area was removed.

Chapter XVIII

THE GENITO-URINARY SYSTEM AND THE SEXUAL FUNCTION (Concluded)

TREATMENT

Disturbances of Sexual Functioning

Treatment of all the neuroses and all psychosomatic conditions requires some treatment of the sexual function. As stated in the introduction the sexual function is almost invariably impaired in the various neuroses and psychosomatic states. So true is this that the degree of sexual impairment often serves as a crude index to the degree of neurotic disturbance. In other words it is one phase of the disturbed personality development and as such demands treatment. Some cases will need more attention to the sexual life than others. Naturally in a neurosis in which actual frigidity or impotence is present, every effort should be made to bring about a cure of this condition. Because, while not in itself the cause of the neurosis, it may constitute the most serious symptom or may add to the total problem of treatment. When a personality disturbance is interfering with sexual functioning it means that one of the important means of drawing emotional sustenance from the environment is cut off and therefore needs treatment along with other aspects of the personality problem, in order to strengthen the emotional resources of that patient. Hence it should be made clear to the patient that impotence and frigidity are not personal peculiarities which must be kept hidden but are fairly common conditions which can be treated psychologically. Even though impotence and frigidity are only two of the many symptoms that may occur in a neurosis, it seemed best, because of their special importance, to discuss their treatment here rather than in the chapters devoted to the general aspects of treatment.

Eliciting History

We suggest the following procedure for eliciting the psychopathology which underlies these conditions:

Obtain complete life history of the patient according to the personality outline (p. 62) but with special emphasis on the following topics:

1. Did the parents seem to be in love with each other?
2. Were they affectionate with each other and tolerant of a demonstration of affection in others?

3. Did the patient receive any sexual education and if so, when?

4. What was the attitude of the parents toward sex matters? [Three general attitudes commonly found in parents: Sexual expression was (a) accepted; (b) condemned; (c) ignored—worst of all!]

5. Were sexual matters regarded as disgusting? Why?

6. Was any care taken in sexual education to separate sexual functioning from the excretory function?

7. Was there any religious attitude in the home which made sexual pleasure incompatible with ethical standards?

8. Were love of the opposite sex and sexual expression associated or not?

9. Were fears cultivated over sexual expression, such, for example, as the evil results of masturbation, the pain of venereal disease, or the shame and disgrace of illegitimate pregnancy?

10. Was sexual indulgence pictured as mean or hateful, disgraceful, or frivolous?

11. Was there any excessive emotional attachment to either parent?

12. Were the social and procreative roles of man and woman, respectively, clearly outlined during the period of psychosexual growth?

13. What evidences are there from scrutiny of the patient's history of social behavior to indicate homosexual love or too much self-love?

14. Was there much, or any masturbation, during adolescence and prior to marraige? If not, what was the reason for its absence?

15. Was there much spontaneous genital feeling aroused through the reading of romantic stories, petting, dancing, or as a result of daydreams about the opposite sex? If not, what reason is given?

Summary

1. What wrong attitudes and feelings exist in the patient which must be changed?

2. What new attitudes and feelings must be learned in order to create the proper attitudes for sexual functioning?

Physician's Attitudes

It is very important that the physician who intends to assist patients in a better sexual adjustment should believe in the importance of a good sexual adjustment for good emotional health. At the same time he himself must not have too many prejudices or condemnations concerning sexual behavior. Otherwise the patient will sense the physician's prejudices or condemnation and will be unable to tell the real truth about himself.

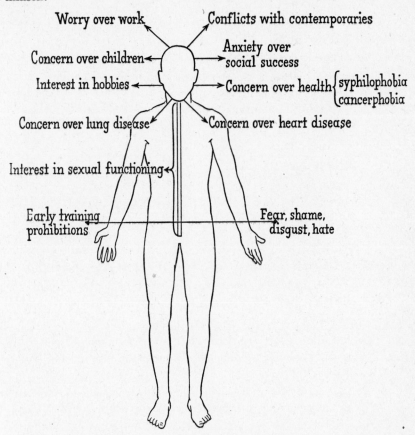

Worry over work

Conflicts with contemporaries

Concern over children

Anxiety over social success

Interest in hobbies

Concern over health {syphilophobia, cancerphobia

Concern over lung disease

Concern over heart disease

Interest in sexual functioning

Early training prohibitions

Fear, shame, disgust, hate

Fig. 8. This diagram is an attempt to show graphically how certain factors may cause impotence and frigidity. Early educational prohibitions to the personality are sufficiently strong to prevent psychic energy from finding its way into the genital function, and this energy is expended to excess in many other channels. To effect a cure, redistribution of psychological energy is necessary. Anxiety and false beliefs must be relieved so that energy can be withdrawn from an area where it is being needlessly expended, such as worry over heart disease or worry over work, and allowed to flow into the genital region.

Contraception

One of the common problems which soon presents itself in discussing any difficulty in sexual adjustment is the matter of contraception. As physicians, we want to know whether contraception is being used and if the method is satisfactory. Is it comfortable, is it reliable, and is there any conflict over its use? It must be admitted that no absolutely reliable

contraceptive exists today, short of the removal of the uterus or both
ovaries. The contraceptive technics commonly used are withdrawal,
vaginal douches, observance of the so-called safe periods, or the use of
some mechanical device. Neither withdrawal nor vaginal douches are
very reliable, nor is the safe period at all reliable for women with irregularity in the menstrual cycle. The mechanical devices most commonly
used are rubber or fishskin protective sheaths, vaginal rubber diaphragms,
cervical caps of metal or hard rubber, jellies, foam tablets, suppositories,
sponges, or combinations of these devices. All of these methods are safe
as far as the patient's health is concerned when used according to proper
instructions by the physician, but they vary as to reliability. While
most vaginal devices are harmless when properly used, intracervical
or intrauterine appliances, on the other hand, may be harmful. Foreign bodies placed in the cervix or within the uterine cavity may cause an
infection, or may set up an irritation which might be a factor in starting
neoplastic growths. Consequently, if the responsibility of contraception
is assumed by the woman it should be by means of some intravaginal
procedure.

The Rubber Diaphragm as a Contraceptive Device. The contraceptive technic which utilizes a flexible rubber diaphragm plus a spermicidal jelly which can be inserted by the woman herself before each coitus,
has now been quite generally accepted as the most satisfactory means of
contraception. The rubber diaphragm covers the cervix of the uterus,
and combined with spermicidal jelly, the safety factor is nearly 100 per
cent. When we say this we mean that studies of many women over a
period of many years have demonstrated its great value when used intelligently. The cases which appear to be failures have been traced to
faulty insertion of the diaphragm, or failure to use the contraceptive
jelly, or to some carelessness on the part of the couple themselves. The
woman must be given a diaphragm of the proper size and be taught how
to insert it correctly. Usually she is made to practice the procedure a
few days and then return and demonstrate to the physician that she can
perform the manipulation correctly. The diaphragm is left in place for
eight hours after coitus, at which time a douche of plain water is used
and the diaphragm removed, dried and kept in a clean place until used
again.

Contraception and Anxiety. There can no longer be any question
regarding the necessity for planned parenthood. This makes it important
that a satisfactory contraceptive method be made available and this in
turn will give married people freedom from what may be termed normal
anxiety in their sexual relations. It is true that some people have scruples
against the use of contraception, but these scruples seem to be diminishing

each year as the importance of human health and happiness are given a more prominent place in our thinking.

There are some women who do not want to use a diaphragm and jelly for contraception because they regard the procedure as too messy, or because they claim that they feel uncomfortable when retaining the diaphragm after coitus. Some women feel that the responsibility for contraception should be assumed by the man through the use of condoms or by withdrawal. They feel that to assume the responsibility of contraception lowers their dignity and makes them appear too interested in the sexual act. Some women claim that they just cannot trust such a contraceptive device. Naturally we have to suspect the motives of these women; they usually have long-standing prejudices against the sexual act itself, and their expressed reasons against contraception are excuses or rationalizations because they wish to do nothing to facilitate intercourse.

Deliberate Accidents. These attitudes are only present in women with some frigidity, and rather than try to convince them about the faulty attitude toward contraception one must take up the more fundamental question of the frigidity itself. Many subtle problems arise. A woman may have strong religious scruples against the use of contraception but overcome them sufficiently to try to use the method. Failure may result from a "deliberate accident." She is either deliberately or unconsciously careless in the use of the method because she cannot circumvent the anxiety resulting from a conflict over a deviation from her life-long beliefs.

The diaphragm and jelly is usually a much more satisfactory contraceptive device for both the man and the woman than the use of a condom. A much smaller surface of foreign material is introduced between the sexual organs, thereby giving both parties more capacity for pleasure.

The Practice of Withdrawal. Withdrawal is an unsatisfactory method of contraception from the standpoint of sexual pleasure and because it is not easy to control, pregnancy may occur. Withdrawal causes a separation of the genital organs at a time when the greatest emotional exchange between the partners should be taking place and therefore often does not permit sufficient sexual excitement in the woman to bring about orgasm. It may produce a feeling of unrest and anxiety in either or both parties, and lead to a state of general dissatisfaction. It is widely practiced but must be condemned.

Some cases of frigidity due to a fear of pregnancy, and without deeper and more complicated psychological background, can be cured by the use of a contraceptive method which the patient can trust. We believe the number of cases in which this can take place is relatively small, but forms, nevertheless, a definite group.

Contraceptive instruction should be a part of every medical school curriculum and a birth control clinic a part of its associated hospital work.

While physicians as individuals have become more liberal in regard to imparting contraceptive advice the medical profession as a whole remains conservative to the point of refusing to recommend contraception except in cases of serious organic disease.

The Fallacy of Pregnancy as a Cure for Neurosis

Moreover, it is not unusual for many organically minded physicians to recommend pregnancy and parenthood as a cure for neurotic illness, instability in the husband, or threatened divorce or separation. This prescription is rarely if ever of value. It is a pretty safe rule that the unstable person will not be helped by becoming a parent, but will usually be made worse as a result of the added responsibility. How often upon taking the history of neurotic persons, and especially women, do we hear, "I was perfectly well until my first child was born. I haven't had a well day since." It is true that some neurotic women will feel better during pregnancy but they pay dearly for their short period of improvement. We discussed the problem under marriage counseling (p. 177) but it should be added that the cost to the child must not be forgotten. Unstable parents usually raise unstable children thus providing the soil for more neurotic illness.

Pregnancy, like marriage, is not to be recommended as a short cut to the solution of involved emotional problems.

Reeducation

While the security provided by a satisfactory contraceptive measure may allay anxiety in a few cases, so that sexual pleasure with orgasm may take place, it is usually true that when a satisfactory sexual adjustment does not take place within six months to a year after marriage some reeducation in thinking and feeling is advisable. Some of the fears must be allayed and some of the false beliefs changed. In a certain number of cases this can be brought about in a few interviews by giving a verbal picture of the full meaning of the sexual act and thereby making it possible for the patient to participate fully, emotionally as well as physically, in sexual intercourse. Many women feel too inhibited in the sexual relationship to make any body movements or to show that they enjoy what is going on lest they be regarded as too sensual, too experienced or guilty of conduct unbecoming to a "nice woman." These beliefs can often be changed sufficiently in a few interviews to permit latent sexual feelings to emerge.

The physician counsellor must be informed on the subject of sex. He must be unprejudiced and unashamed, and able to impart such attitudes to the patient. He should be articulate about sexual matters, since the patient probably has never had the opportunity of instruction on the positive values of sexual expression from someone respected and trusted. If the parents, early in the life of the patient, looked upon the budding sexual emotions with disapproval, threats, and attitudes which label sex as disgusting and dangerous, the physician counsellor may be unable to enliven emotions so stifled or change ideas so fixed. A woman who is young, healthy, and presumably in love should be able to enjoy her sexual life. The physician can be a source of unemotional information, lend his approval as a substitute for parental authority, and impart a philosophy which should help to neutralize the repressive effect of years of exposure to sexual taboos. In some instances this may occur after only a few discussions; in many instances it will take hours of re-education; and in some persons, unfortunately, it cannot occur at all. In these last instances the frigidity or impotence may have to be accepted as an unalterable fact. Counseling may help in this acceptance, but if it cannot be accepted or if life is intolerable a legal rather than a medical solution may be the only resort.

Necessity for Psychotherapy. If no change whatever in the attitude or feeling is brought about after approximately six interviews over a period of two or three weeks, it is probable that any flow of feeling into the genital organs has been so cut off during psychosexual development that a quite marked change in the whole personality will have to be brought about in order to influence the frigidity or impotence. A therapeutic technic is then necessary which by patient, intensive work, will uncover those memories of early life experiences which have led to the faulty attitudes. When the early life memories are uncovered and the emotions associated with them, such as fear, disgust, and hate, are drained off, then the normal feelings and psychological capacity for sexual pleasure are released. Cases illustrating the therapeutic procedure appear later in the chapter.

Infertility in the Female. In a discussion of contraception the question of infertility must also be considered and, indeed, it is a part of the program of the Planned Parenthood Federation to investigate the causes of infertility as well as to look for better technics of contraception. At the very outset it must not be forgotten, as Perloff states, that although it is usually the wife who presents herself to the physician, assuming the responsibility for a barren marriage, the male partner has been responsible for the infertility in 37 per cent of his cases. This the woman often does not suspect; because her husband is potent she assumes that his relation to the problem is not to be questioned.

Perloff emphasizes that the psychological background as well as the medical, gynecologic, and endocrinologic aspects of infertility must be investigated: "One patient was aware that there were fertile and sterile periods during the month; her chief difficulty was that she thought of them in reverse and studiously avoided intercourse during the mid-month. All that was necessary was to inform her of the true facts and she promptly conceived two months later. Another woman . . . was unaware that vaginal penetration was essential in normal intercourse. (Her hymen was found intact twenty-seven months after her marriage.) A short explanation concerning normal sexual practices was all that was needed to cure this patient. A third woman, who had borne a normal child three years previously and who ovulated almost every month, was unable to conceive, although no contraception had been employed for fourteen months. She felt ill and realized that this was in part due to worry over family problems. A frank discussion of these difficulties and better orientation of herself in relation to her family resulted in considerable improvement. She became pregnant shortly thereafter, although no other therapy was employed."

The well-known phenomenon of conception occurring in a previously sterile woman *after the adoption of a child* is very suggestive of psychosomatic influences. Apparently many infantile, dependent women fail to become pregnant because of the necessity for taking responsibility and such women often have infantile or underdeveloped genital organs. A masculine woman may refuse to become pregnant because pregnancy necessitates assuming a feminine role. Here again one often finds structural defects of the genital organs. Unconscious hostility toward the husband apparently may be responsible for sterility in one marriage, while in a later marriage the woman may conceive.

We know of no statistics in relation to frigidity and infertility. While the frigid woman can, of course, conceive, there is probably some relationship.

Perloff considers it likely "that many of the women who conceive after administration of small doses of thyroid extract, vitamin E, vitamin B complex, ephynal acetate, and/or other nonspecific remedies, are examples of the efficacy of psychotherapy in sterility."

Nor must similar considerations in regard to the male be forgotten. The influence of excessive work on the sperm count is illustrated by the case of an interne whose semen was examined at intervals for several months. "While he was on an arduous service and obtained little sleep, the number of sperm in the ejaculate fell to 25 million per ml., the total specimen measuring only 1.5 ml.; whereas during the time he worked in the laboratory and his hours were regular, the number of sperm rose to from 60 to 100 million per ml. with 4 to 4.5 ml. total quantity. The percentage of motile sperm also improved with the change in assignment."

A very precise new test for ovulation, developed by Farris, which depends on the presence of hyperemia in the ovary of the immature rat after injection with the patient's urine, makes it possible to time intercourse during the period when it is most likely to be fruitful. Coupled with this ingenious method Farris has developed a technic of spermatozoa counts which gives a much more accurate indication of the role that the husband plays in the sterility problem.

In connection with this discussion we must caution that a woman should never be told that she cannot conceive except in the case of hysterectomy or the removal of both ovaries. Extraordinary things happen. We have seen a forty-year-old frail creature with an infantile uterus, scanty and irregular menses, and senile changes of the external genitalia, who for years had been trying in vain to become pregnant, finally do so during the course of psychotherapy and without the use of endocrine products.

Psychological Factors in Urological Disorders

Some years ago Menninger discussed psychological factors in urological disease. He introduced the subject by suggesting that even the idea that psychic factors were important might seem presumptuous since the existing knowledge of anatomy, bacteriology, and immunology in this field was so much more complete than the knowledge of psychology. Moreover, thousands of urologically afflicted people are being successfully treated every day without any particular consideration of psychological factors. Nevertheless, he felt that a discussion of the psychological factors had a very practical value. He remarked then, and it is still true, that few psychiatrists are competent to make urological examinations, while few urologists are interested in making psychological examinations. The urologist examines the patient's genitalia, and the psychiatrist examines the patient's emotions, and each comes to his own conclusions. Menninger suggested examining more carefully the respective findings and theories of the urologists and the psychiatrists with respect to the symptoms of importance. He discussed the problem somewhat as follows:

The Urologist's Point of View. The urologists have made certain observations concerning the organs involved in impotence which cannot be disputed. They find, with some degree of regularity, that many patients complaining of impotence show definite congestion and inflammation of the posterior urethra, especially of the verumontanum, and tenderness, enlargement, and congestion of the prostate, either with or without evidence suggesting infection. The interpretation generally given these data by the urologists is something as follows: The prostate becomes the site of a local infection owing to a combination of factors— for example, masturbatory congestion plus infection, or local injury plus streptococcal localization. The resulting inflammatory reaction impairs functional activity (impotence). The impotence causes the patient morti- fication and anxiety—he is driven by this distress to seek medical treat- ment and comes to the urologist. The urologist treats the local condition (by massage, irrigation, endoscopy, chemotherapy, and so on) and it shows improvement. The impotence then (sometimes) disappears, and the theory is substantiated. However, the persistence of both inflam- mation and impotence may be regarded as evidence for the theory of an organic lesion which resists efforts toward removal.

The Psychiatric Point of View. Psychiatrists find that many patients suffering from impotence prove upon examination to have a definite psychological need for this symptom, in spite of their distress about it. In other words, they have unconsciously *wanted* to be impotent in order to satisfy certain unconscious emotional needs. We have already referred to some of the specific emotions which, though they exist only in the un- conscious, exert a contrary and prohibiting effect upon the sexual func- tion. These consist in one or more of the following: (1) fears, especially of punishment or of injury; (2) hostilities toward the love object; (3) conflicting loves, particularly parental and homosexual fixations; (4) rejection of the masculine (or feminine) role with its responsibilities.

The Sense of Guilt as a Psychic Factor. Associated with and de- pendent upon these emotions is a great sense of guilt, and experience has shown that the relief of this sense of guilt by any one of several devices will frequently serve to free the patient from his fears and thus from his inhibitions. The psychiatrists therefore are quite ready to believe that urological treatment frequently cures impotence even when it is of psy- chological origin, but they ascribe the cure not to the structural changes effected by the treatment but to the gratification of the need for suffering always associated with the sense of guilt—for example, guilt over mastur- bation. To simplify the problem let us take this last suggestion of Men- ninger's and suppose that a patient is impotent because of guilt over masturbation but neither he nor the urologist is aware of this fact. The urologist finds the prostate enlarged, pus cells in the secretion, states emphatically that "prostatitis" is responsible for the impotence and treats the patient by prostatic massage and topical applications to the deep urethra. The patient has confidence in the urologist but also pays in time, effort, money, and actual physical suffering. Thus is guilt over his fancied misdeed assuaged. As guilt is relieved and confidence grows impotence is overcome. Thus it is that a reassuring manner and vigorous physical treatment (unconscious psychotherapy) may bring about the cure of a psychologically determined illness when guilt is the basic source of the difficulty. This statement, of course, holds true for many illnesses outside of the urological sphere. Psychotherapy which aims at an understanding and rational dissolution of guilt (and other psychic factors) is more difficult but more fundamental and, therefore, a method of treatment more likely to be permanent.

Psychosomatic Aspects of Venereal Disease. Ruesch commented that while the promiscuous individual often considers venereal disease as a punishment, merely bad luck, or at least a well-deserved warning, the nonpromiscuous individual usually feels hatred and resentment against the person who transmitted the infection, and against the sexual activity which was the source of the exposure. In general, this is especially true of young and inexperienced men who attempt their first intercourse. The basic personality problem which confronts these people is the choice of the partner. Instead of picking a young girl of the same social class, these men resort to prostitutes or otherwise easily accessible girls. Sometimes this behavior is the expression of a dichotomy between affection and sex: Overattachment to the mother and repression of sexual desires directed at her makes all "nice, clean" women inaccessible. When the sexual urge increases, recourse is taken to a prostitute, from whom no affection is expected but merely gratification in the "dirty" matters of sex.

A similar problem is presented in the woman who marries a promiscuous husband. Such a girl is usually frigid and her ambivalent overattachment to her father makes her select a husband who is unlikely to form any emotional attachments.

Dysmenorrhea

It often happens in psychiatric practice that any very intensive treatment directed toward readjusting the emotional health will cure a dysmenorrhea which was not necessarily a presenting symptom. A typical history is somewhat as follows.

Dysmenorrhea

CASE 52

History and Symptoms

A white woman aged twenty-three had begun menstruating at thirteen with no special distress. The menses were regular and she did not refrain from any routine activity during this period. At sixteen she fell in love with a boy of her own age. This love relation was not very happy. There was great depth of feeling which could not be adequately dealt with in the various contacts which she had with him because she felt so guilty about her feelings. She longed to be with the man with whom she was in love but the closer she came in contact with him the more pain (psychic and physical) she suffered. Being close and loving at the same time meant some sensual expression which she could not tolerate. Her body felt tense and uncomfortable and dysmenorrhea began. All through her teens she was unable to be relaxed and carefree in the presence of the opposite sex. She knew she needed them, that they were important in her life, but she did not know how to deal with them in a way that left her physically relaxed. Loving a man conflicted with her ideals. This did not mean that there was conflict over actual sexual intercourse. The ordinary expressions of love such as kissing, or other physical contact without anything so overt as intercourse, gave rise to marked conflict. When dysmenorrhea occurred while in college she often stayed in bed for a day. "I could have managed to get around but I just didn't want to go to classes."

LIFE SITUATION

Reasons for Seeking Treatment

Because of difficulty in concentration and study she came for psychiatric treatment, in the course of which considerable reeducation in sexual matters had to take place. Even though she was twenty-three she still had not achieved a better relationship with the opposite sex. To be kissed and fondled by a man made her "squirm" inside. She did not consciously consider the idea of sexual relations revolting and yet she couldn't feel comfortable when a man made love to her. "It makes me tense and I can't stand it somehow. It has come to the point where I have the same turmoil in my insides as in my head. I guess that is the reason I can't study."

Faulty Education in Sex

It was necessary to tell her, "You have been taught by your father and mother that sexual feeling is wicked and dangerous. They told you this as the only way they knew to keep you from the dangers of sexual promiscuity. They did not intend that these attitudes toward sexual matters should last forever. They took it for granted that as you grew up your attitudes would change and that you would be able to feel and accomplish what the average young woman of twenty-three feels and accomplishes in matters of love." She had to be helped in many ways to feel normally toward men and the inevitable erotic advances which they would make to a girl of her age.

The Progress of Treatment

The conversation and thinking in psychotherapy must be tactfully guided so that the patient is able to see the source of conflict by being helped to think about that aspect of reality which has been neglected. The physician must not proceed faster than the patient can understand, particularly in discussing such subjects as sex and hostility.

Finally after much thought and discussion over a period of several weeks she said, "I'm tired of considering myself a walking bundle of conventions. I'm going to feel like a human being and enjoy life. I don't believe I'll have much to give the world if I don't take something myself." She began to discuss love, marriage, and sensual expression between the sexes, with her admirer with whom she soon became engaged. She felt entirely comfortable and their friendship took on an entirely new meaning. She felt relaxed and happy with him at all times and at the same time the dysmenorrhea of seven years' duration became less and less pronounced and finally disappeared. Asked why she thought the dysmenorrhea disappeared she said, "When I relaxed emotionally I relaxed down there" (meaning her pelvis). "Everything about me flows more freely now. My thoughts are freer, my feelings freer, I feel freer to be a woman in every way, and I guess the symbol of my womanhood, menstruation, flows more freely too. My emotions concerning love and sex do not give me pain and my menstruation no longer gives me pain."

> *Frigidity in a Patient without Deep Conflicts*
> *Good Response to a Short Period of Therapy*

CASE 53

History and Symptoms

A woman of twenty-five who had been married three months consulted a physician about contraception. In the course of being instructed in the use of contraceptives she stated that her sex relations were not as satisfactory as she had hoped they would be. When questioned about her home education in such matters it developed that her mother had made her feel that "nice" women dare not let men know that they feel sexual pleasure, as this would somehow be rather "embarrassing" to the woman and might lead the man to get the wrong opinion of her. Our patient had always been rather shy about exposing herself and had never felt comfortable, for example, in a bathing suit. In spite of her ideas of shame in regard to sexual relations our patient had always been interested in the opposite sex and fantasied rather vividly about the pleasures of sexual intercourse. When questioned about sex play prior to intercourse the patient stated, "I never let myself go. I know I'm married and my husband wants me to have pleasure but it is as if I were waiting for someone to give me permission to go ahead." When she was able to discuss intercourse itself it developed that she did not cooperate in the act with pelvic movements nor did she even draw her legs up in the flexed position. She was instructed to do this and told, "You have every right to derive as much pleasure as possible from your sexual relations. Both your church and your family expect you and your husband to make each other happy in this relationship, as in all of your other relationships, so that you may work together better and be able eventually to pass your happiness along to your children. The happiest children are those that come from homes where the husband and wife contribute the most to each other's happiness."

The patient said, "I guess I needed someone to talk to me like this and make sexual pleasure seem right. I don't know how soon I can overcome all of my shyness in relation to my husband but I'll try."

The Role of the Patient's Personality in Treatment

A week later the patient reported that as a result of the discussion, she had been able to achieve orgasm for the first time since marriage. She said, "I knew what you told me was right even before you said it, but I guess someone had to make me *feel* it would be all right to let myself go that much. It still seems a little wicked when I think of it, but I know it's right and that my husband and I will be much more satisfied with each other now."

In this case an interest in things sexual had already been present, with a belief that a better sexual adjustment should be attained. The mother had not preached hatred of the male nor instilled large amounts of fear and disgust. There was only mild anxiety concerning activity in the sexual act and an excessive modesty, both of which were easily corrected by *reeducation* and *permission* for the patient to let herself go. In other words, the patient had very few unfortunate attitudes which needed correction.

The Authority of the Physician

In the treatment of this patient it should be noted that something took place beyond intellectual enlightenment. This was the patient's utilization of her emotional relation to the physician, who acted both as authority and as a substitute for her parents. It was the physician's attitude as indicated in the formula—"Now that you are married there is no necessity for any prohibitions against sexual pleasures"—that was of equal importance with intellectual enlightenment in helping the patient.

Again let us emphasize that in many cases of frigidity in women or impotence in men which are cured by local treatment or manipulation the same psychological mechanism may be the very factor which brings about the cure. In other words, the physician here too acts as authority and parent, and in his very willingness to treat the impotence and frigidity and thus cooperate with the patient in his aim to achieve sexual pleasure, he is being permissive and encouraging, and is breaking down psychological inhibitions to better sexual functioning.

The more serious cases of frigidity may not come to the physician for treatment. There are several reasons for this. First, as we have said before, unless actual vaginismus exists, the woman can always function in the sexual act whether she is frigid or not. Then, the severely frigid woman is a person who has been educated to eschew sex for so long and to such a degree that she is not likely to dare to ask for any such pleasure or she may just take it completely for granted that she has a personal peculiarity for which nothing can be done anyway. So from a practical clinical standpoint we usually encounter the more severe instances of frigidity only in cases where *other* symptoms have been more distressing and have brought the patient for treatment.

Frigidity with Severe Neurosis, Demanding Longer Therapy

CASE 54

History and Symptoms

A twenty-seven-year-old woman came for treatment because of "fear spells," depression of spirits, irritability, and headaches. She had been married three years and was childless. Her symptoms had become troublesome one and one-half years after marriage. She had been a lonely girl during her teens and had never become very popular socially. She had looked for the sexual relation in marriage to bring more pleasure and to have more meaning than proved to be the case. Her husband was potent and while she enjoyed intercourse during the first year in the sense that she liked being close to her husband and to feel that he wanted her, the vaginal pleasure was minimal and intercourse often left her restless and sleepless. After her symptoms began she tried to avoid coitus; she did not "want to be bothered with it."

Family History. The family history brought out that the patient's mother was a cold, selfish woman, cruel to her husband and children. She nagged and belittled her husband's efforts to earn a living until he finally gave up in despair and perhaps in retaliation lived a life of almost complete idleness after the age of forty.

21

LIFE SITUATION

Lack of Sexual Instruction

The patient had no direct sexual instruction and never dared to ask any questions. She used to hear her mother complaining once in a while about the way men "imposed upon their wives sexually." Her mother always discouraged her from associating with boys but grudgingly permitted her to have a few dates and attend an occasional dance. The mother had always shown a great tendency to criticize our patient, ostensibly in order to prevent her from becoming vain. Actually the excessive criticism on the part of the mother could only be due to hatred and jealousy. As a young child the patient was frequently told how ungrateful she was, and that if her aunts and uncles only knew what a bad child she was they could never like her. When she tried to be friendly with her father she was shamed and scolded and made to feel there was something wicked in her desire to be near her father or sit upon his knee. In her adolescent years the mother told her how unbecomingly she was dressed and commented that she "couldn't see what a boy would want of her." When the girl tried to choose bright and attractive clothes the mother would denounce her as behaving like a hussy and would make her take them back for something more subdued. The patient often hoped that her father would come to her rescue but he seemed to fear his wife's sharp tongue too much.

The Problem of Treatment

Treatment sessions resolved themselves into a discussion of the following problems: (1) the patient's unsatisfied craving for affection, (2) her hostility toward both women and men, (3) her inability to *give* feeling. After about six sessions she said, "I guess I looked for my marriage to bring me all the things I had missed at home but of course that was impossible. My father and mother certainly provided a poor example of a happily married couple. I suppose my mother did not have a happy childhood either but that wasn't my fault. I needed someone to do better for me. I guess I hate father for being so spineless. Why didn't he give me some security and friendship in spite of mother's cruelty and jealousy? I feel as if I now had nothing to give my husband in the sexual relationship. There was a little feeling of love in me in the beginning but it soon gave out. I feel so lonely and helpless at times. That's just the way I felt as a child."

Attitude Toward Treatment. For many months the same complaints went on. She spent much time describing her loneliness, irritability and depression of spirits. She said, "I'm like a whining child. I don't see how you stand it. Why don't you scold me?" We pointed out that it was our function to understand people who had unfulfilled emotional needs and to be trained to accept their demands, since this was the medicine they needed most, *i. e.*, friendship. She began to appreciate and utilize the friendly attitude toward her emotional needs, and after a few more discussions said, "I seem to get something from you. I must cheer up and give more to my husband and everyone else." She began to find that to be interested in someone else and to want to do something for that person made her less lonely and less depressed. At the same time her feelings about sexual matters underwent a change. She said, "I once thought everything my mother said about sex was the truth but I know now it wasn't. Just because mother couldn't be happy doesn't mean that I cannot be. Just because she was sexually frigid doesn't mean that I have to be. Mother wasn't generous and could give very little of herself. I know my husband wants me to feel sexual desire; he wants me to experience pleasure and I now feel I can. It's queer how a person can just tighten up and hold everything in when one's dreams do not come true. I had my dreams but didn't have enough love and good will in me to make them real."

The Results of Treatment

There was little additional explanation necessary. The patient was seen four times weekly and the treatment period lasted ten months. As she related her family history and past experiences the lack of love in the family background and the resulting emotional emptiness became clear to the patient. The unconscious hostility which had been so damaging to her personality became less pronounced. A friendly and understanding person to work with made it possible for her to reach out and absorb from the people in her environment the love and good will she had missed. At the same time that her symptoms began to disappear it became possible for her to experience sexual pleasure with orgasm.

Impotence
Little Modification in Attitude Necessary

CASE 55

History and Symptoms

A man of twenty-five came to a physician six weeks after marriage complaining of impotence. He had been examined by a urologist and pronounced free from organic disease. The patient came from a family in which there had been little sexual instruction of a positive nature. His mother had said, "A woman's body is like a sacred temple and should not be defiled." His father had told him at fourteen that "No gentleman takes advantage of a woman." He did not dare to ask questions on the subject of sex, and very occasional masturbation caused him considerable guilt. At twenty-one he "seemed to undergo a revolt" and began to seek the company of women who were casual in their sexual relations. He associated with such women for three years. He felt guilty about these adventures and always had some anxiety that his family or friends would hear about them.

LIFE SITUATION

Faulty Sexual Attitudes of Husband and Wife

Then he met the girl whom he was to marry and for a year before his marriage his sexual relations ceased. He respected his fiancée greatly and on a few occasions before marriage he wondered if he would be able to enjoy sexual relations with her as he had with other women he had known. Following marriage he had satisfactory sexual relations with his wife for about a month and then found himself growing impotent. He said, "She seemed too good for that sort of thing. I guess it brought to my mind the admonition of my mother that a woman's body was like a temple and shouldn't be defiled. I'm surprised in a way because that idea never occurred to me with the other women." It was explained to him that the other women were more aggressive and casual in their relations with him. They shared responsibility and made him feel that he was not taking anything from them they did not wish to give. Now he felt like a seducer.

Discussion with Wife. We asked to see his wife and talk with her. She was reserved but cooperative. It was clear that she too had had faulty sex education that did not permit her to be very free in their sexual relations. We explained to her that now that they were married she no longer needed to be reserved and inhibited in sexual relations with her husband and that in the face of his difficulty her own inhibitions added to the problem. We suggested to her that she try to become more actively interested in their sexual relations so that her husband would not have the feeling that her reserve was too difficult to overcome. Her response to this suggestion was satisfactory.

In the next session with the husband we explained the relations between his earlier ideas about sex and his present difficulty by saying, "The prohibitions imposed upon you by your parents were meant for before marriage and were not intended to extend beyond the time of marriage. Your sexual organ is still obeying the old prohibitions which are no longer valid. Your wife is just as eager for sexual pleasure as any other woman you have known but her own faulty sex education has not permitted her to make this evident.

Recovery

In the third interview the patient reported that his potency had returned and over a period of three years he has remained well.

Reasons for Impotence in Marriage

This case illustrates a very common occurrence, not generally understood, and that is the fact that the sexual potency of some men after marriage may be much diminished over what it was before marriage. One of the first reasons is that they have sought out women before marriage whose willingness to indulge in sexual relations did not challenge their unconscious fear of inflicting injury. A second reason is that some men have dificulty in maintaining a feeling of romance for their wives. The need for sexual conquest being over with marriage, an important factor in sexual stimulation is no longer active. Lastly, a tendency to marry a "good" woman rather than the woman with whom he has "played" sexually leads to an unconscious association of the good wife with mother, and hence the difficulty in relating himself sexually with a woman representing someone who long ago discouraged his sexual interest.

Impotence
Requiring Considerable Modification of Personality in Order to Overcome the Symptom

---

CASE 56

History and Symptoms

A married man, twenty-eight years old, complained of complete impotence. He had been married one and a half years to a girl one year younger than himself. During the first six months of marriage he had had very weak erections—so weak that he was unable to insert the penis in the vagina. For the past year he had been completely impotent, with very little interest in coitus. At times he felt some remorse that he could not give his wife sexual gratification, but otherwise he was relatively undisturbed about his impotence. Finally he came for treatment because he feared that his wife might seek divorce since he could not give her a child.

LIFE SITUATION

Family Background. He was the second of three children. His father had been a hard-headed business man who felt that his responsibility to his family had been met when he had furnished the money for their home, food, and education. The mother was a capable woman who had been interested in her children to the extent that she wanted them to turn out well. She had, however, been unable to give them much personal individual attention. She took pride in being the mother of a large family, and was pleased when compliments were paid about her good-looking and capable children. However, she was never close to any one of them and shared very little of their fears or ambitions.

Lack of Satisfactory Sexual Education. Although the patient had received a college education he had never been given any education in sexual matters. He had been warned that masturbation would injure his health. The patient remembered that whenever a story having to do with sexual indiscretion entered the family atmosphere either by way of the newspapers or from neighborhood gossip it was alluded to by the parents in hushed tones as "an awful thing." When the patient entered college, the father warned him "not to waste his time and not to get mixed up with women." The patient never attempted to think out very clearly what his father meant by this and obeyed him implicitly. The result was that he went through college getting very high grades and avoiding all contacts with the opposite sex. During his college days he heard his classmates referring to their dates, their petting parties, and occasionally to sexual intercourse. He had an inward sense of pride that he was above such things and that his interests lay only in work. His hobbies were stamp collecting, botanical collections, tennis, and boating. Whenever he heard his friends talking about girls, sex, and love affairs, he thought what a pity it was "that they were so frivolous."

Marriage. It was after leaving college and while serving an apprenticeship in his work that he met a girl to whom he was attracted largely because of her athletic ability. He enjoyed playing tennis with her and then began to see her more often. For the first time he made love to a girl, enjoyed kissing her, and concluded that they had enough in common to make a success of marriage. His thoughts about sexual intercourse were not very concrete, but such as they were, it never entered his head that he would have difficulty in performing the sexual act. Neither did his lack of success in that respect surprise him. At first he looked upon it as a peculiarity which he would overcome.

Necessity for Intensive Treatment. We felt immediately that his interest in sexual matters had been so inadequate and the capacity to function sexually, even under such favorable conditions, was so incomplete that a long period of psychological treatment would be necessary. The patient hoped nevertheless that a few discussions would clear up his difficulty. He was seen once each week, and after four sessions his impotence was still uninfluenced, as were all his ideas on sexual subjects. He therefore began more intensive treatment with sessions four times a week, which gave us a better opportunity to observe his daily thinking processes as well as his day-to-day behavior.

Now when he was asked to unburden himself regarding his thoughts and feelings, it was noted that his ideas and interests did not concern themselves with sexual functioning but always about such other matters as his difficulties at work, his concern over advancement, his dislike of certain business routines, and criticism about the way his wife ran the house. His lack of spontaneous interest in the opposite sex was frequently pointed out to him. It was also explained that his education had provided no information on the very important subject of sex, and that his parents, in whom he had great confidence, had discouraged all sexual activity. We pointed out that he still seemed remarkably obedient to their admonitions even though he had married and was expected to live a normal sex life and to become the father of children. He began to understand that his feeling of antagonism toward his superiors at work was a projection onto them of a hostility which he originally held toward his father.

Relation to Wife. When he was encouraged to discuss his real feelings toward women it was found that he had little affection for them, in fact he was most intolerant of their minds and very disdainful of their bodies. He had never been a close friend with his mother nor with any other woman, and it became clear that his marriage was a rather perfunctory alliance with a woman who, fortunately for him, was a warm and capable person. His chief interest in her was that she kept his house neat and made him comfortable. When his desire really to become a father was questioned he had to admit that he had never liked children, couldn't stand their crying, and actually became angry when his friends who were parents showed off their babies. Finally he understood that his relation to his wife was more like that of a child than of a husband and that another child in the household would be a rival for his wife's maternal care.

History of Masturbation. We learned that prior to marriage he had masturbated only about a half dozen times that he could remember and each time with great guilt. Even so, he had had more pleasure from these acts than he had ever had from intercourse, or rather, from attempted intercourse with his wife. He therefore sought to stimulate his interest in sexual pleasure by masturbation, although he felt himself very childish and disgusting for doing so. He found, however, that he could obtain some erection in this way and absolutely none through any love play with his wife. He talked a great deal about his shame, disgust, and anxiety concerning masturbation, but since this was the only way he could stimulate any sexual feeling or desire he continued the practice.

As time went on he began to see the unreasonableness of his fault-finding attitude toward his wife. He brought her an occasional gift and began to help her with the housework. He became more tolerant toward her desire for a child. His greater consideration extended to his friends with whom he had previously been rather coldly aloof and hypercritical. It was noted by everyone that he was growing more friendly.

Accomplishing Successful Intercourse. After ridding himself of some of his feelings of disgust and shame regarding masturbation he began to achieve some sexual pleasure in this way. Then he spoke of his fear that if he should attempt intercourse with his wife he might urinate in her vagina rather than ejaculate semen. We pointed out that this did not happen in the act of masturbation and therefore no reason existed why it should happen in intercourse. After some reassurance on the part of his wife, he attempted intercourse. For the first few times this resulted in premature ejaculation, but after about three weeks his fears had subsided to such an extent that he was able to maintain erection for a satisfactory length of time. To correct all his distorted ideas and thus permanently to overcome his impotence took a period of many months. When too many inhibiting emotions have been present over such a period of years, long treatment is necessary.

SUMMARY

In this case a serious personality disturbance underlay the symptom of impotence. The change in personality attitudes effected during the treatment were not incidental. They had to take place in order for a sufficient amount of good will to come to the surface to make it possible for him to consider loving a woman. Not only did his love impulses have to be freed but he also had to overcome feelings of fear and disgust in relation to his penis as an organ capable of injuring and degrading the opposite sex.

Premature Ejaculation
Good Response to Superficial Psychotherapy

CASE 57

History and Symptoms

A white man of thirty complained of difficulty in intercourse of a few months' duration. He had been married for a little more than two years and was devoted to his wife. During the last several months they had decided that they would like to have a child and he thought it was with this decision that he began to suffer from premature ejaculation.

The past medical history was negative and the general physical examination showed a well-nourished and well-developed young man who presented no evidence of disease or abnormality. Routine laboratory studies were normal.

The family history seemed negative from the standpoint of the present disorder except for the fact that he described his mother as a nervous woman.

LIFE SITUATION

He stated that he had always had some fear of intercourse and remained continent until marriage. After his marriage to a girl with whom he was very much in love he had enjoyed normal sexual relations but deferred having children until his economic situation would improve. He worked for his father, who had achieved considerable success in the business world and toward whom the patient seemed to manifest great respect mingled with considerable fear. About a year before the onset of his difficulty in intercourse he had been put in charge of a branch of his father's business in another community and there he felt very keenly the challenge of making good. He feared failure and *began to fail in intercourse at about the same time.* This fact was pointed out to him and he immediately saw that there was a connection between his failure in sex life and his fear of failure in business life.

Recovery

In two interviews he had achieved a satisfactory recovery and follow-up at the end of four years demonstrated that he had no further difficulties, and that they were now the parents of a child to whom both were devoted.

Premature Ejaculation, Needing More Intensive Therapy

CASE 58

History and Symptoms

A man of twenty-nine, after one month of marriage, came for treatment for premature ejaculation. He had no other symptoms at the time. He was the third of a family of five. No sexual education had been given to any of the children. In fact, the subject of sex was strictly taboo at all times. The mother of the patient was overly religious and although she attended to the ordinary tasks of life she taught her children that religion came before everything else. According to her teaching there were only two important things in life—work and worshipping God. Demonstrations of affection were frowned upon by the mother. She kept the patient at arm's length herself and in addition always discouraged his contacts with girls. In spite of this he had numerous sexual fantasies about women. He wished that they would surrender themselves to him for sexual pleasure and yet he was sure that none of them wanted to do this. When he first attempted to kiss a girl he was in great anxiety lest she become angry and scold him. He always expected women to repulse and reproach him. On the one hand he was profoundly grateful to women who would love him and at the same time unconsciously quite hostile to them for the attitude of denial which he felt they all held toward him. When he married he was apprehensive as to whether he could function sexually or not. He was not entirely surprised at his symptom ot premature ejaculation. He said, "I can't believe my wife really wants to give herself to me. It seems that I am asking too much. I want sexual pleasure to last longer both for myself and for her but I can't control it."

LIFE SITUATION

The Relation of Emotional Control to Sexual Control

Inquiry into his daily life revealed that he had always been sensitive to the attentions of both men and women. He craved love and friendship and was easily cast down if disapproved of in any way. He remembered that whenever anyone had shown him much praise or affection, or had given him a present, he would cry. "I was always so ashamed of that. As I grew older and people expected me to be strong emotionally I would be weak. I was ashamed of myself for crying then as I am now about this symptom."

As the treatment interviews went on, the patient more and more related his lack of emotional control in social situations to his lack ot ejaculatory control. He said, "When I go to the movies and the hero finally gets what he wants, I cry. I want my wife to give me her body for my pleasure. When she does so I release semen too quickly just as I have always released tears too quickly. It seems to me that I can't stand to get what I want without losing control of myself."

The Importance of Hostility

At this point the patient brought out hostility toward his mother. "If my mother had only given me more love and led me to expect more, instead of constantly preaching and making such an ascetic of me! I am inadequate in making love and I cannot make my wife happy. Perhaps I don't want to, in so far as she represents my mother, but at least I must try to accept pleasure for myself and then maybe I'll be able to give it to her."

After the conscious expression of hostility to his mother he was better able to express his feelings without loss of emotional control. At the same time his ability to maintain erection without ejaculation increased to an entirely satisfactory point.

SUMMARY

In this case fear and criticism and hostility toward the opposite sex were the important psychological trends which needed readjustment. The procedure took sixty treatment hours.

Chapter XIX

THE RESPIRATORY SYSTEM

THE EFFECT OF EMOTIONS ON BREATHING

The respiratory system, like the gastrointestinal and cardiovascular systems, is profoundly influenced by the emotions. "Sighing respirations" are well known in general medicine, and while they are frequently referred to as "shortness of breath" it is generally recognized that they accompany functional illness. When we are frightened we "catch our breath," and under certain other emotional circumstances we breathe deeply. A feeling of "a weight on the chest" is a frequent symbolic representation that the patient has a "load on his mind" which he would like to get rid of by talking to someone about his troubles. "Smothered feelings" also often represent a conversion of repressed emotion which the patient has had no opportunity to talk about. "Ventilating" our feelings often allows us to breathe easier and feel better. A weight on the chest is a frequent symptom accompanying the nocturnal anxiety attack. Many nocturnal attacks of bronchial asthma are preceded by an anxiety dream. Textbooks of medicine are beginning to consider the "mental aspects" of pulmonary tuberculosis, and included in the case histories of this disease are events of emotional significance which have occurred coincidentally with the onset of symptoms. No attempt is made to regard this as a direct cause and effect relation, but physicians are beginning to suspect that some kind of relation does exist. More will be said on this subject shortly.

Analogy to Gastrointestinal Tract

Binger, in an excellent article on "The Psychobiology of Breathing," points out that the respiratory apparatus is genetically and structurally related to the gastrointestinal tract, and that in many ways they seem to function similarly. Embryologically, the pulmonary respiratory apparatus develops from the hind part of the ventral wall of the head gut. He further points out that both systems are concerned with the incorporation of certain substances of the external environment, with the transport of these substances to the tissue cells, and with the excretion of certain products of tissue metabolism. He indicates how both digestive and respiratory systems can be susceptible to similar derangements such as spasms and secretory changes, and that both may act as pathways for the entrance of infectious organisms. He observes that if Alexander is correct in his assumption that the gastrointestinal tract may act out certain emotional trends having to do with ingestion, retention, and elimination, it is conceivable that an organ system so closely parallel embryologically and functionally can exhibit similar responses. Indeed Alexander and Saul analyzed respiratory tracings with special reference to psychological correlations and felt that there was suggestive evidence of a relation between intaking and eliminating tendencies, observable in the mental life, and certain characteristics of the spirograms.

Neurosis and Respiratory Tracings

Christie several years before had made a somewhat similar study in an effort to see whether there was any relation between the type of respiration and the type of neurosis. In speaking of the anxiety neuroses he referred to the fact that *effort syndrome*, while usually classified as a cardiac neurosis, is essentially respiratory and that the invariable symptom is breathlessness, although most patients also complain of palpitation,

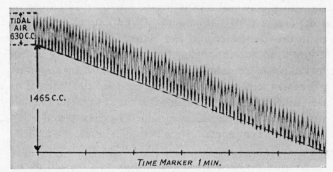

Fig. 9.   Respiratory tracing from a normal individual.   Christie: Quarterly J. of Med. 4: 427, 1935.

giddiness, sweating, and precordial pain, all exaggerated by exercise. He remarked that the breathlessness is reflected by a tendency to a rapid and shallow breathing rather than a true hyperpnea. By inspection of the thorax in a case of effort syndrome he pointed out that it is possible to say that the breathing is rapid and shallow but a respiratory tracing brings out several points which he believes to be even more characteristic of this condition: (*a*) an irregularity of the respiratory level; (*b*) an irregularity of respiratory depth; (*c*) a less marked irregularity of respiratory rate. Some of the examples of respiratory tracings taken from his article are reproduced. He does not, of course, believe that all cases of respiratory neurosis will give a typical respiratory tracing. But he does feel that the respiratory irregularity, if sufficiently pronounced, is diagnostic of a respiratory neurosis. A study of the respiratory curve as

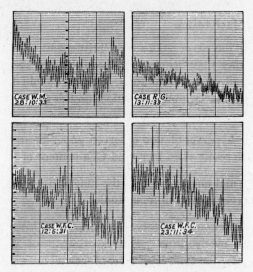

Fig. 10. Respiratory tracings from cases of effort syndrome. Christie: Quarterly J. of Med. 4: 427, 1935.

observed in the ordinary basal metabolic test will often furnish a clue in regard to these matters.

Sighing Respirations in Anxiety States

One of the commonest complaints of the neurotic patient is shortness of breath. When pressed for an explanation such a patient will frequently place his hand over the lower sternum and illustrate by a deep, sighing respiration that he "cannot get enough air." Whether he takes a great number of shallow breaths, or a smaller number of deep breaths, he exposes himself to the dangers of hyperventilation and alkalosis, and even tetany and unconsciousness, as eventual results. There are patients with severe anxiety states who sometimes fear that their breath may be cut off, and they are thrown into a panic. Misinterpretations on the part of the physician increase the patient's fear of heart disease, inability to breathe, and so forth; on the other hand a simple explanation of the mechanics of ventilation and reassurance regarding the absence of disease may accomplish a great deal.

In an analysis of a large number of spirograms Finesinger showed that the incidence of sighing respirations was highest in the group with anxiety states—60 per cent, as contrasted with 21 per cent for normal control subjects. Other neurotic and psychotic disturbances fell in between.

Physiological Mechanisms

After noting the observations by Christie and calling attention to Finesinger's studies that "unpleasant thoughts" are associated with increased depth and rate of respiration, Wolf and Wolff (in a paper previously referred to) made some deductions on this subject from their own observations:

1. That the hyperventilation observed under these circumstances is probably not the result of an increased CO_2 content of the blood.

2. Parenchymal engorgement of the lung is not a factor in the production of hyperventilation in these studies.

3. The production of hyperventilation, or at least its instigation, involves nervous mechanisms. The experiments of Wolf and Wolff suggested ". . . how the contractile state of skeletal muscle in posture and bodily movement associated with various emotional states may be linked with respiration. For example, if a discouraged, dejected individual listlessly approaches a task of lifting a weight or climbing stairs, the act is done so awkwardly that many more than the usual proprioceptive end organs are stimulated, and hyperventilation results. This barrage of afferent impulses may then, directly or indirectly, exert an influence upon the respiratory center. That this is not alone the result of a greater oxygen requirement for muscles inefficiently used was demonstrated by the fact that the oxygen consumption was not increased in proportion to the increased ventilation in these experiments."

4. Increased oxygen requirement in association with disturbing emotions may act indirectly in the production of dyspnea.

Engel and his associates studied the clinical aspects of hyperventilation, which they regard as psychogenic in origin in most instances. They divide the symptoms into those related to reduction in consciousness and those related to tetany. Reduction in consciousness correlates with the degree of slowing in the electroencephalogram while tetany is unrelated to changes in the E.E.G. Reduction in consciousness is associated with giddiness, faintness, lightheadedness, fullness in the head, blurring of vision, and other signs, while tetany appears after much longer periods of hyperventilation and is much less frequent.

Finally, in regard to such mechanisms, Faulkner observed that in a man being bronchoscoped suggestions which produced feelings of insecurity caused the lumen of the bronchi to become smaller in diameter.

FUNCTIONAL RESPIRATORY DISORDERS

Neurotic Dyspnea

CASE 59

A young white woman, twenty-five years old, was first seen in 1934.

History and Symptoms

She complained of "a smothering feeling and an inability to get the proper amount of air." She also said that her appetite was poor, on occasions she vomited, and there had been some loss of weight and strength.

The trouble had begun at the age of eighteen just after she had finished high school in a small western town. For some time she had been aware of enlargement of the neck but now she became nervous, suffered from smothering and choking sensations and a diagnosis of toxic goiter was made. She was admitted to a hospital, was studied for some time, and finally a thyroidectomy was done but the symptoms grew worse instead of better and she was taken to a large clinic, where her family was told that there was no organic basis for her difficulties and that there was no point in being concerned about her shortness of breath. She then came east to make her home with her married brother but symptoms became so pronounced that she was finally brought to Philadelphia and tracheotomy was performed with the insertion of a tube. For the succeeding two or three years she considered herself pretty well but then once more suffered from exhaustion and a feeling that she was not getting enough air. It was at this time that she first came to our attention.

Past History. There was nothing remarkable about her previous health except that she had always been underweight and that the menstrual period had been established late and had been irregular and quite painful.

Family History. Patient was the middle child in a family of four sisters and a brother. The mother and father were both living and well. One sister had chronic arthritis and another had successfully been operated upon for goiter in a large clinic.

Physical Examination

Patient was an undernourished young white woman, who wore an expression of sullen suffering. The blood pressure was normal. There was some evidence of acne on the back and face, and the hands were cold and sweaty. There were no signs of hyperthyroidism. Examination of the mouth and throat showed nothing definite but the patient gagged easily. The breathing space of the nares seemed satisfactory. Aside from the scar of the goiter operation and the presence of a tracheotomy tube, the examination of the neck showed nothing abnormal. Heart and lungs were normal. The abdominal examination showed some generalized tenderness but this seemed a part of the general nervous reaction of the patient because there was no rigidity and no organs or masses were palpable. Knee jerks were excessive but the extremities were otherwise negative. We concluded that there was no gross evidence of disease and that we were dealing with a vagotonic type of individual.

LIFE SITUATION

The patient had been born and brought up in a small town in the far west. The father was very strict in the upbringing of his daughters and would not allow them to go to parties and dances like other girls of their age. Consequently there was often much quarreling in the home because the mother was much more lenient and sympathetic.

Thyroid Enlargement

After she graduated from high school there was some question as to whether she should remain at home or go away to school like some of the other children had and it was during this period that her attention was centered on the thyroid gland and the "toxic symptoms." After her admission to the local hospital her brother and his wife who lived in the east came home for a vacation and the decision was left to them whether she should be operated upon by a local surgeon or sent to a nearby large clinic.

Operations

In spite of the fact that the father could well afford to send her away to a more experienced surgeon the brother decided that it would be satisfactory for the operation to proceed and consequently it was done. As stated above, immediately afterward she became worse and then it was that she came east with this brother and his wife to make her home with them. On the way they stopped off at a large clinic where, according to the patient, the brother was told that it "was all nerves." As a consequence when she developed attacks of breathing difficulty in his home she was treated very unsympathetically and finally at the end of about six months she came to Philadelphia to make her home with an aunt. Then it was that the *tracheotomy* was performed and a tube inserted.

Marriage

Following our examination in 1934, when the patient was reassured about herself, she remained in fairly good health and subsequently married a man "who was very kind and considerate" and constantly solicitous about her health. She remained fairly well until about 1939 when symptoms returned and grew progressively worse. She became convinced that she needed a larger tube "to let more air in" and this was done but her symptoms continued.

Once more she was examined but again no evidence of organic disease was made out. Now it was possible to learn a little more about her as a person.

Hostility

She very much resented the implication that there was no organic disease. In spite of her passive and docile exterior she would look at the examiner sharply and say angrily, "Well, what then *is* causing my breathing difficulty?" It became clear that she blamed the trouble on the "terrible operation" that was originally done on her neck and the scar tissue which she imagined was contracting and displacing the tube to one side.

Resentment for Brother. She also had a great deal of resentment for the clinic where it had been said that her condition was "all mental" and she particularly held her brother responsible for the whole disastrous occurrence that had so wrecked her life. It was only by cautiously introducing the subject of her brother and his responsibility into the conversation that her resentment for him and particularly for his wife came out, because she really felt that it was the wife who had influenced the brother to have her operated upon by the local surgeon so that "their vacation would not be interfered with." It was obvious from her conduct that she harbored a great deal of resentment. Slowly it was made clear to her that her principal symptom was *exhaustion* rather than shortness of breath and that the latter was related to the former. Then it was pointed out that her intense resentment and hostility which she had nursed over this great period of years was largely responsible for her exhaustion because it had sapped her energy. The explanation seemed a satisfactory one because as she *aired her hostility* she was able to breathe better; in other words, she was able to "let more air in" and at the same time she had more energy.

The occurrence which had been responsible for the return of symptoms seemed to be the fact that her brother had ceased to communicate with her and on one occasion she learned that he had been in her vicinity and had not even troubled to call her up. This inflamed her already great resentment.

SUMMARY

A young white woman was first seen in 1934 suffering from exhaustion and breathlessness. She had been operated upon for goiter and then because of shortness of breath tracheotomy had been done and a tube inserted. Later symptoms returned and she felt that the tube was too small to allow enough air to enter but a new, larger tube failed to help her. Physical examination showed no organic reason for the dyspnea and the patient's attention was directed to the exhaustion instead and the explanation was then given that emotional conflict stood in the background of the exhaustion. The emotional conflict surrounded a great deal of repressed hostility for a brother whom she held responsible for her misfortune and when she was able to give expression to her hostility her symptoms diminished, that is, she was able to give herself better ventilation. The problem was an interesting one chiefly because of the complicated psychosomatic situation.

Anxiety Attacks; Hyperventilation; the Taboo of Primitive Thinking; Suggestive Therapy, Schizophrenia

---

CASE 60

A young colored woman, married, aged thirty, was admitted to Temple University Hospital medical service in October, 1938.

History and Symptoms

Chief Complaint. She complained of attacks of breathlessness, weakness, and palpitation. The first attacks had occurred a little more than two years ago. She was then free of attacks and perfectly well for about a year and then they recurred on three or four occasions during the past year. She also complained of frequent vomiting during the last few months.

Description of the Attack. The first attack occurred at night. She woke up with what she described as tremendous shortness of breath and pounding of the heart. She was sleeping on the first floor next to a window; she jumped out and ran up the street, feeling sure that she was about to die. The subsequent attacks occurred chiefly at night. She had been examined on several occasions during or immediately after an attack and attention directed to her heart as a possible cause. Previous medical history threw no light on these attacks. Her father was asthmatic; otherwise, the family history was negative.

Clinical and Laboratory Studies

The intern on receiving ward suggested *hypoglycemia* as a cause and although the initial fasting blood sugar was low subsequent tolerance tests failed to confirm this suggestion. The cardiac department suggested from their study that the patient might have suffered a *coronary occlusion* but there was nothing in the clinical picture to confirm this diagnosis. The gynecologist thought she might be *pregnant* but this was ruled out. General physical examination demonstrated no abnormalities. The blood pressure was 110/70. The temperature remained normal throughout her stay in the hospital. The urine was repeatedly negative; the blood count good; the Wassermann negative. X-ray studies demonstrated a normal chest and a completely normal gastrointestinal tract including the cholecystogram. The basal metabolic rate was minus 2. The vital capacity was 78 per cent. Neurological examination was negative and the eyeground study was normal. Thus, it was felt that we could safely rule out any evidence of organic disease.

LIFE SITUATION

Study of the emotional life revealed the following facts. At about the age of fourteen or fifteen the patient had a long illness during which she suffered from severe pains in the head. Many physicians were consulted but they failed to relieve her. She was finally taken to an "herb" doctor who informed her that someone had "poisoned" her by doing something to a lock of her hair and that was the reason that she had pains in her head. (She recalled that a man, working in the same factory, had removed some hair from her comb.) The cure prescribed was to tie the belly of a live frog against her forehead overnight! The following morning the frog was to be taken to the front door and if he hopped away he would carry her "misery" with him. She was very much upset by the process and very frightened; nevertheless, the frog behaved well and the "misery," so she states, left her, never to return. When sixteen she married but continued to have sexual relations with another man and was *frigid* with her husband. He accused her of her infidelity and she finally left him, whereupon he said to her, "As long as you do not live with me, you'll never do any good." She tried her best to banish this thought from her mind, but, as we shall see, without success.

Powerful Effect of Superstition

The first attack, as described above, occurred one night after she had had sexual intercourse with her lover and it seems reasonable to suppose that this furnished a situation to call forth the curse or "poison" that her former husband had put upon her. The reason that we suggest this is that after complete physical and laboratory investigations had been made upon this patient we informed her that we could find no evidence of organic disease. She thereupon volunteered that this "bad nigger," her former husband, must have "poisoned" her. Asked why she hadn't suggested this idea before she intimated that she had taken refuge in the thought that various doctors had suggested that she really had heart disease and also that the idea of being "poisoned" was so intolerable to her that she had done her best to keep it out of her mind.

Dream Interpretations

A dream suggested some thoughts of unconscious origin to confirm our suspicions. She very often dreamed of snakes. Recently a dream occurred in which she was swinging over a pit where there were many snakes with black tops and white bottoms. To these snakes she associated enemies and "her husband, who hates her." Apparently the dangerous snakes symbolized the husband's "poison" that threatened her. Later she stated that on occasions she had also seen visions and heard voices.

Effect of Spinal Puncture

We did not hope for success in the psychotherapeutic management of this patient but during the course of her study a spinal puncture was done which she concluded had "drained the poison off" and she left the hospital much improved.

Unreliability of Suggestive Therapy

It is of course noteworthy that not only in suggestible people do such physical measures often bring about temporary help. We have discussed this problem in other connections. The point is that so long as the underlying psychological origin of the anxiety is untouched the symptom will return or something else will take its place.

The potency of the *taboo* in primitive thinking as a cause for anxiety probably occurs more often than we have been led to imagine is possible in our present-day civilization. Certainly it was well illustrated in this young colored woman, who must be considered as an early schizophrenic.

EMOTIONAL FACTORS IN COMMON COLDS

While it is generally agreed that colds are due to infection there remains the suspicion that other factors are involved, particularly in the patient who develops colds too frequently. Some patients say they "have a cold all the time," or they "get over one cold, only to get another," or they "have a cold from the beginning of the winter until late spring." Stories like the following are frequently heard. A shy party guest finds himself sitting in a draft and knows that this may cause a cold, yet he is afraid to move lest he call attention to himself, or feels he would be imposing upon his host to ask to have the window closed, or for some other reason continues to remain in a position which endangers his health. Then there is the young woman who rides in an open car on a cold day and wears her most fetching clothes, but at the same time, clothes which are neither comfortable nor suitable for the weather. It is more important for her to make a pleasing impression upon someone than to think of the danger to her health.

These are rather superficial matters and might come under the heading of plain carelessness or foolhardiness. Nevertheless, they indicate that inquiry into the habits of living is necessary in cases of the common cold. The shy, anxious person who dares not move away from a drafty window can be reassured that he will not be despised or laughed at if he seeks to protect his health. The vain person can be shown other ways of gaining favor and prestige than courting a respiratory infection by unnecessary exposure.

More Complex Psychological Problems

When we consider the people who seem to have repeated colds in spite of anything they do, and who may, in fact, be taking excellent care of themselves under all situations, we may find more complex psychological problems related to their indisposition.

Saul and his colleagues reported a study of fifteen patients, treated psychoanalytically for other reasons, who were subject to unusually frequent colds and sore throats. Following treatment every one of these patients had been either entirely free from colds, or had them with conspicuous rarity. No treatment other than psychoanalysis had been employed in any of them.

Clinical Findings. Some of the clinical findings follow: A middle-aged man had a very passive character which had resulted from spoiling in childhood by an overindulgent mother. This passive component of his character was, of course, unconscious, and to keep it concealed, the patient made a great show of independence. When his expectation of receiving what he wanted from others was thwarted in his daily life he reacted with dreams of attacking people with his mouth. His wife noted that his dreams and restlessness were accompanied by severe grinding of the teeth. As a result of these activities his throat, gums, and jaws would be sore in the mornings. At the same time he would react with nasal congestion and secretion. If the thwarting of his desires was severe enough there would be coryza, mild depression of spirits, nausea, constipation, headache, and fatigue. The symptoms would disappear almost immediately following insight into the unconscious mechanisms of his demands on those around him and his rage at being thwarted. For two years following the analysis of this patient there were no more colds, something the patient had never experienced before. Moreover, he was free from a mild soreness of the pharynx which had been persistent for many years. Another patient who had severe colds all winter, had anxiety, restlessness, and hypochondriacal fears of tuberculosis, accompanying each cold. A low-grade fever was almost invariably present. In this case, just as in the man previously mentioned, the colds occurred whenever the patient became distressed and panicky because her intense demand for attention and affection were thwarted.

In some patients *leukorrhea*, diagnosed by the gynecologist as a catarrhal vaginitis, often accompanied the cold. It was felt that the emotional stimuli might be the same for both a nasopharyngeal catarrhal secretion and a vaginal catarrhal secretion. This is an interesting connection when one thinks of the similarity of the lining mucosa and the presence of erectile tissue in both the genital and nasal regions.

Anxiety and Depression

Saul and his coworkers believe that the general feeling of fatigue, loss of energy, malaise, and so forth, so frequently seen in colds, might be the manifestations of a mild depression of spirits and anxiety accompanying the cold rather than the toxic manifestations of the local inflammation.

"Feeding a Cold"

The relation of this type of cold to allergy, rather than to infection, was mentioned but it was thought that whether the cause was a germ, a virus, changes in temperature, allergy, or a combination of factors, it seemed that the emotional situation was the main etiological factor. They thought that the old saying, "Feed a cold—starve a fever," may have arisen because of the fact that these people who had been emotionally thwarted had some of their longings satisfied through eating, and that the eating process, therefore, did more than supply necessary nourishment. The conclusion of this study was that while one must recognize other factors than emotional conflicts in common colds, nevertheless, there may be cases which will be resistant to treatment until some deep personality problem is readjusted.

Relation to Allergy

It is unfortunate that more psychological studies are not available of the common condition, *vasomotor rhinitis*, which is a kind of perennial hay fever. Elsewhere reference will be made to the general problem of the Relation of the Emotions to Allergy and again the studies of Saul and his coworkers will be quoted. Probably many of their observations concerning hay fever apply equally well to this condition.

Usually vasomotor rhinitis is regarded as a purely allergic problem but its relation to sinusitis is important. Formerly it was often regarded as *sinusitis* and numerous operations were performed, usually without benefit. Now it is recognized that vasomotor rhinitis frequently precedes sinusitis. By blocking of the nasal passages drainage is interfered with and sinusitis may follow. What is not recognized is that emotional factors are just as important as allergic factors in its etiology (p. 715). This is a subject to which Wolff and his associates have devoted considerable attention.

EMOTIONAL FACTORS IN PULMONARY TUBERCULOSIS

Anyone who has carefully studied pulmonary tuberculosis realizes that there is more to the etiology of this disease than a constitutional factor and the presence of the tubercle bacillus. Two additional factors are undernourishment and fatigue. It has not been sufficiently stressed that there are emotional patterns which are related to eating habits, appetite, and nutrition, and that these may be responsible for the underweight with which many cases of pulmonary tuberculosis begin. Furthermore, anxiety may prevent adequate sleep and rest. Finally, the shallow respiratory excursion seen in certain anxious personalities may play some role in this disease. These and other emotional factors should be considered in the etiology of pulmonary tuberculosis.

High Incidence of Neurosis

It has been frequently observed by physicians and nurses working in tuberculosis sanatoria that there is a high incidence of neurosis in people suffering from this disease. So often the neurosis is attributed to the disease but, as suggested above, the neurotic constitution may be present before the disease starts and indeed may be a factor in the etiology. In other words, neurotic symptoms during the course of tuberculosis are the result of neurotic trends present in the personality previous to the disease and only accentuated by it. The restrictions imposed by sanatorium life and the experiences of chronic illness, of course, add their complications. Intensive psychiatric treatment of the neurosis accompanying many cases of incipient tuberculosis would do much to hasten cure and to insure that the cure lasted, by bringing about a more efficient utilization of the patient's psychic energy.

A strong need for love and protection seems to be present in some of the cases which have been studied, the same trend which has been found in cases of disease of the upper gastrointestinal tract. One patient may have been overworking in order to obtain satisfaction for this emotional need, meanwhile taking poor care of himself, while another patient may have reacted much more passively, readily submitting to the slightest indisposition, but in either case the relation of this emotional need to the total picture of the disease must be given more attention by general medicine. Certain aspects of this problem are understood and brilliantly described by Thomas Mann in *The Magic Mountain*.

Personality Study

A study by Hartz illustrates the relationship of some deeper psychological mechanisms to the development of tuberculosis.

A nineteen-year-old girl had pneumonia in December 1940. She returned to school in January 1941, felt well, told no one of blood-spitting which occurred in February. X-ray in May showed extensive tuberculosis.

Following admission to a sanatorium and pneumothorax in July 1941 she did well, but a year later developed anxiety attacks.

The patient was the only child of very diverse parents. Her father was a self-made man with slight schooling. He was sports editor of a local newspaper, and contributed to several widely read sports magazines. The patient's mother was well educated, timid and retiring, and dominated by the aged grandmother. The patient resented the grandmother's strict rule but there was no trouble until the mother's first mental depression, which occurred when the patient was ten. During this time the mother remained secluded, nursed by the grandmother. This marked a turning point in the life of the ten-year-old daughter. She clung to her father, became very much interested in everything that he did, and ignored the mother as much as possible. The girl's activities in school became a mirror of her father's activities, and he seemed to welcome this identification.

Busy with clubs, cheerleading, and dramatics, she was never at home and thus avoided the demands of her mother. There was a frenzy in her activities. Three weeks before the onset of her pneumonia in December 1940, she was exhausted but kept going. Anxiety to be out of her home explained her neglect to mention the blood-spitting. She was secretly rather glad when she was told she had tuberculosis. The mother reacted to this news with another depression, and was unable even to correspond with the daughter. The girl's anxiety attacks, which may have aggravated her tuberculosis, grew severe when she learned that her mother was getting well enough to visit her. When the mother arrived she suggested at once that the girl leave the sanatorium and come home with her.

The problem was solved by the girl, who, in the presence of both parents, suddenly voiced her resentment of her mother's behavior. This was followed by the disappearance of the patient's anxiety symptoms. The patient left the sanatorium a few months later, but after being home with her mother she had a return of symptoms and eventually a spread of the disease to the other lung.

Social Readaptation

Coleman and his associates failed to observe any personality factors which appear to have etiologic significance in tuberculosis, but they were impressed with the relationship between personality trends and prognosis. Discussing all phases of the care and management of the tuberculous patient, they emphasize that medical care should include:

1. orientation of the patient to his illness,

2. evaluation of organic and psychologic factors and their interaction,

3. a plan of treatment to include organic and psychosocial factors,

4. a period of social readaptation, with regard for psychosocial as well as organic limitations. They look upon psychiatric insight not as an occasional need but as of continuous importance in any program of comprehensive care in tuberculosis.

Social Work and Tuberculosis

Largely through her work in tuberculosis the social worker has become recognized as an indispensable member of the medical team. Her position was securely established as a result of the broader approach to illness and disease achieved through the medical experiences of World War II. Where tuberculosis is concerned she enters into every phase of treatment, hospital admission, and home care. Spencer explains that "family problems may arise during hospitalization which are harassing to the sick person and may impede his recovery. It is the [case] worker's responsibility to deal with these problems, frequently in cooperation with some other agency. Such situations may be due to the following causes: the lack of continuous correspondence from the family, the lack of a regular allowance, fears based on poor familial relationships, the threat which the illness presents to the patient in relation to his status in his home and community, and guilt arising from the inability to be a provider. In addition there are more deep-seated motivations, such as: realization of an unconscious drive to be sick in order to abandon family, job and community responsibilities; hostility toward a member of the family, who may be imagined as an instrumental agent in the inception of the illness; and restlessness as a result of the enforced relinquishment of normal social outlets and experiences with the family.

"The same or opposite reactions in the family picture may be noted and dealt with by the community [social] worker: anxiety caused by illness of one of its members; fears of infection of another individual of the group, generated by a knowledge of the disease and enhanced by the necessity for a checkup of every other group member; hostility towards the patient for having brought the disease into the home; acknowledgement, conscious or otherwise, by mother, father or siblings that they may have been in some way responsible for the patient's breakdown; rejection of the patient as a cause or result of the disease and bringing into consciousness of this rejection by the necessity for hospitalization; overcompensation for relief at the removal of the patient, expressing itself either in the attitude of being unwilling to face separation or in the anxiety manifested regarding the patient's progress."

Speaking of the service in a tuberculosis hospital, Spencer concludes that a comprehensive social service and vocational therapy department is an important factor, not only in the arrest or cure of the tuberculosis, but also in the stabilization of the personality to the end that the patient may remain well.

In a more recent paper from the same institution Axelrad emphasizes that the social worker's approach must be integrated with the total plans formulated jointly between the physicians, social worker, and guidance counselor. She calls attention to the fact that staff members specifically trained to deal with the psychological difficulties of the patient need good medical orientation and the reverse is equally true, that is, staff members responsible for the physical care of the patient must have a psychological orientation.

Excessive fear of tuberculosis is a common clinical problem. It occurs both in those who have never had the disease and in those who have recovered from it.

Tuberculophobia—Healed Tuberculosis; Neurotic Invalidism; Hospitalitis; Character Problem

---

CASE 61

History and Symptoms

An intelligent, single, white woman complained of pain in the right lower quadrant of the abdomen and in the right loin; pain in the precordium referred down the left arm; shortness of breath and tightness in the chest; an ache in the throat with bleeding from the throat and soreness on talking or coughing; severe headache; nausea and vomiting.

The patient stated that her entire life had been "*one long succession of illnesses,*" starting with whooping cough in 1912, when she was six years old. About the age of twelve or thirteen, according to her medical advisors, she developed tuberculosis. She was ill and weak for the next five years and at the age of eighteen had a *tuberculous left kidney removed.** No microscopic pathology was done but the surgeon informed her that it was a badly diseased kidney. She then developed *tuberculosis of the bladder,** with frequency, burning, and hematuria, which she said was cured in about two years. At this time she insisted that she also had evidences of pulmonary tuberculosis but stated that nothing was done

---

* These diagnoses were given by the patient and could not be confirmed.

until the age of twenty-two when she went to a private sanatorium for seven months. She was studied at this time from the standpoint of intestinal tuberculosis but a gastrointestinal X-ray series was negative.

In spite of this background of illness the patient continued to work and attend college and finally completed her education at the age of twenty-seven. She had frequent breakdowns and hospitalization during this period. Then she developed a pain in the right side of the abdomen and right loin and was generally run down and weak. She felt "miserable and was worried about her right kidney." Studies were done which were reported negative but a diagnosis of *chronic appendicitis* was made. In spite of her illness she worked and managed to hold an excellent position. At the age of thirty, in March, 1936, she went to another private sanatorium in the southwest, suffering from "general asthenia." She had "slight fever, low blood pressure, was very thin and rundown." At this institution she gained weight and her general health improved considerably. She remained there for three months. There was no evidence of active tuberculosis and a tuberculin test was negative. She did, however, have severe *gastrointestinal symptoms* such as nausea and vomiting. Sometimes these symptoms would come on in the middle of the night "for no apparent reason."

Fever and Fatigue. The next medical episode was "painful swelling of the glands in the neck" accompanied by extreme fatigue and a fever of 100° F. The temperature was especially elevated in the premenstrual period. She maintained her weight, however, and returned to the sanatorium where she remained until the end of April, 1937. Here, in spite of the fact that she continued to hold her weight (in fact, gained up to 127 pounds, which is the highest that she had ever been), she did not feel well and developed pain in the joints and some limitation of motion. The glands in the neck, she stated, remained large and tender in spite of sun treatments. She developed black spots in front of the eyes and on one occasion had a violent attack of diarrhea for which no cause could be found. She felt that she was worse than she had ever been. Her back and right arm were the only regions of the body in which she had no pain!

Many Diagnoses and Numerous Forms of Treatment. In the spring of 1937 she entered a general hospital, where she was thoroughly studied. She remained until September and then continued to visit the outpatient department for another three months. The gastrointestinal department made a diagnosis of *brucellosis* on the basis of a positive agglutination test, and the gynecologist made a diagnosis of *ovarian cyst.* An *exploratory laparotomy* was done and a multiple cystic right ovary was found and removed, also part of the right tube and the appendix. She said that the appendix was found to be normal. The chest department made a diagnosis of *old fibrotic tuberculosis* with many calcified hilar nodes. She was treated by *brucellin injections* twice a week for the entire summer but felt no better at the end of the summer. By December she was somewhat improved but still dissatisfied with the diagnosis and visited a special tuberculosis clinic. No definite conclusions were reached here and she was made quite ill by *sun treatments*. Now she had much intestinal pain, fever, frequency of urination, and loose bowel movements. She also suffered from frequent sore throats, colds, fatigue and joint pains, and attacks resembling "grippe." From this clinic she went to another for treatment of brucellosis. Here she was told that she had no brucellosis and that the diagnosis was "chronic tuberculosis in an unlocated area." She returned to the first clinic for further rest which continued until the end of June, 1938, but by the end of the summer she became very fatigued, had an attack of "grippe" lasting three days, and this was followed by *marked exhaustion*. She was generally wretched, now was bothered with much intestinal gas and great thirst, returned to the first clinic and was told the stool examination showed the presence of *staphylococcus*. Then she developed backache; the pain was severe over the entire spine and she became very nervous with a sensation of falling just as she was about to go to sleep. She also had marked shakiness in the legs. Then she had what she called *"heart attacks"*—sharp precordial pain referred down the left arm. In December, 1938, she noticed bright red spots of blood in her stool. Returning to her home in March, 1939, she continued to lose weight, became very weak, and had "terrible headaches." She went to a small hospital—her weight at this time was 87 pounds—and finally was admitted to Temple University Hospital.

The *menses* began at fifteen and had been very irregular until the removal of the cystic ovary in May, 1937. Since then they had been quite regular.

Family History. The mother died of tuberculosis at the age of twenty-nine. Her illness began with cervical adenitis and she had been sick for several years before her death. The patient was eight years old at the time. The father was fifty-nine and was said to have had a minimal tuberculosis at the time of his wife's death. The patient had one sister, age thirty-one. She was said to have had "some kind of kidney infection, not tuberculosis."

Physical Examination and Laboratory Studies

After this rather remarkable history of ill health we were surprised to be presented with a patient who did not seem ill aside from being very thin. She was quite tall and weighed only a little more than 100 pounds but her color was good. The fingers were not clubbed and there was no dyspnea. Temperature had been slightly elevated on occasions, 99.2° or 99.4° F., but the pulse and respirations were not increased. Examination of the head and neck showed nothing remarkable. There was a small lymph node at the angle of the jaw on the left side, but the cervical nodes generally were not enlarged. The thyroid gland was not enlarged. The cardiovascular system seemed perfectly normal, the blood pressure within normal limits, and the lungs showed evidence of an old healed lesion at the right upper lobe. The vital capacity was normal. The abdominal examination seemed normal. There was no special tenderness or rigidity and no organs or masses were palpable. The arms and legs were normal; certainly there was no evidence of chronic arthritis.

It was important, of course, for us to decide whether tuberculosis was present. All of the evidence was in favor of an *obsolete tuberculosis*. X-ray studies of the chest showed a healed fibrotic lesion in both upper lobes and a calcified lymph node at the right hilum. The urine was perfectly normal and the urogram showed a normal kidney on the right side, so that we could exclude urinary tract tuberculosis. The blood count was good, the Wassermann test was negative, and the blood sedimentation rate was within normal limits. Gastrointestinal studies proved negative.

We concluded that there was no evidence of active tuberculosis nor indeed of any other infection.

This really remarkable history of prolonged ill health seemed so out of keeping with the paucity of physical findings that we at once were led to inquire into the life situation to see if that might throw light on the illness.

LIFE SITUATION

It would take a long time to recount all of the details of this unusual life history. Unfortunately we must confine ourselves to the most important trends. After hearing this patient's story we could not help thinking that here was an intelligent, well-educated, attractive young woman who seemed to have some demon of destruction within her which, by its own force, or by allying itself with the tubercle bacillus, had worked against her on one occasion after another as if determined to prevent her from attaining success and happiness.

Family Problems

We have said that the mother died when the patient was eight years old. The family had always considered that the mother had married beneath her station. The patient's father was a man of good stock and fair background, but he had never measured up to the high standards set by the mother's family. Since the father was not approved of, his offspring was also not accepted, and the patient early in life made a resolve that she would work to bring to herself the approval of her mother's family. She held to this resolve firmly but barely won this recognition at about the age of thirty, after a great deal of time and energy had been spent in the pursuit of culture, education, and the obtaining of a position of importance. In achieving this recognition she had attended many colleges and had more than one degree. Her special interest had been psychology. She had traveled extensively, usually in search of health.

Personal Goal

During all this effort she had been held back many times by long periods of illness. In all she said that she saw at least a hundred and fifty physicians. Apparently none of them thought of a possible correlation between this girl's striving attitude and her illnesses! She stated that the things she always wanted most were love, a home, a husband, and security. As we understood her inordinate ambition we saw that it was hardly possible for her to have had the things she declared that she wanted, because this kind of personality, in the first place, could never have been satisfied with the love and attention of one man. She had enjoyed traveling and she felt that marriage would have meant settling in one place and quite possibly leading an obscure life. It was not hard to see that obscurity was something that this girl could never tolerate. She strove to satisfy her love needs by being an unusual student and receiving the attention and praise of many persons, particularly for her intellectual ability. She was attractive and had taken pride in her physical appearance, but this pride was small in comparison to that which she felt in her intellectual achievements.

Difficult Personality

As we studied her life story and her attitudes we saw that all of this girl's aggression had not been turned into healthy channels, but that there was a large quantity of it which spilled over to annoy and prejudice people against her. For instance, on the ward she had been very haughty and demanding, and obviously did not consider herself in the same class with the other ward patients. It was true that she had had a large experience and had certain abilities well above those of the average ward patient. That she was, however, on the same plane with them financially was to her merely a source of irritation, and she could not bring herself graciously to accept equal attention with them. She was so demanding as to bring a few disciplinary remarks from the head nurse. This had a most unusual effect upon her, and as she put it, "It caused her world to fall in upon her." In spite of her illnesses she had held a few good positions, on one occasion earning as much as $4000 a year. She had been helped financially by her uncle and had been loaned money by various schools which were impressed by her ability. She had been able to live nicely and command a great deal of attention and service. However, since we expect a person of the world to be able to meet a real situation with more equanimity than this patient did, her reactions, therefore, only indicated both the sensitivity and the hostility in her make-up.

Symptoms of Emotional Origin

The patient had had many gastrointestinal symptoms of both the upper and lower gastrointestinal tract with no evidence of an organic lesion to account for them. She also had "heart symptoms," a description of which corresponded almost exactly to that of an anxiety attack with palpitation. While there was definite evidence that tuberculous infection had been present in this girl's body, the nature of the gastrointestinal and heart symptoms indicated that they were of emotional origin. The fatigue of which she complained, also had been due in large part to the emotional tension under which she was suffering.

This patient had never permitted herself any heterosexual relations. She had not been uninterested in the advances of men, but she said that she never considered physical relationships with a man an important factor in her plan of life. She seemed to have been afraid that any feelings of this sort might lead to marriage, "settling down," and abandonment of her avid search for culture, knowledge, and prestige.

Possibility of Latent Psychosis

We thought that we were dealing with an unusually severe kind of neurotic personality; so severe, in fact, that numerous symptoms of illness had been the price paid for keeping in check emotions which could not be brought into consciousness. These emotions were primarily those of love and hate, but we believed the latter to be present to such a degree as to furnish the energy for a psychosis if a superficial or clumsy attempt were made to remove some of her symptoms. The patient had become more and more incapacitated until she wondered if she would ever be able to work again. Significantly she said, "If I must become an invalid then I must learn to do it gracefully." She had become quite discouraged in the six months prior to admission and while outwardly gay she talked of death and the end of things.

TREATMENT

Prognosis

Here we felt was too big a problem for a general medical man. Just as the physical problem in itself was very complicated so this young woman's personality structure was complicated. However, just as we have said that the general practitioner must be prepared to understand and treat the simpler neurotic problems which he meets, he must also be able to recognize his limitations and realize that a patient like this one is probably best off in the hands of a skillful psychiatrist. We could say this not only because incapacity was out of proportion to physical disease and therefore on a psychological basis, but also because that psychological basis in turn was deeply rooted in the character of this patient. Moreover, we were not very hopeful that after her many years of invalidism and her deep fixations on organic problems a great deal could be done for her from a psychotherapeutic standpoint.

Major Psychotherapy

Certainly the ideal treatment in this case was intensive psychiatric therapy. Treatment might release certain psychic symptoms, either in the form of depression or even of schizophrenia. This might sound like too drastic a kind of treatment but if such psychological potentialities resided within this patient, then she was doomed to suffer from many physical symptoms and be rendered economically inefficient until the cure of her emotional illness had been brought about. While temporarily she might be made psychologically sicker it would probably be for an eventual greater good. It was a major psychiatric operation but one which we felt was necessary in this case.

When a patient suffers from many symptoms over a period of years, in the absence of evidence of physical disease to account for them, and has also failed in social and economic adaptation, she should be regarded as a problem for major psychotherapy.

Follow-up

The patient remained in the hospital for a period of about six weeks and our conclusion at the end of that period was "no evidence of organic disease—pronounced psychoneurotic invalidism." A short time later she was admitted to a private sanatorium where she remained for a period of about two months. Here, too, physicians were unable to find any evidence of active tuberculosis or any other infectious disease but the patient remained unconvinced and through the influence of wealthy friends was finally admitted to still another tuberculosis sanatorium where she remained at the end of a year. She triumphantly informed us that in this institution they were of the opinion that she did have organic disease "even though it was obscure" and so we see our prophecy borne out that the long period of invalidism and the tremendous fixation upon organic disease, made it impossible for this patient to accept any treatment that did not play into her unconscious need to remain ill.

SUMMARY

A young white woman had led a life of chronic invalidism with repeated hospital admissions and many medical experiences. Tuberculosis had been present but was healed. Incapacity was out of proportion to disease.

Major psychotherapy was advised but the patient was so strongly fixated on ideas of physical disease and so unconsciously desirous of remaining sick that nothing could be done for her. When last heard from she was continuing her career of invalidism.

Another tuberculophobia case with slight fever was less complicated and responded better to treatment.

Tuberculophobia—Fatigue and Slight Fever; Marriage Problem
Fair Degree of Recovery

CASE 62

History and Symptoms

A young woman complained of fatigue and slight fever. She had been told that there was "something suspicious in her lung," whereupon she consulted a specialist who examined her thoroughly and told her that he did not *think* that she had tuberculosis. Nevertheless, the slight fever continued, and with the conviction of tuberculosis still present, she remained at rest in bed for one year. During that period she complained chiefly of fatigue and occasional mild diarrhea with a good deal of mucus in the bowel movements.

Physical Examination and Laboratory Studies

Physical examination and x ray studies failed to disclose evidence of organic disease, and discussion brought out the following story.

LIFE SITUATION

During the winter prior to her illness she was keeping company with a young man and the townspeople took it for granted that they were engaged. The following summer, while she was considering the question of the marriage date, she became irritable, lost weight, and felt ill. In September she had what she called "an attack of ptomaine poisoning" following a dietary indiscretion. It was during this attack that the fever was discovered and the suspicion arose that the lungs were affected.

Rest in Bed

She then gave up her work and spent practically a year in bed. During this period the young man remained as attentive as ever, but she told herself that it was not fair to him to continue her engagement. She argued with herself in the following fashion: In view of her continued illness, she felt that it would be better to give him up; that she would not be strong enough to marry, to have children, or to do housework. She had many more "reasons" why she should not marry. For one thing, both a brother and a sister had been unhappily married and were divorced. She also felt that her mother needed her, that she was happy at home, and did not like to leave. She informed us that her husband-to-be did not have enough money to marry but, on further discussion, there seemed no question that he would adequately support her.

TREATMENT

Different Approach Necessary

It seemed to us that a different approach to her problem was indicated. Instead of agreeing with her that she must exercise caution and that it would be better for her to put marriage out of her mind "until she was well," she was told that there was no physical evidence to indicate organic disease; that her slight fever was due not to any lung trouble but simply to a slight bowel disturbance which, in turn, was very closely associated with the worry and stress incident to the problem of marriage. We carefully avoided the term "colitis."

Then she was told that her illness represented an unconscious effort on her part to escape the responsibilities of marriage, and that all the points she raised about not getting married were simply self-deceptive rationalizations to assist her in escaping this responsibility. She then admitted that shortly after her engagement "she had a premonition that she would get sick." She was told that it was necessary for her to face the fact that she must either marry or not marry, and that she could not go on as she was going. Shortly afterward she announced that she would decide upon a marriage date. Following this resolution she became worse than ever. Her menses became irregular, she was fatigued all the time, had pain in the back, and became upset if there was any variation from her usual routine. Finally she forced herself to marry. Adjustment to marriage was difficult but at the end of a year she reported that she was fairly well. She still had considerable fatigue but did not worry about tuberculosis and no longer took her temperature.

This did not mean that all her troubles were over. Often there are grave problems ahead for the emotionally immature person who marries. This phase of the problem will be discussed later.

SUMMARY

A young white woman, following a slight bowel disturbance, discovered that she had fever. Suspicion was aroused that she might have tuberculosis and she spent a year in bed. Conflict over marriage stood in the background of the illness and partial recovery followed her marriage.

Chapter XX

THE RESPIRATORY SYSTEM (Concluded)

BRONCHIAL ASTHMA

Asthma is a well-defined clinical condition that has been recognized since the days of antiquity. Thomas Willis described the disorder in detail in 1679 and stated that "the Ancients allowed the cause of it to be only obstruction of the bronchi," but he himself referred to "the default partly of the lungs and partly of the nerves appertaining to the breathing parts" (Major). In fact he held that every inveterate case of asthma was a mixed affection due to a combination of the two causes.

Diagnosis

The diagnosis of a typical attack of bronchial asthma is seldom difficult. So-called cardiac asthma may present difficulties, and occasionally also obstructive lesions of the larynx, trachea, or bronchi. But the differentiation from cardiac asthma is the only one that usually offers a serious diagnostic problem. One of the reasons is that cardiac examination is difficult during an attack of asthma because of the distress of the patient and the loud noises in the chest. If there has been no history to suggest an affection of the cardiovascular system and the general physical examination discloses nothing that would incriminate the heart, the problem is usually not difficult, especially in the younger age group. It is in the older age group with evidence of hypertensive-arteriosclerotic cardiovascular disease that difficulties in differential diagnosis arise. However, if the history is carefully taken and the cardiovascular examination complete, including tests of circulation time and venous pressure, the differential diagnosis can usually be made.

Etiology

It is the etiologic diagnosis of bronchial asthma that presents difficulties. A *Psychosomatic Medicine* monograph was devoted to psychic factors in bronchial asthma, representing a number of studies by French, Alexander, *et al.*, from the Chicago Institute for Psychoanalysis. In this monograph, from which a great deal of the following material will be taken, Rappaport and Hecht present an admirable discussion of the clinical features of this disorder. In discussing the etiology they state, "Assuming that a careful history of the asthmatic seizures or the exami-

627

nation during an attack indicates that the presenting complaints are those of bronchial asthma, the following procedures stated in the order of their importance are used to determine the etiologic basis for such attacks: (1) history and physical examination; (2) skin tests; (3) environmental and dietary studies.

"The history obtained from the patient and his relatives is the most important single means for this study. Its value is directly proportional to the experience and diligence of the physician. While many cases fall into easily classifiable groups as seasonal, environmental, or infectious, a large proportion are unclassifiable problem cases. These require a diligent, persistent search for causes by an experienced physician. Even a thorough preliminary history obtained at the first visit often fails to reveal a clue to the causes of the attack, and it then becomes necessary to continue this form of inquiry during subsequent visits. If the patience of both doctor and patient holds out, this type of inquiry may last for many months during which other procedures supplement the search for causes. Skin tests, physical and laboratory examinations, environmental surveys of the home and of the place of occupation, the habits of the patient, and various dietary studies are the important steps in such a study." They go on to say that "despite these and a number of other means ol search for specific causes of the attacks, a large proportion of patients with asthma still remain etiologically unclassifiable. These are generally grouped under the broad term of *intrinsic asthma*. The following are among the factors that predispose to such attacks: bacterial sensitization from an obscure respiratory or distant focus or from a preceding infection such as pertussis; endocrine disturbances including the vague but well-known description of 'exudative diathesis'; 'vagotonic'; physical allergy, including heat and cold sensitivity; tissue electrolyte disturbances with special reference to the metabolism of calcium, potassium, and sodium; and finally, but not of least importance, emotional disturbances. Most of these factors are considered predisposing rather than primary causes for precipitating or aggravating the attack of asthma."

Emotional Factors in Bronchial Asthma

In the past twenty years or more many observations have been made and articles written on the relation of the emotions to bronchial asthma. Neurotic trends were recognized, but as in other "organ neuroses," were generally held to be due to the disease rather than causally related to it. It was noted that the sufferer from asthma often seems to make the most of his attack by drawing attention to himself and, by his distress, disturbing those around him to the utmost. Now, however, we recognize that the gain through such behavior is only secondary. The psychological factors that are important lie far deeper in the unconscious mental life, have no such thinly disguised purpose, and reveal themselves only after patient study.

McDermot and Cobb, in a clinical survey of fifty cases of bronchial asthma, studied each case from a psychiatric standpoint. They summarize their study as follows:

1. Thirty-seven of the fifty cases studied seemed to have an emotional component in the asthmatic attacks.

2. The thirteen "nonemotional" were predominantly young males.

3. Twenty patients reported that the first attack was emotionally precipitated.

4. Thirty-one reported that later attacks were often emotionally precipitated.

5. Thirty patients showed neurotic traits other than asthmatic, usually of a compulsive character.

6. Only 20 per cent of the "emotional group" were benefited by somatic therapy, while 54 per cent of the "nonemotional group" were benefited. Likewise in the "neurotic group" only about 20 per cent were helped by drugs and biological products, while 50 per cent of the "nonneurotic group" were helped.

Personality Structure of Children Suffering from Asthma

British investigators have been keenly interested in the psychological study of asthmatic patients. Strauss studied the psychogenic factor in asthmatic children and felt that a very large percentage were both overanxious and insecure. This anxiety often reflected the personality of the parents, who, in many cases, were themselves overanxious and insecure, and therefore would be expected to arouse a similar response in the children. He felt that the asthmatic children fell into two groups. The first were children who had been very much wanted by their parents, such as an only child or the first boy to be born in a family of girls, or vice versa; while the other group were definitely unwanted children whose parents were overcompensating for their unconscious hostility toward the child.

Rogerson, Hardcastle, and Duguid also worked predominantly with children who presented the "asthma-eczema-prurigo syndrome." They report that out of twenty-three "no less than seventeen of the children were fussed over and overprotected by their parents to a pathological degree. This was not just a slight abnormality of parental attitude, it was pathological to a degree which made one feel that if these children had not been brought to the hospital with asthma or prurigo they might easily have been referred on account of the nervousness engendered in them by this situation."

Attitude of Parents. This overprotective attitude of the parents was due to varying causes. In one case the overprotectiveness on the part of the mother was understandable, owing to the fact that she had lost several children and the patient was the only surviving boy. In several cases the children were born very soon after marriage; in two cases they were incident to forced marriages. In such cases the conscientious mothers were torn between a desire to love and cherish the children and a feeling of not really wanting them, which latter feeling, however, was so repugnant to their social ideals of maternity that they found great difficulty in bringing it to conscious expression. As a result of this ambivalence the mothers attempted to cherish and protect the children all the more strongly in order to overcome the feelings of guilt which the real attitude toward the child tended to produce.

The Asthma-Prurigo Personality. They conclude: "In fact, if we might be permitted to generalize from this small group of cases we might speak of an asthma-prurigo personality. The characteristic of this 'asthma-prurigo' personality which our patients have shown may be summarized as follows: high intelligence on verbal tests with a poorer performance ability, marked overanxiety and lack of self-confidence, considerable latent aggressiveness and egocentricity."

Psychic Conditioning. The authors raise the question, which they leave partially unanswered, as to how far some of these characteristics may be "the result of difficulties produced by the disease itself in the patient's relationships with others." It would seem quite possible that the excessive anxiety of these children and their parents' overprotective attitudes may be in part a reaction to the disability caused by illness. A severe asthma attack with its acute threat of suffocation is obviously a terrifying experience to both the child and its parents and it is not surprising that children who suffer from asthma should develop feelings of helpless anxiety and insecurity and a tendency to cling to their parents, nor that the parents should develop an overprotective attitude toward them merely as a reaction to the fear of the asthma attacks themselves. On the other hand, the examples cited above make it plain that in a number of the cases reported in this study the overprotective attitude of the parents existed prior to the onset of the asthma and had also a deeper motivation, such as need to overcompensate for not really wanting the child or the fear of losing the only surviving child after several other children had died.

Rorschach Studies. Then there is some evidence from Rorschach studies on asthmatic patients which suggests that the personality disturbance existed before the onset of the disorder. The Rorschach method (see p. 101), a projection test of the personality, has been widely used in recent years and seems to be one of the outstanding methods of personality evaluation. Schatia, who analyzed the Rorschach records of forty patients suffering from bronchial asthma, confirmed an impression gained by a number of analytical workers that asthmatics tend to have compulsive personalities without evidence of phobia or compulsion. Dunbar called attention to this fact in 1938, and Felix Deutsch made similar observations from psychoanalytic study.

Therapeutic Efforts. That the overprotective attitudes of the parents and the excessive anxiety of the children probably also have some part in the causation or at least in the aggravation of the asthma itself is indicated by the results of Rogerson's therapeutic efforts, which were directed primarily to encourage greater independence in the child and a less inhibiting and overprotecting attitude in the parents. In accordance with their concept of the personality disorders associated with asthma, they attempted by psychotherapy to modify the attitudes of both the child and the parents. They tried on the one hand to induce the parents to adopt a less solicitous attitude toward their children and to allow a greater degree of independence; on the other hand they attempted to diminish the anxiety of the child and to encourage the child itself to adopt more independent attitudes. In a considerable proportion of the cases, the effects of this sort of treatment were very satisfactory even when the child remained in the home environment in which the asthma attacks had been severe.

The Site of Selection for Organ Neuroses

Gillespie, also of London, expressed his belief that "an idea may become the affective stimulus which elicits the asthmatic response just as much as pollen or horsehair." He believes that asthma furnishes a striking test of what needs to be emphasized in the education of the medical student; that the body and mind are one, or at least that their interaction is so close that no examination of a patient should neglect some consideration of what is going on in his mind. He felt that not only could psychological factors in the shape of emotions or ideas elicit individual attacks, but that these factors could also act in a continuous fashion to produce a state of tension which every now and then would reach the stage of explosion expressed by a paroxysm of asthma. Why the organism should choose asthma as a special mode of expressing mental unrest, he thought, depended upon constitution, a preexisting fear of lung disease, a preexisting disease of the lungs, a conception of breathlessness, or an imitation of asthmatic attacks which the patient had witnessed. Felix Deutsch has also been interested in the choice of organ in organ neuroses. He suggests that many affections of the respiratory tract in childhood, coinciding with excessive emotional dependence upon the mother, formed a combination which might result in asthma. Thus the early affections of the respiratory tract plus its use for the expression of conflicting tendencies throughout childhood would create a personality of a specific structure. The mothers in these cases usually encourage the dependence and at the same time suppress the aggressive tendencies in such children; hence, the conflicts underlying this interaction between mother and child form the background for asthma.

Dunbar, in 1938, after an intensive study of asthmatic patients was not convinced that asthmatic patients undergo a "somatic preparation" in terms of early respiratory disease, such as croup, whooping cough, bronchitis, and the like, any more frequently than patients who develop heart disease, diabetes, or some other disorder. She felt that in any psychosomatic disorder the choice of organ was dependent upon a complex combination of psychic and somatic factors playing different quantitative and qualitative roles in the total make-up of the different individuals.

Parent-Child Relations

In the cases of asthma studied by Dunbar the struggle of separation from the mother was an important emotional problem. In the case of a woman, asthma and coughing began after her marriage, which involved leaving her mother, the coughing being in part an expression of aggression. The same dilemma and the same result appeared in the case of a man. Dunbar noted that the hostility in these patients seemed constantly on the point of being carried into action, and hence the patients were in constant terror. There seemed to be little intervening between fantasy and actually doing what was fantasied. Another noteworthy observation was an alternation between symptomatology in psychic and somatic spheres. One of the women became hypomanic and homicidal in the periods when she was free of asthmatic symptoms, whereas in the men there was depression in the asthma-free periods.

Further Psychoanalytic Observations

We have previously stated that the most comprehensive work on this subject has been carried out at the Institute for Psychoanalysis in Chicago. The work was first reported in a paper by French, which later appeared in monograph form. Twenty-seven cases were studied. The cases chosen were nearly all patients in whom *allergic hypersensitivity* had been previously demonstrated by means of allergic history and skin tests, this work having been judged by an experienced allergist.

Variability in Personality Traits. Reviewing the cases from a psychological point of view, the first impression was that the sufferers from asthma varied considerably both in their personality traits and in the type of emotional disturbance for which they sought treatment. A number of the patients had been particularly good children and in adult life their behavior was characterized by an urge to help and give to others. Some of the children, on the other hand, were brought to treatment because of their particularly aggressive behavior. In one of the adult patients and in one of the children the picture was that of a compulsive character with mild compulsive neurotic symptoms. An asthmatic man sought treatment originally on account of conscious homosexual impulses.

Common Features. However, in spite of these differences, the cases showed certain common features. In several it was found that the patient would have an attack when he was exposed to a situation which might estrange him from a parental figure, usually the mother. This might occur in an actual life situation or might be portrayed by dreams. The attack of asthma occurred at the point where the defenses failed and the patient was suddenly exposed to the conflict between an actual life situation and the fear of losing the mother's love. These emotions would become transferred to the physician in the course of treatment, and the patient's fear of losing the good will of his physician took the place of his original fear of losing the mother's love. Over and over again these patients would become blocked just at the point where the unconscious material was leading up to a confession, which represented an attempt at reconciliation with the mother figure. They would be afraid to confess and would develop an attack of asthma. As long as the technic of winning reconciliation with the mother by confession was successful, the patients appeared to be protected from asthmatic attacks. When the confession got "choked in the throat" an asthmatic attack occurred in its place.

Relation to Crying. There was much to suggest that the asthma attack is really a sort of equivalent of a cry of anxiety or rage which has been inhibited and repressed. For some reason, in the situations which provoked asthma attacks the child was unable to cry. Some of the patients stated they had not cried for years, and others boasted they had never been afraid. In some of the treated cases it was observed that as the asthma attacks ceased, attacks of crying appeared in their stead. Such replacement of asthma attacks by crying was particularly apt to occur as insight was gained into the cause of the attacks.

Threatened Loss of Mother's Love. The fear of temptation, and the loss of love threatened by yielding to the temptation, seemed to occur particularly in relation to the mother. Frequently, in the family histories, it was noted that the mother was overprotective to the child and bound the child to her in a dependent relationship but at the same time rejected the first signs of the child's genital interest. This created a situation in which the first early strivings of genital sexuality became a temptation which threatened to deprive the child of the mother's love, upon which it was so dependent. It was striking with what frequency the mothers of these patients played the double role of being at one and the same time seductive and prohibitive. Four of six adult male patients had continued to sleep with their mothers until the age of puberty or even later.

Aggression. The situation which threatened loss of the mother's love did not arise out of sexual temptation in every case. Pregnancy in the mother or the birth of other children seemed to play a role in precipitating asthma attacks. The possibility of another child, or the actual presence of another child, was a definite threat of the loss of the mother's love, and this in turn stirred up aggressive impulses, both toward the mother and toward the younger child.

Other Defenses. Defenses other than confession were utilized by the patients. Some were overobedient, seeking to avoid rejection in this way. Still others utilized sickness and suffering for gaining sympathy and affection. It was noted that symptoms such as rheumatic pains or headaches would tend to protect the patient from an attack of asthma. In the case of a male patient, an attack of asthma resulted in his being taken into his mother's bed. It was noted that many asthma patients were particularly prone to attacks of asthma at times when they were in conflict as to whether or not to leave some mother figure. Similarly, during psychological treatment, it was observed that asthma attacks tended to occur predominantly on weekends or during the periods just preceding some separation from the physician.

SUMMARY

To summarize this material concerning the emotional background of attacks of asthma French concluded that asthmatic attacks tend to be precipitated by situations that threaten to separate the patient from some mother figure. The separation feared may be actual physical separation; more frequently it is the danger of estrangement from the parental figure due to some temptation to which the patient is exposed. In such a situation the asthma attacks seem to have the significance of a suppressed cry.

In this connection Alexander added that in some asthma histories we learn of the peculiar, childish habit of breath-holding. To be sure this habit may occur also in nonasthmatic children. The background of breath-holding, however, seems to be always the same: A spiteful protest against the environment, something like a hunger strike, "If I do not get the protection I want, I will not breathe." Alexander continues, "The other emotional factor in the asthma attack expresses just the opposite tendency. The patient suppresses an expiratory function, crying, by which he would express his protection-seeking attitude toward the mother. This suppression of crying represents the opposite tendency, the wish not to give in to the dependent attachment to the mother."

"Thus, the asthma attacks, like a hysterical conversion symptom, express both opposing tendencies: the protest against separation and the protest against wanting to reestablish a dependent relationship to the mother by crying. This conflict seems to be the deepest and most primitive substratum of the asthma attack."

Psychic and Allergic Factors Complementary. Finally French and his colleagues concluded that *psychological* and *allergic* factors probably stand in a somewhat complementary relationship to each other in the etiology of bronchial asthma; that in some cases asthma attacks may be precipitated by allergic factors alone, in others by emotional factors alone, and in still others the combination of allergic and emotional factors seem necessary to bring about an attack.

The following case is cited to show the interplay of complex factors in the pathogenesis of bronchial asthma and to indicate certain treatment problems.

Asthma
Typical Conflicts; Danger of Self-analysis

CASE 63

History and Symptoms

A healthy-appearing, young white woman was first seen in June 1946. She reported that she had had severe asthma since early childhood and that in the more than twenty years that she suffered from this disorder she had known only a few periods of real freedom. These were the period during which she was away at school, and her two pregnancies. She also had eczema as a child and on a few occasions since, and vasomotor rhinitis which had been quite bothersome in recent years.

History of Allergy

The mother suffered from migraine and had asthma in her early years, and a brother had hay fever. The father had died of "heart disease" in 1942.

The patient reported that eczema began in early infancy and that asthma occurred at about the age of two; this was confirmed by the mother. When the asthma became quite severe about the age of seven she was studied in a large hospital where allergic tests were made for the first time. These tests were repeated frequently afterwards, the last time three years ago in the course of a complete study at a well-known clinic. Certain foods were denied the patient which she says she eats with impunity during the periods when she is free of asthma.

Physical Examination and Laboratory Studies

Physical examination showed a robust young woman with no evidence of eczema, rhinitis, or asthma at the time of examination. She appeared to be in good health, and no evidence of organic disease was detected. Routine laboratory studies were negative.

LIFE SITUATION

She was an obedient child who was taught cleanliness early. Brought up in a small community where the parents were in comfortable circumstances, she enjoyed all of the material possessions that a child could want. In fact she reported that her father, a tense, nervous, and domineering person "gave gifts instead of understanding." He demanded exacting obedience and the patient resented his treatment of her as well as of the mother. The father was so emphatic in his instructions to the young girl regarding men that she was constantly warned about the dangers of murder and rape. Pity for the mother, the mother's air of martyrdom and her threats of withholding love, forced the child into a submissive attitude. She tried to make up to the mother for the way the husband treated her.

Disturbed Relationship to Mother

She looked to the mother for approval, was very dependent upon her and yet, as she reached later childhood, found difficulty in accepting gifts from her. She felt that there was something wrong about doing so and this feeling has continued to the present time. Apparently accepting a gift was an indication of the dependence against which she struggled. When she went away to school, for the first time she became free of asthma for a long period and the asthma would recur only when she returned home at vacation time. In the junior year she was assailed with doubt regarding her choice of career but was afraid to change because of the mother. In order to solve the problem she became engaged, married the following year, and immediately became pregnant, "in order not to have to finish school." She was well during the pregnancy but a few weeks after the birth of the child asthma began again and she then decided to leave home and move to Philadelphia. The father objected but she left anyhow. Shortly afterwards he died of "heart disease." She felt no grief, "only a slight guilty feeling," and merely expressed the thought that "if she had not left this might not have happened."

Emotional Factors

Sexual intercourse, which had been painful before the birth of the child, continued to be unsatisfactory. She became concerned about the frigidity and decided to consult a physician but again asthma interfered. After another period of hospital observation failed to help the patient, she and her husband decided to move south. She did not, however, do well there and they ran into great difficulties, with the husband trying to earn a living and take care of the sick mother and child. The patient came north to visit the mother, who had remarried, so that she would no longer have to worry about the mother "being alone," but the asthma continued. When her child was three she decided that because she had been well during pregnancy another pregnancy would be helpful. True enough she again felt completely well during the second pregnancy but again developed severe asthma shortly afterwards. Now the husband's difficulties were redoubled because he not only had to work harder to earn a living but had a very sick wife and *two* young children to look after.

The patient went from doctor to doctor until finally one of them suggested that emotional factors must have something to do with her illness. For the first time she began to think of her illness from that standpoint and, recalling that during her school days she was entirely comfortable away from home and sick as soon as she got home, she concluded that her relationship to her mother must be the reason.

Self-Analysis

Now as the patient "thought the problem out for herself" she went through a very bad period. She was sleepless and despondent, had a "terrible, queer, detached feeling"—as if she were in another world; suffered from dizziness, pressure on the head, blurred vision; had fears that she would lose her mind or commit suicide and was unable to be alone with the children for fear that she might harm them. Her physician was in constant attendance and she poured out to him many of the thoughts regarding her life and her relationship to her parents, husband and children. She spoke of resentment against the father, of her hated dependence upon her mother, and of a nameless resentment against the husband "as though she would like to throw a knife at him." At the same time she admitted that he was an extremely able person and an excellent husband. If anything "he was too good" to her. She decided that she had been escaping from life and that with the doctor's help she would learn to face things. Now her black moods came and went and at times she felt exhilarated. For the first time she was able to achieve orgasm in intercourse. She felt like a different person: as if "a new personality was emerging." She described this new person as more adult, possessing a great deal of self-confidence. For several weeks she continued in this mood and was quite free of asthma but then, for reasons that she did not understand, her chest tightened up again and she became as ill as before. The couple decided to leave Georgia and on the way north by automobile she was very ill, causing the husband a great deal of distress and effort as he looked after her and the family.

Conflict of Love and Hate

After establishing herself in Philadelphia she very quickly improved as she was encouraged to talk about her life situation. Almost her whole conversation centered on the topic of her relationship with her mother and just as she described her life up to this year as one of affection and devotion to the mother, now her sentiments were just the reverse. She could find almost nothing good to say about the mother. In an interview with the mother we did not gain the impression that she was mean or malicious but it was apparent that because the mother had been deprived of love as well as material things in childhood she was determined to see that her own child was loved, protected and denied nothing. Thus she overprotected the child, confided in her regarding her loveless marriage, and made the girl too dependent upon her by threatening her with loss of love. These were the conclusions that the patient had reached in her self-analysis.

She described the mother as an infantile person who had encouraged the child's dependence, overprotected the daughter to satisfy her own emotional needs, dominated her by threatening loss of love and by an attitude of martyrdom, withheld help when it was necessary, and gave gifts that were not wanted.

The patient had some insight, however, because she spoke of desiring a better relationship to the mother with neither the affection she had felt before nor the hostility which she now feels. The mother would call on the telephone and say that she was going to visit the patient and the patient would develop an attack of asthma immediately upon hanging up the receiver. The mother would send gifts that the patient found either impossible to accept, or if she did accept them she promptly lost them. On one occasion she lost a valuable piece of jewelry and felt no remorse. This quixotic behavior was not confined to the mother, however, because on one occasion the husband gave her a twenty-dollar bill which disappeared the next instant and was found in the baby's play-pen. The husband recovered it and handed it back to her, telling her to be careful, and the next moment it was gone again. This time it was found in the waste basket.

Dreams

Her dreams dealt with frustration (for example, being tied up in a car that could not get up a hill, or in a plane that could not reach its destination). About the time that she was trying very hard to get established in a home she had a dream of "buying a house with a fence around it. In order to get the house she had to take the fence." In the face of this very obvious symbol she was asked what fenced her in and her reply was her illness, her mother, and housework. She was trapped in her adult life as well as in her childhood by the dependent relationship upon her mother, which she hated but from which she could not escape. It seems significant, however, that all the time that she was freely expressing her hostility for the mother she was free from asthma except for very minor attacks occurring in direct connection with the mother's visits, presents, or telephone calls. The husband observed that when the mother visited them the patient "withdrew from him, not only sexually but in every way."

SUMMARY

A young woman suffered from asthma which began at the age of two. Eczema preceded the asthma and vasomotor rhinitis occurred in recent years. There was a family history of migraine, asthma, and hay fever. Allergic factors apparently were not important in relation to the patient's illness; psychological factors seemed to be. Such was her dependency upon the mother's love and her fear of estrangement from the mother that she married and became pregnant in order to solve a conflict in regard to finishing school rather than confess to the mother her inability to pursue a course which she no longer wanted. On another level and untouched by therapy was her disturbed relation to her father which revealed itself in her relations with her husband.

When for the first time, at the age of twenty-six, it was suggested to her that emotional factors might have something to do with her asthma, she went through a period of self-analysis which apparently precipitated a near-psychotic reaction. The self-analysis brought into consciousness a deeply submerged *hostility to the mother* so that the patient, who had previously felt only affection and respect, now could hardly abide the mother. A physical contact such as a kiss or an embrace revolted her. But whereas in the period of conscious devotion (and repressed hostility) she suffered almost constantly from asthma, in the period in which she expressed her hostile feelings she has been comparatively well. That she has not been entirely well may be attributed to other factors, constitutional as well as psychological; then too, she cannot adequately ventilate all of her hostility by talking. To make an adult of her would be a difficult job because of her deep infantile attachment to the mother; only prolonged psychoanalysis could hope to accomplish such a task. Since that is impossible we must get along with less and it is hoped that this may result in some permanent benefit even if "cure" is not brought about.

Bronchial Asthma
Vasomotor Rhinitis; Paranoid Personality; Improvement from
Combined Social-Psychiatric Approach

CASE 64

History and Symptoms

A white man, fifty-two years old, first applied to the medical out-patient department of the Temple University Hospital in October, 1937. He complained of attacks of shortness of breath which resembled bronchial asthma, but the diagnosis was in doubt for some time. He also complained of frequent head colds and a constant discharge from the nose which he described in considerable detail, telling us all about the amount and character of the material and just what level in his head it was coming from and all of the peculiar sensations associated with it. Not only did he describe his symptoms in the greatest detail but he launched upon irrelevant discussions, waving aside any questions from his physician, and insisting upon telling his story in his own way. As a consequence many physicians in the outpatient department lost patience with him and probably for this reason were a little more prone to refer him to other clinics than is ordinarily done. As a consequence he was shunted from one clinic to another and accumulated a very thick chart. (*A thick chart usually means a complicated case and often one difficult to handle.*) However, we finally came to the conclusion that he was suffering from true bronchial asthma; in fact, one of the outpatient physicians saw him in an attack.

The department of *allergy* was unable to establish any specific allergic diagnosis and the *nose and throat department* sent us this interesting statement after examining him on a number of occasions: "We can detect no evidence of nasal or sinus pathology. There is no reason for treating this man in this department. It is regrettable that he suffers to the extent that he does but the conclusions that he reaches regarding his bodily function do not make sense. We feel that he should be handled as a sort of a psycho! *It will not help matters to poke things up his nose even though he likes it.*"

Family History. The patient came from a New England family of healthy stock and long lives. His father and mother were still living but had been separated since he was a child. The mother was in California and the father in New England. An aunt, of whom the patient was very fond, died in 1925 from "asthma and heart trouble." The patient married in 1912 at the age of twenty-four. His wife had four children.

LIFE SITUATION

He had always been a salesman earning a living on a commission basis. Conditions were satisfactory for him up-until about 1926 and 1927 when financial matters became difficult, and about the same time while in New England he developed asthma and hay fever. Up to this time he had been very well but since that time he suffered repeatedly from frequent colds and asthma. He concluded that the atmosphere in New England was intolerable and he left his wife and family and established himself in New York State. There he said that he was free ot asthma for a period of about three years and then he returned home. At that time, for some minor traffic violation, he was put in the county jail and much to his chagrin, his wife did not bail him out. This made him very angry and he again left his wife and family in 1933, came to Philadelphia, renewed his acquaintance with a woman he had previously known, and then established a home and had three children with her. Whether they were married, we were not quite certain. He insisted that each time he went back to New England to visit his folks, he got a severe attack of asthma and believed that it had something to do with the atmosphere or the water in the vicinity.

Personality Study

Because of his difficult personality and also because his physical symptoms did not improve with the regular medical treatment, he was referred to the psychiatric department and there they also had their difficulties with him. They found that he shifted rapidly from a discussion of his illness to his personal and economic problems, was alternately friendly and resentful, constantly complained of employers who were unsympathetic to him, and alternately flattered the hospital and condemned it because it had not made him feel better. After a number ot interviews the psychiatric department was unable to make any headway with him. He still felt that treatment should be directed to some portion of his body and refused to believe that emotional factors had anything to do with his illness. He placed much of the blame for his difficulty on the world economic situation rather than on his own inadequacy. On the surface, he appeared very confident and overbearing but he quickly became petulant and was easily moved to tears. The psychiatrist suggested that his bombastic attitude, his reproaches of those in authority, and his sensitiveness indicated that he might be in danger of developing a marked persecutory trend; in other words, paranoid characteristics were already very prominent in this man.

Home Visits

The patient was placed under the care of a senior student who visited the home. It was felt that because he had done so poorly in the outpatient department perhaps some additional information could be obtained from the home visits that would be helpful in understanding the illness. The student arrived at the patient's home in time to talk to his wife before the patient had returned and found her to be an intelligent and hard-working person who was trying, but not very effectively, to meet her difficult problems. She seemed to understand her husband's difficulties and was well aware that he was able to do more than he did. She seemed to realize that he was a great braggart, always waiting for some big thing to turn up, meanwhile neglecting the smaller ways of making a living or of looking after the little details about the house that might make it more livable. They were living in very poor quarters, as would naturally be expected of a patient on public assistance, but the student noted that there were many things about the house that could have been improved had the patient been willing to do so. The place was drafty and poorly heated and it seemed possible that many of his colds could be blamed upon this physical fact. "He just couldn't be bothered fixing the apartment."

The student held out to him the possibilities of getting a commission salesman's job with a friend of his that would be more likely to assure him of making a living but the patient was not to be bothered "with such little things." He wanted big stuff! He considered himself a remarkable salesman but rarely went out to do any selling because of his poor clothes and lack of an automobile and the fact that changes in weather affected his asthma. He constantly complained that his employers did not understand him, were unfriendly and unsympathetic.

Wife's Attitude

His wife was very free in her criticism of him while he was absent, but was very docile as soon as he returned. In a later interview she explained that he often flew into tantrums and on some occasions had struck her. She had a fairly good education and always earned a satisfactory living as a secretary but never since she married had this man been able to support her and the children. The student noticed that he had not taken his medicine and accused him of the fact in his wife's presence, which embarrassed him somewhat. We felt that this was a tactical error.

Relation to Social Agencies

The patient had been on public assistance ever since he came to Philadelphia but recently he had had an opportunity to visit New England and not knowing that the public assistance regulations would not permit him and his family to absent themselves from the city beyond a certain interval he lost his relief status and because of that fact applied to the Family Society for help. The Family Society is a private social agency in Philadelphia which makes an effort to help people with social problems but does not have certain funds for assistance purposes. They were able to help the family out and finally after a conference with us, were able to reestablish them on public assistance. The case worker of the Family Society found the patient to be a dependent individual with an infantile attitude toward his wife, and told us of an additional complication.

An Unwanted (?) Pregnancy

The wife had expressed a fear that she might become pregnant again, adding to her already difficult problem, and as a consequence had been sent to the Maternal Health Clinic for contraceptive advice. There she appeared to be an intelligent person but in spite of that fact was unable to master the instructions in the use of a contraceptive device. This appeared strange to the attending physician at the Maternal Health Clinic. It was only a short time after this visit that she spoke of the fear that she was actually pregnant again and this fact seemed well established because she had all the signs and symptoms of early pregnancy even though she had been given some medicine by her husband to act as an abortive agent. Whereas she had previously seemed very anxious about pregnancy, now that it was established she seemed to accept it not only with resignation but apparently with some satisfaction. Thus we were led to be suspicious about the whole situation in regard to this pregnancy and wondered if it might not signify that although she seemed anxious not to become pregnant she may have actually contrived, unconsciously, to become pregnant, for some such reason as to maintain her relationship with this inadequate person with whom she was living. This may sound strange but the fact is that while she constantly talked about leaving him and going back to her mother it was obvious that she did not intend to do so and even though she had suffered great hardships and even blows and humiliation at his hands, she still said, "Well, we will wait and see what turns up," as though he might change in his attitude at this late date. Therefore, it would seem that there was something irrational about this pregnancy. It was, of course, interesting from another standpoint and that was, what effect it would have upon him and his asthma because we felt that his dependent attitude toward his wife, and inner longing for even greater dependency, might be threatened by the pregnancy. The case worker was concerned to know how to deal with the family in order to be most helpful to them.

Follow-up

The patient continued to visit the outpatient medical department and at the end of a year we could report that he had not had any asthmatic attacks but he did continue to complain about his nose and relied upon a mild solution of ephedrine used as nasal drops and which he felt gave great relief. It was likely that here, as in many cases thought to be "sinus-itis," there was some nasal obstruction due to *vasomotor rhinitis* and that this affliction, like bronchial asthma, had a psychosomatic background. Certainly to regard it as "catarrh," "sinusitis," or even wholly from an allergic standpoint does not constitute a satisfactory approach.

Unfortunately this man's peculiar personality allowed little room for help from psychotherapy so that the best we were able to do was to offer him a friendly atmosphere, to reassure him and, with the help of social agencies, bring about certain changes in his environment.

So often we hear the statement made by patients "there's nothing the matter with me that money wouldn't cure" and this patient fervently believed that such was the case. We knew, however, that his difficulties would only assume another form if he were fortunate enough to have money. His personality was so distorted by *paranoid tendencies* that he would find it impossible to get along with people. Such recognition is, of course, very important to the physician in order that he may decide how such a patient will react to his care and what the ultimate prognosis may be. We were willing to continue to see him not because we felt that a great deal could be done but because we felt that *something* could be accomplished. This is in line with our belief that no case is absolutely hopeless; that if we pursue the psychosomatic approach thoroughly there is always something that can be done.

SUMMARY

A middle-aged asthmatic with a paranoid personality was benefited by the combined efforts of psychiatrist and social worker. His difficult personality made it impossible to accomplish far-reaching changes. Nevertheless, the asthma improved as his general life situation was bene-fited by the friendly, cooperative efforts of understanding people.

Chapter XXI

THE CENTRAL NERVOUS SYSTEM

Anxiety resulting from mental conflict may affect the central nervous system itself just as it affects other systems of the body. Insomnia, weakness and faintness, vertigo, numbness and tingling of the extremities, ringing in the ears, various ocular and visual phenomena, headaches including a large component of the disorder migraine, and even a certain element of the syndrome of epilepsy are some of the results of such anxiety.

INSOMNIA

Insomnia is a frequently encountered symptom. A victim of this disorder may state that he has trouble going to sleep, sleeps only a short time, and then awakens early. Or he may awaken frequently during the night, toss about restlessly, have disturbing dreams, and awaken unrefreshed and too fatigued to do his work.

The amount of sleep needed for each person varies. Some people get along on five to six hours nightly but they sleep soundly and awake refreshed. Most people never sleep so well for the first night or two upon changing arrangements, such as a different bed, or sleeping in a pullman car, or sleeping where there are unfamiliar noises. But, of course, we are not referring to such conditions when speaking of chronic insomnia.

Insomnia and Anxiety

It is always important to inquire about sleep in taking a medical history. *Sleeplessness* is not just a symptom to be met with sedatives. Rather it is an indication of anxiety within the individual and the proper approach to the problem is to try to discover the cause of the anxiety. Unless sleeplessness is caused by pain, organic lesions of the central nervous system, or advanced systemic organic disease, it may be considered a neurotic symptom and as such deserves the same careful attention as other symptoms due to emotional conflict. As with other neurotic symptoms people frequently make a fetish of their sleeplessness and surround it with all kinds of exaggerated importance. Every physician is familiar with the patient who insists "that he has not slept a wink" and yet the nurse reports that he has had a fairly good night. Some physicians are unwise enough to set traps for such patients and confront them with evidence to prove that they are mistaken. This is never a satisfactory approach to a neurotic symptom. It only increases the patient's unconscious determination to make the most of the illness, and he will seek another outlet for his anxiety. The proper way to approach the symptom is to listen attentively to the description of the horrors of the night but not to be too concerned and hence by this very attitude help the patient place the symptom in its proper perspective. Then an effort to understand the personality of the patient, in its relation to the life situation, may suggest a solution of the conflict and thus allay the sleeplessness.

Insomnia Not an Isolated Symptom

Many of our readers are familiar with an acute anxiety situation which will disturb sleep, such as concern over a sick child, an important pending business deal, the physician's very sick patient, the lawyer's important case. The anxiety here is a more rational anxiety, however, than we see in people suffering from chronic insomnia. In the case of chronic insomnia the patient may insist that he does not worry or that he has no problems. But it is the job of the physician to reveal to the patient the problem which is causing him anxiety. This anxiety, often borne of infantile insecurity, may be the result of misunderstanding in the management of sleep during early childhood. The child who is unable to sleep because of anxiety, may be disciplined for being "bad," whereupon the insomnia is increased. He feels insecure as a result of the unfriendliness around him, as well as from his own hostility. Then, in adult life, although the same individual may have every outward reason to feel secure, he cannot sleep because he is inwardly prepared through his residue of experience (unconscious) to expect catastrophe.

Treatment

Lack of inner peace and security may cause enough tension to require psychoanalysis. But sometimes a few simple suggestions will help to encourage sleep.

1. Try to relax for at least one hour before bedtime with quiet music or an unexciting, easily read book.

2. Avoid too much physical activity just before bedtime. Plan to have tooth-brushing, bathing or other toilet duties done an hour before bedtime in order to avoid being "waked up" too much in case drowsiness comes.

3. Resting quietly in bed is better than turning and twisting with annoyance because sleep does not come. Sleep must be wooed, not fought.

4. All sleep is to some degree restless. The quiet period without motion during sleep averages twelve minutes. Hence waking at intervals does not necessarily mean a "bad night's sleep."

5. Just as the neurotic person fears to exert himself when he feels tired lest he do himself harm, so the person who sleeps with difficulty may look forward with apprehension to the activities of the following day if he has less than his usual allotment of sleep. These fears are groundless. People differ greatly in the amount of sleep they need; often five or six hours will do as well as seven or eight.

6. To be resigned to the disturbance in the sleep function—to accept it and neither fight it nor fear its consequences may be a great help.

7. If seemingly insoluble problems tend to keep you awake, seek good counsel and start on the road to a solution.

8. Remember that rest alone will repair, to a large extent, the effects of fatigue. To be satisfied with rest, without demanding the anaesthesia of unconsciousness, requires fortitude, but this in itself is often an important step in overcoming insomnia.

It must be said that insomnia rarely occurs as an isolated symptom. It may be the most troublesome symptom but there are always other symptoms of emotional origin. The following case illustrates this point.

Insomnia

CASE 65

History and Symptoms

A single professional woman came to her physician because of insomnia and crying spells. She reported difficulty in going to sleep, restless tossing, and early awakening. She could not at first give any reason for these symptoms. Inquiry into her life history revealed that she was the youngest in a family of three with an older brother and sister, both married. The father had been an ineffectual business man and the mother a kind but colorless woman with "few definite ideas about life." As a result the patient had entered into professional work which she had followed with a moderate amount of interest until her illness began. At nineteen she had been infatuated with a man but the affair did not last long. She had had dates and was fairly popular with men but she never seemed eager to marry and have a home and family of her own. The result was that she felt she was no longer young and had failed to find what she had hoped for in life. When we asked what she hoped for, she replied, "I'm ashamed to say I don't know. That sounds ridiculous because in my work

I have to see that people have a plan of living that brings satisfaction. But I guess I never thought of that for myself."

LIFE SITUATION

Psychological Background of Insomnia

We urged her to try to state what she wanted to get from life. She said, "Well, I suppose I wanted to be more important to someone than I am at present. I feel I'm only a cog in a machine, a rather impersonal machine at that. I thought professional women got a lot of glory and attention but all I seem to get is responsibility. Probably what I want is a husband and home of my own and my own children. Then at least I can feel that my efforts are invested in something permanent." She then made the often-heard complaint that she had never met a man whom she could love. We asked her, "Have you ever thought specifically about marriage and living a day-to-day life with any of the men you have known?" She admitted that she had not placed her ideas of love upon any one man but still had in the back of her mind the idea that the man who would awaken her to the idea of marriage was yet to come and would have something special to recommend him. He would be unusually handsome or unusually rich or otherwise be apart from the ordinary men she had met. We said, "It looks as if you needed to be shaken out of an adolescent dream state. You have already passed men by who could make you happy and it is time you looked around you and began to take an interest in your available chances of happiness before it is too late. You have been anxious, as if pursued by something and that something has been *time*. You have been unable to relax and rest, as if there was some important thing you should be doing or thinking about. There is! But if you turn your attention to your emotional needs for physical love, home and family you will find that you can relax and rest."

TREATMENT APPROACH

As we said, insomnia is a signal of anxiety or distress but the cause may be unconscious. We must make the patient aware of his problem and set him consciously at work upon it. We saw our patient five times at weekly intervals. A male friend who had been mildly interested in her for some time began to be more responsive to her as soon as she began to realize what they could mean to each other. She was hesitant at first about the "niceness" of physical love-making with "just anybody." We pointed out, "Some degree of physical love-making is accepted in every community. You, like every other girl, must be willing to give your affection to some man in your community. To save it for a movie hero is not good judgment since there are only a few of them and most of them stay in Hollywood. Your friend is not just anybody. He is a respectable, well-thought-of man and you must respect him." This was followed by some discussion of love-making and sexual values which she had not received in her home, and upon which she had not informed herself. The result was that she came to be less self-centered and more able to interest herself in other people. She stopped crying and began to sleep better, and eventually made a successful marriage.

SUMMARY

We see from this case (and it holds true for others) how thoroughly we must enter into the life situation in order to elicit the cause of anxiety. Sedatives may occasionally be given the first few nights until the life problem is known and thrown into relief. But as we begin to understand the emotional background of the sleeplessness and set the patient to work remedying the situation we see an improvement in the insomnia.

WEAKNESS AND FAINTNESS
[See also **Vertigo**, p. 688]

We often hear these two symptoms spoken of in one breath. "I feel so weak and faint," the patient states. While they may be symptoms of physical disease, they are also frequently present in emotionally unstable individuals and are part of the neurasthenic syndrome. Fainting is apparently due to cerebral anemia as a result of a sudden autonomic imbalance, the emotional stimulus for which may be a frightening scene or an unpleasant sight. The autonomic action results in flight through unconsciousness. It is well known that fainting occurs not infrequently in nurses and medical students in the first part of their course when they do dissections, watch operations or postmortem examinations. But it is also a common occurrence in every walk of life in individuals who are emotionally unstable or who have not had the proper conditioning to blood, injury, filth and other unpleasant facts of life.

Significance of the Symptoms

Aside from the fainting which occurs in obvious physical disease and the once-or-twice-in-a-lifetime fainting of the average person, a history of "fainting spells" requires careful study. Many cases are found to be instances of *petit mal* and require the special management of the epileptic. Others are probably close to *malingering*. These "weak spells" or "fainting spells" are often used by self-centered people as a club over other people in the environment. They sit down or lie down, throw the head back, close the eyes, and thus many an argument is won. If it happens, and it often does, that they have been told about "a weak heart," they put their hand to the region of the heart as they throw back their head and close their eyes and thus, as the central character of the drama, they achieve an almost invincible position. These people never actually become unconscious. They are emotionally immature and so sensitive that if anything is said or done to hurt their feelings or if they are threatened with loss of love, attention, or prestige they feel the inner sensory discomfort of *anxiety*. They may be enraged but lack the ability to express this rage directly. The pain or rage is shunted into the autonomic nervous system; possibly they feel a little palpitation, breathlessness, or perhaps only the mild discomfort of anxiety which ordinary individuals go through every day but which these people stand so poorly; and they announce that a "weak spell" or a "fainting attack" is coming, go through the motions described and usually get the situation changed to their satisfaction.

The Mechanism of Syncope

In a valuable study of syncope, Romano and Engel follow Alexander in differentiating between hysterical conversion and vegetative neurotic symptoms. (p. 51). Classifying their patients with syncope into two groups, they pointed out that in vasodepressor syncope the loss of consciousness is preceded by rather striking clinical manifestations, including pallor, sweating, sighing respirations, hypotension and sometimes bradycardia, while in hysterical fainting consciousness is lost without any demonstrable changes in circulation or respiration.

While the similarities are rather superficial both conditions are psychogenic, that is to say, they are caused by chronic repressed or, at least, unrelieved emotional tension. The mechanisms involved, however, are fundamentally different, both psychodynamically and physiologically. The hysterical conversion symptom is an attempt to relieve an emotional tension in a symbolic way; it is a symbolic expression with a definite emotional content. This mechanism is restricted to voluntary neuromuscular or sensory perceptive systems whose function it is to express and relieve emotions. A vegetative neurosis consists of a psychogenic dysfunction of a vegetative organ which is not under control of the voluntary neuromuscular system. The vegetative symptom is not a substitute expression of the emotion, but its normal physiological concomitant.

Vasodepressor Syncope

In the application of this concept to fainting, Romano and Engel cited a patient with vasodepressor syncope in whom emotional experiences were accompanied by certain changes in the circulatory system which led eventually to loss of consciousness. These physiologic changes were clearly demonstrable in the form of pallor, sweating, changes in respiration and pulse, and in falling blood pressure leading finally to cerebral anemia and marked distortion of the electrical activity of the brain. The physiologic mechanism suggested flight. The concomitant emotional experience appeared to be that of anxiety overwhelming the ego and preventing other compromise compensatory defenses.

Vasodepressor syncope could be initiated by a great variety of stimuli such as venous puncture, facing threatening situations, and so forth. Indeed it is common upon first exposure to a new and threatening situation.

Hysterical Fainting

They contrasted fainting of hysterical patients in which there is a notable lack of change in respiration, circulatory dynamics and electrical activity of the brain during periods of unconsciousness. In other words, the absence of any alterations of electrical activity of the brain in these hysterical patients clearly distinguished them from the fainting which results from cerebral anemia. The specific hysterical structure of the neurosis manifests itself by the symptom of fainting as an attempt to express repressed sexuality in a symbolic manner.

Hysterical Fainting

CASE 66

A white girl of nineteen was first seen in early 1946 complaining of frequent fainting spells which had been occurring about once a month for the past year under various circumstances of "crowds, excitement, overwork, heat, et cetera." The patient fainted while relating the history and we observed that there were no circulatory changes. She simply rolled her eyes and slumped in her chair.

Previous health had been good, except for rather severe dysmenorrhea and she thought that more fainting spells occurred about the time of the period.

Physical Examination

Physical examination showed a healthy appearing girl with no evidence of organic disease. Routine laboratory studies were also normal.

LIFE SITUATION

The patient and an older sister and brother were brought up very strictly. Before she could go out on a date the father would give her a lecture about sex. When the patient was about eleven the brother became delinquent, later was apprehended for rape, and committed to a penal institution. With the background of her strict upbringing and this lamentable experience, the patient eschewed all thought of sexual matters and led a very narrow and prudish existence.

About the time that she was graduating from high school, and "excitement ran high," she developed the first fainting attack. She had known for some time that her parents were troubled but didn't know quite what about and forbore to speak of it, but about this time learned that her sister's husband had left because of her "fast" behavior and the sister had returned home. Now the patient expected more trouble.

One night "after having had her hair done" she was reading a book and the chapter closed with a woman falling off a cliff and at this point the patient fell out of her chair in a faint. Dreams followed that she was "falling or running away from something" and in her discussions it seemed very clear that her fainting was her response to sexual temptation, the danger of "a moral fall."

Treatment

Bringing this material into the open, encouraging her to talk about her brother and his sexual defections, her sister's behavior, and her father's early admonitions regarding the dangers of sexual transgressions, together with better instruction in these matters, brought about considerable improvement so that one year later she was able to report that she had been free of attacks for a period of more than six months. In addition she was better adjusted socially and found more pleasure in the company of men.

Weakness and Fainting

CASE 67

History and Symptoms

A woman of fifty, married and childless, came for treatment of what she called "heart attacks." They came on suddenly and produced weakness and faintness, and the patient believed that she would die. She insisted on never being alone. She had been the only child in the family of an educator who "loved his students but didn't know his daughter was alive." Her mother had been a semi-invalid most of her life. Our patient did well in school and college but never could make and hold friends. Even after marriage she did not do any better at this even though her husband was friendly and sociable. She tried to interest herself in cards but could not. She tried to participate in the work of civic clubs but never felt popular or wanted. She was always sexually frigid and had only one pregnancy which ended in a spontaneous abortion at the end of two months.

LIFE SITUATION

In her late thirties, she began to be concerned with her health and had an appendectomy, tonsillectomy, and frequent treatments for "sinusitis" as well as for "colitis." Her "heart attacks," so-called, began shortly after she heard that her husband was having a love affair with another woman. Having already failed, she knew that she had not the ability to hold him if she were symptom-free, so partly consciously, partly unconsciously she was trying to hold his interest and sympathy through her weakness and her fainting spells. Her husband understood this in part but still he remained in her power.

TREATMENT

We said before that some of these cases are "close" to malingering. Not that they are always consciously deceitful. There is always an element of belief in the reality of their symptoms and yet the mechanism is often not deeply buried in the unconscious. It can be fairly quickly exposed and, as in this case, the logic of behavior is so clear that the patient cannot long deny it. They need the friendly support of their physician's understanding and tolerance to encourage them to give up behavior which is due to emotional immaturity. Antagonism and condemnation only make matters worse. In the above case it was necessary to have a thorough medical study, which found no evidence of organic disease. In particular the heart was found to be normal. Then, as we have discussed elsewhere, it was necessary to say, "Your heart is not weak. It is perfectly normal and therefore you can exercise normally." This was essential in order to make an effective attack upon the already entrenched invalidism. We gave the patient assurance that she possessed a sound body and we asked her to use it as such. Then we allowed her to see the background of her life situation, which induced a more tolerant attitude and a better acceptance of her status, and her fainting spells subsided. "She couldn't feel sure that they wouldn't return"—but we pointed out that this was merely a warning that she wasn't sure that she could keep up her efforts at tolerance and good will. Nevertheless her improvement continued.

HEADACHE

Headache is probably one of the most common symptoms confronting physicians in their daily practice. It has been estimated to be present in 50 per cent of patients, being exceeded in frequency only by constipation. Both symptoms are often regarded in the same way, namely as an inherent part of the body pattern and the person takes it for granted that no relief can be obtained. It is true that some headaches are very refractory to treatment. The causative factor is difficult to locate and a therapeutic program that is not aimed at the causative factor is unlikely to bring relief.

Etiology

Headache occurs both as a result of physical disease and in association with emotional disorders. Among the well-known physical causes are organic brain lesions, vascular disorders, and toxic factors; for example, brain tumor, meningeal irritation, hypertension and uremia.

Most chronic headaches that are not migrainous or posttraumatic are "functional" and here psychic factors are all-important. Nor for that matter can psychic factors be disregarded in the first two groups. These will be discussed. Among the alleged causes which, in many instances, have only the remotest relation to headache, are constipation, eyestrain, focal infection, low blood-pressure, and "sinusitis."

These headaches may be located in the frontal region, in the occipital region, directly on top of the head, on either side, or "all over." They may be dull or sharp, constant or intermittent. They may appear at the time of some emotional stress or more often in the absence of surface anxiety.

Constipation. Probably the most frequently assigned cause of headache is constipation and it is very obvious why this should be so. On the assumption that "obstruction or accumulation" leads to absorption of toxins from the gastrointestinal tract which may prove poisonous, and that a symptom of such poisoning is headache, a great many sufferers from headache are addicted to the laxative, enema, or colonic irrigation habit. We cannot say that there is no such cause of headache but certainly it is overemphasized both by the laity and the medical profession and also exploited by drug houses from the standpoint of advertisements for laxative preparations and by institutes for colonic irrigations. Every physician has had the experience of observing patients who are constipated for many days and do not have headaches. They are also familiar with the headache victim whose headache disappears magically just as soon as the bowels move—too soon for a physiological mechanism to be responsible.

Eyestrain. There was a period only a few years ago when the *eyestrain cause* of all kinds of illness enjoyed a great popularity in the medical profession. It gave way to the focal infection concept in medicine but is still frequently held to be responsible for headaches. Again, as in the case of constipation, we believe that it is possible for eyestrain to be responsible for headache but not nearly so frequently as people think. Hardly ever do patients present headache as a chief symptom that they have not had their eyes refracted and glasses recently changed. It is almost as rare to see a patient suffering from repeated headaches who has not recently been *refracted* as it is to see a patient with arthritis who has not had teeth or tonsils removed. But just as in the latter instance, the arthritis is rarely benefited, so in the former instance, the headache usually persists. The subject will be discussed at greater length in chapter XXIV (p. 732).

Focal Infection. Any obscure illness is very apt to be blamed upon *focal infection* but fortunately the wave of enthusiasm for that concept of the cause of disease, which resulted in the removal of countless thousands of teeth and tonsils, is coming to a close. While the idea still enjoys a certain vogue in rheumatic disorders, it is no longer common for physicians to order tonsils removed or teeth extracted because of a headache.

Sinusitis. Physicians ought to know that sinusitis is not the commonest cause of headache. A great many patients refer to their headache as a "sinus headache" and indeed so common is this idea that patients habitually refer to the fact that their "sinus" is troubling them again, instead of saying, "I have a headache." First of all, to have a sinus headache one must have sinusitis. As discussed elsewhere, we have at last discovered that vasomotor rhinitis is not in itself sinusitis nor is a "postnasal drip" necessarily an indication of sinusitis. Again we must beware of a little thickening of the mucous membrane, so often reported by x-ray, as an indication that sinusitis is responsible for headache.

A genuine sinus headache is usually localized in one region, is periodic in character, occurring at intervals during certain times of the day, and usually is accompanied by localized tenderness. Even the so-called "vacuum headache" has these characteristics. Therefore, vague headache without the demonstration of definite sinusitis should call for a thorough psychosomatic study before it is definitely decided that it is of sinus origin.

Low Blood Pressure. The concept of *low blood pressure* as a disease entity or a cause of symptoms, almost takes precedence over high blood pressure, and the latter is acknowledged to be one of the commonest disorders of civilized life. When patients present ill-defined symptoms or an illness of obscure origin and the physician finds that the blood pressure is low, he is very apt to assign this as a cause, and from that point on, the patient speaks of "my low blood pressure" in the same way that he speaks of a "sinus headache." But the relationship is just as indefinite. The truth of the matter is that in recent years we have come to understand that low blood pressure is often a sign of longevity and therefore, rather than being a sign of ill-health, it is an evidence of sound physical structure.   Once again, a little bit of fact is responsible for a great deal of fiction.   There are instances of true *essential hypotension* in which postural circulatory changes take place and here the circulatory disorder may undoubtedly be responsible for headaches. Again, there are rare instances of adrenal disease in which the blood pressure is unnaturally low and may be responsible for certain symptoms. But the majority of patients who suffer head discomfort and blame it upon low blood pressure are really attributing the headache to a cause which does not exist.   The blood pressure may be low but it should be interpreted as an indication of probable longevity rather than as a sign of disease.

Headache of Emotional Origin.   Therefore, in the absence of definite organic disease which is known to produce headache, the physician should be aware that the common cause of "reflex headaches," so-called, is emotional stress, conscious or unconscious.   The results of fitting glasses, treating the sinuses, irrigating the colon, etc., for headaches of psychic origin are only temporary if they give any relief at all, and the time has come for the physician to realize what the layman has known for a long time—namely, that there are many life situations which produce anxiety which, in turn, expresses itself as headache.   This has been well enough recognized for the expression to have crept into the language that a vexatious wife is a "headache" to her husband, a difficult customer is a "headache" to the salesgirl, or the irate boss may be a "headache" to his employees.

Mechanism of Headache

From available data, including observations of patients undergoing surgical procedures on the head and subjected to mechanical stimulation of the intracranial contents, Wolff stated that there are six basic mechanisms of headache from intracranial sources:

1.   traction and displacement of the longitudinal sinus and contributing veins;

2.   traction of the middle meningeal arteries,

3.   traction of the circle of Willis and its branches;

4.   direct pressure upon cranial nerves V, IX and X and cervical nerves I and II;

5.   inflammation in or about any of these structures; and

6.   distention and dilatation of intracranial arteries.

The cranium, the brain itself, the parenchyma of the brain, most of the dura and the pia-arachnoid, the ependymal lining of the ventricles and the choroid plexuses appear to be insensitive.

Intracranial Pressure

Headache associated with altered intracranial pressure, high or low, is due to traction on pain-sensitive structures. Brain-tumor headaches arise from local traction upon adjacent sensitive structures, or from distant traction by extensive displacement of the brain. The histamine headache is a function of dilatation and stretching of cerebral arteries and surrounding tissues; the rise in intracranial pulsations in this situation has been demonstrated, together with the fact that the headache can be abolished by raising the intracranial pressure. Similarly, in headache induced by typhoid vaccine, an increase in arterial pulsations has been recorded and if intracranial pressure is purposely raised, a decrease is accompanied by abatement of the pain. Probably headaches associated with acute infections, sepsis, et cetera, are attributable to the same mechanism.

Arterial Pulsation

The soft tissues covering the skull, particularly the extracranial arteries, are pain-sensitive. It is from distention of cranial arteries, chiefly though not exclusively the external carotid, that migraine arises, and procedures that constrict these arteries and reduce their amplitude of pulsation will diminish or terminate the headache. The headache associated with hypertension seems to be on a similar basis, bearing no direct relation to the level of blood pressure, and susceptible to influence by agents that decrease the amplitude of pulsations of the cranial arteries. Here it is the contractile tone of the arteries which is of major importance; distention and headache occur in the hypertensive subject if this contractile state is impaired.

Muscular Contractions

Tension headaches, says Wolff, together with those on a vascular basis, constitute 90 per cent of the headache problem. These headaches may be psychogenic; they may arise from factors setting up contractions in various muscles of the scalp and neck, experienced most conspicuously as posterior headache or a "band-like" sensation. Such muscular contractions can be recorded electromyographically. The posttraumatic headache, too, is usually on a muscular basis. In the last analysis, no headache is imaginary: Emotions are quite capable of producing true headache, by their repercussions in the muscles or vessels from which the painful sensations arise.

Character of Pain

Generalized and bizarre headaches, such as the feeling of pressure on the top of the head and the "tight band" around the head are usually regarded as of psychic origin but Friedman and associates uttered a word of warning against making a diagnosis of psychogenic headache purely on the basis of the patient's description of the distribution and character of the pain. They illustrated this by the following case.

"A white female nurse, age twenty-two years, had been suffering from headaches for two months. These were described as a feeling of pressure throughout the head or in one or another part of it. They were occasionally accompanied by nausea or even vomiting and were usually relieved by aspirin. Two days before entry into the hospital, the headache grew worse, and the patient felt tired and listless. During the recent severe headaches, the patient screamed at times, was emotionally upset and even seemed confused but if she was spoken to she could always be roused and brought into contact. When the history was taken it was learned that she was dissatisfied with her present job, and that she had left her previous, congenial one just before the onset of her headaches. She lived with her family and was under considerable emotional tension, both because she disliked her stepfather and because the other members of her family disapproved of her fiancé.

"Physical and neurologic examinations were negative except for questionable blurring of the disk margins. Roentgenograms of the skull and lumbar puncture did not reveal any abnormality. An electroencephalogram was diffusely abnormal, more on the left than on the right. Since visual-field studies showed enlargement of the blind spots, a pneumoencephalogram was attempted, but the ventricles failed to fill. A ventriculogram then revealed dilatation of the entire ventricular system, and at operation a *medulloblastoma* was removed from the left cerebellar hemisphere."

Diagnostic Test

As a simple diagnostic aid in the examination of patients who complained of headache at the time of the examination, Friedman practiced the simple procedure of local infiltration of the scalp with procaine hydrochloride or isotonic solution of sodium chloride. This procedure usually brought relief within a few minutes after injection of either solution when carried out on patients with psychogenic headaches but patients with headaches due to migraine or cerebral tumor were not relieved.

Posttraumatic Headache. A great deal of work and much writing has been done concerning patients with symptoms persisting after head injury but many such patients continue to be misunderstood and badly handled. Ross and McNaughton pointed out that every head injury involves trauma, both physical and psychic. The physical effects are exerted on the meninges and the brain. Meningeal contusion and meningeal adhesions may be directly responsible for a localized type of headache mediated largely through the nerve supply to the dura from the fifth nerve. This may clear up spontaneously if there are no other factors in operation. It may persist, however, for anatomical reasons and require surgical interference, or the headache may persist for emotional reasons.

Many of the localized headaches appear to wax and wane with the presence and absence of fatigue and emotional stress, suggesting a relationship to cerebral functioning rather than to meningeal adhesions. Other effects include some intellectual impairment and some emotional instability with severe injuries, and at least temporarily after less severe injuries. These factors are interlinked with the psychic effects of the trauma, the previous personality of the individual, and the situational factors in operation after the injury, to produce an emotional disturbance which may result in any of the symptoms of headache, dizziness, fatigability, irritability, lack of concentration, and other mental symptoms so commonly present in psychoneurotic patients.

Mechanism. Simons and Wolff stated that between one third and one half of all persons who injure their heads sufficiently to warrant hospitalization develop chronic posttraumatic headaches. They studied sixty-three such patients, all of whom were known to have no epidural, subdural, subarachnoid, or parenchymatous hemorrhage at the time of observation. The vast majority of patients with posttraumatic headaches that persist or recur for long periods of time after head injury have no such intracranial abnormalities to explain their headaches. Utilizing the electroencephalogram as an indication of muscle potential, they concluded that such headaches result from sustained contraction of the skeletal muscles of the head and neck associated with the occurrence of sustained resentment, anxiety, frustration, tension, and fear, and are sometimes augmented by noxious stimuli arising from abnormal healing and scar formation within these extracranial soft structures of the head and neck. In many instances the amount of muscle contraction is minimal but it is probably the basis of complaint because it is sustained and because of an abnormal preoccupation with the head.

They concluded that, as to the basic pathophysiological mechanisms and symptomatology, chronic headaches which follow trauma closely resemble other headaches which accompany and follow stress and untoward life situations but which are unrelated to head trauma.

Kozol reported a detailed study of 101 civilians with acute head injuries. His method was a statistical analysis of fifty symptoms based on personality traits before and after the injury. Correlations were made with the nature and estimated severity of the acute cerebral trauma and with various potentially complicating factors, such as associated bodily injuries and various possible sources of psychological stress (litigation, occupation, and financial and marital difficulties).

A good portion of the posttraumatic psychiatric symptoms appeared in the patients with previous psychoneurotic personalities. No close correlation was found between the severity of the acute injury to the brain and the severity of the sequelae. A high correlation was found between the sequelae and persistent complicated sociological factors, such as continuing compensation, pending litigation, occupational stresses, and persistent associated bodily injuries, and the severity and persistence of psychiatric sequelae. The conclusion was drawn that given psychiatric sequelae cannot be ascribed to one particular cause or to any particular group of cases, because the etiological factors are specific for each case. Such studies as this are valuable in demonstrating again that the significant feature in any case stems from the underlying psychodynamics and is rarely correlated with a descriptive diagnosis based on a particular outcome of the basic dynamics.

Diagnosis. After calling attention to the necessity for a study regarding the presence or absence of skull fracture, and of neurological findings, the duration of coma, the amount of blood in the spinal fluid, the treatment given, and special tests such as x-ray, electroencephalogram, and psychological procedures such as the Rorschach method, Ross and McNaughton emphasized the study of situational factors as well as the previous personality background.

How was the patient's life situation altered by the accident and what other environmental circumstances are present which may be relevant? Does he fear the continuation of impaired mental power? Does he feel a threat to his earning power? Does he feel that he is deserving of pension or compensation? Are there any legal complications? Are unpleasant duties and responsibilities avoided because of the symptoms? If military service is involved what is the individual's attitude to the service and to his duties? Are there any concomitant reasons for anxiety or personality conflict? Was the individual working under an intolerable strain before the accident? These are questions which must be asked subtly, through indirect and tactful discussions, following up whatever leads are offered. They cannot be asked by direct query. When the proper approach is used, however, it may indicate what the patient's real "headache" is at the time of examination apart from his predisposition or the physical effects of the injury.

Treatment. Treatment should consider the whole person, and prophylaxis to avoid the psychic concomitants is the best guarantee against the development of posttraumatic symptoms.

The treatment of the patient who has already developed posttraumatic headache and dizziness and is seen some weeks after the injury, begins with the thorough investigation already outlined. This is the first step needed in order to reassure the patient and in order to understand the personal situation which needs attention. The mere ventilation of the emotional problems may contribute to a cure, although generally further psychotherapy and situational therapy are needed, as well as palliative drug therapy.

According to Ross and McNaughton a measure offering greatest promise, especially for the compensation case, is "occupational therapy merging into therapeutic occupation" (Denny-Brown). "If the individual who has reverted to a child-like dependent attitude as a result of the accident, demanding a financial recompense for a real loss of personality security, can be persuaded to learn again how to become a mature and independent adult earning his own way, both he and the institution from which he would have obtained his pension will benefit. Pension claimants are rarely satisfied with their awards, and this resentment, together with the hope of further compensation, serves to aggravate the symptoms. In contrast with this it should be possible to fit injured individuals into employment which suits them and which reestablishes their self-respect and sense of security. How much better, both psychotherapeutically and financially, if compensation and pension boards would devote to rehabilitation the funds now going into partial disability pensions. Both the brain-injured individual and the psychoneurotic, as well as the patient with a little of both, could benefit from a reeducation program helping them to make the best use of their resources. Surely it would be more just to the injured war veteran or the handicapped industrial worker to establish the principle that he deserves a secure job and not a dole."

Headache of Emotional Origin

CASE 68

History and Symptoms

A young farmer complained of severe headaches which were situated generally over the entire cranium. They had been present for about a year's time and had been unresponsive to drug therapy and dietary changes. He was the youngest of five children, having two older brothers and two older sisters, all married. The *father*, also a farmer, had considered himself a very religious man. He had attended church regularly, prayed with fervor, and taught Sunday school, but at home he had been a tyrant who rarely spoke to his wife and when he spoke to his children it was only to reprove them. He had died of pneumonia two years prior to our seeing the patient. The *mother*, equally devoted to religion, was just as incapable of practicing its precepts in her daily life. She, like the father, was never affectionate with the children, never praised them, never took their interests seriously. She seemed to feel that if through scolding, threats, or cajolery she could get our patient to church, all would be well. He had completed high school and had been working on the farm for his mother ever since, but his dissatisfaction with life was growing and his headaches were making it almost impossible for him to carry on.

LIFE SITUATION

Absence of Organic Disease

Physically and neurologically he showed no sign of organic disease. He was seen twice a week over a prolonged period. He soon made clear his hostility toward his mother and father for their unsympathetic attitudes. He was particularly angry because they pretended to be so good, "talking about the love of God, the need for man to pattern his life after the tolerance of Christ, and preaching the need of love of one's fellow man." He added, "If they had been that cold and cruel and unfeeling toward others without acting in the name of Christianity I might have stood it. But the hypocrisy of it all, which they could not seem to see, nearly drove me mad. When father used to come home from prayer meeting and start scolding me for some minor or imaginary offense it used to hurt me and sometimes I would cry to myself. But since he has died and mother goes on the same way I can't cry. I only suffer and hate and get these intolerable headaches."

Social Adjustment

His social adjustment was poor because all women seemed to him as his mother and sisters had been, *i. e.*, "critical, fault-finding, and wanting something all the time and having nothing to give." Nevertheless he had a conscious longing for a woman's love, although he had masturbation fantasies in which he was cruel to women. He had so much guilt and anxiety about these fantasies that he could speak about them only with great difficulty. We said to him, "Since you feel that women have been cruel and indifferent to you it is natural that you think of retaliation. This retaliation happens to be combined with your sexual feelings and fantasies but do not be distressed too much by this. Speak of it freely and you will see that some separation will take place between your ideas of love and your fantasies of hate."

Expression of Hostility

He despised the farm and hated going to church and finally got the courage to discuss these attitudes with his mother. She tried to make him feel ashamed but because of his discussion of these matters in an uncritical atmosphere he had gained courage and would not let himself be dissuaded by her. The result was that finally she rented the farm and he got a job in the city. He liked this better, and for the first time his headaches were less troublesome. In the first few weeks of treatment his headaches were so bad that while talking about his parents and their injustices to him he would hold his head in his hands, sway from side to side, and beg to be taken to the hospital and have some operation done upon him, "any operation. . . There must be something in there, a brain tumor or something. My hatred for things that have happened to me is intense but it can't be producing all this." We urged him to be patient and keep up the struggle.

Marriage

After leaving the farm he suffered from loneliness for which he sought relief in feminine companionship. These friendships always ended disastrously because he always expected the girl to be kind beyond reasonable possibilities. He wanted her to be a normal, active, friendly girl and yet make up to him in affection all that his mother had failed to give him. He could not bear to have her ask anything in the way of a favor from him and he was very sensitive to the slightest trace of disinterest in him. We said to him, "Remember, you have been a deprived person both as a child and as a young man. While you feel that you have missed a great deal and have much coming to you in the way of affection and regard, you must recognize that it cannot be all one-sided. Any girl expects from you a cheerful demeanor and some consideration of her desires. If you can forget yourself a little and think of the girl you will be rewarded by her gratitude."

He finally saw the point of this discussion and at the end of about two years met a girl whom he wanted to marry. By this time his headaches had entirely disappeared and he was reasonably happy at his work. He married and in the two years since then he has been symptom-free and happy.

MIGRAINE

There is a variety of headache which comes in attacks, often periodically, is usually one-sided (hemicrania), and is frequently accompanied by one or more of the following phenomena: scotomata or other visual disturbances, nausea and vomiting, constipation or diarrhea, urine retention or frequency of urination, and general or one-sided chilliness, numbness, and pallor. The attack is often preceded by some kind of an "aura" and may be followed by fatigue and depression, although again the contrary may occur—the patient may be lively and energetic once the attack is over.

Clinical Features

Migraine has been called a familial headache, thus indicating the hereditary factor. It has also been called the "sensory type of epilepsy," indicating that the two conditions are related. Migraine attacks in women frequently occur just before the onset of menstruation and often cease after the menopause. The attacks may occur as often as two or three times a week or as infrequently as once a year. Usually no definite interval between attacks is noted. The condition is most common in persons between the ages of fifteen and thirty-five. A visual *aura* may precede the attack; the eyes may feel hot and painful and the lids begin to droop with a feeling of heaviness. There are sensations of flashing lights and zig-zag bright lines, contraction of the visual fields, and other visual disturbances. Dizziness and ringing in the ears, strange odors and taste disturbances may also occur. Dizziness and soreness of the scalp may be present, accompanied by a sensation of "pins and needles" in the extremities. Once the head pain of migraine has developed any stimulation such as slamming of the door, noises from the street, or glaring lights will increase the pain. In at least one-third of the cases of migraine psychic disturbances are common. These are anxiety, drowsiness, and confusion, sometimes amounting to disorientation.

Mechanism

There are various theories as to how these phenomena are produced— phenomena which apparently are due to circulatory disturbances mediated by way of the autonomic nervous system. It is well recognized that this system is markedly affected by emotional influences. The headache is thought to be due to spasmodic contraction, followed by dilatation, of the smooth musculature of the cerebral blood vessels. These vascular spasms in turn apparently cause ischemia and edema, which irritate the brain and its centers. The stimulation of these centers disturbs other systems, particularly those under the control of the vagus nerve.

In the course of aviation medicine experiments, Engel and associates have made some observations about a migraine-like syndrome complicating decompression sickness. They describe the scintillating scotomas, the focal neurological signs, and the headaches, which emphasize the similarity between this syndrome and clinical migraine and suggest that the mechanisms are similar. Their studies confirm the observations of Wolff on the mechanism of the neurologic prodromes of migraine and suggest the identity of the two. The characteristics of the neurologic disturbances suggest that they originate in the cerebral cortex and probably result from spasm of cerebral arteries. Moreover, the authors discovered a high incidence of migraine-like headaches in the subjects who were susceptible to this decompression syndrome, indicating that a predisposition to this particular type of vascular reaction is an important factor. They accept the interpretation that the scotomas and other neurologic symptoms result from cortical ischemia due to spasm of intracranial arteries, but insist that the headaches result from dilatation of pain-sensitive cranial arteries. The headache was not associated with any changes in the electroencephalogram; this is consistent with experience of others in the study of clinical migraine.

Personality Features

Apparently these mechanisms can be set in motion by psychic stress related to the personality structure of the patient with migraine. In a review (Weiss) of twenty-four patients studied from a psychosomatic standpoint we were impressed with the features that they shared in common: a *compulsive character*, an inability to express hostile impulses adequately, a high incidence of various degrees of impotence among the men and frigidity in the women, and the patient's willingness to blame his headache upon the bowel, the sinuses, or "something he *et.*" To the last we usually answer "No, it is probably something you *met*," but because of this association to the gastrointestinal tract and the willingness of the patient to blame the headache upon a disturbance in bowel function he usually becomes addicted to the laxative or enema habit while, for the same reasons, his physician endorses the allergic approach. Blaming the disorder on the sinuses is also very common, so common in fact, that the patient often uses the expression "I've got my sinus again" rather than to say that he has a headache.

Emotional Immaturity

In a study by Touraine and Draper of fifty migrainous patients it was suggested that there exists a characteristic constitutional type in which the skull shows acromegaloid trends, the intelligence is outstanding, but the emotional make-up is retarded in development. They observed that the headache was characteristically repeated in the same pattern for each patient and recurred in similar circumstances. Situations necessitating the individual to stand alone, such as loss of home protection or the assumption of adult responsibilities, marked the beginning of the headaches. Headaches were observed to come through the maternal line with the factor of unconscious imitation of the mother important in causation. Thus an effort must be made to differentiate factors of *true heredity* and *pseudoheredity*. They found that there was an emotional attachment to the mother which could not be resolved. This resulted in retarding the process of emotional maturation so that arrest occurred at some point short of mature psychosexual adjustment. They concluded that the migraine attack was a syndrome comparable to any neurosis and the fact that migraine responded to such a variety of treatments spoke in favor of a psychic etiology. They felt that the psychological approach offered the most in research and therapy.

Relation to Hypertension

A recent article by Gardner, Mountain, and Hines observes that migraine occurs very frequently in association with hypertension. Their study, conducted at the Mayo Clinic, indicated that migraine occurred approximately five times more frequently among patients with hypertension than in a control group without hypertension. This suggests a common factor in the pathogenesis of the two conditions. It is well known that vasoconstriction plays an important role in producing an attack of migraine as it does in the production of hypertension. The study also indicated that the association of migraine and hypertension is intimately concerned with *heredity* factors common to both conditions. They suggest that the common denominator in the two conditions may be influenced by genetic factors which particularly concern the inheritance of a certain type of personality. Once more we would call attention to the fact of pseudoheredity (unconscious imitation dating from childhood) which conceivably could operate in migraine but hardly in hypertension.

They refer to the study of migrainous patients by H. G. Wolff, who emphasized that the patient with migraine often demonstrates unusual ambition, is meticulous and exacting, and frequently proves himself to be a hard driver with the ability to accomplish much in a short time. These are also the characteristics of the personality noted in many patients suffering from hypertension.

Psychoanalytic Observations

Fromm-Reichmann treated eight patients with migraine by intensive psychotherapy. Of these, five were cured, two were improved, and one remained uninfluenced. She found that they were all people who had a marked hostility, of which they were not consciously aware, for some person to whom they were closely attached. Realizing that many ordinary headaches are also a conversion of anger or hatred, Dr. Fromm-

Reichmann asked herself why the ambivalence of feeling (conscious devotion and unconscious hostility) is so intense in the migraine patient, or in other words, why it is so necessary to repress the negative feelings. The question of why the head is chosen as an area for expressing the hostility also interested her.

Unconscious Hostility. She thought the answer to the first question lay in the fact that so often the migraine patient comes from a conventional family with strong solidarity and strong family pride. Aggression against each other is strongly forbidden. If one member dares to express hostility against another he is punished by exclusion and thus loses the protection of the family in the struggle of life. The fear of such a punishment is enough to keep him in line and keep his hostilities repressed. Then when anger is aroused and cannot express itself adequately either by words or direct action the individual takes it out upon himself, so to speak, in an attack of migraine. He punishes himself for the destruction he would like to visit upon another. Why the head is chosen as the organ to "take the punishment" seemed to be on the basis of rivalry with the intellectuality of the person to whom the sufferer is attached. It is as though in his impotent rage, he could "dash his brains" against a solid wall. We submit, from previous discussion, that identification as well as rivalry may play a part in the choice of the head as a site for the expression of this form of "body language."

Rorschach Tests

A careful study of migraine by means of the Rorschach method, using control groups (Ross and McNaughton) fails to confirm the clinical finding of repressed rage but does corroborate the personality features, namely: persistence toward success, difficulty in sexual adjustment, perfectionism, conventionality, intolerance, and in general, obsessive-compulsive features. They found that these personality features are associated with migraine to a greater degree than would be accounted for by chance.

Medical Observations

Alvarez, more recently, discusses the treatment of migraine somewhat as follows: It is often thought that migraine is the result of some disorder in the gallbladder or liver, the teeth, tonsils, or appendix, and the patient is examined from head to foot. It is not caused by such conditions, but is due to some sort of "storm" in the brain or in the sympathetic nerves regulating the caliber of the blood vessels of the brain. Patients tend to blame the liver for their so-called bilious spells, but actually instead of producing migraine, disease in the liver commonly protects the patient from having the headaches. In cases of migraine the digestive tract is normal enough; it is upset by the storm that comes down the vagus and perhaps the sympathetic nerves, a storm similar to that which causes the vomiting of seasickness and Ménière's disease. Alvarez goes on:

"The physician should carefully study the details of the lives of these sufferers, for often serious problems may be avoided. Sufferers from migraine are generally unusual persons with a characteristic tense personality. They are commonly above average in intelligence and nervous drive, and they are particularly reactive to emotion and particularly sensitive to stimuli of all kinds. They are often too conscientious in their work, and they worry and take life too seriously. Often they lack stability and self-discipline; they stay up too late, and they do not use the brain wisely. Some are a bit psychopathic and have difficulty in adjusting to life. In a considerable percentage of cases the trouble is brought on by unhappiness, family squabbles, and sexual incompatibility."

The following cases are selected to demonstrate some of the points which we have discussed.

Migraine; Thought to Be Allergic; Good Response
to Psychotherapy

CASE 69

A Jewess of twenty-eight was raised in an orthodox home where, however, in her own words, religion was applied with a light hand. She married a man who observed the orthodox tenets of his religion with an almost fanatical zeal. Although migraine headaches antedated the marriage they now became very severe and occurred quite regularly on Saturdays.

The patient came from a family that was highly intellectual, but quite psychopathic. She considered herself scholastically the black sheep, although she was really a very intelligent girl, self-educated, and had accomplished a great deal for herself. The headaches were attributed to "sinus trouble."

Death of Mother

The mother died of bronchial asthma about the time that the patient's headaches began. The patient stated that she had a "sense of relief" because the mother had been so ill with asthma. Then the father remarried a rather ignorant woman (the patient's own words) in sharp contrast to the patient's own mother, and apparently this had something to do with the patient's determination to get married herself.

A fear of developing asthma because of the mother's illness was accompanied by a great fear of cancer, a real cancerophobia. Just before we saw her, she had had an anxiety attack and since then she had been nervous, weak, and depressed.

Allergy Tests

She had been studied by allergists who, because of the occurrence of the headache on Saturdays, suggested that something in the orthodox food rituals might be related to the attacks. So she was subjected to skin tests, and to a number of elimination diets which, however, failed to help her.

Husband's Fanaticism

Much of her conversation had to do with her husband. She said that his whole life was religion; that his fanatical traits were especially marked on Saturday, the sabbath day; that he rushes her to get ready for that day and that she doesn't like to be rushed. There must not be a spot of dust for the holy sabbath. On one occasion he spoke to her about the fact that he couldn't love a woman who didn't see eye to eye with him on his religion. She resented this, saying, "His love of religion is enslaving me. If love is based on ritualistic observance, he can keep it. He says he can only love me if I give up my rebellious ways. I want to worship in my own way. He forces his religion on me and he won't compromise."

Sexual Frigidity

In addition to that fact, just when she was so irritated and fatigued by preparation for the Sabbath, it was invariably on Friday nights that he asked for sexual intercourse. There is a special preparation for intercourse among those who observe the orthodox tenets: The woman has to immerse herself completely in a tub reserved for that purpose. She very much resented this preparation. She was frigid in intercourse, failed to obtain any satisfaction, and regularly on the night or the morning following she developed her attack of migraine. Before this was called to her attention she herself observed that when she was away for the summer, she didn't have migraine; in fact, she noted, "When I am away from home, I don't get migraine on Saturdays." When we pointed out her inability to express hostility directly and hence the mechanism of body language she replied that "hers was very eloquent."

She spent the summer away from Philadelphia. On her return, after having been free of migraine, she became irritable and depressed, complained of a heavy head, spoke about the boredom of facing another winter, said that she felt alone even when her husband was at home.

Improvement

Finally, with our persuasion she decided to get herself some employment. We suggested that she try to find something that would fall in with her husband's interests. She got a job teaching, and derived a great deal of satisfaction from it. Her migraine improved during this period. The anxiety of the cancerophobia came up again. We discussed that with her. She said, "Yes, people sympathize with the headache, but not with anxiety. Even my husband walks around on tip-toe when I have my headache."

SUMMARY

A young married woman with typical migraine, thought to be allergic, failed to respond to the usual medical and dietary measures but obtained considerable relief from brief psychotherapy which permitted her to achieve a better personal and social adjustment.

Migraine; Childhood Asthma; Psychological Conflict in Regard to Mother
Help from Superficial Psychotherapy

CASE 70

A married, white man of thirty-five was first seen in the spring of 1939.

History and Symptoms

He complained of migraine headaches of about a year's duration and fatigue of about six months' duration.

The headaches were typical and at first had occurred every few weeks but more recently had been occuring about every week. Fatigue appeared gradually but became very pronounced. Further inquiry revealed that on rare occasions many years before he had had milder attacks of similar headaches. From about the age of nine until fourteen he also suffered from bronchial asthma, which disappeared completely.

He had been married for four years. There were no children.

Family History. The father had been killed in an accident when the patient was ten or eleven. The mother was living and well although she suffered from hay fever and asthma and also somewhat similar attacks which she termed "sick headaches." A sister two years younger was living. She was subject to attacks of fatigue and nervousness. There was no other history of migraine or allergic disease within the family. The patient reported that his father's family were known as high-strung and irritable people.

Physical Examination and Laboratory Studies

The patient was a well-nourished and healthy-appearing young man. The chest cage was small, and the hips were heavy. The general physical examination otherwise was negative. The cardiovascular system seemed normal and the lungs were clear and resonant throughout.

The routine laboratory studies were within normal limits and basal metabolism was minus 3. Blood sedimentation rate was normal. Routine allergy tests disclosed no special reaction.

He had been placed upon various test diets, various kinds of medicine and endocrine products, especially thyroid, but the headache and fatigue had become steadily worse.

LIFE SITUATION

The patient considered himself a normal child but had suffered from *enuresis*. The childhood asthma which followed whooping cough interfered somewhat with his schooling. After the father's death the mother had a small income from insurance and the children were assisted in their education by contributions from the family. After graduating from high school he went to business school, then had a clerical position in a manufacturing plant which, however, did not interest him. Meanwhile he cherished the ambition of becoming a musician and studied music at night. He continued to live with the mother although they were not congenial. The mother had urged him to study teaching and frowned upon his interest in music, predicting that he could not make a success in this field.

He felt that he must continue with a position that he did not enjoy in order to help contribute to the mother's support but at the same time considered the mother a spendthrift who invested her small income badly and "could live well enough on it alone if she had to." On one occasion he separated from the mother and established his own apartment "in order that he might pursue his musical education to better advantage" but felt guilty about leaving the mother and returned again the following year to live with her although he found her more irritating than usual and was conscious of a growing antagonism. "He could not bear to touch his mother physically and at times found her revolting and repulsive."

Marriage

At the age of thirty he married a girl of the same age who was also a musician. This was done against his mother's wishes. While the mother later became reconciled to the marriage there was always an undercurrent of dissatisfaction which flared into open discussion now and again.

After the marriage, although his own income was barely enough for their needs, he continued to contribute small amounts toward the mother's support even though the mother never made direct demands. The patient felt that if the mother were only wiser about spending he would not have to contribute to her support and of course did so very reluctantly. Yet he felt guilty when the mother confessed herself in financial difficulties if he did not contribute. On one occasion in the spring of 1938 he got in a row with the mother over a problem having to do with the mother's squandering funds. He became so enraged that he refused to speak to the mother and they continued to be bad friends for the next six months. It was during this time and especially around the Christmas period that *headaches* first appeared and, as he later said, he felt guilty about not spending Christmas with his mother, which had always been his habit hitherto.

RESULTS OF TREATMENT

From this point on it became more and more clear to the patient that the conflict with his mother stood in the background of his migraine headaches and that when he became enraged and could not give vent to his rage, the headache promptly appeared. It was very obvious that he had a conflict in relationship to his mother and that while he felt that it was his duty to help her he keenly resented the necessity for doing so. On further discussion of music as a career it seemed clear that his heart was not in it and that this too had represented an effort to succeed in something that the mother opposed just as the marriage itself represented an escape from the mother to a person (musician) to whom the mother objected.

As his relationship to his mother became clear and he was permitted to discuss the situation without criticism on our part, he had fewer headaches and when they occurred they were less intense. Now some of his conflicts in regard to other matters made their appearance and it was discovered that his relationship to his wife was not entirely satisfactory and that there had been considerable indecision over the question of having a child. Nevertheless, the airing of the main conflict with the mother seemed to help the patient a great deal.

SUMMARY

A young man suffering from typical migraine had no evidence of organic disease. He seemed to derive much benefit from a discussion of a conflict in relation to his mother.

EPILEPSY

In discussing symptom pictures related to the nervous system we must include the problem of epilepsy, which seems closely related to migraine. We approach the subject of epilepsy with less certainty than some of the other psychosomatic entities, being aware of how little is known of its real etiology and how resistant it may be to treatment. However, our chief reason for including it is to bring to the attention of the physician the necessity for treating the personality problems of the patient who has seizures as well as restricting his activities and giving him drugs. The social-personality problem of the epileptic is often overlooked. Only the seizures are treated and the personality that has to live and try to work out a destiny with such a handicap is ignored.

Predisposition

Recent information indicates that the most fundamental factor in seizures is a predisposition in the nature of a cerebral dysrhythmia which can be demonstrated in *brain waves* measured by electroencephalographic tracings. Brain damage, physicochemical disorders in the body fluids, and emotional disturbances play their individual role in producing unconsciousness and the muscular activity of the seizure. From our own experience and from references to the literature it would seem that a certain number of patients with convulsive seizures respond well to minor psychotherapy; a few have been benefited by major psychotherapy; and in others even intensive psychotherapy has failed to break up the convulsive mechanism even though a greater emotional equilibrium has been achieved.

The discussion of the treatment of epilepsy has been divided into three phases by Lennox. He speaks of the physical, the pharmacological, and the psychological-social fronts.

Treatment

Physical Treatment. On the physical front he stresses a common-sense regularity of life without being either too dependent upon or too careless of rules. He believes that both physical and mental activity are indicated since activity seems to function as an antagonist of seizures. The greatest benefit is derived from activities which combine muscular exercise, intellectual interest, and rest. He makes the point that anxious parents, whose minds are filled with visions of accidents of bodily injury to epileptic children, should consider the small chance of an attack occurring when the child is in a dangerous position and the large chance of invalidism and psychological damage as a result of oversolicitude and overprotection. Unless a ketogenic diet is being used, the patient should eat the diet of the rest of the family. Plenty of rest and adequate elimination are, of course, indicated.

Drug Treatment. On the pharmacological front Lennox names three useful drugs: bromides, phenobarbital, and dilantin sodium. He warns that some patients are not helped by medicine no matter how much is taken and that sedative medication which stops seizures but slows up the body and mind to too great a degree is a failure. Likewise he suggests that an effective drug should produce some composure of the abnormal waves of the electroencephalographic record as well as stopping seizures. Drugs are only palliative; it is doubtful if they ever act as a cure in themselves.

Social-Psychological Treatment. The social-psychological front is important. The very diagnosis of epilepsy is in itself a shock to the patient and his family, who have usually hoped that the condition was only a "fainting spell" or the result of a digestive disturbance. A diagnosis of a condition which, with all its handicaps, may persist throughout a lifetime is news which is difficult to break to a patient or family. But once it has been proved it is better to face the situation than to take the attitude that it may disappear at any time. One's life work has to be shaped around the condition, so it is much better to know the whole truth. The physician may emphasize to the patient that the seizures are not a threat to life and that various treatments are available but that time may be needed to find the best regimen for him. He can be reassured that while life with seizures has real difficulties one can still be happy and useful. Any feeling of shame or inferiority on the part of the family regarding epileptics must be dealt with, in order that the patient has at least the support of his family in meeting some of the inevitable prejudices in the world outside the home. *Neither the family nor the patient should be led to hope that seizures will disappear with puberty, marriage, motherhood, or any other life epoch.* The patient should be frankly told (not at one consultation, of course), some of the problems associated with the illness and prejudices that he may meet; and his life should be so ordered that he may be most useful to himself and to society. In other words, while some social and psychological protection to the epileptic may be given, he should, in so far as possible, assume the obligations and responsibilities of the other members of the family. This applies to children and adults alike.

About 10 per cent of epileptics who are outside of institutions become too dull mentally to be employable. About 10 per cent have difficult personalities, being stubborn, irritable, suspicious, and opinionated. Other physical disabilities may complicate the problem. Altogether perhaps a third of adult epileptics are not proper subjects for training or regular employment. The remaining two thirds can give a good account of themselves if each case is considered individually.

Marriage in Epilepsy

A frequent question which may be asked of the physician is in regard to the marriage of those suffering from seizures. Connecticut has answered this question by a law which punishes by imprisonment anyone who contracts such a marriage, if the wife is of child-bearing age, and even punishes, by fine or imprisonment or both, anyone assisting in such a marriage. Records of the brain waves by means of the encephalograph show that many people have cerebral dysrhythmia who never have seizures. The person with cerebral dysrhythmia and seizures should take pains to marry a person who registers normal brain waves. Such a marriage reduces the chances of having a child subject to seizures.

Heredity

In other words in epilepsy there is a tendency to hereditary transmission. This varies from person to person and if the family history is not already too heavily weighted with psychopathic individuals or other epileptics and if he or she marries a person registering normal brain waves on the encephalographic tracing, the chances of having an epileptic offspring are not great. In fact two dysrhythmic individuals, even though seizure-free, might be more likely to produce an epileptic offspring than the union of an epileptic and a normal person. Sufferers from migraine are greater potential "carriers" of epilepsy than is commonly recognized.

Lennox provides further information on this subject in a letter to the Journal of the American Medical Association, answering an author who felt that the only hope of eliminating epilepsy is by birth control among epileptic adults. "Brain wave studies indicate that for every epileptic patient there are probably twenty or more nonepileptic patients who nevertheless are carriers of this or an allied disorder. Therefore, childlessness of all persons with epilepsy would eliminate only 5 per cent of epilepsy. Prohibitions applied to a person with epilepsy apply with equal force to one-half of his relatives and to something like 10 per cent of the whole population. Again the probability of having affected progeny depends in part on whether the person whom the epileptic person marries carries a predisposition to epilepsy. The marriage of two normal carriers of this disorder is more dangerous than the marriage of an epileptic person with a noncarrier. Logically brain wave tracings of both partners to a marriage should be secured if the physician is to offer specific advice to an individual. Even so he should consider the possibility suggested by unpublished observations that unusual, so-called 'abnormal' frequency of waves may be associated with high attainment or genius. Many implications of electroencephalography are as yet unexplored."

The psychological help to the person suffering from seizures may vary from an occasionally friendly talk to intensive psychotherapy. The following case is illustrative.

Epilepsy

CASE 71

History and Symptoms

A man of thirty-nine was first seen in a psychiatric hospital where he arrived in *status epilepticus* following a series of convulsions. When he became conscious he was eager to relate his history. He was a friendly, good-looking man, appearing younger than his years, who had suffered many hardships. His mother had died when he was one year old and his father was a shiftless alcoholic who had left him to be cared for in a series of foster homes and by distant relatives who did not want him. He was ambitious to have an education but found it difficult to apply himself. Very often money saved for his education would be spent on a pleasure trip instead.

LIFE SITUATION

Marriage

His first seizure occurred at the age of twenty-two. At times there were as many as ten to twelve in twenty-four hours. At other times he might go for a number of days without them. He lost many jobs and began to be seclusive. Then he met a girl who fell in love with him. She thought that what he needed was a woman's love and care and they were married. But he was unable to appreciate the friendship and love of this warm-hearted person who worked and most of the time supported him. When we first saw him he was twenty-nine and unemployed. He seemed anxious to receive help from psychotherapy. In spite of his apparent eagerness to cooperate it was evident, in the therapeutic relationship, that he wanted all the help given *to* him.

Psychotherapy

When we asked him to write an autobiography he put this off for weeks although he had nothing else to do. However, he volunteered, "My seizures are a punishment for my laziness and my disinterest in other human beings." He knew from experience that if he would speak to someone during the aura preceding the attack he could often prevent a seizure. In spite of this he would ignore the aura and lapse off into unconsciousness. We said to him, "We know you have had a deprived childhood and have missed the personal interest, friendship, and guidance of capable and loving parents but you have a good wife and we all want to help you. If you are ambitious and want to enjoy the prestige and pleasure of occupying a place of usefulness in the world you must stop being sorry for yourself and start doing something for the people around you." As a result of emphasizing this point of view and showing him exactly how he could please his wife and his physician he became more alert and cheerful.

Employment

He obtained work in an office as a draftsman. We made a contact with his employer, who agreed to be patient, and he held this job for eight months. He had an occasional seizure at work but most of them came at night. Aside from being late to work in the morning following such a seizure he did tolerably well. He was at first elated at having the job but frequently lapsed into his old attitude that people did not appreciate his efforts. He deplored his meager education and complained that the job had no future. We would tell him, "Happiness and usefulness in this world do not depend entirely upon education, large salary, or high position. You could have those things in greater degree than you have now and still not be satisfied. You must learn to appreciate what you have." Then for another period he would be satisfied.

Change of Position

He was still ambitious to learn more, especially in the mechanical world. We pointed out the risks in this field and the greater intolerance of employers, but he insisted that he must try it. Finally he lost his draftsman's job and then felt that he must try engineering. His wife succeeded in getting him placed but in his third week he had an attack of petit mal in the engineering school and was dismissed. Then he obtained a job in a chain restaurant—work with which he was already familiar from years before. By application to work his wife had been able to save a little money and, with a friend who knew the restaurant business, she planned to open a little restaurant of their own where his occasional seizures would not bring up the constant fear of dismissal.

Results of Psychotherapy

In this case we treated the emotional problems of the epileptic and his wife. We did not abolish the seizures but we felt that by combating despondency and a tendency to withdrawal in the patient we did succeed in reducing their number. We "kept him going," so to speak, by encouragement, by helping him to work out his plans, and by urging him to show greater friendliness and more appreciation for what he had.

DELIRIUM

Delirium refers to the mental symptoms associated with somatic disease. It may be gradual in onset or appear suddenly as a psychotic episode in a patient with advanced physical or metabolic disorder. Often it is associated with drug intoxication, febrile states, and advanced cardiac and renal diseases.

Generally the term is used to cover grossly disturbed behavior arising under the circumstances indicated above but Romano and Engel think that the term should apply to a much larger group of patients in whom the symptoms may appear very insidiously and are not so striking. After calling attention to the various noxious stimuli that bring about delirium, Romano emphasized that the most important variable is the nature of the personality structure which is reacting to the stimulus. Patients who are experiencing considerable anxiety in connection with their physical illness; patients who through language difficulties or superstition are apt to misinterpret events connected with the illness; patients of advanced age, with preexisting cerebral vascular disease; and patients of limited intellectual endowment: these three types are the ones apt to succumb to delirium.

Symptoms

The early signs of an impending delirium are: inability to sleep; increased frequency of frightening dreams and nightmares; irritability; occasional misinterpretations of people, objects, shadows, and noises; loss of appetite; and increased motor restlessness. Recognition of the primary disturbance, that is, the disturbance in consciousness, which can be tested by having the patient subtract serially, may aid in early diagnosis. At this stage, treatment may be successful in avoiding the development of the full-fledged delirium.

Electroencephalographic Study

Studies by Engel and Romano of fifty-three patients with delirium of varying cause, intensity, and duration revealed E.E.G. abnormalities in all patients who had disturbances in consciousness. These changes were found to be reversible to the extent to which the clinical delirium was reversible. Psychologic data showed a direct correlation between the electrical abnormality and the disturbance of consciousness but there was less correlation with the more personal aspects of behavior, namely, the character and expression of anxiety, the content of thought, and the nature of sense deceptions.

"The mere presence of abnormal brain waves in the electroencephalogram of a person with disturbances of behavior does not establish a relation between the two," they say.

Treatment

The underlying physical or chemical disorder must be treated first. Adequate food and fluid intake should be maintained. Sleep may be obtained by use of the continuous tub bath at neutral temperatures, but most hospitals are not equipped for this procedure, and there is need to use a noncumulative, nontoxic chemical sedative such as paraldehyde or chloral hydrate. A low bed rather than sideboards is a good precaution-ary measure to prevent injury. The room should be kept well lighted at night to avoid shadows and misinterpretations, and tactful attendance and explanation of procedures to patients may aid considerably in avoid-ing further anxiety.

Although general hospitals should have facilities to care for such cases, most do not, and it may be necessary to transfer such a patient to a psychiatric hospital.

ORGANIC BRAIN DISEASE SIMULATING NEUROSIS

The situation which so many doctors fear—of missing an organic lesion and labeling the patient a neurotic—may actually occur. The problem sometimes occurs in connection with *brain tumor*. However, it must be remembered that the presence of an organic brain disease does not exclude the possibility of previous personality difficulties. In many patients with organic disease of the central nervous system the neurotic symptoms which make their appearance depend upon two interrelated factors—the previous personality trends plus the destruction of brain tissue. For example, a patient with a strong element of suspicion in his personality make-up may show an exaggerated suspicion of relatives and friends as a mental symptom of central nervous system syphilis. In other words, personality difficulties in an obscure case should not blind one to the necessity of a careful neurological examination, perhaps in-cluding thorough visual field examination, x-ray of the skull, and en-cephalogram if necessary.

The following cases have been selected to illustrate this topic.

Brain Tumor and Functional Symptoms

CASE 72

History and Symptoms

A white woman of fifty was admitted on October 21, 1940, com-plaining of *headaches* and *convulsions*. She had had three previous ad-missions to the hospital. The first was in January, 1939, when she was admitted directly to the ophthalmology service stating that she had begun to lose vision in the left eye and that she had had a similar occurrence in the right eye two years before. A diagnosis was made of *acute optic neuritis* of the left eye and *postneuritic optic atrophy* of the right eye. The only other point noted was that she had been told of *high blood pressure* three years before. The general physical examination was declared to be negative. She was treated with typhoid vaccine intravenously and her vision improved but at that time it was pointed out that there was some evidence of tetany which was confirmed by positive Chvostek and Trousseau signs as well as by calcium-phosphorus determinations, blood calcium 5.5 mg. and phosphorus 7.4 mg. The neurologist concluded that there were no definite signs indicating a focal cerebral lesion but suggested the necessity for a skull examination. There was no evidence of abnormality in the examination of the skull by x-ray. Special x-ray studies of bone suggested a high calcium content of the femur.

Second Hospital Admission. She was readmitted in April, 1939. Now the medical history stated that ten years before nausea, vertigo, pallor, and headache occurred in attacks lasting several hours and terminated by vomiting. A diagnosis of *migraine, spontaneous hypoparathyroidism, and optic neuritis* was established and the following notes were made by the resident physician:

"For the past ten years the patient has had attacks of nausea, vertigo, pallor, and headaches, lasting several hours and terminated by vomiting on an average of one every two months. For the past four years the patient has had fleeting muscle cramps in sides, legs, hands, and pharynx on countless occasions. When hands were affected they assumed a typical tetany position. Two and one-half years ago the patient felt 'an explosion' in her head. Several days later she noticed cloudy vision in her right eye. Her vision became gradually more impaired. Ten weeks ago the same thing happened to the left eye. For the past year the patient has had momentary twitching of the muscles of the extremities, abdomen, and face on numerous occasions. She had amenorrhea during the past four months but then had an apparently normal period. Noise and progressive deafness in the left ear began fifteen years ago."

Physical Examination and Laboratory Studies

Ears—impairment of hearing in the left ear. Both drums were slightly retracted and somewhat dull in appearance. Eyes—fundi showed pallor of each disc; the right more than the left. This resulted from previous optic neuritis. Nose—slight amount of purulent discharge of both nasal chambers. Nasal mucosa congested and hyperplastic. Maxillary sinuses did not transilluminate well. Chvostek sign negative. Trousseau sign negative. Growth of hair over chin and upper lip. Extremities—triceps and patella reflexes hyperactive bilaterally.

Gastric analysis revealed a moderate hypoacidity curve. No evidence of pyloric obstruction. Serum calcium and phosphorus estimates:
April 18—calcium 7.1 mg., phosphorus 6.8 mg.
April 24—calcium 7.23 mg., phosphorus 6.4 mg.
April 26—calcium 7.7 mg., phosphorus 6.6 mg.

Clinical Course. No treatment was given until April 22. From April 20 until she left the hospital the patient had mild muscular cramps and muscular twitchings. On April 22 calcium lactate therapy was instituted. On April 25 dihydrotachysterol, i. e., A. T. 10, was administered.

Final Diagnosis. Hypocalcemia and optic neuritis.

Third Hospital Admission. The next admission was in August, 1940, when in addition to the other complaints, which apparently had been controlled by calcium and A. T. 10, the patient had had an attack two weeks prior to this admission which resembled a *Jacksonian seizure*, that is, she had convulsions, loss of speech, and apparently loss of consciousness as well. Spinal fluids studies and x-ray of the skull were normal. The audiometer test showed left ear deafness and the Barany test showed some disturbance which was not typical of an intracranial lesion. The x-ray of the skull was again quite normal. She was discharged with the same diagnosis as before plus menopausal syndrome.

Fourth Hospital Admission. On the last admission she stated that in addition to the seizures previously described, there had been three *convulsions* consisting of movements of the left hand and arm, then movements of the head, rigidity of the body and spasm of the muscles of mastication, incontience of bladder and bowel and unconsciousness. Following the attacks, which lasted a few minutes, she slept for ten to fifteen minutes. In addition she spoke of weakness of the left arm and leg, right-sided headache, and deafness of the left ear.

Physical Examination and Laboratory Studies

The patient was an obese, middle-aged woman. The skin was course and dry. There was considerable hair on the chest, breasts, and chin so that the patient said that she had had to shave one area of the chin for the past twenty-five years. There was impaired vision of the right eye and deafness of the left ear. Examination of the heart and lungs was normal and there was nothing particular to be noted in the abdominal examination. Gynecological examination was negative. The resident physician thought that the left arm showed impaired motor power and that the tendon reflexes were hyperactive on the left side as compared with the right. There was no evidence of a Babinski sign. In an effort to rule out an intracranial lesion a spinal tap was done which showed a pressure of 24 mm. but the spinal fluid otherwise was negative. Neurological consultation one week later found that there were no significant central nervous system signs of abnormality aside from the high spinal fluid pressure and that the emotional state of the patient at the time might have had something to do with that. It was suggested that the tap be repeated in the operating room under sedation and that if it was checked as high further studies could be done at the time. Once more the x-ray of the skull was negative. The eyeground examination confirmed secondary optic strophy of both eyes. X-ray of the right femur for bone calcium evaluation suggested that now it seemed to be within normal range as contrasted with the previous study. Now calcium studies were 10 mg. and phosphorus 5.1 mg., phosphatase 5.3 mg. (Bodansky units). Another calcium was 8.9 mg. and phosphorus 6 mg. The blood Wassermann was negative; the blood count good; urinalysis negative.

Nothing has been said about the emotional aspects of this illness but here was a complicated clinical problem in which the neurologist suggested that the psychiatrist see the patient and the psychiatrist insisted upon a complete neurological study!

LIFE SITUATION

This woman was born and brought up in a small village in Russia. Her father died when she was young and she soon acquired a stepfather who was none too kind. She had very little formal education. There was always a great deal of worry about money and how the family would exist at all under the prevailing conditions. When the patient was fifteen the family came to America and she married at nineteen, after four years of factory work. She had four children in ten years. They ranged in ages from twenty-nine to nineteen. The husband was proprietor of a neighborhood clothing store. Having so little formal education, it was a great transition in this woman's life, with her background of a small Russian village, to begin bringing up four children each of whom was struggling for recognition on the American scene. Problems arose about which she felt inadequate. Some of these were: the children's going to school and their association with other children; their further education; their choice of vocations, and their marriages. All this made life here with its responsibilities very perplexing and very productive of anxiety.

Method of Expressing Anxiety

She had a special way of reacting to anxiety which was different from that of many other patients whom we have seen. Instead of feeling anxious inside she projected her anxiety in the form of hostility. If the children had any questions or difficulties for which she did not have a solution she scolded them for their stupidity. If they did not progress as successfully as she wished she threatened them with her disfavor. Often she reacted rather violently. She would cry and scream and have a tantrum when things went too badly. She had very little knowledge about life and could not help these children in their personal problems. All this had made for considerable anxiety and a good deal of friction between her and the children. This had resulted in some harm to the children's personalities and two had to have help from a psychiatrist. She continued to worry even though the youngest child was nineteen and all were doing fairly well. It was interesting that when she really no longer had to worry about the children she was worrying about herself, wondering whether she was going to have difficulty in keeping the friendship of her children for the rest of her life, and especially worrying about money. She always had to be worrying about something. So that in this patient anxiety existed over a long period but no anxiety attacks occurred and there were no anxiety-producing symptoms of a conversion nature. Her ability to work and carry on had been pretty good if we disregarded her manner of doing it and its effect on others. In spite of worry she had struggled on. In addition to anxiety there was some tendency to depression.

In *summary*, we may say that the patient was in the menopausal period of life and presented a rather bizarre clinical picture in which there were no definite findings from a neurological standpoint and many symptoms which apparently originated in the emotional life of the patient. It must be emphasized that the optic atrophy of the previous neuritis definitely was held not to be due to an intracranial lesion. It seemed to be rather tacitly assumed that psychogenesis and menopause were somehow responsible for the clinical pisture and it was only the psychiatrist's insistence that led to the final vigorous prosecution of the diagnostic study. An encephalogram was done which showed a *large intracranial mass lesion* occupying the right frontoparietal region!

We need hardly say how often brain tumors in the frontal region fail to manifest themselves by positive neurological findings and how often indeed peculiar and quixotic behavior is for a long time the only evidence of the growing tumor.

Blaming Illness on Menopause

The first point to be noted is that we all have a tendency to blame too much on the menopause and that the diagnosis "menopausal syndrome" always ought to be looked upon with suspicion and certainly no physical study and no psychological study should be neglected because a woman happens to be in that period of life. All too frequently it happens that it is only that the menopause acts to bring out latent disease or disorder, that is, either a physical disease now comes to light for the first time, although it has been making inroads very silently for a long time, or a personality difficulty which might have been quite obvious to the perceptive physician now breaks out in a more definite form. This, of course, is also true of psychosis which occasionally appears at this time.

The second point that we must emphasize is that personality or emotional difficulties appearing for the first time after the age of forty must be looked upon with suspicion from the standpoint of organic disease. As we have said before, almost invariably neurotic difficulties are mirrored by the personality long before middle life is reached.

The Psychosomatic Approach

The third point is that in our usual approach to a complicated diagnostic problem we attempt to establish a diagnosis by the orthodox approach of the ordinary facts of medical history, physical examination and laboratory tests. On this basis we either make the mistake of never giving up the possibility of physical disease ("If we are only thorough enough it will be discovered") and thus continue to investigate the patient with one test after another until the neurotic difficulty is forever fixed; or we make the other mistake, which arises in the same way, of concluding, because physical signs are negative, that the disorder is functional, without building up the latter phase of the diagnosis by personality study. On more than one occasion, we have seen such a "functional diagnosis," established by exclusion of organic disease, prove to be wrong *because the personality study had not been done*. Once more then we come to the conclusion that every diagnostic study must be a bilateral one, that is, the physical and psychological phases of the problem must be considered simultaneously.

Study of the Patient from a Specialty Standpoint

One of the difficulties about specialization in medicine as it has been practiced in America is that the patient is so often studied only from the standpoint of the specialty involved. When a patient with a complicated problem, in which one symptom related to a specialty stands out prominently (as for example the eye problem in the case we are considering) is admitted to a special service of a hospital, the patient's history is apt to be taken from the standpoint of the specialty represented instead of having a complete medical history and a complete medical diagnosis. It must be constantly emphasized in the teaching and practice of medicine that no matter what the presenting symptom is or how narrowly confined to a specialty it seems to be, the only safe rule is to take a complete medical history, in which psychological factors are given equal weight with physical factors. Only by adopting the points of view just discussed can we finally get rid of the either-or concept in medicine and substitute for it the psychosomatic concept, that is, how much of the problem is physical, how much is psychological, and what is the relationship between the two.

SUMMARY

A middle-aged white woman presented a complicated clinical picture without definite evidence of organic disease so that the problem was tacitly assumed to be emotional on the basis of the menopause. The psychiatrist insisted, however, that the clinical facts could not be accounted for on the basis of the personality study and subsequent observations proved that the patient had a brain tumor of the right fronto-parietal region.

Operation disclosed a large, inoperable glioma and the patient died within a few months after the operation.

Organic and Psychic Disease Coexisting
Silent Gallstones; Cholecystectomy; Arteriosclerotic Parkinson
Disease; Atypical Depression; and Conversion Hysteria

CASE 73

History and Symptoms

A white woman, aged fifty-two, was admitted to the Temple University Hospital in January, 1938.

In March, 1937, the patient had had a cholecystectomy because there was x-ray evidence of stone in gallbladder, although there was some discussion as to whether her symptoms were really due to the gallbladder pathology. Upon awakening from anesthesia she felt pain in the right heel and several days later clonic movements of the right foot and hand as well as involuntary twitchings of the second, third, and fourth toes of the right foot. Neurologic examination at that time showed: all deep reflexes hyperactive; an abortive type of clonus bilaterally; bilateral Hoffman. The clonus was explained as being on a functional basis and the examiner had the impression that this was mild psychoneurosis of the hysterical type.

The patient dated all of her complaints from the operation for removal of gallbladder which was done ten months before this illness began. Difficulty in using the right hand and the right foot continued. Generalized weakness and tiredness, pain in the back, nervousness, and a change in disposition occurred.

The difficulty in using her right hand had persisted and increased since the operation until she could not sew or knit or prepare food. Careful questioning of the patient and the family brought out the fact that this difficulty was apparent and noticed at least a year before the operation, though it was not so pronounced. The patient complained that her right hand was very weak, the fingers were flexed and trembled upon effort, the third and fourth often spread involuntarily, and the hand felt "as if it was dead."

After the operation she complained that she was a different person; she had no interest in pleasurable activities or social affairs, and no longer felt happy or talked and laughed as she used to. She had no patience to do her household tasks and suffered from marked weakness and fatigue. She had lost 24 pounds in ten months.

Family History. The family history was negative. She had been married thirty-one years and her husband was living and well. She had two children, one a son who had just begun business in another part of the city, and the other was a daughter who had a very pronounced strawberry birth mark on her face.

Physical Examination and Laboratory Studies

The examination showed unmistakable evidence of a mild degree of Parkinson's disease. There was a suggestive masklike facies. Tongue was coated and protruded with tremor. Thoracic kyphosis and lumbar lordosis. Tenderness to percussion hammer over cervical and thoracic spine. Pain sensation increased over both scapulae and in midline of back; delayed deep pressure sensation over cervical and thoracic vertebrae. Right hand showed flexion of fingers, tremor, positive finger-to-finger test, and positive Hoffman. Deep reflexes of upper and lower extremities were increased bilaterally and equally. Gait: round-shouldered; body stiff, right arm flexed and held to side with absence of associated movements; turned en masse. Physical examination essentially negative otherwise. The blood pressure was 162/90 and varied somewhat but on the whole was lower than this first reading. The temperature and pulse were normal. Cardiovascular system seemed normal. X-ray of cervical and thoracic spine were normal. Gastrointestinal x-ray studies were normal. Gastric analysis showed normal acidity values. Urine was negative; blood count was good; blood sugar, normal. Calcium and phosphorus were normal. Serology was negative.

LIFE SITUATION

The patient was born and spent her early life in Russia. Shortly after coming to America she married a man who had always had to struggle to make a very poor living and she denied herself many things in order to educate her son and daughter. She had just succeeded in establishing her son in a small business and was very concerned over her daughter's marriage because she had misgivings as to whether it would prove successful. She cried a great deal in discussing her daughter's handicap. She also felt that she was a burden to her son who had just established himself in business and had to support his parents as well as earn his own living.

Findings Preceding Operation

It seemed clear that organic neurological findings had preceded the operation and that since the operation there had appeared an atypical depression in which there was a large element of conversion of the anxiety into somatic discomfort as in hysteria.

In thinking of the mechanism one would feel that:

1. The operation offered a convenient date around which to focus certain symptoms which were already in the process of development.

2. Depressive patients have compulsive personalities that are only happy when working and struggling. Hence once she realized her life ambition of getting her daughter married and her son set up in business she could not bear to enjoy the result of her effort.

3. In addition to the guilt associated with her success there was also a sense of loss associated with her son's removal to another part of the city. Her illness had resulted in getting her daughter back home. She undoubtedly wanted her son back too even though she consciously would renounce such a suggestion!

The *sense of loss* and the *guilt* were probably the two most important causes for her depression (which was the most important thing to be treated).

Lack of Psychological Preparation for Surgery

The case is cited to illustrate the points noted in the beginning of this report, that is, the danger of operating on a patient who is psychologically unprepared—and especially when the operation is one not definitely indicated. In the present case there was already an organic neurological disorder antedating the onset of symptoms at the time of the operation; then the operation precipitated the psychoneurotic depression. The case itself illustrates the necessity for a psychosomatic evaluation of the patient in whom both psychic and physical disease coexist. Either viewpoint alone is insufficient to explain the illness.

SUMMARY

Illness followed an operation for silent gallstones. Unnecessary operative interference in a patient with a "pathological curiosity" (silent gallstones), arteriosclerotic Parkinson's disease, and a depressive personality precipitated neurotic illness.

Chapter XXII

EAR AND EYE

PSYCHOSOMATIC ASPECTS OF EAR DISORDERS

Vertigo

Vertigo is a symptom. The term "dizziness" is often used synonymously, as are the terms "giddy" or "light-headed," to describe sensations which vary from the slightest sensation of confusion to the most intense vertigo. Simonton, in a review of this subject, states that vertigo may vary in degree from a fleeting sensation of rotation, barely perceptible to the patient, to a sensation of violent rotation by a force so strong that the victim is immediately thrown to the ground. Consequently, when a patient complains of dizziness the physician must secure an accurate description of the sensations which the patient has experienced, a detailed statement of associated symptoms and definite information about conditions which predispose to or precipitate the symptom described as "di ziness," before he can evaluate its significance.

Differentiating Vertigo and Syncope. Patients commonly confuse vertigo with syncopal states of varying degrees and refer to all such sensations by the terms "dizzy" or "giddy." Distinction must be made between the two symptoms, because vertigo implies a disturbance of equilibrium, syncope a transient cerebral anemia. The diagnosis of the symptom of vertigo requires a sensation of rotation which is not present in cerebral anemia. Hypersentitivity of the carotid sinuses or petit mal epilepsy may be confused with vertigo by the patient.

Nystagmus and the past pointing reaction are almost constant accompaniments of vertigo, and nausea or vomiting, or both may be present in severe attacks.

Ménière's Syndrome. Ménière's symptom complex is a condition of unknown cause characterized by recurring attacks of vertigo, nausea, and vomiting, associated with tinnitus and deafness of the perceptive type. The term "pseudo-Ménière's disease" has been used to indicate instances of severe recurring vertigo of unknown causation in which evidence of cochlear dysfunction is not exhibited. An infinite variety of treatments has been advocated for this condition, such as limitation of salt and fluids; and the Furstenberg regimen, which consists of a diet entirely free of sodium with the substitution of ammonium chloride to maintain the chloride level in the body. Recently nicotinic acid and thiamine hydrochloride have been tried, just as they have been in almost every obscure disease, but without striking results. Therapy with histamine is said at times to produce immediate relief of the attack of vertigo. Intracranial division of the acoustic nerve or its vestibular fibers has also been recommended. Very little attention has been paid to emotional factors in the so-called pseudo-Ménière's disease.

Relation to Anxiety States. Vertigo, ringing in the ears, and numbness and tingling of the extremities are phenomena which often result from psychic stress and usually occur together. Frequently they are not the early symptoms of an anxiety state, for they occur only after anxiety attacks have continued for months or years. The early symptoms of anxiety are usually expressed through the cardiovascular, respiratory, gastrointestinal, and genitourinary systems. Only as the emotional illness progresses does it include symptoms referable to the central nervous system itself. So little is this understood that when psychosomatic disease has affected the nervous system, giving symptoms such as the above, some rare condition is usually thought of to explain them. Among these are Ménière's disease, labyrinthitis, hypoglycemia, brain tumor, and peripheral neuritis. Careful neurological examination will rule out disease of the nervous system. A patient often fails to receive a satisfactory diagnosis even though the physician finds the neurological examination negative. The physician continues to think that "there must be neurological disease somewhere." This means that either he does not believe emotion can produce symptoms referable to the nervous system or that he does not trust his findings. We have said that the diagnosis of psychosomatic disease is not a matter only of the exclusion of physical disease. In addition to the psychological study, tests aimed at exclusion of organic disease prepare the way for a psychotherapeutic program.

Sexual Tension. This group of symptoms tends to occur in the hysterias, particularly anxiety hysteria, although it may be present in neurasthenia as well. Strange as it may sound they are related to fantasies arising out of repressed sexual tension. This sexual feeling and the associated ideas are not easily brought to consciousness.

The following cases represent special phases of the mechanism and treatment of vertigo.

Vertigo

CASE 74

History and Symptoms

A married white women, twenty-nine years old, was admitted to the hospital on September 17, 1940. She complained of dizziness and nausea; pain in the right ear and in the right side of the head; pain in the right arm and right leg, and an occasional pain in the right loin.

Present Illness. She said that she was well until the birth of her first child ten years ago. During the delivery "there was a loss of much blood" and following that she developed a pain in the coccygeal region which lasted about a year and then disappeared. Soon after this there was pain in the heart region which lasted for several months and still occurred occasionally. A short time later she noticed a tendency to fall to the left. There was no nausea or vomiting. Spells occurred at intervals and were followed by periods of weakness. They occurred suddenly without warning and had been increasing in frequency and severity. She had never actually fallen during one of these episodes. Asked for an accurate description, she said that she felt as if she was "sinking into the ground." At times she felt as if her surroundings were revolving and at other times as if she herself was revolving.

Mental Reactions. In the last few years she had had peculiar mental reactions, described as an impulsive desire to strike someone or to take her own life. She had to throw away a knife for fear she would attempt suicide. She was greatly disturbed by crowds, having the feeling that she might become sick.

A year ago she had severe pains in the coccygeal region again and at that time she was told that she had scoliosis and shortening of the right leg, so that a lift was prescribed for the left foot.

Medical Experiences. She had been to so many physicians that she couldn't remember them all. One said, "something wrong with the heart", another said, "a sinus condition," another that she had "curvature of the spine," and another that the "right leg was shorter than the left"; still another that there was "something wrong with her equilibrium." She had had injection treatments and x-ray treatments and, in fact, almost every type of medical treatment.

Five years ago she had an abdominal operation because of the pain in the left side; the appendix was removed. Tonsillectomy was done three years ago for the same complaint for which she was admitted to the hospital on this occasion.

Marriage and Pregnancy. She was married twelve years ago—"I married young, that's half my trouble"—and she had two children; one was ten, the other two years old. She really did not want any children after the first but had another pregnancy *for therapeutic reasons*, "to help her condition," but it failed to do so; on the contrary, she had been worse since.

Family History. Father and mother were living. The father was well but the mother has had some kind of eye condition and a kidney operation for stone. Three sisters and two brothers were all well. Her husband was well and working but was discouraged by her long illness. Their social life was limited because of her illness.

Physical Examination

The patient was a tall, thin woman but fairly well-nourished and the general physical examination showed no departure from normal. Specifically the cardiovascular system seemed perfectly normal and the blood pressure was within normal limits. Examination of the head and neck seemed normal; the lungs were clear and resonant; and the abdominal examination showed no tenderness or rigidity. The extremities were normal.

Laboratory Examination and Other Studies

Because of her many head symptoms and particularly because of the "disturbance in equilibrium," we asked for a *neurological consultation.* This showed no evidence of organic disease A *Barany* or vestibular examination was done and the result of this suggested that the patient was suffering from a "bilateral atypical toxic labyrinthitis." Examination of the ears by the otology department showed no evidence of disease. X-rays of the skull and cervical region were normal. X-rays of the lumbosacral spine and pelvis showed no evidence of abnormality. Routine laboratory studies—urinalysis, blood count, Wassermann and Kahn reactions—were normal. Temperature, pulse, and respirations were normal.

Summary of Physical Studies

Here, then, was a young woman who had been practically invalided for the past eight years. She had gone from doctor to doctor and clinic to clinic. It was obvious that the problem had not been understood and indeed we may say, it had been very badly handled. An enormous number of suggestions regarding physical disease had come her way and were still coming and this was a phase of the matter with which we had to concern ourselves.

LIFE SITUATION

Nature of Symptoms

There were two groups of symptoms. First, those symptoms relating to the body itself, and secondly, the symptoms relating to the personality, attitudes, and fears of the patient. Let us discuss those relating to the mental side of the illness.

The first symptom of this type began about eight years ago with an anxiety attack while the patient was attending a street carnival. She described this as a strange, aching sensation beginning in the lower part of her body and ascending toward her head. She had a feeling "that she was going to pieces," accompanied by apprehension and dread, and rapid, forceful pounding of the heart. She felt weak, thought she was going to faint, and had to be helped home. This was a fairly typical *anxiety attack;* we have spoken of their frequency and the errors in diagnosis that are made. Not only are fully developed attacks erroneously diagnosed but anxiety is such a commonplace thing that it appears in various degrees or minor manifestations such as "shaky knees," "all-gone feelings in stomach," "dizziness and vertigo," etc. Almost invariably the physician fails to recognize the anxiety attack as a psychogenic illness and instead looks for a physical cause. Hence such episodes are constantly called heart attacks, gallbladder attacks, hyperinsulinism or hypoglycemic attacks, neurocirculatory asthenia, and thyroid disease; in fact, a hundred different designations are given for an anxiety attack. We must be on the alert to discover this very common disorder and to differentiate it from organic disease. It is, of course, possible that the differential diagnosis may be difficult because, for example, hypoglycemic attacks sometimes have mental symptoms just as anxiety attacks are sometimes associated with low blood sugars. We have had the experience of patients who were supposed to be suffering from hypoglycemic attacks when they really had anxiety attacks because the blood sugar was normal or above. (See p. 535.)

Significance of Anxiety Attacks

Instead of casually dismissing such an attack one should regard it as a dangerous symptom. Such attacks rarely occur only once in the life of an individual. Anxiety attacks tend to occur with increasing frequency as they did in this patient. She had another within a few days and soon attacks began to occur both day and night. During the night she would wake up with a start and find her heart palpitating. She would be almost crushed by an apprehension and dread that something was going to happen and she would have to waken her husband. He would prepare some sodium bicarbonate or some sedative mixture for her and after a period of time she would be able to sleep again. Simetimes the attacks were the result of a frightening dream and sometimes they occurred without any memory of a dream having taken place. She often felt that she would die during one of these attacks and required a great deal of reassurance from her husband. Finally, after a year or two she was able to take care of herself when the attack occurred. She allowed her husband to sleep while she sat up in bed and waited for the discomfort to pass away.

Physical Results of Anxiety

Anxiety begins as a psychological phenomenon but it has many somatic reverberations. In small quantities it causes increase in the heart rate, sweating, and some mild discomfort throughout the body. In larger quantities it affects respiration, the function of the gastrointestinal tract, and sometimes the urinary system, and brings about marked weakness and distress over the entire body. As the anxiety attacks progress other mental phenomena enter the picture. Our patient began to be depressed, she cried a great deal, and became sexually frigid. She was *afraid to go out on the street alone* lest an attack occur. She finally became unable to ride in a subway, trolley car, or bus. On her best days she was able to walk a block or two with the children, but on her worst days she had to stay at home. Then she was unable to do the work in her home because of the fear that she would fall down and be forced to lie there totally helpless. Moreover, she had developed a fear of knives and other sharp instruments lest she use them to hurt her children, her husband, or some friend, or to kill herself. She also had the impulse to hurl herself in front of a subway train. All these fears regarding traveling alone, of doing harm to herself or others, we recognize as the *phobias* which act as defenses against the unpleasant sensation of anxiety.

Marriage and Childbirth

Having discussed some of the features of her anxiety, let us return to the life history of this patient. She was the third of seven children. The father was a laborer. His interest in his children did not go far beyond their actual material support. He was not cruel or unkind, but at the same time was not very close to his children, especially the patient. The mother was an average mother of Italian-American extraction. The patient said that she was never on particularly good terms with her mother. The patient described herself as a lonely, sensitive child; a day-dreamer. The mother did not seem to know the needs of a growing young girl and during the second year in high school the patient ran off to get married. She stated that she wanted to have a little freedom and through her marriage she thought she could obtain it. Her husband had always been a steady worker and was quite devoted to the patient. Even though the patient had more freedom as a result of her marriage she had not been able to utilize it very well. She was not married long before her first child was born, and soon after that her illness began.

The First Anxiety Attack

The family history and marital history did not reveal anything so very different from that encountered in the case of many other young women who have married and remained well. We may discuss now what we have learned from an intensive study of similar cases of anxiety hysteria: What causes anxiety? It is a sense of insecurity, a feeling that through lack of love or through some danger the individual is going to suffer. We know that in this patient the attachment to the parents was lacking in real warmth and affection because the parents were unable to impart those ideas which give a child the security to get through life without anxiety. We cannot say exactly what stimulus precipitated the first attack while the patient was attending the street carnival. It is not easy to elicit the cause of an anxiety attack even when the patient is seen following his first experience with this distressing symptom. When asked what they were thinking of at the time, or what may have frightened them, patients will usually answer that they do not know. They will be telling the truth, for we must always remember that these ideas are unconscious.

Sexual Impulses

We have said before that the primitive anxiety in children is caused by a fear of being left alone. As the individual grows older his hostile and sexual impulses inevitably threaten him with fear of reprisal or fear of loss of love. In women particularly a forcible repression of the sexual impulse is very common, and they feel that the release of a sexual thought will bring them into a dangerous situation. In this patient we cannot help but wonder if her presence at the street carnival caused some forbidden romantic ideas to come dangerously close to consciousness and thereby released the first anxiety attack. At any rate, we do know that it was the first time that the patient forcibly felt a threatened disintegration of the ideas and feelings which had kept her relatively secure and comfortable. The description given by the patient who has anxiety attacks is really quite correct when she says she is "going to pieces." Her ego-integration is going to pieces and she feels herself slipping out of that relationship to the world in general and to human beings in particular which makes for security.

Symbolism of Anxiety

We have talked about the symbolism of symptoms, that is, how symptoms often express through a kind of body language what the individual is unable to express in words or actions. We might add that the expression "going to pieces" also seems to be symbolic of the disintegration of the personality. In this connection it is interesting that physicians frequently make an effort to help these patients by slapping them on the back and saying, "Pull yourself together, man." Unfortunately, this is not a thing that is easy to do because the impulses that are responsible for the disintegration of the personality are unknown to the patient and his will-power is not a strong enough instrument to overcome these impulses. We may also say that vertigo can be the symbolic representation of insecurity. Because of *inner* insecurity the patient shows *outward* instability and hence becomes dizzy.

It is unfortunate that proper attention could not have been paid to this illness at the time it began. All the treatment that she received for her bodily symptoms was not only of no avail but convinced the patient that she had some obscure bodily illness.

TREATMENT

Treating the Physical Symptoms Instead of the Anxiety

When anxiety and the symptoms accompanying anxiety are present it is a therapeutic error to treat the symptoms and ignore the anxiety which is the real causative agent. This patient was treated for heart disease, thyroid disease, sinus disease, disease of the vertebrae, disease of the eyes. She was treated by x-ray therapy and by orthopedic appliances. None of these treatments was aimed to combat the anxiety in any way. In a disease such as pneumonia, the physician knows that his main task is to help the body overcome the positive agent, the pneumococcus, or whatever organism is causing the lung infection. During the course of pneumonia the patient may have headaches, backaches, muscle soreness, and other symptoms. However, the physician does not busy himself with adjusting glasses, treating the thyroid, manipulating the back, or trying to effect an adjustment of a short leg. He knows that if the infection can be successfully combated the accompanying symptoms will disappear. The problem is analogous in anxiety hysteria. If the physician will concentrate his attention upon relieving the anxiety the accompanying symptoms will disappear. This emphasizes that in our present-day medical set-up the outpatient clinic and the general hospital ward are bad places for such patients. They come into contact with too many unfortunate suggestions that do harm so far as their personality is concerned and it is almost impossible to protect them against these suggestions.

Treatment of Anxiety

The treatment of anxiety hysteria has been considered in Chapter IV. Here we will mention only a few points that apply particularly to this patient. We have discussed the nature of anxiety. It signifies a defect in the relation of the patient to other human beings. He fails to feel their interest in him and their presence no longer reassures him. No matter how old the patient may be he is reduced to the state of the two-year-old child who has lost his mother in a department store.

Childhood Anxiety

The child has lost his attachment to someone he trusts to protect him from the dangers of a world strange to him. We do not necessarily mean that all children, if lost in a crowd, would go into a panic of anxiety. However, we can readily connect the phenomenon of anxiety with children since it may take considerable development before a child has acquired a group of sound ideas about the nature of reality so that he can feel safe in it. The individual who falls ill with anxiety attacks, whether it be at fifteen or thirty-five, has been rather loosely attached emotionally and ideationally to other human beings and when his anxiety attack occurs something of this attachment has broken down. The therapeutic approach of the physician, therefore, must be to repair this damage by making the patient aware of what is wrong and then getting him to act and think in a more mature way. This is not an easy task and requires a great deal of patience and hard work on the part of both physician and patient. In the first place, no one likes to be told he is afraid; no one likes to admit he is weak and dependent. It is much more respectable, to the patient's way of thinking, to assume that he has heart disease or gastrointestinal disease or even Ménière's disease than to accept the statement that he has an emotional illness and is being made sick through fear. One needs only to look at the way the patient with anxiety seeks the protection and reassurance of other people to see what his needs are, and yet it is remarkable how often this escapes the notice of the physician.

The anxiety and panic of very young children is usually due to the separation from the reassuring friendly adult. As the child grows older anxiety is often stimulated by ideas of hostility or ideas of sexual activity for which the child so often receives threats of withdrawal of love or actual physical punishment. The role which these factors play can be determined when we investigate the conditions under which anxiety attacks occur.

Hostility and Sexual Feelings

At any rate, after careful physical study, the patient who is having anxiety attacks with their accompanying somatic symptoms needs to be reassured that there is nothing wrong with his organs but that they are malfunctioning as a result of his emotional disturbance. By questioning the patient about his attitude to those around him during both his childhood and his adult life we are able to see why the patient remains aloof from close friendship. It may be that close friendships are avoided because they have forbidden sexual significance or it may be that they are avoided because of hostility felt against others.

Our patient told us that she had a poor relationship with her mother and, in defiance, left home at a very early age. From this behavior and because of her fear that she would use power destructively we could be sure that there was considerable hostility within her personality. These attitudes had to be altered so that the patient understood that she need not be afraid of her thoughts or her impulses. When this has been achieved the patient can live more normally socially and will be able to utilize the good will of those around her. In this particular case such treatment would take a long time and unfortunately could not be arranged in our clinic. Her physician was properly advised and it was our hope that he would be able to carry on.

No Danger to Others. Although she had hostile impulses, indicated by her fantasies of attacking people and her fear of knives, there was no reason to believe that this patient would really harm her children or anyone else around her. Sufferers from anxiety hysteria are usually not dangerous to others. They have built up their defenses against hostile or violent impulses so that the latter are unlikely to break through. They injure only themselves by developing an increasing number of symptoms or further isolating themselves from life in order that none of their hostile impulses can be acted out. The murders and other acts of violence that one reads about in the newspapers are done by persons with other types of emotional sickness such as schizophrenia, paranoia, manic-depressive psychosis, and psychopathic personality.

SUMMARY

A young woman with dizziness due to anxiety was thought to have "labyrinthitis." The psychological mechanism is discussed and treatment suggested.

Certain treatment principles are indicated in the following case.

Vertigo

CASE 75

History and Symptoms

A married woman of twenty-six was troubled by attacks of anxiety with palpitation of the heart, difficulty in breathing, a fear of "going to pieces" and fainting in the street; and with these attacks dizziness would occur and numbness and tingling in the extremities were felt.

After physical examination had ruled out organic disease and after getting to know the patient we said to her, "These symptoms occur in people who are holding back two strong emotions—those of hate and sexual desire. Since this is true of others perhaps it may also be true of you." At first she could not believe that such feelings were present and said, "Even if they were I don't see how they could make me feel this way." However, she was quite incapacitated by her symptoms and was willing to talk about herself.

LIFE SITUATION

She was the youngest of two sisters and as a child had shown "terrible tempers," which disappeared when she went to school. She was frightened by very strict parents into avoidance of everything pertaining to sex. She was ordinarily a shy person but during treatment these "terrible tempers" of childhood reappeared. Shortly after this a great deal of sexual feeling began to emerge. She day-dreamed about being picked up on the street by men and taken to a hotel room. When sexual feelings were about to emerge she would complain of dizziness, and numbness and tingling in her extremities.

Sexual Fantasies

Because of these sexual fantasies the patient was terrified to be alone on the street. We said, "You must not feel that thinking of a thing and doing it are synonymous. You must trust yourself more. At any rate we trust you. In spite of your sexual thoughts we do not believe you would acquiesce to seduction." As a result of exposing these thoughts plus re-education her symptoms diminished but it took months for them to disappear.

OCULAR AND VISUAL DISTURBANCES

It has been said that the ophthalmologist is in a position to see a great many symptoms that are due to emotional conflict. The eye is an organ of orientation but it is also the receptor of stimuli that satisfy many needs. Much that is forbidden can be taken in by way of the eye. The eye is most important in learning the secrets of sex and if sex has been too strongly tabooed during the childhood period the unconscious needs of the adult may determine a functional disturbance in the organ whereby he comes in contact with so much that is forbidden. Moreover, the eye not only absorbs pleasurable stimuli; magic and erotic power are supposed to emanate from the eye so that there are additional reasons why, in the unconscious, the organ is closely related to sexuality. Persons so disposed, who have seen something which they consider improper, may react with squinting, blepharospasm, watering of the eyes, or hysterical blindness. As Freud expressed it in one of his early papers, "If the sexual component-instinct which makes use of sight—the sexual 'lust of the eye'— has drawn down upon itself, through its exorbitant demands, some retaliatory measure from the side of the ego-instincts, so that the ideas which represent the content of its strivings are subjected to repression and withheld from consciousness, the general relation of the eye and the faculty of vision to the ego and the consciousness is radically disturbed." Or, as he later states in the same paper, it is as if an accusing voice had uplifted itself within the person concerned, saying, "Because you have chosen to use your organ of sight for evil indulgence of the senses, it serves you quite right if you can see nothing at all now," thus giving its sanction to the outcome of the process. Any threat to the safety of the eyes in such persons may result in serious anxiety.

Anxiety and the Eyes

In certain anxiety states there may be bizzarre complaints related to the eyes and vision. Patients frequently say that electric lights appear to have a ring around them, that they are divided into sections, or that they appear as if the light were being looked at through a screen. Others complain of pain or itching in the eyeballs in the absence of organic disease. The treatment of these bizarre sensations is treatment of the underlying neurosis, which is usually a severe one. These sensations in the eyes or symptoms related to vision are similar to vertigo and paresthesia. Usually they represent late symptoms in a severe anxiety state although they are not generally thought of as symptoms of anxiety. Too often the physician thinks only of ocular or central nervous system disease, overlooking the possibility of a psychogenic disorder.

Hysterical blindness is a common symptom, occurring in one or both eyes or in various fields of each eye. Many cases have been "cured" by hypnotism or the profound suggestion of electrical treatments. Such "cures" are usually only temporary, however, because the underlying neurosis has not been modified. Real psychotherapy, in which the patient participates intellectually and emotionally, is necessary if we are to do more than temporarily abolish the symptom.

Asthenopia

Rutherford defines asthenopia as "a syndrome in which the visual discomforts that attend prolonged close work are accompanied by feelings of fatigue and reflex manifestations remote from the eye. It can be classed as a psychoneurosis because of its mechanism and symptomatology. The term "eyestrain" may be reserved for those cases in which visual discomforts are brought on by prolonged close work, are limited to the eyes, and promptly disappear when close work is discontinued." *Hence, the wise ophthalmologist recognizes that the patient with asthenopia needs a change in his outlook upon life rather than a change of his lenses.* Even when a headache has been attributed to "eyestrain" and actually cured by fitting glasses, it does not necessarily prove that the headache was due to a minor error in refraction. The elements of suggestion and transference, discussed in the treatment chapters, must be evaluated.

Night-blindness

Night-blindness is a disturbance of light perception which results in difficulty and occasionally an inability to adapt the vision to faint illumination. In a study of fifty-two soldiers with this disorder Wittkower and associates found no ocular cause for the night-blindness and in particular could find no indication of vitamin A deficiency as an etiological factor. However, "nervous" habits—nail biting; speech disorders; food-fussiness; morbid fears, such as excessive fear of darkness and fear of injury, especially to the eyes; conflicts over aggressiveness; and abnormal prying interests—were commonly seen, and long antedated the onset of the disorder.

Forty-three patients had definite evidence of neurosis; the chief characteristic was a life-long history of overdependence. Stressing the importance of sexual conflict in the early development of these patients Wittkower thinks that it is not surprising that the blindness is limited to the night when we consider that night is predominately the time for sexual expression and darkness is the best ally of the criminal aggressor. In other words, if the sexual curiosity of childhood centers in the eyes and has to do especially with trying to see in the darkness and the conflict is repressed because it is forbidden, then it is conceivable that under the stimulus of seeing in the dark, symptoms will occur.

Miners' Nystagmus

In a study based on incapacity among miners, Halliday discussed, among other conditions, miners' nystagmus. This type of oscillation, found only among miners, was regarded as a disease and was sometimes associated with such symptoms as movement of objects, headache, giddiness, and night-blindness. Inasmuch as it was a compensable condition when its incidence increased, a committee was appointed to study the disorder. The committee concluded that deficient illumination was the essential factor. Again the incidence rose. Culpin had already suggested that that it was a psychoneurosis and Halliday called attention to the fact that although insufficient illumination was held to be responsible for the disorder the incidence increased ten-fold during the period when the physical environment generally was undergoing a progressive improvement as regards lighting, ventilation, and hygiene. He concluded that miners' nystagmus is mainly, if not entirely, a psychoneurotic disorder with symptomatology centering on the eyes, the symptoms being fixed on the visual organs as a result of such psychological factors as suggestion, "knowledge," compensation, and fear of blindness.

Incidentally, this is one of a series of observations which form the background for a sociodynamic approach to psychosomatic problems. Halliday has recently published a book on this subject.

Central Angiospastic Retinopathy

Just as general physicians became more aware of the psychosomatic concept as a result of medical experiences in World War II, so was ophthalmology influenced. Harrington commented that the precision of diagnostic and therapeutic procedures available to ophthalmology has led to a conspicious neglect of psychic factors in ocular disease. He feels that prolonged but reversible psychologic disturbance can eventually give rise to irreversible organic disease in the eye just as in other body systems. Among other conditions he discussed central angiospastic retinopathy. This clinical entity begins acutely as a grayish edema of the macula which may vary from the faintest haziness with loss of foveal reflex to a disciform, sharply outlined, flat, serous detachment of the macula. As the edema subsides, a redistribution of retinal pigment gives a mottled and irregular appearance to the macular area. Frequently there are numerous discrete, punctate yellowish dots around the fovea. The pigmentary disturbance is followed by a gradual loss of substance in the fovea and the development of a sharply outlined, punched-out, slightly irregular and usually minute hole in the macula. Visual disturbance in the stage of edema is usually pronounced. This may be followed in the end stages by complete or partial restoration of central vision.

At the same time that Harrington was making his observations Zeligs reported on this condition among navy personnel and marines. He concluded that spasm of retinal blood vessels is induced by emotional factors. In discussing Harrington's paper, Zeligs stated that the ophthalmologist cannot treat such patients merely by asking them to abstain from smoking or by prescribing some antispasmodic drug, but rather that they should be given the opportunity of psychotherapy.

Glaucoma

Attacks of primary glaucoma have been precipitated by emotional upsets. Schoenberg cited cases in which the attack seemed to be connected with accidents or with the death of a member of the patient's family, worry over ill health, or financial losses. Inman has referred to primary glaucoma as an organ neurosis and proposed the term "angioneurotic edema of the anterior eye."

Certain it is, stated Harrington, that there are many aspects of glaucoma which cannot be explained by the old mechanical theories of aqueous drainage. "More and more evidence is being accumulated to show the close relationship between the intraocular vascular circulation, the secretion of intraocular fluid and the autonomic nervous system. The susceptibility of the autonomic nervous system to emotional shock is well known."

In a study from the Chicago Institute for Psychoanalysis of thirty-six glaucoma cases Piers found in twenty-four of them a close connection between glaucoma attacks and specific emotional events to which these individuals were especially sensitive. In nine cases the original attack was precipitated by witnessing an accident which resulted in injury or death to someone with whom the patient had intense emotional ties. In the majority of the other cases, where such acutely traumatic upsets did not occur, there nevertheless were found chronic emotional conflicts involving the patient and one or more of his dependents.

A forty-four-year-old woman who had had an operation for glaucoma on one eye was studied psychoanalytically. A daily chart of the eye tension was kept; later biweekly readings of the ocular tension were made. From the beginning of the psychoanalysis it was obvious that the patient was laboring under intense anxiety. A relation was found between ocular tension and emotional tension; the ocular pressure rose whenever aggressive, hostile feelings with the comcomitant anxiety were intensified and fell during periods of relative freedom from anxiety.

Treatment

Among the few ophthalmologists who understand the ocular neuroses, the best advice regarding their management comes from Derby: "A diagnosis of neurosis is not hard to arrive at, but once it has been made one should be prepared to spend some time on the patient or, if not, to send the patient to someone else who will. One must gain the patient's confidence or no results will be obtained; a hasty, superficial examination will not inspire confidence. Once one is sure of the diagnosis, I think that the best procedure is to put all the cards on the table, tell the patient frankly what is the matter, and explain to the best of one's ability and as simply as possible how the trouble developed. Pain, as is well known, can become a habit; and as we all use our eyes constantly for one thing or another during our waking hours, the habit pain repeats itself frequently. . . . Most people can grasp the fact that the use of the eyes should be a subconscious function, that it is only when we are conscious of them that we suffer from discomfort, and that the only way to get rid of this discomfort, is to get the eyes back to the subconscious level. To do this depends largely on the patient's own effort. He should use the eyes, not rest them, and disregard discomfort; when the eyes feel especially uncomfortable they should be used. Such discipline will almost always effect a cure if the patient has confidence in his physician and has what is vulgarly termed 'guts.' I freely confess that in earlier days I supported these measures sometimes with prism exercises, sometimes with graduated reading (Dyer's method). Now I rarely use either but depend solely on the mental effect of a careful explanation of the trouble. It is far more dangerous to tell a patient to rest a healthy pair of eyes than to induce him to use them. Many a sensitive patient has been made hypersensitive by the prescription of rest and dark glasses; the potential psychoneurotic becomes an actual one. Our aim in this, as in other fields of medicine, should be prevention, and we can nip many a beginning neurosis in the bud."

Changing Lenses. We refer here again to Derby: "There is entirely too much changing of lenses a fraction of a diopter or a few degrees of axis among us, and naturally so, because it is the path of least resistance. I believe that we ophthalmologists should take more pride in not prescribing glasses and in changing a minimum of glasses, than in the number of prescriptions we issue."

Chapter XXIII

SKIN DISORDERS AND ALLERGIES

PSYCHOSOMATIC ASPECTS OF SKIN DISORDERS

Recent years have witnessed an increasing interest in the relation of the emotions to disorders of the skin. The skin, like the eye, is an organ of expression. Both the eye and the skin, including the hair, are said to sparkle and "glow" with vitality or to be dull and lifeless. The skin, like the eye, is important as a point of contact between the inner and outer worlds.

Blushing, pallor, and sweating are well-known skin phenomena which express behavior such as excitement, embarrassment, shame, fear, and anger. But beyond these very obvious reactions we are interested to know whether definite skin lesions may also express behavior; in other words, whether emotional factors may be responsible for more permanent changes in the skin.

Attitude of Dermatologists

The general opinion of dermatologists in this regard is exactly similar to the attitude toward psychosomatic problems encountered among other specialists and general physicians as well. This has been discussed elsewhere. It is well expressed by Sulzberger in his recent book, "Dermatologic Allergy," wherein he states that there is no proof for "nervousness" as causal in the production of a dermatosis. "In our material, we have gained the impression that these occasional instances of 'nervousness' were (1) purely coincidental, (2) concomitant (*i.e.*, psychoneurologic disturbances caused by the same factor or factors which produced the dermatologic manifestation), or (3) clearly the entirely comprehensible result of and the normal reaction to the dermatosis and its 'maddening' itching, loss of sleep, and continuous worry about disfigurement, about the future, about economic and other personal and related conditions." Continuing, Sulzberger points out that "the older designations of neurodermite, neurodermatitis, angioneurotic edema, etc., have nothing to do with the present meaning attached to the words 'nervous,' 'neurogenic,' 'neurotic,' etc."

Concept of Multiple Causation

Stokes, on the other hand, has stood in the forefront of the dermatologists who accept psychosomatic influences in the etiology of skin disorders. In a recent review he and Beerman have this to say on the general topic of the attitude of dermatologists toward this subject: "Dermatologists and allergists, like all new groups in the specialisms of medicine, pass through a stage in which they resist liaison with their neighbors in other fields of medicine, as one of the unconscious devices for establishing their individual autonomy and identity. The accustomedness of the dermatologists to the visible and structural which, in the field of skin diseases, is a constant temptation to superficial thinking as well as an advantage in study and classification, is a possible factor in the reluctance with which the psychogenic problems have been admitted to the fold of causes in diseases of the skin. A highly objective, highly 'ocular' speciality in which enthusiasm for the photographic, and dominance by the photographic type of mind is a natural consequence of the character of the material, tends perhaps to be slow in acquiring a functional viewpoint either in diagnosis or research.

"One might almost say that until relatively recently only self-infliction, recognizable by the bizarre and unclassifiable physical outlines of the lesion, was admitted to the field of the psychogenous in diseases of the skin. There is also recognizable in medicine in general, a disposition to think in terms of sole causes rather than complex interacting factors. This sole-cause attitude of mind has perhaps an admirable cutting edge in exposing the etiology of a relatively unknown group of ailments; but it must give place ultimately to a viewpoint which recognizes multiple causation and interrelations as equally fundamental with, if not more fundamental than the single isolated cause. The psyche rarely appears in dermatoses as a sole cause, and for that reason has met with more difficulty in acceptance, perhaps, than have fungi, body cells, and so forth."

With this viewpoint of *multiple* causation in regard to psychosomatic skin disorders, as well as other psychosomatic conditions, we are in complete agreement.

Neurodermatitis

A large amount of the case material of the dermatologist is made up of the "eczema-neurodermatitis" group of disorders. Often they are difficult problems, refractory to treatment. The question of multiple etiological factors, acting in complementary fashion, is important in regard to them.

In connection with the controversy of "nervous eczema versus contact dermatitis," we cite very briefly a case that is now old in the literature but which has some keen and critical comment that is still pertinent.

Rattner reported the case of a young man who two weeks after his marriage developed an acute dermatitis on his face and neck and the upper half of the body. He had a psychoneurosis and anxiety state. The dermatitis was assumed to be neurogenous. It was subsequently shown that this acute dermatitis was excited by perfumed cosmetics which his wife used.

For sixteen years this patient had had recurrent attacks of eczema, all of which were considered to be seborrheic dermatitis. Then, superimposed on this seborrheic habitus, the acute dermatitis was found to be a sensitization dermatitis. The importance, if any, of the neurogenous component, Rattner went on to say, could be estimated only by inference, whereas positive patch tests were tangible evidence that the irritant was at fault.

We had some correspondence with Dr. Rattner about this case and he said that the diagnosis of neurogenous dermatitis was made by a dermatologist in another city, only after a thorough search for irritants had failed. Another capable dermatologist concurred in the diagnosis. The patient then consulted a neuropsychiatrist who agreed that there was a psychoneurosis, but felt that the dermatitis was a thing apart.

We shall not give further details of the correspondence, except to say say that the patient eventually got himself into the predicament of going to a psychiatrist for treatment of his skin and to a dermatologist to look after his psychological disturbance!

"Nervous Eczema." Dr. Pusey commented about the foregoing case: "We are witnessing an intense agitation of the subject of nervous eczema. Dr. Rattner's case illustrates the pitfalls into which we are apt to get in following this lead. Here is a case which seemed made to order for the diagnosis of eczema of nervous origin. The sexual element is exaggerated, the psychic factors are all there, including, as is usually found in such cases, a readiness of the patient to accept the emotional origin of his trouble. The background is perfect and it takes but a few bold strokes of the sympathetic artist to give a striking picture of a neurogenous or psychogenous eczema. But what do the unsentimental facts show when they are worked out? The patient is sensitized to perfume and that is what is exciting his attacks. Many similar cases of nervous or other systemic origin which have vanished into thin air when they are traced down to their local irritations must occur to everyone with a large experience in skin disease.

"The insistence on the importance of nervous factors as a cause of eczema and many other dermatoses is a backward step into the old maze of conjecture, out of which we have been trying to find our way for more than a century. Each revival of the conjecture gives us a new set of terms, but the idea remains the same. Forty years ago they were treating neurasthenia by cutting off prepuces, correcting defects of vision and removing other actual or imaginary causes of reflex irritation to cure eczema. Then they called them 'eczemas of reflex nervous origin.' Now we are psychoanalyzing them and calling them psychogenous and neurogenous eczemas. The words are new, but it is the same old tune. The ideas are remnants of the old hippocratic humoral pathology which has obfuscated our views for twenty-five years."

"*Multiple Factors.*" To continue with Pusey, "One of the chief businesses of dermatology since it has been able in the last hundred years to study more accurately the physical and chemical facts of pathology has been to show in respect to one disease after another that these diatheses are broken reeds, extremely tempting and appealing in one way or another, according to the predilections of the individuals, but in the end broken reeds. When the diathesists are confronted with a case which they would have of a nervous origin but in which there has been demonstrated an external cause which excites the eruption and without which the eruption would not exist, they are wont to take refuge (and now it will be recognized why we are quoting this in such detail) in the explanation that the irritant is actually one of the causes, and that their theory still holds good because there are emotional or both factors in the case which may be contributory.

"That sort of reasoning," he states, "is begging the question. The same facts apply to every pathologic condition of specific origin that can be conceived. A longer list of predisposing causes can be offered for tuberculosis. One could even get up a list of respectable causes for scabies. But these predisposing facts in themselves are not the cause of the disease. You may emphasize them and elaborate them. You may indulge in all kinds of intellectual and physical gymnastics, but they alone are impotent; without the definite, specific cause, disease does not occur. And it may be added in the case of irritant dermatitides, without the discovery of the cause, treatment is likely to be ineffective."

Psychosomatic Approach. We will not carry the discussion further, because we have demonstrated Pusey's point of view and the point of view of a great many dermatologists today. For the sake of discussion let us take a case of fungus infection of the feet recently reported by Harris. This is a condition that is often complicated by an allergic reaction.

A virile-appearing, handsome, twenty-four-year-old marine had spent 210 days in naval hospitals during a two-year period of service, most of this time because of recurrent fungus infection. Personality study revealed a severe anxiety neurosis manifested by a great many psychosomatic complaints, very low self-esteem, and an unmistakable feminine trend in job preference. When the data were discussed with him he admitted bisexuality. Apparently the stress of constant stimulation and threat of exposure kept him in a state of anxiety. He was given sufficient insight to understand the mechanism of his trouble: homosexuality—anxiety state—excessive sweating of hands and feet—inability to cure the fungus infection in the presence of constant moisture.

Incomplete Presentation. This case of course cannot serve as an example for a complete presentation of the controversial problem because no one would contend that there is a specific relationship between this patient's personality and the fungus infection. And yet this is truly a psychosomatic problem from the standpoint that psychic and physical factors act in a complementary fashion to produce the disorder and that only by the utilization of psychological as well as physiological technics can we understand the illness. But of course the real problem in regard to psychosomatic medicine is whether there is a specific relationship between the personality and the skin disorder, and the dermatologist wants to know whether psychogenic influences can be responsible for an actual dermatosis. The following case is intended to illustrate, not prove, this proposition.

Neurodermatitis; Good Response to Psychotherapy

CASE 76

History and Symptoms

A woman of fifty had typical neurodermatitis behind the ears and the back of the neck, sometimes extending to the arms. In addition she suffered from asthma, migraine, and hypertension. The migraine had begun in adolescence, the asthma and skin trouble had been present for perhaps fifteen years, and hypertension had been discovered in the last several years. In the beginning the migraine had been associated with menstruation which was irregular and painful. During high school she had suffered from "anemia" and had to give up school in her third year because of "fatigue." She had been free of headaches in the last several years. (She related that her physician had said "either they would wear me out or I would wear them out.") But the migraine apparently was replaced by the other difficulties. The patient had given up many of her household and social activities because she was "too nervous." She slept poorly and blamed it on the irritation of the skin. She had been studied in many excellent clinics and the diagnosis of neurodermatitis was well established. Allergy studies and eliminating diets had not proved helpful.

LIFE SITUATION

The patient had been brought up in a small midwestern town by wealthy parents. The father was a benevolent tyrant, the mother a neurotic and overprotective person. The patient was married at twenty-seven to an inadequate man who never made a satisfactory living. She had known him for four years but had to wait until her older sister married before she could marry. Then her marriage was disturbed by the mother's final illness and the mother's death took place a short time afterwards. The patient had had three pregnancies but only one child, a daughter now married and living in another city.

Husband's Impotence

The patient had always been frigid and in the last several years the husband had become completely impotent and there was a great deal of resentment on the part of the patient. She thought that her husband was unfaithful and in an off-guard moment blurted out that "she hated him."

After about ten years of marriage the father died and a great deal of trouble arose in the settlement of the estate. There was a quarrel between two brothers who have not spoken since and the patient played a buffer role between them, her sympathy being with the younger brother, who suffers from a heart ailment. She feels that he was cheated out of his fair share of the estate. Because they are a close-knit family living in a small community she is constantly reminded of and humiliated by the family quarrel.

Treatment Not Directed to Skin

She became aware of the fact that her feelings had much to do with her illness and that she had retired into herself, nursing the family problems. Attention was directed to the life situation rather than just to the skin, the asthma, or the high blood pressure. In fact nothing was done as far as the skin was concerned (it was largely ignored) while attention was centered on the main life problems of resentment against an inadequate husband, the highly charged tension of the family schism, the retirement from life's activities, preoccupation with symptoms and the attendant neglect of personal appearance.

Improvement

As she learned to express her feelings and saw her problems in a somewhat different light, her attitude changed both toward her illness and toward the family situation. She was encouraged "to carry on in spite of symptoms." This meant doing more work, such as needlework and cooking (which incidentally kept her hands busy so that she bothered her skin less). It also meant going out more socially "in spite of the appearance of the skin." Her improvement was reflected in all aspects of her personality. She became more reassured, lost twenty pounds of her excessive weight, "spruced herself up as she came out of her shell," and took up many of her former life activities.

The clearing of the skin coincided with the other improvements and a checkup two years later found her in good shape even though she had returned to her former environment.

SUMMARY

A middle-aged woman with typical neurodermatitis presented additional features to establish a psychosomatic diagnosis. Dermatologic and allergic treatments failed to help her. Treating the personality, rather than the skin, seemed to account for marked improvement.

Acne

Not only is the manipulation of the skin in acne an important aspect of the emotional disturbance but the relation of the psyche to the disturbance itself has been hinted at from time immemorial. The very fact that the disorder is so prevalent in adolescence suggests that it is related to the active psychosexual development during this period.

The vulgar explanations that are often given regarding the occurrence of acne in youngsters and the common belief that marriage is a cure for acne vulgaris are further indications of this line of thought. Clinical experience suggests that females with acne, who also have menstrual disturbances, undergo an improvement in the appearance of the skin as the menses become more regular. As in many of the other problems that we have been considering it seems probable that both endocrine and psychological factors are important in this condition.

Severe Acne—Improvement with Psychotherapy

CASE 77

A white girl of twenty-five was first seen early in 1946.

History and Symptoms

Her face was badly scarred from severe acne of five or six years duration. She had had numerous treatments, including x-ray. Fatigue was pronounced, the menses were regular but painful, and for about three or four years she had suffered from vasomotor rhinitis.

The family history was negative except for two younger children who also had acne, one quite severely.

Physical Examination

The general physical examination disclosed no evidence of organic disease and routine laboratory studies were within normal limits.

LIFE SITUATION

The patient was raised in a small community. After graduating from high school she obtained a secretarial position in which she had remained until very recently. About the age of twenty she had an offer of marriage from a young man with whom she had kept company for about a year but she felt that she was not ready for marriage, "that she was needed at home." Shortly afterwards the young man married and the acne became worse about this time. Her life was rather dull and monotonous and she restricted her social activities more and more because of the facial eruption.

Quite unexpectedly her employer, who was many years older than she, began to make advances with the plea that his wife was ill. She discouraged his attentions but was obviously excited by them. She was in a great conflict about whether to continue with her job but finally resigned and left home to consult a physician in another city. There she lived with relatives and for a time felt greatly relieved but the episode with her employer recurred in her thoughts repeatedly. She expressed great resentment toward him, obviously because he had turned to her only "because his wife was ill."

Sexual Conflicts

With great reluctance, after many interviews, she stated that she had indulged in masturbation as a child, felt terribly guilty about it, and confessed to her clergyman at the time of a revival meeting. He explained how common the practice was and that there was no sin attached to it but she could not relieve her guilt and sought him out again and again to repeat over and over the story of her "bodily abuse." She had the erroneous idea that one could develop venereal disease in this fashion; secretly she had Wassermann tests on numerous occasions and now desired another.

Social Activities

Now she went through the same situation in regard to making friends. Her attitude was that if her face would only heal she would have more confidence in making friends but again we said to her, "No, you must not wait for your face to heal, you must go out and make friends in spite of your acne. You will find that they do not care and as you establish more friendships, getting your interests out instead of in, we think your skin will undergo further improvement."

Gradually she made friends, extended the range of her social activities, and at the same time gratefully acknowledged that her face was considerably better.

SUMMARY

A young woman with severe acne of the face was involved in sexual conflicts carrying much guilt. As she overcame these conflicts and gained confidence in herself, her skin cleared although no local or systemic medical treatments were used.

Urticaria

Urticaria is a disorder in which allergic factors are at times clearly recognizable but at other times obscure. It is the puzzling, chronic cases to which "multiple causation with important psychic component" applies.

Stokes and colleagues in a study of 100 cases of urticaria found a familial and hereditary background in 60 per cent of the cases compared to only 25 per cent in a control group. Constipation, and other digestive disturbances, including abnormalities of the biliary tract, were commonly present. Positive reactions to scratch tests for allergic conditions were obtained in 64 per cent of the cases. The most common allergic concomitants of urticaria were hay fever and vasomotor rhinitis.

Etiology. They grouped the possible causal factors as follows: familial predisposition, personal allergic status, gastrointestinal disturbance, infection of all types, idiosyncrasy to drugs, and what they termed "the psychoneurogenous component." Seventy-five per cent of the cases showed one to three causes, the largest proportion of the cases exhibiting two causes other than the psychogenic. In seven cases the psychogenic background seemed to be the sole etiological factor. The principal psychogenic elements were: the tension make-up, neuroticism, the worry habit, shocks, family troubles, and finances. They felt that the psychoneurogenic background lay in a personality type rather than in external impinging circumtances. Concerning treatment, improvement seemed to increase as a wider range of causes, including the psychogenic factor, was considered. Additional observations on urticaria will be discussed in the section on allergy.

Pruritus

Klauder has emphasized the role of psychogenesis in itching. He finds that a considerable percentage of all patients with pruritus, particularly those with pruritus vulvae and pruritus ani, are psychoneurotic. Other symptoms of psychoneurosis are present and may be elicited from the history. In the vast majority of patients with pruritus vulvae and pruritus ani, local examination fails to disclose a physical cause.

Pruritus Ani

Pruritus ani is also regarded by many other dermatologists as having a strong psychogenic component. The anal region is particularly sensitive to stimulation. In many patients with this disorder satisfaction from sexual intercourse is diminished or absent, while scratching of the anal or perineal regions may be associated with a sensation similar to orgasm. In some patients it seems to serve the purpose of a substitute for masturbation. It is well known that stroking and manipulation of the skin produces a feeling of pleasure which arises from the stimulation of the sensory nerve endings. Some parts of the body are supplied with more nerve endings than others and these are more likely to be manipulated. This is of course particularly true of the genitals. We discussed in our first chapter that when a young child has discovered the greater degree of pleasurable sensation derived from the manipulation of the genitals he handles that part more than others and this phenomenon has been called masturbation. If the child is punished too severely for this act he will cease manipulating the genitals and may turn his attention to other parts of the skin surface.

Pearson reports the case of an eleven-year-old boy who had an itching eruption of the feet. Each day while bathing he would hold his feet under hot water from the faucet until they became numb. He also rubbed and picked at the thickened skin. He had been doing this over a long period of time and was reluctant to confess the habit. Psychological study showed that the manipulation of the skin of the feet was a substitute for handling the genitals. The boy volunteered that when he rubbed his feet he had an erection. He also noticed that they itched worse when he was left alone with his sister with whom, at an earlier date, he had had some sexual play. Pearson also reports the case of an adult who had a persistent iching and infection of the scrotum which he would not allow to heal because of the neurotic necessity of squeezing, picking, and manipulating as a masturbation substitute. Occasional patients admit that they derive more pleasure from the scratching of the perineal region than from the act of sexual intercourse. One of our patients would develop pruritus when he was in a temporary period of impotence.

Hostility and Skin Disorders

Both Menninger and Ackerman have cited cases of dermatitis in which there was a great deal of repressed hostility in addition to the sexual component. The skin lesions served not only a sexual purpose but also served as a punishment for the hatred which they had held toward a parent. In a study of self-mutilation and self-imposed injuries inflicted upon the skin, Menninger discovered that quite regularly the unconscious motive for such attacks depended upon (a) impulses relating to the expression of otherwise inexpressible hostility toward someone or something in the environment, (b) impulses relating to the punishing of self in response to the sense of guilt which such hostility engendered, and (c) the erotic capitalization of the suffering in a masochistic way. In addition, of course, there are the obvious conscious motives of secondary gain, such as the sympathy and attention which the patient obtains.

Necessity for Psychotherapy

Saul made some observations regarding pruritus ani during psychoanalysis. One young man complained of attacks of pruritus ani which occurred regularly when he was in the company of older men who were personally interested in him. The patient's association showed clearly that passive and homosexual wishes were aroused by these situations. He occasionally indulged in anal masturbation and stated that he used the pruritus as an excuse for this indulgence. His pruritus was sometimes relieved by a satisfactory defecation, which likewise may give much sensual satisfaction. French, in a communication to Saul, told of a woman patient who similarly had a strong desire for anal gratification by inserting the finger in the anus at the time of scratching. Her pruritus was cured by helping her to achieve a greater capacity for genital satisfaction.

Thus it would seem that, in addition to physical causes, pruritus ani may represent a perversion of sexual desire, that is, an itching for satisfaction which cannot be achieved in genital sexuality. The treatment, of course, is not so simple as to advise sexual intercourse, but consists of an attempt to remove the inhibitions to the normal flow of sexual energy through the genital channels. This may occur from superficial psychotherapy but it usually requires many psychotherapeutic sessions at the hands of a skilled therapist.

In a discussion of seborrheic dermatitis Wittkower has this to say: "Whereas the effort syndrome patient is predominantly concerned with problems of honor, morality and religiosity, the peptic ulcer patient preoccupied with bread-and-butter problems, the patient suffering from colitis with cleanliness and tidiness, difficulties in social contacts are the most prominent feature in seborrheics. It looks as if the seborrheic patient not only feels ostracized because of his skin affection but also is prone to develop his skin affection because he feels—and has always felt—ostracized. Whatever the psychological and physiological dynamics of the disorder may be, the malady disturbs his social relationships still further and relegates him in many cases to the position of a pariah. Though outwardly protesting against this state of affairs and actually suffering through it, the seborrhoeic may inwardly accept the affliction as being well deserved."

This dynamic situation must be borne in mind in treating such patients.

Many other psychosomatic considerations apply to skin disorders, for example, the psychological material concerning the asthma-prurigo syndrome which has already been discussed under Bronchial Asthma in Chapter XX, p. 627. Additional references will be found in the section on Allergy.

Necessity for Physical Studies

Nor must we forget, as Sulzberger has pointed out on many occasions, that we must be very skeptical about accepting the coincidence of emotional factors and symptoms as a proved casual relationship. For example, a spinster of forty-seven who had had her uterus removed and then began to itch and scratch was referred by her physician as a case of "nervous itching." There were many aspects of her life situation, besides the fact that she was a spinster of forty-seven and had just lost her uterus, to suggest a background for nervousness, but the appearance of the skin indicated the necessity for further physical study and after a prolonged search one of our colleagues found unmistakable evidence of scabies.

THE RELATIONS BETWEEN EMOTION AND ALLERGY

Allergy and psychosomatic medicine have much in common. The allergic population and the neurotic population are so numerous that they must overlap. Therefore, if for no other reason, these disorders exist together in many people.

Applied in an empirical way for many years, both subjects were established on a scientific footing at the turn of this century and both saw a more complete integration into general medicine after World War I. Utilized to some extent by many practitioners, both subjects must become a part of the understanding of all physicians. In order to accomplish this, increased facilities must be established in medical education for undergraduates and graduates. But they have more in common than that: Both have been exploited by irregular practitioners when orthodox medicine has disdained to endorse them, and both have potentialities for doing harm as well as good.

In addition to these aspects which they have in common, there is an intimate relation between them. Psychosomatic medicine would seem to have a special application to allergy. It has long been recognized that emotional factors entered into problems of allergy but up until recently we have lacked any exact methods of measuring these effects.

This is one of the problems with which Abramson concerned himself in a detailed discussion of the subject.

It is generally admitted that there is a high incidence of neurosis among allergic individuals, so high indeed, that we must pay particular attention to the personality of allergic patients to see whether we cannot find psychic factors that are fundamentally important in the background of the illness and also important from the standpoint of precipitating attacks. Because allergic problems are so often thought of as hereditary let us suggest that *pseudoheredity* is also important and must be distinguished from true heredity. We are thinking of the condition that we have discussed previously, namely, the manner in which a child can absorb the behavior pattern of some member of the household to whom it is intimately attached and then in later life, without consciously realizing it, imitate the illness of that particular person. Because the person is a blood relative we often think of this relationship as an hereditary one when it is in truth an environmental problem dating back to the earliest days of infancy.

The Psychosomatic Point of View

As previously stated, a person gets sick for a variety of reasons, physical and psychic. In other words, it is usually not one thing that determines illness, but rather multiple factors acting together. As Halliday points out, in our approach to illness we must think:

1. What kind of *person* are we dealing with? (inherited and acquired characteristics, physical and psychologic).
2. What has he *met*? (germs, allergens, or emotionally disturbing events).
3. What has *happened*? (the physiologic mechanism or pathogenesis of the disorder).

For example, allergic responses occur when a prepared organism, possessing certain physical and psychologic characteristics, meets certain elements, physiologic and psychologic. In some allergic disorders a single preponderant factor may be largely responsible, as for example in pollen hay fever. In others, such as asthma, there are frequently multiple interrelated factors, allergens and psychic disturbances, which act in a complementary fashion to produce the disorder. (p. 62, chap. III).

The Common Cold

In an article devoted to the subject of emotions and allergy, Saul suggests a hypothesis as to the mechanism of emotional factors in hay fever and in allergy in general. Attention has been called to his observations upon common colds in patients who were being treated by psychoanalysis. The colds occurred in situations in which the patients suffered intensification and frustration of passive receptive wishes, usually with a prominent oral component, that is, in which the wishes for love, attention, care, and help from others were represented in the dreams and associations largely in the form of being taken to dinner, receiving gifts of candy, and otherwise being fed. These colds sometimes disappeared dramatically with insight into these situations or with alleviation of the frustration. This suggested that these colds were not primarily infectious, but that they were perhaps allergic, related to the coryza of hay fever. Saul has repeatedly observed the occurrence of colds in patients when their analyses had to be temporarily interrupted, for example by the absence of the analyst for a week or so. He has also observed that colds occurred regularly in several patients who were very passive, dependent persons, when they forced themselves to do sustained work. In this regard they approximate the hay fever mechanism.

Hay Fever

Wilson introduces the subject of structural and instinctual conflicts in cases of hay fever by suggesting that "man's assumption of the upright position was the beginning of greater utilization of the visual and auditory sensibilities and a lessening of olfactory perceptions. This produced a corresponding increase in the visual and auditory acuity, accompanied by a diminution in olfactory sensitivity. It is a well-established fact that primitive vertebrates rely primarily upon olfactory perception for the maintenance of existence and as the stimulus for reproduction. Danger, food, and sexual stimulation are all perceived by the olfactory centers before perception takes place in either the optical or auditory spheres."

Personality Study. He then reports a psychoanalytic study of seven cases of hay fever (five female and two male patients). The material presented by these patients during psychoanalysis led him to the assumption that the psychological component of the hay fever symptom is a result of unsuccessful olfactory repression. Probably the first and most important factor in determining this unsatisfactory repression is that of unsatisfied, thwarted, and inhibited sexual curiosity. The failure or refusal of parental figures to enlighten and instruct the child who is attempting to satisfy and master his sexual curiosity leads to a displacement and an increase in preoccupation with other bodily functions—particularly elimination. This function is intimately associated with odors: breath, perspiration, urine and feces. When parents and other persons in authority place a strict taboo upon the sexual curiosity, while at the same time they encourage the child to become preoccupied with the excretory functions, this displacement readily occurs.

Parent-Child Relationships. The mothers of his patients were all sexually inhibited women, who had themselves been reared and brought up according to strict, mid-Victorian patterns including a strict taboo of anything sexual. The fathers of these allergic patients maintained complete aloofness to their children's curiosity along sexual lines. Wilson does not infer that children reared in such an environment are predestined to hay fever. The parent-child relationship that he has indicated is fairly common, both for children who develop other types of neuroses as well as for children who make fairly satisfactory psychological adjustments. What he does try to demonstrate is that these patients were reared in an atmosphere that was conducive to the repression of sexual curiosity and at the same time encouraged the indulgence of olfactory perception.

Displacement of Sexual Interest. A study of the material collected during psychoanalysis of seven patients convinced him that the psychological component in hay fever is based upon a displacement of sexual curiosity from the visual to the olfactory sphere. When this occurs the eyes and nose (the organs of sexual curiosity) assume the character of sexually stimulated genitals with congestion and increased mucous secretion. This results in a diminution of both olfactory and optic sensitivity.

Interaction of Psychic and Physical Factors. Wilson concludes that analysis of unconscious material makes it possible to hypothecate the specific psychological factors in patients suffering from hay fever. The interplay between these inner conflicts, attempts at their solution, and the external agents (specific pollen allergens) which precipitated the actual hay fever attack remains unknown. Patients who, as a result of their psychosexual development, have substituted olfactory for visual sexual curiosity may, because of this, become more sensitive to pollens. Olfactory curiosity that has never been relieved may be considered to be a constant irritant to the mucous membrane of the nose. An added irritation from an external agency such as pollen may produce an attack. It is possible that there are cases in which the local sensitivity alone, in the absence of psychological stimulation, may be sufficient to precipitate an attack. It may be assumed that sometimes, when the psychological stimulation is increased by the mobilization of repressed sexual tension, this alone may suffice to produce an attack of rhinitis. This would explain the resistance to pollens that was obtained by patients who had undergone analysis. When the genital inhibitions and the chronic psychological stimulus were eliminated the pollen irritation could no longer precipitate an attack.

Asthma

More material dealing with emotions and allergy was provided by observations on psychoanalyzed asthma patients made by the same group working at the Chicago Institute of Psychoanalysis (French, *et al.*) This material was referred to in the discussion of bronchial asthma (p. 634). It will be recalled that the close attachment to the mother was the central feature. The asthma occurred regularly when this was suddenly threatened.

Urticaria

Two young women, both with severe prolonged generalized urticaria, have been analyzed by Saul. In both of these cases the central feature was deprivation of parental, but primarily of maternal love in childhood, with consequent strong masochistic attachment to the father. In one case the mother died when the patient was two years old and the patient was exploited by the father. The stepmother received almost no love or regard from either of them. The other girl's parents overtly preferred the other children and treated her as the ugly duckling or Cinderella of the family. The attacks of generalized urticaria occurred regularly and exclusively when the first patient's longings for love were intensified and frustrated. The second patient had attacks under the same conditions. In these cases the longings for love were expressed in dreams largely in the form of wishes to be admired, to be beautiful, and to have fine clothes. Both patients wanted to be dancers; the first acted in amateur theatricals and the second modeled for artists.

Exhibitionism

The evidence, though meager, suggests that where the wishes for love are in the form of exhibitionistic desires and related to the skin, and where there is a heightened skin eroticism, this operates as one determinant of the skin as a site for the symptom. Wilson's paper discussed the choice of the nose as the site of the symptom of hay fever as determined by repressed olfactory sexual curiosity. The hypothesis as to the site of the symptom in asthma, as described in the asthma study, is that the asthmatic attack replaces a cry, which is stimulated by the threatened loss of the mother's love or by the separation from her, but which is repressed. In the urticaria cases, weeping relieved the attacks and apparently could replace them, it being an alternative mode of expression for the feelings of frustration.

General Theory

This leads Saul to suggest a general theory as to the mechanism of emotional factors in allergy. In all these studies of symptoms of an allergic nature in which emotional factors were found to play a role, the central emotion related to the symptom was a strong longing for love, basically for the mother's. This suggests that intense, unsatisfied longing for love affects the individual's allergic sensitivity. This longing is of the infantile, dependent kind of the child for its mother. It further suggests as a hypothesis to be tested, that when this longing is especially intensified and frustrated or threatened with frustration, the allergic sensitivity is increased and the symptoms appear.

The Child's Longing for the Parent

Of course such longings are important in everyone but they apparently bear a special relationship to allergic symptoms. In contrast to this allergic group, for example, are functional cardiac cases which serve as a control group. Studies of emotional factors in essential hypertension indicate as the chief emotional tendencies related to the symptoms, not libidinal longings as in these allergic cases, but hostility and struggle with an unsolved conflict situation. This difference in the emotional background of the allergic symptoms, as opposed to essential hypertension, may be of significance for the fact that these two conditions are generally believed to occur only very infrequently in the same individual. The following excerpt is taken from Saul:

"The situation appears then to be as follows: The emotional factor which is important for the allergic symptoms in these particular cases is libidinal longing probably basically of the nature of the child's for the mother. This longing must of course come to expression in specific ways and involving specific body sites in each case. The choice of these particular sites must be determined by specific psychological and biological factors. There is nothing mutually exclusive about these, for allergic individuals usually present symptoms in different organs at one time or another. The specific factors determining the site of the symptoms in the asthma cases are apparently: 1. the sudden threat to the attachment to the mother, and 2. the repression of the consequent tendency to cry out. Further study may reveal further specific elements. The specific factors in cases of the common cold of the type described above have not been worked out in detail but the evidence suggests that one of these is the frustration of the oral components of the longing. Wilson's paper has demonstrated the specific factors involved in localizing the libidinal longings in his hay fever cases to the nose, namely, the suppression of the olfactory sexual curiosity, which was found to express not an adult genital sexuality but an immature, dependent, demanding attitude. Not enough cases of urticaria have been studied to reveal the specific elements of the skin as the site for the symptom but the three analyzed cases all showed a relationship to the repressed longing which did not achieve genital sexual expression and which apparently resulted in a high degree of erotization of the skin (as seen in strong exhibitionistic tendencies). In all these allergic cases in which the emotions appear to play a role in the production of the symptoms, the central factor related to the symptoms was intense libidinal longing and certain specific factors involving the status of the longing. Its manner of frustration and mode of expression determined the bronchi, upper respiratory passages or skin as the particular sites for the symptoms."

Psychological and Allergic Factors. To continue from Saul:

"The observation of the relationship of intense, repressed, frustrated longing to allergic sensitivity provides a theory which takes account of both the psychological factors and the pollen sensitivity, for according to this concept the one complements the other. The situation is this very simple one, that the emotional state leads to physiological changes which either 1. imitate the allergic symptoms, or 2. render the tissues more sensitive to allergens, or 3. do both; and conversely an individual who is allergically sensitive on presumably an entirely organic basis might conceivably through the very fact of this sensitivity more readily produce symptoms which are psychologically determined. For example, a patient may have seasonal attacks of hay fever due to pollen sensitivity, entirely apart from his emotional state. However, if his longings increase, his hay fever may become more severe. Further, if the repressed frustrated longing becomes sufficiently intense, then the symptoms may appear on this basis alone. An individual in whom certain tissues are constantly stimulated and sensitive because of his emotional state (like a congestion of the nose from a chronic tendency to cry for mother, or of the skin from a chronic tendency to blush) may well be more sensitive in these tissues to irritating allergens. Conversely, it is easily conceivable that an individual whose tissues are irritated by allergens will react more sensitively in these particular sites to emotional stimuli.

"It must not be forgotten in all these discussions that when we refer to psychogenic factors we do not mean certain intellectual ideas of the patient, but on the contrary, the emotions, which are powerful and eminently biological. The child's longing for the parent and its anxiety when left alone are deeply biological; they are concerned with the individual's very existence, and when such deep-seated emotions are aroused, they produce far-reaching biological changes."

Personality Trends

Now the question arises: Are these various disorders related to one another and to the personality of the patient? Studies demonstrate that they have certain features in common which correspond to the clinical picture of a vegetative neurosis and meet the previously discussed criteria for a psychosomatic affection. In other words, there is a positive family history; evidence for childhood neurosis or psychosomatic disturbance; the personality structure of neurotic character; exacerbation at crucial life periods in connection with specific life situations; demonstration of specific behavior on exposure to a conflict situation, such as may occur in a medical interview; and improvement by the hyposensitization of psychotherapy or the avoidance of the trouble by avoiding a provocative situation. Although the work that has been done on the question of the specific relationship of personality to disease is impressive it cannot be regarded as conclusive. Nevertheless certain trends within the personality seem to favor certain disturbances.

In regard to this question Saul, in a more recent paper, calls attention to the fact that it is the oral form of attachment to the mother—consisting of a mixture of impulses, desires, and feelings which become interwoven with the sucking and later the eating mechanism—that enters into psychosomatic gastrointestinal problems, while other biological mechanisms and forms of attachment to the mother seem to be important in the allergies. These are the dermal and the respiratory. In other words, in many persons the form of attachment to the mother as seen in fantasies, dreams, and real life is not, as in many instances of gastrointestinal disorders, strongly "oral," but consists rather in a desire for shelter. The longings are represented not by wishes to be fed and all that this can imply emotionally, but rather in wishes to be sheltered and protected. Such persons often gravitate to modes of life which gratify such tendencies. Perhaps it could be said that, given a choice, they would prefer snug housing to good food. Here, too, can be points of weakness and fixation, to form a physiological pathway for the attachment to the mother and become interwoven with powerful feelings and longings. When the relationship to the mother, with all of its significance to the child (and later in life, unconsciously to the adult) is threatened, or when a person is under stress, the longings for help or consolation are expressed in various combinations or forms in different persons: wanting to be fed, wanting to be carried or led, wanting to be snuggled and and sheltered, and so on, reflecting the oral, ambulatory, dermal, respiratory, and other mechanisms and forms of attachment to the mother. The impulses may be *gratified* by personal relationships, sexual or sublimated, which reestablish in some degree the relationship to the mother. The gratification may be *sublimated* (oral: eating and drinking; respiratory: talking and crying; dermal: baths and massage). The impulses may be *repressed* so that symptoms appear when the tension disturbs organ function. Of course oral as well as dermal and respiratory trends can exist in the same individual. But Saul states that it is the person in whom the dermal and/or respiratory mechanism has some weakness, or is a point of fixation, or in whom the attachment to the mother predominately takes these forms, who seems to be predisposed to skin and respiratory allergy.

He concludes, "The dermal and respiratory mechanisms, trends, and relations to the mother are analogous to the oral ones. They are fundamental to an understanding of psychological functioning. Preliminary observations strongly suggest that they play a role in the skin and respiratory allergies similar to that of the oral ones in the gastrointestinal disorders."

Cooperative Therapy

In addition to the treatment aspects already discussed in the sections dealing with asthma, migraine, and so forth, recent cooperative efforts by an allergist (Miller) and a psychotherapist (Baruch) dealt with twenty-two patients, seven of whom were children. In all cases the history of classical allergic symptoms was confirmed by positive skin reactions to various allergens. Recognizing that clinical allergy must be practiced with constant awareness that psychogenic factors influence physical results, the authors utilized both individual and group psychotherapy in dealing with their patients. Repeatedly they observed that the fluctuation of symptoms paralleled the degree of freedom with which a patient expressed his feelings and that the intellectual appreciation of the dynamics involved was not important to the patient. Marked improvement was observed in nineteen of the twenty-two allergic patients. Miller and Baruch feel that allergic symptoms express hostility, mask a feeling of guilt or anxiety, and at the same time represent attempts to gain sympathy.

Conclusions

The allergic and the neurotic populations are so large that they must overlap. If for no other reason, therefore, these disorders will exist in the same individual. But in addition, personality studies suggest a more intimate connection—a specific relationship between neurotic character structure and allergic disorder—possibly representing parallel manifestation of the same basic fault, the one discharging on the level of psychic representation through thoughts and feelings and the other on the physiological level by means of disturbances in organ functioning.

Psychosomatic study of an allergic problem, therefore, utilizes separate technics, psychological and physiological, applied simultaneously; and diagnosis must be established not only by exclusion or evaluation of physical factors but with additional positive evidence of personality disorder meeting certain psychosomatic postulates. This will demonstrate that in a given case physical and psychological factors act in a complementary fashion to produce the disorder; in one instance specific physical factors may predominate, in another instance specific emotional factors. The latter seem to be determined by certain trends within the personality, for just as oral attachments seem to determine gastrointestinal disorders so do respiratory and dermal attachments (to the mother) apparently determine respiratory and dermal allergic manifestations (Saul).

The allergic disorders seem to fall for the most part into the group of organ neuroses that can be termed vegetative (Alexander), representing early and profound deviations of personality development. What role the constitution may play cannot be determined, since no methods are available to delimit constitutional and acquired factors. One can, however, evaluate physical and psychological factors, and proper management depends on such evaluation. Then psychotherapy plus the allergic approach will mean better treatment for the individual with an allergic disorder.

Chapter XXIV

DENTISTRY, ARTHRITIS AND ORTHOPEDIC PROBLEMS

PSYCHOSOMATIC ASPECTS OF DENTISTRY

Of all branches of medicine, dentistry has perhaps been the one most separated from the psyche. The word "dental" has come to be associated with the idea of "mechanical": fillings, extractions, dentures, appliances, and devices. It is the purpose of this discussion to point out that we cannot divorce a man from his teeth. In other words, not everything dental is synonymous with "mechanical." The cliché "the very idea of going to the dentist stops the toothache" is an indication that psychosomatic influences enter into dental practice.

Poor oral hygiene is not limited to people in the lower income brackets who cannot afford dentistry; it occurs as well in the middle and upper income brackets, for the reason that the patient is afraid to go to the dentist—he is afraid of being hurt. Many people have great anxiety about physical pain, and while they are very ashamed of it, they can do nothing about it. The idea of being stuck with a needle for a blood count or a Wassermann test fills them with dread. After being hurt by a dentist's drill they have great difficulty in returning for treatment.

Another reason for avoiding the dentist is that the loss of teeth may have a greater significance than just the association of pain or discomfort. Losing a tooth, according to an old adage, means "losing a friend," but it also means, in the unconscious thinking of many people, loss of strength and loss of virility. Of course, there is the conscious idea of the effect on the appearance, but quite aside from the idea of a possible alteration in the appearance is the idea that the wearing of dentures is a sign of old age. This is true not only of women, but of many men. It is one of the reasons that many chronic illnesses of psychosomatic origin can be traced to a dental operation, or the fitting of dentures and the failure of the patient to adjust himself to them.

Dental Problems of Childhood

A partial answer to this problem is for the parent and the dentist to cooperate in persuading children to regard dental treatment as sensible and necessary and something with a minimum of discomfort, rather than as an ordeal. Many adults exaggerate how painful a visit to the dentist can be so that the child comes to fear the dentist's office as a modern torture chamber.

Adults should therefore avoid conveying to the child the idea that a visit to the dentist is going to be painful, and visits should be started before painful procedures have to be carried out. This gives the dentist and the child an opportunity to get acquainted and enables the child to find out that the visit can be fun rather than torture. If early in the life of the child parents do their part and the dentist does his, there will be less neglect of dental hygiene because of fear.

Once the child is in the dentist's office he should not be babied by either mother or dentist. Often the child will sit in the chair and be content to be alone with the dentist, and the mother can remain in the waiting room. It is bad practice for the mother to hover about inquiring if her child is being hurt. Suggestion is worked in subtle ways and if the parent and dentist assume the child will behave like an adult he will often do so, whereas if they expect him to be afraid and to refuse to co-operate he may also readily do this. If a child refuses to cooperate it is not wise to use force unless a real emergency exists, for the combination of force and pain will cause him to dread the next occasion all the more and be the means of establishing an attitude which in later life means dental neglect.

Thumb-Sucking

While this subject is discussed in more detail elsewhere (p. 154) it has special significance for the dentist and especially the orthodontist because of the problem of deformity. The orthodontist feels that malocclusion must be avoided at all costs but, with Binger, we must ask ourselves if malocclusion of the personality is not more serious than malocclusion of the teeth. The need to get solace and comfort from sucking is the most powerful craving of early life and when it persists into later childhood it means that this symptom is answering a bodily need that is imperative. If it is met with forcible restraint (for example, by the use of mechanical devices or worse yet by shame and ridicule) the craving simply seeks another outlet which may be more serious so far as the developing personality is concerned than a continuation of the practice of thumbsucking.

Relation of Dentistry to Emotional Aspects of Surgery

Just as in childhood the dentist is feared, so does the opposite situation sometimes exist in the adult patient. He may be all too amenable to the idea of losing his teeth. Indeed, he may derive a certain perverse satisfaction from having teeth extracted. As Menninger states, these are the people addicted to polysurgery. As may be imagined, they are psychoneurotic. When they have some physical discomfort, having heard of illnesses being cured by the removal of "foci of infection," they become their own diagnosticians and often conclude that a tooth or several teeth should be removed. Like the patient who wants his tonsils or appendix removed, they usually manage to get the operation done.

There are some powerful unconscious impulses at work in these people that cause them to be so persistently illogical. First, the idea of a "focus of infection" makes them feel that they harbor something "unclean." The idea that "toxins" (impurities) are being discharged from an "unclean" (infected) area and entering the blood stream causes them anxiety. Their whole attitude is one of "Out with it!" as soon as possible and they will not rest until the tooth, the appendix, or even the gallbladder is out. Often the patient is assisted in his desire by a dentist or a physician who is not certain of the advisability of the operation, but feels that "it will do no harm." That it will do harm has been demonstrated by numerous case reports of confirmed invalidism.

Another unconscious motive in this sacrifice of organs is to help get rid of a sense of guilt. This sense of guilt usually dates back to childhood and resides in the unconscious mental life, so that such patients do not realize that they are trying to assuage guilt when they periodically suffer the pain and make the sacrifice of having something removed, be it from the mouth, abdomen, or pelvis.

A man of forty-four, studied in February 1945, complained of pain in the left chest which he suspected was due to heart disease. At first he said that his trouble had begun in January 1944 following an indiscretion in eating. At that time he had consulted a gastroenterologist, who explained his trouble as due to a spastic colon and treated him on this basis. Later when he developed pains in the left chest he was referred to a cardiologist, who told him that he did not have heart disease. But the patient saw a report which was sent to his physician and this stated that "he should be watched because of a family history of heart disease." This was sufficient to reinforce his suspicion of heart disease. His physician told him that his trouble was "all in the head," which annoyed him, and that he "probably ought to see a psychiatrist," which annoyed him further.

In reviewing his history it was noted that chest pains had really begun in 1937 at the time of a business crisis. Then during a period of several years he had worked very hard, eaten irregularly, and smoked a lot, and he felt that this was the real basis of his gastrointestinal disturbance. In the background of his trouble was long-standing difficulty with his wife who was not "sympathetic" and advised him only to "stay away from doctors."

In 1941, at the suggestion of his physician, six teeth were extracted. He felt "nervous" for a long time afterwards and became very angry that the teeth were removed and at the necessity for wearing a bridge. He blamed the dentist for unnecessary surgery and was very vindictive toward him. He continued to regard the denture as a foreign body. (He could not get used to it, and "felt burned up every morning" when he put the bridge in his mouth.)   Moreover it served to remind him of the fact that his father had died of heart trouble not a long time after the son had urged him to have some dental extractions. We allowed him to talk over this situation on more than one occasion until his guilt was somewhat mitigated.

We satisfied him as to the absence of organic disease; showed him the relationship between his life situation and his symptoms, particularly his identification with his father and his hostility for the dentist; and urged him to adopt his prosthesis as a part of himself. On this basis he made considerable improvement.

Psychologic Preparation for Surgical Operations

It is necessary for the dental surgeon, just as it is for the general surgeon, to be on guard with such people lest he play into their hands by performing useless operations. If it were just useless, it would not be so bad, but it adds to the misery of the patient and eventually results in criticism and trouble for the surgeon. Both the general surgeon and the dental surgeon must learn that there is such a thing as psychologic preparation for operations, just as there is a physical preparation. Surgeons are always so careful to prepare their patients physically for operations. They would not think of performing a major operation without knowing that the cardiovascular-renal system had been surveyed, but they almost never give any consideration to the personality of the patient: how much anxiety is present, and what the effects of a surgical experience may be as far as the personality is concerned. We recently had in the hospital ward an elderly woman who had a huge enlargement of the thyroid gland, which was removed because it was pressing upon the trachea. She had had discomfort, but not severe dyspnea. The anatomic problem loomed large in the clinical picture, but the patient was very apprehensive before the operation and after the operation she became frankly psychotic. As it turned out, we wonder whether perhaps she would not have been better off with the lump in her neck. Similar instances occur in dental surgery.

An attractive single woman of thirty years complained of fatigue, nervousness, and constipation. She had had the same symptoms at seventeen and her physician had said that the illness was due to focal infection and he ordered all of the upper teeth extracted. This was during the period when the theory of "focal infection" was so enthusiastically endorsed by the profession that the removal of teeth and tonsils proceeded at a prodigious rate. Every obscure illness was held to be due to focal infection. If we could pile together the teeth and tonsils that have been unnecessarily removed from patients with illnesses of emotional origin, we would have an imposing monument to an era of overcredulity in regard to a significant American contribution to medicine—the theory of focal infection. What sins we have committed in its name!

The removal of the upper teeth in this young woman, despite the fact that a very satisfactory denture replaced them, was a circumstance that affected her whole life, coloring her reactions in all of her personal contacts. She became extremely sensitive about her mouth and thought that everybody was looking at it and making remarks about it. She developed marked feelings of inferiority. These feelings interfered with her position and with her marriage. It is impossible to conclude that it was unnecessary to remove her teeth, but from her description of them it seems probable that it was a radical and unwise procedure. Nor do we wish to contend that her sense of inferiority was entirely determined by this circumstance. Undoubtedly, she had some such feelings to begin with, but the surgical operation added to her problem and burdened her whole life.

Atypical Neuralgia

Many pains about the head, face, and neck are wrongly assumed to be due to dental pathosis. Teeth are extracted or sinuses operated upon, when a careful analysis of the pain would show that atypical neuralgia due to "focal conflict" rather than "focal infection" is present. A study of the life situation rather than a search for "foci of infection" is the proper approach.

For many reasons it is advisable to proceed cautiously in the case of the patient who is eager to have a surgical operation, either general or dental. The mouth is an area around which a great deal of interest and pleasure are centered during infancy and childhood. Likewise, it is an area around which fantasies of hostility are likely to occur. The child identifies himself with the animal who attacks and destroys with the mouth. He thinks of himself as doing likewise, and then has guilt and anxiety over his destructive thoughts. These fantasies often remain buried in the unconscious mind of the adult and then come to the surface when psychologic conflicts arise.

Personality Structure

Binger pointed out that the mouth, quite aside from its utilitarian attributes is, psychologically speaking, directly or symbolically related

to the major human instincts and passions: to self-preservation, to cog-
nition, to love and sexual mating, to hate and the desire to injure or kill.
From the standpoint of psychopathology this is of the greatest importance.
Since the mouth represents the organ for the expression of certain instinctual cravings it is charged with a high psychological potential. Therefore, when operations are performed on this area reactions occur which
may seem irrational and bizarre to those who look upon the mouth simply
as an organ for taking in food. The human infant puts everthing in its
mouth. In other words, it tests out its environment in this fashion, and
the sucking impulse, which appears at birth, and continues long past
weaning is an important method of deriving emotional satisfaction. In
addition to chewing there survives in man a tearing and biting impulse.
Again to quote Binger, "Darwin pointed out that in states of rage, the
teeth are not only clenched and ground together, but the corners of the
upper lip are drawn back and the teeth bared—which he thought remarkable, considering how seldom they are used by men in fighting.
This attribute of the human mouth is now largely transferred to its verbal
offerings. We speak of 'sharp' words, 'biting' wit, or 'mordant' humor
. . . Other functions, gustatory and olfactory, properly belonging to the
mouth, may be conferred on our utterances which are described as
bitter,' 'sweet,' 'acid' 'pungent'—even 'foul'."

Nor should the mouth as an organ of love be forgotten. Love, genetically, is closely related to sucking and swallowing. A doting mother,
cooing over an infant, says: "I could just eat you up." Such terms of
endearment as "sweetheart" and "honey" indicate that the object of
our affections is conceived of as a dainty morsel. Binger goes on, "In
any case the lips and tongue and buccal mucosa are highly erogenous
zones and throughout life retain an important pleasure-giving function.

"Suppressed, controlled and redirected though they may be, these
atavistic traits, that is, these impulses to use the mouth for purposes of
attack, for example, remain in all of us, and can be easily revived. For
our personalities are built up of archeological layers and our earlier experiences and tendencies have left in us living, though perhaps dormant
traces, not merely dead bones and pot shares. These traces possess a
dynamism which affects our health, our relationships and our destiny."

Binger refers to the menopause as a period of life when dental operations are apt to promote unexpected reactions. A woman often feels
that a denture is the last straw in her already wounded vanity and self-
esteem. Depressions, long periods of invalidism, and even attempts at
suicide may be preceded by dental operations. Men, too, have their
hypochondriacal preoccupations. Tarachow reported a patient who went
from one dentist to another insisting that he had a tooth cavity which
needed filling. None of the dentists was able to find a cavity. This

preoccupation developed shortly before the man was to be married, and was a symptomatic reflection of his fear of being found wanting in his approaching role in marriage. In a sense he was looking for help to be bolstered against his sexual fears. The repair of the defective tooth really meant a repair of his defective masculinity.

Commenting that the fatigue state is often the result of heavy emotional expenditures, Ryan states that persons who tire easily may be suffering not from the results of dental foci but from emotional toxemia. He advises dentists to keep this in mind in making diagnoses and planning treatment. He does not suggest that the dentist assume the role of the psychiatrist before he passes judgement on a pulpless tooth. Nor does he recommend that in any situation the dentist attempt to function as a psychiatrist. To have the psychosomatic point of view is not the same as attempting to practice psychiatry. Just as physicians and surgeons are urged to think in psychosomatic terms and to integrate this point of view with other treatment methods, so should the same situation prevail for dentists. "Psychosomatics," Ryan states, "is an adjunct to dental diagnosis and practice, not a substitution for other procedures."

Thus we see that the work of the dentist may have a significance far beyond the superficial, purely mechanical ideas that are usually associated with dental procedures. If the dentist becomes a little more aware of the structure of the personality, in the same way that he is now aware of the structures in the mouth, he may avoid many unfortunate occurrences. The teeth can no more be divorced from the personality of the patient, so far as psychosomatic medicine is concerned, than can any other part of the body.

CHRONIC ARTHRITIS

Chronic arthritis is perhaps the oldest of all known diseases. Harbin, in Champion's book, states, "The word 'cripple' is derived from the Anglo-Saxon word, 'creep.' The word 'dwarf,' used sometimes in referring to a cripple, is closely akin to the Sanskrit word 'Dhvaras,' meaning 'evil one incarnate.' Convinced that the cripple embodied an evil spirit of ill omen to the community, that he would never be an asset to their armies, and that he was likely to become a social burden, our forefathers ostracised him, sacrificed him to their gods, or abandoned him in his infancy. The Romans later, however, made the first recorded provision to care for cripples. Pope Gregory, in 590 A. D., included them in his classifications of infirm and destitute to be supported by public funds. However, it was not until 1832 in Munich that the first institution, the Royal Bavarian School and Home for Crippled Children, was established; in the United States the first institution was the Hospital for the Ruptured and Crippled which was open in New York City in 1863."

Focal Infection

Rheumatism, the term that is generally used in lay circles, includes all forms of aches and pains in the muscles and joints, as well as arthritis. In this discussion we are not referring to acute arthritis, which may be due to many different organisms. For example, the gonococcus may attack a joint and when it does it produces a very serious acute inflammation which may leave the joint crippled after the disease subsides. This is a true example of a focus of infection with dissemination to a distant area which is quite different from the prevailing concept in American medicine of "focal infection." It is the latter which has been so overexploited particularly in regard to chronic rheumatism. European medicine never paid so much attention to the idea. Consequently, Europeans did not sacrifice quite so many teeth or tonsils on the altar of this concept. It was because medicine felt so helpless in dealing with this disease and because there was often such obvious indication of an infection that the concept of focal infection was so eagerly grasped. One almost never saw an arthritic who had not lost his teeth and his tonsils, and had various other areas in his body attacked on the presumption that infection flourished there. Fortunately, that is not quite so true today. But even when medicine was attacking arthritics most vigorously from the standpoint of removing their "foci of infection," it recognized at the same time that there were other factors of importance in the disease.

Polypharmacy

There is hardly any therapeutic process in medicine that has not been utilized in the treatment of arthritis. All kinds of drugs have been used. Harry Gold has listed the commoner agents that have been recommended by various writers at various times for the treatment of arthritis:

    I.   General
          1. Rest
          2. Foci of infection surgery
          3. Diet
   II.   Physical therapy
  III.   Orthopedic procedures
  IV.   Vaccines and nonspecific proteins
   V.   Drugs

          1. Arsenic
          2. Iodine
          3. Salicylates
          4. Cinchopen
          5. Aminopyrine
          6. Quinine
          7. Digitalis
          8. Strychnine

9. Cod-liver oil
10. Vitamin D
11. Liver extract (Vitamin B complex)
12. Vitamin C
13. Nitrites
14. Ortho-iodoxybenzoic acid
15. Bee venom
16. Colloidal sulfur
17. Sulfanilamide
18. Colchicine
19. Acetyl-b-methylcholine
20. Endocrine materials (Pregnancy)
21. Radium
22. X-ray treatment
23. Laxatives
24. Mineral waters
25. Local injections
26. Therapeutic jaundice
27. Dehydration
28. Intravenous alterative therapy (salicylates, iodides, colloidal sulfur)
29. Autochemotherapy
30. Gold salts.

He continues, "I know of few subjects in therapeutics which seem to be in a more unsettled and unsatisfactory state than the treatment of arthritis. It does not seem possible to chart the progress in this field by other than a horizontal line with repeated spikes representing new therapeutic ventures. The rise of the spike represents the 'passive faith' which is so common a reaction to new agents or procedures and the fall of the peak represents 'aggressive skepticism.' In few therapeutic fields do we find such sharp contrasts of views concerning matters which should be matters of fact. One arthritis specialist working with a new compound reports dramatic results and another complete failure." As an editorial concerning the treatment of arthritis stated, "...almost any form of treatment seems to produce about 20 per cent of claimed cures or arrest of cases, 30 per cent of improvement and 50 per cent of failure."

Whether gold salts, now being reported as so successful, will represent another "spike" remains to be seen. Because of the difficulties in dealing with arthritis, such patients are exploited by quacks and irregular practitioners. One has only to witness, for example, the countless thousands of people who visit shrines and faith healers. Most of these people are suffering from some form of chronic arthritis. Many magical shrines are famed for the piles of crutches that have been thrown away by cripples, who, for the moment, consider themselves cured but most of whom have to buy more crutches after they get home.

Social Implications of Chronic Arthritis

Most chronic arthritis is something quite apart from the crippling of one joint by a specific infectious agent. The end result of chronic arthritis is apt to be much more serious in the degree of crippling. The two great types are rheumatoid, or arthritis deformans, also referred to as chronic infectious arthritis and osteo-arthritis, the chronic hypertrophic variety. These are the common forms of chronic arthritis that are responsible for so much disability and because they are so widespread and so frequent, especially among the poor, they enter very importantly into the problems of unemployment and dependency. In fact, one may well say that the interrelation of chronic disease and social dependency is nowhere better illustrated than in chronic arthritis. Chronic arthritis makes for social dependency and social dependency adds to the problem of chronic arthritis.

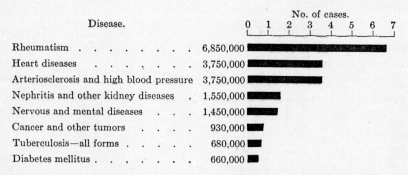

Disease.		No. of cases. 0 1 2 3 4 5 6 7
Rheumatism	6,850,000	
Heart diseases . . . . , . . .	3,750,000	
Arteriosclerosis and high blood pressure	3,750,000	
Nephritis and other kidney diseases .	1,550,000	
Nervous and mental diseases . . .	1,450,000	
Cancer and other tumors	930,000	
Tuberculosis—all forms	680,000	
Diabetes mellitus	660,000	

Chart 3.—Estimated prevalence of specified chronic diseases in the United States, 1937. (Osgood: A. J. M. Sc. 200: 429, 1940. Lea and Febiger.)

Clinical Features

Rheumatoid arthritis often resembles an infectious disease. That is to say, it frequently begins with fairly acute manifestations—redness, swelling of the joints, and fever, and other constitutional symptoms that frequently accompany an infectious disease. It may begin acutely and then gradually subside only to recur. Or it may begin insidiously and run a progressive course, both forms leading to considerable destruction of the joints and, hence, crippling. It is a disease which frequently attacks the small joints first and the larger joints may follow. Eventually the disease may be so crippling that the patient becomes bedridden, or confined to a chair. Rheumatoid arthritis is quite common in the younger age groups, whereas the second form is a disease of the older age groups. Of the two, rheumatoid arthritis is less well understood from the standpoint of etiology and less amenable to treatment.

Sociological Factors

Cobb, Bauer, and Whiting, in an effort to throw light on this subject, studied fifty patients with typical rheumatoid arthritis from a social and psychological point of view and concluded that there was a significant relationship between life stress and the arthritis in over 60 per cent of the patients (Chart 4). Their study was conducted by means of life charts

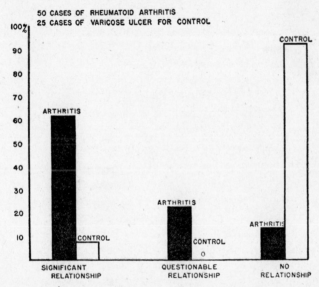

Chart 4. Temporal relationship between the environmental stress and the onset or exacerbations of rheumatoid arthritis. It will be noted that a significant relationship was encountered in a large number of the arthritic patients and rarely in the control group (patients with varicose ulcers). (Cobb, Bauer and Whiting: J. A. M. A. 113: 668, 1939).

one of which is reproduced here and which shows the chronological relation between different events in the patient's life. The severity of the arthritis is indicated in black in the middle column of the life chart. Thus one can tell roughly how often the environmental burdens occurred at the time of the onset of the arthritis or in relation to an exacerbation of the arthritis. The authors state that in some instances the patient himself emphasized this relationship in telling his own story. They do not regard this method of study as psychologic in any deep sense but rather as a sociological approach. They comment, "This study was undertaken in order to determine whether or not there existed a temporal relationship between environmental stress and the onset or exacerbations of rheumatoid arthritis. It was thought that, by employing a relatively

Year	Medical Data	Arthritis	Social Data	Age

CASE #13 ♀   HOSPITAL – #264864   DATE : 1936

BORN IN ITALY

Year	Medical Data	Arthritis	Social Data	Age
1898			ADOPTED IN FAMILY OF 11 CHILDREN	1
1902			NOT VERY HAPPY	5
1907			SCHOOL	10
1909			CAME TO UNITED STATES · SCHOOL	12
1913			MARRIED · LIVED WITH MOTHER	16
1914			OWN HOME · FIRST CHILD BORN	17
1915			SECOND CHILD BORN · HUSBAND OUT OF WORK	18
1916	ARTHRITIS OF ANKLE FOL- LOWING THIRD PREGNANCY		THIRD CHILD BORN · UP IN 1½ DAYS · MOVED · LITTLE WORK FOR HUSBAND	19
1917			MOVED FROM DAMP HOUSE · HUSBAND WORKED OCCASIONALLY	20
1918	ARTHRITIS WRIST & KNEES		SECOND CHILD DIED · FOURTH CHILD BORN · "NOT WELL"	21
1919	HOSPITALIZED			22
1920	REMISSION		FIFTH CHILD BORN	23
1921	EXACERBATION · REMISSION		SIXTH CHILD BORN	24
1922	EXACERBATION			25
1923	WRIST OPERATION		FOURTH CHILD DIED	26
1924	HOSPITALIZED · SEVERE EXACERBATION		HUSBAND ILL WITH TUBERCULOSIS	27
1925			HUSBAND IN TB SANATORIUM SEVENTH CHILD BORN · UP IN 3 DAYS	28
1926	IMPROVING		HUSBAND WENT TO COLORADO · RELIEVED	29
1927			MOTHER'S AID RECEIVED · NOT SO WORRIED	30
1928			HUSBAND IN COLORADO · LIVING EASIER	31
1929			,,	32
1930			,,	33
1931			,,	34
1932			,,	35
1933			,,	36
1934	EXACERBATION · HOSPITALIZED		MOTHER'S AID STOPPED · 1 SON WORKING · COULDN'T KEEP 5 CHILDREN ON $13.00 A WEEK	37
1935			ON PUBLIC WELFARE · NO FUEL · SON OUT OF WORK	38
1936	MARKED MALAISE AND FATIGUE		NOT ENOUGH FOOD AND FUEL · DESPERATELY WORRIED AND VERY TIRED	39

Chart 5.   Life chart of arthritic patient.   (After Cobb, Bauer and Whiting: J. A. M. A
113: 668, 1939.)

simple method such as the Meyer life charts, the synchronism between
social and medical events might become apparent if it existed. Examination of the life charts reveals that such relationships are demonstrable,
whereas they might have been overlooked had they been recorded in the
conventional medical record.   Our failure to elicit similar temporal relationships in the control series adds to the probability that such relationships represent more than coincidences. Certainly the results obtained from
this relatively simple study suggest that more detailed psychologic studies
should be made.   A statistical analysis of more detailed studies on a large
series of cases, correlated with the many other factors, should make it
possible to evaluate more correctly the exact etiologic role of such environmental and psychic factors in rheumatoid arthritis.   Irrespective of
the results obtained a better definition of the host of this chronic disease
and the many environmental factors (social and otherwise) with which he
has to contend will result." (Chart 5).

Those authors conclude that "Environmental stress, especially poverty, grief, and family worry, seem to bear more than a chance relationship to the onset and exacerbations of rheumatoid arthritis. The relative importance of these factors in the etiology of rheumatoid arthritis can be established only by a much more detailed psychiatric study on a large group of such patients."

The Social Worker and Arthritis

Speaking of the care of the patient with rheumatoid arthritis, Margolis states that the physician who would assume full responsibility for treating such patients must be an internist in the fullest sense of the word, combining psychotherapy with physical measures. Moreover, the psychotherapy will have to be based on more than intuition; at least the rudiments of psychodynamics must be understood. In addition, the medical social worker occupies an important role in treatment. He defines that role as follows: "By discovering the causes of blocking to the acceptance of recommendations for medical care and eliminating them, the case worker may really start the patient on his course. Discussions that allow the patient to vent his hostility reduce emotional tension that might otherwise be going into diseased joints. For the reticent, sensitive patient, the worker may serve as a liaison, helping the patient through the trying experiences of meeting and talking with the doctor. The worker also helps the patient express his fears about his disease and its effect on his future plans. She offers constructive help as the individual becomes ready to move ahead step by step when his physical activity is increased, when he becomes capable of leaving for short walks, when he is allowed resumption of employment, which may mean the return to an old job or taking on a new one, in which case still further emotional adjustments may be required.

"There are also the problems of family adjustments. The patient often needs help in his interpersonal relations with his family, and the latter, in their reactions to the patient and his illness. Inadequate and perhaps unable to face the situation, and confused by the illness and its burdens, the family may wreck all plans for the patient's rehabilitation unless they have the guidance and help of a skilled social worker.

"These and many other aspects of the medical social worker's job must be integrated within the framework of the therapeutic problem as a cooperative venture in which the worker utilizes the physician's medical recommendations and in which they pool their psychologic understanding to bring about the best results attainable.

"Although the medical social worker carries the major responsibility for giving social case work help to the arthritic patient who is under the

care of the hospital or clinic, community social workers also have a large
and fertile field for constructive help in this problem. In many communities they are the only ones available for such help, especially when
they are serving arthritic clients not under the care of a hospital but
rather receiving medical supervision from a private physician.

"The fact that many patients with rheumatoid arthritis come from
the lower income groups must mean a large prevalence of arthritic clients
in the case loads of community agencies. Therefore, not only medical
but community social workers as well should be informed about what
medical science has to offer to the arthritic patient."

Commenting upon the role of the social worker Schless shows that
the case work method utilizes the patient's conscious feelings about the
illness but is based on an understanding of the unconscious motivation
for behavior. "Accepting the difference between herself and the psychiatrist, the social case worker shares with the patient that difference and
confines the scope of her helpfulness within the limit of the realistic services she offers."

Emotional Factors

Jelliffe, a pioneer in psychosomatic medicine, was one of the first
to call attention to the importance of the psychic factor in arthritis. It is
gradually being recognized that the emotions have something to do with
the disease but what part they play is not understood. The prevailing
view is that if a person develops such a painful and crippling disease,
it is no wonder that he is nervous. The opposite point of view would be
that the cart is placed before the horse in this attitude—that arthritis is
largely due to a response to certain strong emotional influences which
arise within the individual and influence the function of the joints. Then
there are those who traverse the middle road and feel that it is neither
wholly one nor the other, but that many factors are at work of which the
psychic factor is only one—sometimes important, sometimes not, and
sometimes missing altogether. This is our belief.

Personality Studies

In a detailed study of selected cases of rheumatoid arthritis, Thomas
found that in many cases "the rule was to find that for years the patient
had been neurotic, then an unusually severe conflict developed, and in
the midst of this struggle arthritis appeared. The sexual adjustment of
most of the patients was inadequate; the women usually thought sex
disgusting, and many were so reticent that it was impossible to obtain
any details."

Johnson, Shapiro, and Alexander in a preliminary report of the psychodynamic findings in thirty-three patients with rheumatoid arthritis

found impressive similarities in the nuclear conflict situations and in the general personality structure of the women patients, of whom there were twenty-nine.

In adolescence many were of the athletic, tomboy type, but in adult life showed a strong control over their emotional expression. (Halliday also stressed this tendency to control and self-restriction.) They manifested the so-called masculine protest reaction with a rejection of the feminine role. Often they had passive and compliant husbands. In addition to a rejection of the feminine functions the patients showed an excessive masochistic need to serve others, which acted as a discharge for hostility and a denial of their own dependency.

The general psychodynamic background is a chronic, inhibited, hostile aggression relieved by discharge through these character trends.

While the precipitating factors of the disease covered a wide range of events, analysis of what these events meant to the patient provided certain formulations:

1. Circumstances which increase the unconscious rebellion and resentment against men.
2. Events which tend to increase hostility and guilt feelings.
3. An intensified masculine protest reaction as a defense against fear of sexual attack.

The same authors conclude that the majority of these patients learned to discharge hostility through masculine competition, physical activity, and serving, and also through domination of the family. When these methods of discharge are interrupted the increased muscle tonus resulting from the inhibited aggression and defense against it apparently precipitates the arthritis. But, they continue, this constellation of psychodynamic factors is found so commonly in patients who do not suffer from arthritis that additional etiological factors, still unknown, must be postulated. They suggest that these factors are probably somatic: inherited, traumatic, or infectious. They found that their patients improved as they became better able to receive help in analysis.

Rorschach Studies

An interesting consideration by Booth of the Rorschach method in regard to hypertension, arthritis, and parkinsonism indicates that the personality characteristics in chronic arthritis are reflected in some statistical features of the scores, but that this is not the case in hypertension. Booth thinks that significant differences can be established between L (locomotor arthritis, parkinsonism) and V (vascular hypertension) responses, but that they are indicative not of disease but of two different types of human attitudes. In other words, form and functioning of the body, in health as well as in disease, persistently express aspects of the basic personality structure. He suggests that the L and V types seem to represent opposite extremes of attitudes required by western cultures: on the one hand the emphasis on competition, on the other the emphasis on the emotional dependency of a protective social environment. The psychological interpretation of the findings suggests to Booth that arthritis and parkinsonism patients are dominated by an urge for individualistic, independent action while patients suffering from arterial hypertension have a tendency toward dependent relationships in the form of identification with their social environment.

Summary

We believe that there are, within the individual, certain emotional factors that may express themselves through tension and spasms of the voluntary muscular system and thus influence the working of the joints. In other words, if there are numerous interacting factors such as predisposition, fatigue (which may also be psychologically determined), specific infection, and perhaps even other factors, then arthritis may develop.

OSTEOARTHRITIS

Current theories regard the cause of osteoarthritis as senescence and trauma, and the fact that no obvious psychosomatic changes in glandular secretion or muscle contraction are demonstrable to explain the development of bony overgrowth, make it seem difficult to establish a relation of life situation and emotion to this disorder.

Irvine decided to get a brief life story on a number of cases of systemic osteoarthritis with special reference to childhood emotional trauma, early neurotic traits, circumstances associated with the onset of the arthritis, and evidences of emotional disturbances during the course of the disease. In the investigation of fifty cases, an opportunity was also found to observe whether there was a parallelism of emotional disturbance and progression or arrest of the organic disease.

Irvine found that noxious emotions, especially fear, anxiety, and grief, of unusual severity and duration, are important in the genesis and persistence of activity of systemic osteoarthritis. Widespread, progressive and persistently painful osteoarthritis as well as many lesser lesions (such as Heberden's nodes) were found to have a background of severe emotional trauma shortly prior to the onset of the arthritis, often in a psychic field sensitized by trauma in early life.

When the emotional state improved in such cases, the arthritis became less painful and progression of bony overgrowth ceased. The severity of the emotional disturbance and that of the activity of the arthritis were usually parallel.

NONARTHRITIC RHEUMATISM ("FIBROSITIS")

A common problem in the practice of internal medicine is the patient who complains of aches and pains in the muscles and joints, and chronic fatigue. Often there is slight fever but otherwise the physical examination and laboratory studies are negative. Attention is focused on this slight rise in temperature and the patient undergoes repeated and prolonged studies from the standpoint of obscure infection or endocrine dysfunction. Formerly such patients were often thought to be tuberculous; later rheumatic infection, with much attention to the heart, was suspected; nowadays chronic brucellosis is the most frequent diagnosis. In the course of the many physical and laboratory studies slight deviations from normal are detected and additional diagnoses are made which add to the patient's concern. She sees herself crippled by arthritis or heart disease and anticipates being a burden to her family. In addition to the many physical and physiotherapeutic measures that are used in treatment, rest and more rest is urged upon the patient, which perpetuates the invalidism and leads to greater restriction and a more impoverished life. This kind of story continues, sometimes for years, often with prolonged periods of hospital observation and sanatorium stay.

Clinical Findings

These observations are based (Weiss) on a study of forty patients encountered in a larger study of 200 patients with chronic fatigue, because so-called psychogenic rheumatism is only an aspect of the chronic fatigue problem. Of the forty patients only five were men. Physical findings of significance were uniformly absent. Sixteen patients had slight fever, always less than $100°$ F., and in only two was there slight elevation of the sedimentation rate. Laboratory evidence for chronic brucellosis seemed positive in only one patient. Otherwise there was nothing to suggest infection and the temperature disturbance was regarded as an unimportant phase of the disordered constitution.

Psychological Symptoms

Psychosomatic study, meaning the simultaneous application of physiological and psychological technics, proved the presence of psychopathology rather than tissue pathology. Hysteria was encountered in sixteen patients, anxiety states in eleven, hypochondriasis in two, and two suffered from psychotic depressions.

Psychological symptoms most frequently encountered were poor sleep and poor sexual adjustment, and a marital conflict was the most frequent underlying problem. Significant emotional conflicts were found which were apparently responsible for the fatigue, but the special feature associated with muscular aches and pains was the presence of chronic resentment of which the patient was usually totally unaware.

Psychodynamics

The muscles serve as a means of defense and attack in the struggle for existence; thus internal tension is most easily relieved by muscular action. When the external expression of aggression in the form of muscular action is inhibited by repressing forces, then muscular tension may result which is felt by the individual as pain and limitation of movement and is often erroneously interpreted by the examining physician as fibrositis or muscular rheumatism. When we say to these people that their aches and pains and fatigue are due to the fact that they are always in a state of tension, that they do not know to relax, even at night, and that because their muscles are taut they are crying out in protest with aches and pains, it makes sense to them and provides a stepping-stone for them to begin to talk about their emotional problems.

Instead of calling this psychogenic rheumatism, fibrositis, or even muscular rheumatism, the most suitable diagnostic term, as Flind and Barber point out, is the psychiatric diagnosis applicable to each case because it is the psychopathology which is chiefly responsible for the syndrome and it is by means of psychotherapy that we can deal with these patients most effectively.

Previous Studies

Halliday deserves credit for opening up the whole subject of the psychosomatic aspects of rheumatism in his studies on the insured population of Scotland. In a survey of 1000 consecutive cases he found that 15 per cent were certified with a diagnosis of rheumatism and of this group 70 per cent were nonarthritic and were usually referred to as cases of fibrositis. Occurring mostly in males having dangerous occupations, rheumatism was found to be a major cause of incapacitating sickness.

Boland and Corr found psychogenic rheumatism to be the most frequent cause of disability in 450 consecutive cases diagnosed as arthritis or allied organic conditions in an army general hospital. Approximately one third of the patients in the entire series were considered incapacitated because of psychic difficulty. The sedimentation rate was normal in all cases and in one third of the cases there was a history of invalidism or semi-invalidism from rheumatism in one or more members of the immediate family.

An outstanding characteristic in their patients with psychogenic backache was persistence of disability in spite of prolonged bed rest. They emphasize this feature of the disability when they cite the patient with advanced active rheumatoid spondylitis who was found pushing another with pure psychogenic backache to the post-exchange in a wheel-chair.

Instead of cautioning rest and more rest, which only permits these people to "stew in their own juices," we recommend that they "carry on in spite of symptoms" and this they will often be able to do once they have divorced their pain from the fear of arthritis, heart disease, cancer, or what not. Once neurotic pain is divorced from a fear of organic disease, it is remarkable how rapidly it will disappear or diminish. As soon as possible we try to get them away from injections of vitamins and hormones, from sedatives and even physiotherapy, or if some of these measures are continued we make it clear to them that they are being used in a supplementary capacity and that the cure lies in emotional reeducation. Halliday has called attention to physiotherapy and fixation of symptoms in his insured patients and we see the same thing in private and hospital practice. It is of course sometimes necessary to make certain concessions to the previous organic miseducation which the patient has had. We cannot go too quickly in changing our approach from disease to disorder, from the idea of doing something for the patient to having him do something for himself, from education along physical lines to the necessity for emotional growth. The essence of psychotherapy, which should be a part of the equipment of every physician, is not to go faster than the patient is prepared to go.

In connection with *physical medicine* one more word ought to be said, and that is on the problem of belts, braces, and supports. So often we find these patients wearing sacro-iliac or abdominal supports when what they need is *inner* support. Instead of trying to bolster them up with a crutch what we ought to do is try to develop their inner emotional security so that they will not have to lean on supports or braces, or for that matter on their physician.

ORTHOPEDIC PROBLEMS

It took the medical experiences of World War II to persuade us that the emotions enter importantly into orthopedic problems. Heretofore the specialty of orthopedics had been just about as divorced from psychological considerations as dentistry. Statistics previously quoted from W. C. Menninger (p. 54) showed that disorders of the musculoskeletal system ranked high among the psychosomatic problems in military medicine.

A South American book on psychosomatic medicine by Zeno and Crespo devotes an important chapter to this subject. There they refer to the accident habit, which we discuss in this section.

The Low Back Problem

The problem of the patient with low back pain has been with the medical profession since our first great ancestor pulled himself from the four-footed to the upright position. The low back takes all the strain. It is one of our points of least resistance. It is like the poor—it is always with us. And very much like the poor, it is apt to be shoved away into a corner so that we will not be bothered by seeing it. Thus Stimson, who saw how frequently low back pain was an incapacitating factor in the British Army, as it was in the American Army, refers to the fact that it is also a common problem in civilian medicine.

Working at New York's Presbyterian Hospital, Stimson saw the problem as follows: "If the patient had a proved orthopedic lesion such as a spondylolisthesis, a protrusion of the nucleus pulposus, or a compression fracture, he fitted well into the orthopedic or fracture clinic. But if he had a pain in the back with negative x-rays for these orthopedic lesions, medicine didn't want him, arthritis didn't want him, and he certainly didn't fit into the fracture or orthopedic clinics. There really was no place for him. This procedure of handling patients with low back pain did not seem right. As far as the patient was concerned, he or she still had a pain in the back, and no one seemed to be doing very much about it. At best, these patients were sent down to the physical therapy department for diathermy and massage three times a week. *ad infinitum.*"

The Low Back Clinic. On the basis of the above observations a combined clinic for the handling of low back pain was set up. The personnel of the clinic consisted of a physician, a neurosurgeon, a member of the physical medicine department, a psychiatrist, a rheumatologist, and three members from the fracture service. Gaston reported the working classification of three hundred cases from this clinic as follows:

Posture	60
Osteoarthritis	57
Acute low back	30
Congenital anomalies	27
Neuropsychiatric	26
Miscellaneous	23
Myositis	18
No back diagnosis	14
Rheumatoid arthritis	13
Diagnosis deferred	10
Herniated discs	9
Coccygodynia	5
Compression fractures	3
Scoliosis	2
Gluteal bursitis	2

He reports that the largest single group in the neuropsychiatric category was the returning servicemen.

Commenting further on this material Stimson states, "The posture group consists quite largely of women who have borne one or more children, who have very weak abdominal muscles, and who have low backache at the end of the day. We find that we can do a great deal for this group, thanks to the cooperation of our physical medicine specialist, who is present at every session of the clinic. Exercise, proper beds, et cetera, have done wonders, and these patients are already among our most grateful."

Treating Patients Rather Than X-rays. In these days when we are seeing so many patients whose backs have been operated upon in an effort to relieve them of pain, in much the same way that formerly so many abdominal exploratory operations were done, that is, in a vain effort to remove a pain from the body that actually resides in the spirit of the individual, it is well to remember that no area of the body lends itself to such misinterpretation of x-rays as does the low back area. Chamberlain cautions as follows: "A great many variations, and deviations from the so-called *normal*, are visualized by x-ray films, and are quite meaningless from the standpoint of the etiology of the patient's pain. To ascribe a patient's low back symptoms to an enlarged transverse process of a fifth lumbar vertebra, or to some hypertrophic spurs and fringes at some of the joint margins, is to jump to an unwarranted conclusion. Careful studies have shown that many of these positive x-ray findings are very poorly correlated, or not correlated at all, with the presence or absence of low back pain."

Stimson also comments on this subject: "Some of the arthritic patients come in with x-rays which show marked osteoarthritic spurs, lists, and scoliosis. (We are learning not to treat x-rays, but patients.) A nice woman, of about fifty-two years, came into the clinic. She said she had had a little pain in her back for the past four months. She had one of the most appalling x-rays of an osteoarthritic spine that I have ever seen, but she had only this mild backache over a short period of her life. Other patients have a great series of symptoms, and x-rays which show only mild changes. We are finding that we can relieve the osteoarthritics, especially in the older age groups, with proper fitting girdles."

She concludes that patients whose workups are negative and whose x-rays are essentially negative present the real problem but with the help of a physician, a psychiatrist, and the physical medicine expert, most people can be helped.

Camptocormia. An exaggeration of the low back problem, occasionally encountered in military medicine, has been referred to as camptocormia, or the "functional bent back." Sandler reported on this condition as did Hamlin. Such soldiers often walk like anthropoid apes. Sometimes they are bent over so that the trunk and head almost parallel the ground. Obviously they cannot be soldiers in this posture and yet no organic disease can be discovered to account for the condition. Sandler observed that on the surface these soldiers often appeared affable and genial but were given to explosive outbursts of hostility and aggression. From a therapeutic standpoint camptocormia proved to be a most difficult problem. In the majority of them only discharge from the service effected a cure.

Intractable Pain Syndromes

In a psychosomatic study of eighty patients whose activities were limited either by absence or disease of an extremity and/or chronic intractable pain, Kapp and Rosenbaum noted that fifty-one patients had some type of chronic, severe, intractable pain and of these seventeen had phantom limb pain. Many had had a variety of neurosurgical procedures without obtaining relief.

Phantom Limb. The initial emphasis of the study dealt with the postamputation phenomenon of phantom limb. Here the concept of a pain body-image describes the specificity of the site of pain in the limb (phantom or real) where the pain does not seem to be related directly to the current injury. Rather, it appears to be associated with pain experienced in the past by the patient or by a person with whom the patient has identified. Such previous pain and the injury associated with it is invested intensely with emotional significance for the patient. At times the type and local area of the pain appear to resemble an hysterical conversion symptom. Other workers agree that phantom limb is a consequence of the proprioceptive body-image which every individual develops in childhood.

Intractable Pain. Kapp and Rosenbaum write, "Every person has a 'pain memory' which is gradually built up by the painful experiences suffered and witnessed by the individual since early childhood. There are certain individuals who re-suffer previous pains in an effort to relieve some current interpersonal difficulty. Such pains represent a neurotic manifestation. They are sometimes associated with demonstrable autonomic nervous system discharges which accompanied the original pain, and become part of the neurotic symptomatology. Trivial injuries or disease often are the precipitating factors in the initiation of such neurotic pain and trophic reactions. We found that a majority of our patients with phantom limb pain and minor causalgia had such reactions.

"A number of patients were observed who developed chronic intractable pain syndromes after industrial accidents. They were bitter, hostile, mistrusting people with whom the therapist had to establish a warm positive relationship before relief could be expected. This we attempted to do in a controlled hospital environment by gratifying the patients' frustrated dependency. Only then could therapy be directed toward resolving the intense hostility intimately attached to the painful syndrome."

CHART 6. MAIN CAUSES OF DISABILITY AND DEATH

Disability		Number
1. Accidents		9,700,000*
2. Rheumatism and Arthritis		6,850,000**
3. Heart Diseases		3,750,000**
4. Arteriosclerosis and high blood pressure		3,750,000**
5. Cripples		2,600,000***
6. Nephritis and other kidney diseases		1,550,000**
7. Nervous and Mental Diseases		1,450,000**
(Mental cases in mental hospitals	487,237	
Total mental cases	697,023)	
8. Cancer and other tumors		930,000**
9. Tuberculosis, all forms		680,000**
10. Diabetes Mellitus		660,000**
11. Syphilis		590,604†
12. Gonorrhea		282,815†
13. Blind		250,000‡
14. Deaf		120,000‡
15. Malaria		58,917†
16. Hookworm		12,756†

* National Safety Council, 1943.
** Psychosomatic Medicine, P. 506, Estimated prevalence of specified chronic diseases in the U. S. 1937. (Osgood: A. J. M. Sc. 200; 429, 1940 Lea and Febiger.)
*** U. S. Health Report, 1935.
† U. S. Public Health Service, 1943.
‡ Social Work Year Book, 1943.

Deaths		Number
1. Heart Diseases		394,915
2. Cancer and other tumors		163,400
3. Childbirth		158,563
Neonatal deaths	72,122	
Stillbirths	79,174	
Maternal deaths	7,267	
4. Diseases of the nervous system and sense organs		136,924
Cerebral Hemorrhage (excluding birth injuries)	105,391	
Cerebral embolism and thrombosis	10,461	
Hemiphegia	4,037	
Meningitis	2,254	
5. Kidney diseases		100,443
6. Accidents		94,500*
7. Pneumonia: bronchial, lobar, unspecified		63,633

8.	Tuberculosis, all types..................................	57,690
9.	Diabetes...	33,971
10.	Arteriosclerosis......................................	24,342
11.	Syphilis...	16,345
12.	Suicide..	16,117

U. S. Bureau of the Census Vital Statistics: Special Reports, Vol. 19. No. 3. January 10, 1944.

Prepared by the Albert and Mary Lasker Foundation, Inc.

The Accident Habit

A glance at the chart which accompanies this text shows that among the causes of disability in this country accidents rank first and in addition are an important cause of deaths—100,000 in 1946 according to the National Safety Council. It is estimated that the 10,400,000 disabling injuries of 1946 cost $5,600,000,000.

Dunbar made a systematic study of patients admitted to a large hospital in an effect to determine the role that emotional factors play in illness and decided to use fracture patients for a control, thinking that they would represent the most "normal" group that could be found in the hospital. She was surprised to find that they were far from "normal" so far as emotional factors were concerned and that, indeed, it was this aspect of their personality that had to do with the accident. Dunbar found that others had been working on this problem and that many authorities were agreed that the majority of accidents are linked to the personalities of the victims. She tells of a public utility company which operated a large fleet of trucks and became seriously alarmed at the rate of accidents. After a futile effort to determine the cause they fell back upon the simple expedient of shifting men with bad accident records from the driver's seat to other work. In this way they reduced their accident rate to about one fifth of what it had been, so far as the trucks were concerned, but they found that these same men, instead of smashing up their vehicles, were injuring themselves at work or at home.

The National Research Council, which had made a study of this company as well as of three others, reported that the automobile accidents and personal injuries of more than 2000 drivers tended to accumulate side by side.

Personality Study. Dunbar found that the hospital group with accident-proneness are generally impulsive people who concentrate upon daily pleasures with little interest in long-term goals. While their illness rate is below that of the general population their accident rate is high. They are usually extremely resentful of authority, often on an unconscious level, and an unusually large proportion of them had neurotic traits in childhood. These traits often expressed themselves in the form of walking and talking in their sleep, in persistent lying, stealing, and truancy. Later these tendencies disappeared, apparently replaced by the accident habit. The decisiveness of the accident-prone person is part of a drive for independence and self-reliance in a situation of the moment rather than as a part of a planned career or program. Dunbar finds that when this personality pattern is set beside those of other groups of the population, it turns out to match precisely that of the juvenile delinquent and the adult criminal. "The behavior characteristic of the persistent breaker of laws is virtually identical with that of the persistent breaker of bones right up to the point where the one commits a crime and the other has an accident." One group carries the early record of lying, stealing, and truancy into a broader field and becomes a criminal, while the other begins to hurt himself instead of the community.

Treatment for patients with the accident habit involves a deep understanding of all the factors which enter into their accident-proneness. The following case illustrates the many factors that may enter into a "purposeful" accident, determined by unconscious motivation.

A Purposeful Accident

CASE 78

History and Symptoms

A very obese, hypochondriacal, middle-aged, white woman had been obsessed for several years with the idea that she had cancer of the throat and despite the reassurance of many physicians who had studied her carefully, she continued to believe that "there must be some physical basis for the pain and burning sensation in the back of the throat." She also had a great fear of infection, was meticulously clean about her home, and was forever washing her hands. She was very insistent about having something done for her throat and she herself would make topical applications of irritating solutions until, on many occasions, bleeding occurred. Even this did not satisfy her need for suffering so that she finally succeeded in persuading a dentist to remove her perfectly good teeth. She encountered less difficulty in sacrificing her tonsils. Both operations gave temporary relief but the symptoms returned worse than ever.

LIFE SITUATION

She was so fixated upon her physical symptoms that it was impossible to accomplish more than the most superficial investigation of her life situation. The only digression she would make from a discussion of her physical symptoms was to upbraid her local physician for fancied mistreatment and insulting behavior. He had sent her for a general diagnostic survey but continued to supervise her care. She spent a great deal of time criticizing him for a lack of interest in her condition and for the "contemptuous way" in which he treated her. Nevertheless, it was obvious that underneath the surface hostility there was a very positive attachment to her physician which was indicated by her continuing under his care and by such statements as: "she had great faith in his scientific ability; on occasions he had been very kind to her; and her children and her husband were devoted to him."

She was a very religious person and went to church every morning seeking help for her illness. We had refused to help her to decide whether to leave her local physician, and so on one occasion when she felt that she had been more than ordinarily mistreated by him, she went to church to seek help in making a decision on two related questions: first, whether finally to quit her physician and seek another and secondly, whether for financial reasons it would be better to give up a health insurance policy which provided nursing service in case of a confining illness. She had carried this costly policy for a long time without realizing benefits and now her funds were low.

On the particular morning in question she prayed for help in making these two decisions. As she left church she noted that it had been raining and while ordinarily, because of her overweight, she took special precautions in descending stairs, "she was not as careful as she should have been" and on reaching the third of three steps, slipped on a wet spot, fell and fractured the left ankle. As she explained on the telephone the next day, "she got her answer quicker than she thought." She seemed in a cheerful frame of mind as she told with evident satisfaction, that her physician had immediately responded to the call after this accident.

Comment

Aside from the purposefulness of the accident the marked ambivalence for her local physician was the striking feature of this case. Just as many neurotic people take up much time in criticism of some member of the family, just so did this woman express herself toward her physician. On the surface she was markedly hostile and yet she continued under his care and obviously held him in great respect and even with some evidence of underlying affection. He found the patient a very disturbing factor in his practice and confessed that when it was necessary to see her, "it made a wreck out of him." When the psychological background of this relationship was explained to him, he found matters a little easier, but needless to say, was pleased when the patient finally made up her mind to place herself under the care of an older physician who had "taken care of her in childhood." Because, to conclude the story related above, once the fracture had healed, she was back once more with her old throat complaint and criticism of her local physician.

The ambivalent relationship to her physician, so excessive in this particular instance, is a very important element in the doctor-patient relationship, as yet not understood in general medicine.

Low Back Problem
Improvement with Brief Psychotherapy

CASE 79

History and Symptoms

A young man of eighteen was discharged from the service because of pain in the low back area. He said that he had sprained his back two years before, doing heavy work; he was in bed for a week. He gave up the job but has been troubled on occasion ever since. Later while in school he tried to play football but "the back seemed to go out of place." He thought he had a curvature of the spine and consulted an osteopath, who gave him a lift for his left shoe. He continued to be troubled some but was admitted to the navy in April, 1946 saying nothing about his back difficulties. Two weeks later he began to limp, could not sleep because of the pain, and spent about two months in the hospital until he was finally discharged.

Past History

He had been a healthy youngster, always highstrung. There were no serious diseases of any kind.

Family History

Both parents had lame backs. The mother suffered from "sacroiliac" and the father had low back pain and was nervous. The father's mother had suffered from involutional psychosis with paranoid trends.

The mother confessed that she had had some difficulties in her marital life but "had tried to protect the boy from knowing about them." She felt guilty because she took a job "instead of giving him the proper care." The mother had marked social anxiety and the father suffered from many phobias and prejudices. The patient was an only child and the home life had overprotected him and failed to train him for adaptation to discipline or hardship.

Physical Examination

The general physical examination showed no evidence of organic disease and, although his movements seemed restricted, orthopedic examination was negative and special x-ray studies showed a normal low back. The right lower extremity was said to be one centimeter shorter than the left.

Personality Study

The patient had an anxious appearance. Being studied psychologically meant to him that he was being accused of malingering and much of his conversation during the first interview had to do with protestations that such was not the case. We assured him that nothing of the kind was intended, that we were only interested in finding the cause of his disability in order to cure him, but he seemed less interested in cure than in keeping the record clear "that he was no weakling." He was repeatedly reassured and toward the end of the second interview, when he began to understand that many strong personalities developed symptoms of this kind under stress, he became more amenable to education in the relation of emotion to symptom-formation.

Then a new conflict appeared. He had volunteered for the service, developed symptoms, and been discharged. The war was not over and there was rumor that certain discharged persons with his rating would be drafted back into service. This he dreaded. He had disliked the discipline and missed his home environment and the idea of a return to service was very disturbing. He said, "That would break my back for sure!" We convinced him that being drafted was impossible because the screening process in his area was very effective and that the policy was clear that men with his trouble were not wanted. With reassurance he relaxed, and asked if return to exercise would hurt him. We convinced him that not only would it not hurt him but it would be good for him. He then took up exercise which involved full use of the back muscles and in six weeks he was free of symptoms and has remained so for two years.

Psychotherapy involved: resolving his shame of being psychoneurotic, his fear of returning to service, and his fear of doing himself harm from exercise; and helping him to understand how his family background had failed to give him the "backbone" to adapt to the strains of life in the service.

PSYCHOSOMATIC ASPECTS OF PHYSICAL MEDICINE

There is great need for psychosomatic study in physical medicine. Many problems exist to which such studies might contribute valuable information.

What are the elements of the physician-patient relationship that enter into these problems, and can they be evaluated? What personal elements enter into the question of massage? Is the ordinary positive relationship between patient and physician (or attendant) heightened by the factor of actual physical manipulation? What are the feelings of warmth, security, and protection that may be created and which in many instances seem to support the patient by reminding him of an earlier relationship to a parent or protective figure?   On the reverse side of this picture is the question of physical therapy giving too much gratification so that the patient unconsciously may be encouraged to hold on to an illness.   Here is an important aspect of the subject that needs illumination, when it is found, for example, that the patient tends to utilize the treatment as a substitute for making an adjustment to real life.   Are there certain personalities in which massage works and others in which it does not?   It would seem likely that there may be elements in the personality structure that find massage "too stimulating," rather than relaxing.

Spas

What are the elements of suggestion that enter into spa treatment? If they were properly evaluated would it not help us in the development of spas in the United States?   It has always been suspected that this motivating force entered into spa treatment and it may even be that with our determination to advance scientific medicine in the United States there has been a neglect in the development of spas.   European spas were always looked upon with some suspicion by the American medical profession.   If we could evaluate this factor and utilize it scientifically would it not help us in the spa development which is occurring in this country?

What we must do is try to decide how much benefit may be due to physical therapy and how much to emotional factors.   Perhaps we have reached the point where we can apply fairly precise measurements to both.

Physician Relationships

There is another aspect of the problem that is very important and that is the question of the relationships between general physicians, including psychiatrists, and specialists in physical medicine.   One group has looked upon the other with suspicion.   The general physician or the psychiatrist has had the experience wherein his patients being treated in commercial institutions for the application of physical therapy have been influenced by suggestions that were harmful; for example, the state of the circulation, the pulse, the condition of the blood pressure ("too high" or "too low"), the question of bowel function ("autointoxication"), the matter of muscle tone, and so forth.   Specialists in physical medicine, influenced by their training in organic disease and by methods of physical measurement, have perhaps not been fully informed regarding the principles of psychodynamics evolved in recent years which permit scientific applications of psychotherapy.   Certainly many specialists in physical medicine have been reluctant to accept patients with psychological ills, apparently because they do not wish to "contaminate" their specialty by applying it for purely suggestive purposes. Studies of the kind that we have in mind might go a long way toward resolving these problems.

Still another question in this connection is whether physical therapy and psychotherapy are incompatible in the same patient (in psychosomatic affections). For example, if a muscle group is painful and this discomfort is on the basis of spasm resulting from tension is there more than one way of relieving this tension? Can the methods be applied at the same time or are they mutually exclusive? The psychiatrist may feel that emotional factors are responsible for the tension and that the only way to make the patient face the necessity for discussing these emotional factors is to approach the problem from a purely psychological standpoint. He may feel that if a physical name is given to the affection ("fibrositis," for example) and he allows the patient to undergo physical therapy it may "fix the neurosis" and make it impossible for the patient to appreciate that psychological forces are responsible. The physical therapist often feels that because it is simple to apply physical measures to get relief from muscular tension that there is no point in doing more. Perhaps these problems could be settled from the kind of study that we have suggested.

Practical Suggestions

Watkins and Finesinger attempt to answer some of these questions in a discussion of the psychiatric aspects of physical medicine. They caution against prolonging passive procedures, such as massage and hydrotherapy, and recommend that the patient take up exercises and more active procedures, such as occupational therapy. In planning occupational therapy they encourage the patient to work independently as soon as possible.

These authors call special attention to the necessity for avoiding unnecessary physical contacts such as patting the patient or holding his hand. Such gestures suggest a social situation and tend to change the professional relationship. They also give some good advice about what to say and what not to say in dealing with the patient in a physical medicine relationship. They avoid probing for information, avoid giving the patients lectures on physiology as well as psychology, avoid making promises that cannot be kept. They try to use reassurance in moderation. Wisely the authors recognize that the therapist often praises the patient to relieve his own insecurity or because he does not know what else to do. Consequently they try to avoid flattering patients. Nor (and this is a good point for medicine in general) do they respond when patients attempt to flatter them. They prefer to have a relationship with a patient characterized by attitudes of earnestness, honesty, and cooperation in working toward alleviating the patient's suffering.

Nov. 5, 1955

APPENDIX

Orientation Chart for Teaching Psychosomatic Medicine

In an effort to outline some of the basic concepts in the field of psycho-somatic medicine Levine, of the University of Cincinnati, has devised a chart which he has very kindly permitted us to reproduce. The four groups used in the chart do not cover the entire field of somatic mani-festations but they include the majority of psychosomatic reactions of interest to the internist.

The outline provides a frame of reference with which internal medi-cine is familar, that is, the general concepts of hysteria and hypochon-driasis, etc. In the setting of such a frame of reference, and with an understanding that the basic patterns are to be used flexibly rather than as hard and fast "disease entities," the internist can learn something about the specificity of psychodynamic problems in the field of general medicine. Thus he can acquire a feeling for the sick person as an in-dividual with specific problems that may produce definite bodily re-actions.

NEUROTIC DISORDERS

Names of neuroses in which somatic manifestations predominate	Typical Clinical Picture, or Examples of Clinical Manifestations	Are the Manfestations Signs (i. e. Observable by Another Person) or Symptoms (i. e. Subjective Sensations, Not Observable by Another)?	Patient's Attitude to Disorder	Is the Symptomatology Diffuse or Circumscribed?	Type of Sense Organ Involved	Type of Motor (or Efferent) System Involved
Hypochondriasis	Diffuse complaints; aches & pains in many areas	Symptoms	Extreme concern	Diffuse; the discomforts are in many areas and systems	Enteroceptive predominantly	Autonomic
Hysteria	Hysteric paralysis; hysteric convulsions; hysteric blindness	Almost always sensory or motor signs; some exceptions, e. g. hysteric pain	Often very indifferent; occ. dramatize	Usually limited to specific functional area; may shift subsequently	Exteroceptive predominantly	Voluntary (central) in most cases, since voluntary system serves areas which are under central control & can be used unconsciously purposefully in solution of conflict; some exceptions, e. g. in hysteric pseudocyesis
Anxiety Neurosis	Anxiety attacks, with fear of death, precordial discomfort, tachycardia, palpitation, etc.: between attacks, or in cases without specific attacks, anxiety overactivity of cardiac, respiratory gastro-intestinal & other systems	Vegetative signs plus symptoms	Often extreme concern	Usually diffuse, since fear is associated with responses in many areas of autonomic activity	Enteroceptive predominantly	Autonomic
Organ Neurosis	Peptic ulcer, hypertension, asthma, etc., insofar as they are psychosomatic in origin	Signs of specific visceral disorder; some (e. g. peptic ulcer) with symptoms; some (e. g. hypertension) may be without symptoms	Variable	Usually limited to one viscus or visceral system	Enteroceptive predominantly	Autonomic

*Levine, Maurice: An Orientation Chart in the Teaching of Psychosomatic Medicine. Psychosomatic Medicine 10: 111 (March) 1948.

IN INTERNAL MEDICINE

Does the Etiologic Mental Conflict or Impulse Have a Potentially Conscious or Conceptual Relation to the Specific Organ Involved?	Types of Psycho-Dynamics	Sample Contrast When Same Symptom Appears in All Four Neuroses, e. g. Headache	Can Irreversible Somatic Changes Appear?	Depth of Etiologic Problem and Psychotherapy	Does the Existence of the Disorder Lessen the Central Conflict or Alleviate the Anxiety?	Chief Problems in Differential Diagnosis
Probably not	Narcissism; severe masochism; concealed persecutory delusions; secondary gains; (note that hypochondriasis not clear, either as clinical entity or in dynamics)	Headache as one of innumerable complaints of aches & pains	None known	May be superficial, but safer to assume it is deeper and to avoid anxiety-producing therapy	No (except secondarily, e. g. the gain of sympathy may lessen some of the complaints)	Organic disease associated with marked complaining; early paresis; early schizophrenia; depression; concealed paranoid development; malingering
Always, e. g. peeping conceptually related to eye & so to blindness	Dissociation; conversion; solution of specific problem by loss or change of somatic function of related area; symbolism; occasional identification; conflicts related to phallic (and oral) periods; secondary gains	Headache based on identification with parent who had headaches or fractured skull or "stroke"; headaches based on "memories" related to the head, e. g. childhood punishment of blows to head	Usually none—in rare instances some irreversible changes, e. g. shortened tendons in hysteric contractures	Often superficial and amenable to superficial therapy, unless there is concomitant severe hysteric personality or marked secondary gains	Yes—this is the unconscious purpose or meaning of most hysteric phenomena, e. g. onset of hysteric blindness lessens conflict over peeping & alleviates the related anxiety	Various organic, esp. neurologic, diseases, esp. multiple sclerosis and brain tumor; hysteric psychopathic personality; traumatic neurosis with inhibition of function (due to fear of external situation rather than to internal fear as in hysteria); malingering
No—e. g. peeping conflict may lead to anxiety attack, with predominant cardiac manifestations, without conceptual relation of peeping with the heart	Partial failure of defenses against impulses or conflicts of any variety; failure of defenses is based on accentuation of impulse (e. g. through temptation) or lessening of defense mechanisms; tension is primitive defense vs. anxiety; somatic manifestations are the accompaniment or partial expression of anxiety and of tension	Headache as result of scalp or neck tension, when tension is result of anxiety	None definitely known; some evidence that severe anxiety plays a role in coronary disease	Varies from quite superficial to very deep, including psychotic formations; psychotherapy dependent on specific conflict, ego-strength, environmental situation, etc.	No—the anxiety becomes manifest, but there is no relieving expression of the conflict-producing urge and no new strong defense against it, as in hysteria	Infectious disease, etc., with marked neuroendocrine reactivity; cardiac disease of organic etiology; hyperthyroidism; organic g. i. disease; psychotic disorders with manifest anxiety; character disorder underlying the neurotic symptoms; panic state; malingering
Sometimes yes, e. g. peptic ulcer often related to impulse to be fed & helped; sometimes not, e. g. hypertension often based on hostile impulses which conceptually are not related to blood vessel function	Acute emotional impulses are normally associated with specific physiologic concomitants; when the impulses are chronic, the physiologic concomitants are chronic & hence pathologic; e. g. chronic rage may lead to chronic elevation of B. P.	Migraine, in which (possibly) hostility leads to local vasoconstriction & painful vasodilatation	Yes; emotional conflicts lead to peptic ulcer formation, stenosis, etc., possibility chronic psychogenic hypertension leads to structural change	Variable, according to conflict, personality and specific disorder	No—the stomach hyperactivity or the hypertension is a concomitant of the impulse and has no alleviating value as a convulsion has in hysteria; (some evidence that asthmatic attack alleviates some emotion and therefore is closer to hysteria)	Comparable systemic diseases predominantly of organic etiology; organic factors combined with psychogenic; concomitant or underlying psychosis

REFERENCES

CHAPTER I

THE CONCEPT OF PSYCHOSOMATIC MEDICINE

Allbutt, T. C.: Visceral Neuroses. P. 17. P. Blakiston's Son and Co., Phila., 1884

Barr, D. P.: Ann. Int. Med., 27: 198, 1947.

Bennett, A. E.: J. A. M. A., 130: 1203, 1936.

Dunbar, F.: Psychosomatic Diagnosis, pp. 696-697, Paul B. Hoeber, Inc., New York, 1943.

Freud, S.: Collected Papers. Vol. I, p. 76. Internat. Psychoan.Press, N. Y., 1924.

Friess, C., and Nelson, M. J.: Am. J. of Med. Sci., 203: 539, 1942.

Halliday, J. L.: Brit. J. M. Psychol., 19: 367, 1934.

Hamman, L.: Ment. Hyg., 23: 177, 1939.

Macy, J. W., and Allen, E. V.: Ann. Int. Med., 7: 861, 1934.

CHAPTER II

PERSONALITY DEVELOPMENT AND PSYCHOPATHOLOGY

Abraham, K.: Selected Papers on Psychoanalysis. Hogarth Press, London, 1927.

Alexander, F.: Psychoanalysis of the Total Personality. Nervous and Mental Disease Publishing Co., N. Y. and Wash., 1930.

Alexander, F.: Modern Attitudes in Psychiatry, Columbia University Press, New York, 1946.

Alexander, F.: Ten-Year Report, Institute for Psychoanalysis, Chicago, pp. 8, 9, 10, 1932-1942.

Alexander, F.: Psychosom. Med., 5: 205, July, 1943.

Brill, N. Q.: Bull. U. S. Army Med. Dept., 5: 383-384, April, 1946.

Ferenczi, S.: Further Contributions to the Theory and Technique of Psychoanalysis. Hogarth Press, London, 1926.

Freud, S.: Collected Papers. Vols. I-IV. Hogarth Press, London, 1934.

Freud, S.: Three Contributions to the Theory of Sex. Nervous and Mental Disease Publishing Co., N. Y. and Wash., 1916.

Freud, S.: Psychopathology of Everyday Life. The Macmillan Co., N. Y., 1919.

Freud, S.: New Introductory Lectures on Psychoanalysis. W. W. Norton and Co., Inc., N. Y., 1932.

Freud, S.: The Problem of Anxiety. W. W. Norton and Co., Inc., N. Y., 1936.

Freud, S.: Civilization and Its Discontents. Jonathan Cape and Harrison Smith, N. Y., 1930.

Glover, E.: Medico-Psychological Aspects of Normality. Brit. J. M. Psycholo., 23: 152, 1932.

Gregg, A.: Address at the Amer. Psychiatric Assoc. Meeting, New York, N. Y., May 22, 1947.

Jones, E.: Collected Papers on Psychoanalysis. Hogarth Press, London, 1923.

Menninger, K.: Bull. Menninger Clinic, 7: 36, 1943.

Menninger, W. C.: Psychiatry in a Troubled World: Yesterday's War and Today's Challenge, The Macmillan Co., New York, 1948.

Menninger, W. C.: Somatization Reactions as Seen in Mental Hygiene, Bull. U. S. Army Med. Dept., *5:* 640-642, June, 1946.

Mirsky, I. Arthur: The Biology of Diabetes Mellitus in Man, Presented at the Institute on Psychosomatics, University of Nebraska, Feb. 11, 1948.

Saul, L. J.: Nerv. Child, *5:* 332, 1946.

Saul, L. J.: Emotional Maturity: The Dynamics and Development of Personality, J. B. Lippincott Co., Phila., 1947.

Selye, Hans: The General Adaptation Syndrome and the Diseases of Adaptation, J. Clin. Endoc., *6:* 117, 1946.

Stephen, K.: Psychoanalysis and Medicine. Cambridge University Press, London 1933.

CHAPTER III

PSYCHOSOMATIC DIAGNOSIS

Alexander, F.: Psychosom. Med., *5:* 205, 1943.

Booth, G.: Psychosom. Med., *10:* 1, 1948.

Deutsch, F.: Psychoanalyt. Quart., *8:* 354, 1939.

Dunbar, H. F.: Psychosomatic Diagnosis, Paul B. Hoeber, Inc., New York, 1943.

Garrett, Annette: Interviewing: Its Principles and Methods, Family Welfare Association of America, N. Y., 1942.

Grinker, R. R., and Spiegel, J. P.: Psychosom. Med., *6:* 123, 1944.

Halliday, J. L.: Lancet, *245:* 692, 1943.

Harrower, M.:
   (a)   Arch. Neurol. and Psychiat., *43:* 859, 1940.
   (b)   Montreal Neurological Institute, Reprint No. 195.

Jelliffe, S. E.: J. A. M. A., *94:* 1393, 1930.

Kemple, C.: Psychosom. Med., *7:* 85, 1945.

Kilgore, E. S.: J. A. M. A., *97:* 93, 1931.

Kubie, L. S.: Psychoan. Quart., *13:* 503, 1944.

Levine, M.: Proceedings of The Brief Psych therapy Council, The Institute for Psychoanalysis, Chicago, Illinois, Oct., 1942.

Levy, D. M.: Am. J. Dis. Child., *69:* 7, 1945.

Mittelmann, B., Weider, A., Brodman, K., Wechsler, K., and Wolff, H. G.: Psychosom. Med., *7:* 220, 1945.

Rapaport, D. and Schafer, R., Manual of Diagnostic Psychological Testing, Vol. 2, Josiah Macy, Jr. Found., N. Y., p. 27, 1946.

Ripley, H. S., and Wolf, S.: Psychosom. Med., *9:* 269, July-August, 1942.

Sherrington, C.: The Brain and Its Mechanism, Cambridge Press and The Macmillan Co., 1933.

War Department Pamphlet, pp. 21-35, Government Printing Office, Washington. D. C.

CHAPTER IV

TREATMENT—GENERAL PRINCIPLES OF PSYCHOTHERAPY

Cockerill, E. E.: Bull. of the Johns Hopkins Hosp., *80:* 86, 1947.

Deutsch, F.: Psychoanalyt. Quart., *8:* 354, 1939.

Dunbar, F.: Am. J. Psychiat., *95:* 1277, 1939.

Gayford, M.: Personal Communication, May, 1947.

Halliday, J. L.: Brit. M. J., *2:* 11, 1938.

Hertzman, J.: J. Social Case Work, *27:* 299, 1946.

Kilgore, E. S.: J.A.M.A., *97:* 93, 1931.

Margolis, H. M.: J. Social Case Work, *27:* 291, 1946.

Ross, W. D.: Psychosom. Med., 7: 80, 1945.
Ross, W. D., and McNaughton, F. C.: Psychosom. Med., 7: 73, 1945.

CHAPTER V

TREATMENT—"NORMAL" PROBLEMS IN PSYCHOTHERAPY

Boas, E. P.: The Unseen Plague—Chronic Disease. J. J. Augustin, N. Y., 1940.
Giberson, L. G.: Clinics, Vol. 2, No. 3, J. B. Lippincott Company, Philadelphia, 1943.
Kroger, W. S., and DeLee, S. T.: Am. J. Obst. & Gynec., 51: 544, 1946.
Overholser, W.: Med. Ann. Dist. Columbia, 10: 1, 1941.
Steinberg, A., Pastor, N., Winheld, E. B., Segal, H. I., Shechter, F. R., and Colton, N. H.: Psychosom. Med., 8: 176, 1946.
Stieglitz, E. J.: Technology Review, p. 358, June, 1941.
Wolf, A. W. M.: The Parents' Manual. Simon and Schuster, N. Y., 1941.

CHAPTER VI

TREATMENT—SPECIAL THERAPEUTIC PROCEDURES

Ackerman, N. W.:Psychosom. Med., 8: 118, 1946.
Alexander, F.: The Medical Value of Psychoanalysis. 2nd ed. W. W. Norton & Co., N. Y., 1937.
Harrower, M.: Amer. Soc. for Research in Psychosom. Problems, Atlantic City, May 4, 1947.
Jelliffe, S. E.: J.A.M.A. 94: 1393, 1930.
Kubie, L. S.: Practical Aspects of Psychoanalysis. W. W. Norton & Co., N. Y., 1936.
Main, T. F.: Bull. Menninger Clinic, 10: 66, 1946.
Wolberg, L. R.: Hypnoanalysis, Grune and Stratton, New York, 1945.

CHAPTER VII

TRAINING IN PSYCHOSOMATIC MEDICINE

Barr, D. P.: Ann. Int. Med., 27: 200, 1947.
Deutsch, F., Kaufman, M. R., and Blumgart, H. L.: Psychosom. Med. 2: 213, 1940.
Margolin, S.: Personal Communication, 1947.
Menninger, K. A.: (a) The Human Mind. 2nd ed. Alfred A. Knopf, N. Y., 1937; (b) Man Against Himself. Harcourt, Brace & Co., N. Y., 1938.
Romano, J.: J. A. M. A. 117: 664, 1941.
Saslow, G.: An Experiment with Comprehensive Medicine, Psychosom. Med., 10: 165, 1948.

CHAPTER VIII

THE CARDIOVASCULAR SYSTEM—FUNCTIONAL DISORDERS

Aring, C. D., and Bateman, J. F.: J.A.M.A., 109: 1092, 1937.
Bishop, L. F., and Bishop, L. F., Jr.: Am. J. Med. Sci., 182: 19, 1931.
Conner, L. A.: J.A.M.A., 94: 447, 1930.
DaCosta, J. M.: Am. J. Med. Sci., 61: 2, 1871.
Dunn, W. H.: Psychosom. Med., 4: 333, 1942.
Freud, S.: Collected Papers. Vol. I, p. 76. Internat. Psychoan. Press, N. Y., 1924. 1924.
Friedman, M.: Functional Cardiovascular Disease, Williams and Wilkins Co., Baltimore, pp. 24, 51, 1947.
Hamman, L., and Wainwright, C. W.: Bull. Johns Hopkins Hosp., 58: 109 and 307, 1936.

Harrison, T. R.: Am. Assoc. Advancement Sc., Pub. 13, p. 231, 1940.
Harrison, T. R.: Am. J. Med. Sci., *207*: 561, 1944
Jones, M. and Mellersh, V.: Psychosom. Med., *8:* 180, 1946.
Kilgore, E. S.: (*a*) J.A.M.A. *177:* 258, 1941; (*b*) Am. Heart J., *5:* 9, 1929.
Lewis, T.: The Soldier's Heart and the Effort Syndrome. 2nd ed. Shaw and Sons, Ltd., London, 1940.
Mainzer, F. and Krause, M.: Brit. Heart '., *2:* 221, 1940.
Menninger, W. C.: Southwest. J. Med. and Surg., *21:* 281 and 324, 1937.
Oille, J. A.: Canad. M.A.J., *45:* 1, 1941.
Ross, W. Donald: Psychosom. Med., *7:* 80, 1945.
Wendkos, M. H.: Am. Heart J., *28:* 549, 1944.
Willius, F. A.: Proc. Staff Meet., Mayo Clinic., *13:* 11, 1938.
Wittkower, E., Roger, T. F., and MacBeth Wilson, A. H.: Lancet., *240:* 531, 1941.
Wolf, G. A., Jr., and Wolff, H. G.: Psychosom. Med., *8:* 293, 1946.

CHAPTER IX

THE CARDIOVASCULAR SYSTEM—EMOTIONAL FACTORS IN ORGANIC HEART DISEASE

Dunbar, F.: (*a*) Emotions and Bodily Changes. 2nd ed., p. 210. Columbia University Press, N. Y., 1938; (*b*) New York State J. Med., *36:* 1, 1936.
Romano, J.: J.A.M.A., *177:* 664, 1941.
Sprague, H. B.: J.A.M.A., *112:* 2384, 1939.
Wolfe, T. P.: Am. J. Psychiat., *93:* 681, 1936.

CHAPTER X

THE CARDIOVASCULAR SYSTEM—ESSENTIAL HYPERTENSION

Alexander, F.: Psychosom. Med., *1:* 173, 1939.
Alexander, F., and Saul, L. J.: Psychosom. Med., *1:* 139-153, 1939.
Allbutt, T. C.: Abstracts, Tr. Hunterian Soc., 1895-96; Diseases of the Arteries Including Angina Pectoris, London, 1915.
Ayman, D.: (*a*) J.A.M.A. *95:* 246, 1930; (*b*) J.A.M.A., *96:* 2091, 1931.
Ayman, D.: M. Clin. North America, *28:* 1151, 1944.
Ayman, D. and Pratt, J. H.: Arch. Int. Med., *47:* 675, 1931.
Barker, N. W.: (*a*) Proc. Staff Meet., Mayo Clinic, *8:* 284, 1933; (*b*) J.A.M.A., *106:* 762, 1936.
Binger, C. A. L.: Bull. New York Acad. Med., *21:* 610, 1945.
Binger, C. A. L., Ackerman, N. W., Cohn, A. E., Schroeder, H. A., and Steele, J. M.: Personality in Arterial Hypertension, The American Society for Research in Psychosomatic Problems, N. Y., 1945.
Bright, R.: Guy's Hosp. Rep., *1:* 338, 1836.
Corcoran, A. C. and Page, I. H.: J.A.M.A., *116:* 690 (Feb. 22), 1941.
Cushing, H.: (*a*) Bull. Johns Hopkins Hosp., *50:* 137, 1932; (*b*) J.A.M.A., *99:* 281, 1932; (*c*) Arch. Int. Med., *51:* 487, 1936; (*d*) Am. J. Path., *9:* 539, 1933; (*e*) Am. J. Path., *10:* 145, 1934.
Dunbar, F.: (*a*) N. Y. State J. Med., *36:* 423, 1935; (*b*) Am. J. Psychiat., *92:* 1095, 1936; (*c*) Am. J. Psychiat., *91:* 541, 1934; (*d*) Emotions and Bodily Changes. Columbia University Press, N. Y., 1938; (*e*) Psychoan. Quart., *8:* 18, 1939.
Fahrenkamp—cited by Dunbar (*d*), p. 228.
Fishberg: Hypertension and Nephritis. 4th ed. Lea and Febiger, Phila., 1939.
Gardner, J. W., Mountain, G. E., and Hines, E. A., Jr.: Am. J. M. Sc., *200:* 50, 1940

Goldblatt, H.: For complete bibliography, see: Experimental Hypertension Induced by Renal Ischemia. Harvey Lectures, vol. 33. Williams and Wilkins, Baltimore, 1937-38; also Surgery., *4:* 483, 1938.

Griffith, J. Q., and Lindauer, M. A.: Am. Heart J., *14:* 710, 1937.

Grollman, A., Williams, J. R., Jr., and Harrison, T. R.: Report before the American Society for Clinical Investigation, May 1, 1939. In J.A.M.A., *115:* 1169, 1940.

Gull, W. W., and Sutton, H. G.: Tr. Med. Chir., *55:* 273, 1872.

Herrick, W. W., and Tillman, A. J. B.: Arch. Int. Med., *55:* 643, 1935.

Hines, E. A., Jr., and Brown, G. E.: Proc. Staff Meet., May Clinic, *7:* 332, 1932.

Huchard: Traite Clinique des Maladies du Coeur et de l'Aorte. 3rd ed. Paris, 1899.

Janeway, T. C.: Arch. Int. Med., *12:* 755, 1913.

Kesilman, M.: M. Rec., *154:* 16, 1941.

Menninger, K. A.: (*a*) Bull. N. Y. Acad. Med., *14:* 198, 1938; (*b*) Man against Himself, p. 378. Harcourt, Brace and Co., N. Y., 1938; (*c*) Bull. New York Acad. Med., *14:* 198, 1938.

Moritz, A. R., and Oldt, M. R.: Am. J. Path., *13:* 679, 1937.

Moschcowitz, E.: Am. J. Med. Sci., *158:* 668, 1919.

Page, I. H.: J.A.M.A., *110:* 1161, 1938.

Page I. H. and Corcoran, A. C.: Arterial Hypertension: Its Diagnosis and Treatment, Year Book Publishers, Chicago, 1945.

Page, I. H., Helmer, O. M., Kohlstaedt, K. G., Kempf, G. F., Gambill, W. D., and Taylor, R. D.: Ann. Int. Med., *15:* 347, 1941.

Palmer, R. S.: New England J. Med., *216:* 689, 1937; *215:* 569, 1936.

Robinson, G. C.: Ann. Int. Med., *11:* 345, 1937.

Saul, L. J.: Psychosom. Med., *1:* 153, 1939.

Schulze, V. E., and Schwab, E. H.: Am. Heart J., *11:* 66, 1936.

Smith, H. W., Goldring, W., and Chasis, H.: J. Clin. Investigation, *17:* 263, 1938.

Stewart, H. J.: Bull. New York Acad. Med., *14:* 681, 1938.

Trueta, J., Barclay, A. E., Daniel, P. M., Franklin, K. J., Prichard, M. M. L.: Studies of the Renal Circulation, Blackwell Scientific Publications, Oxford, England, p. 156, 1947; also Chas. C Thomas, Springfield, Ill., 1948.

Von Basch, S.: Ueber latente Arteriosclerose. Vienna, 1893.

Weiss, E.: J.A.M.A., *120:* 1081, 1942.

Wolfe, T. P.: Am. J. Psychiat., *93:* 681, 1936.

CHAPTER XI

THE GASTROINTESTINAL SYSTEM

Alexander, F.: Psychoanalyt. Quart., *3:* 501, 1934.

Dwyer, M. F., and Blackford, J. M.: Radiology, *14:* 38, 1930.

Eusterman, G. B.: J.A.M.A., *107:* 1232, 1936.

Friess, E. C., and Nelson, M. J.: Am. J. Med. Sci, *203:* 539, 1942.

Macy, J. W., and Allen, E. V.: Ann. Int. Med., *7:* 861, 1934.

Rivers, A. B., and Ferreira, A. E. M.: J.A.M.A., *110:* 2132, 1938.

Robinson, G. C.: Bull. Johns Hopkins Hosp., *68:* 203, 1941.

Stevenson, G. S.: J.A.M.A., *94:* 333, 1930.

Wilbur, D. L., and Mills, J. H.: Ann. Int. Med., *12:* 821, 1938.

Wilbur, D. L., and Washburn, R. N.: J.A.M.A., *110:* 477, 1938.

CHAPTER XII

THE GASTROINTESTINAL SYSTEM (Continued)

Alvarez, W. C.: J.A.M.A., *114:* 1301, 1940.

Brown, P. W.: Proc. Staff Meet., Mayo Clinic, *7:* 651, 1932.

DaCosta, J. M.:   Am. J. M. Sc., *89:* 321, 1871.
Daniels, G. E.:   Psychosom. Med., *2:* 276, 1940.
Dunbar, F.:   Emotions and Bodily Changes.   2nd ed. P. 301.   Columbia Univ. Press, N. Y., 1938.
Heintzelman, J. H. L., and Evans, F. A.:   Am. J. Med. Sci., *201:* 651, 1941.
Murray, C. D.:   Am. J. Med. Sci., *180:* 239, 1930.
Sullivan, A. J.:   Am. J. Digest. Dis. & Nutrition.   *2:* 651, 1935.
Tumen, H. J.:   Northwestern Med., *41:* 42, 1942.
White, B. V., Cobb, S., and Jones, C. M.:   Mucous Colitis.   Psychosom. Med. Monograph I, 1939.
White, B. V., and Jones, C. M.:   Ann. Int. Med., *14:* 854, 1940.

CHAPTER XIII

THE GASTROINTESTINAL SYSTEM (Concluded)

Alexander, F.:   Psychoan.   Quart., *3:* 501, 1934.
Alvarez, W. C : Am. J. Surg., *18:* 207, 1932.
Beattie, J.:   Canad. M.A.J., *26:* 278, 1932.
Cushing, H.:   Surg., Gynec. & Obst., *55:* 1, 1932.
Daniels, G. E.:   Med. Clin. of North America, *28:* 1944.
Donavan, E. J., and Santulli, T. V.: Am. J. Dis. Child., *69:* 176, 1945.
Eusterman, G. B.:   J. M. Soc.   New Jersey, *36:* 1, 1939.
Guthrie, K. J.:   Arch. Dis. Childhood, *17:* 82, 1942.
Kapp, F. T., Rosenbaum, M., and Romano, J.:   Amer. J. Psychiat., *103:* 700, 1947.
Keller, A. D., Hare, W. K., and D'Amour, M. C.:   Proc. Soc. Exper. Biol. & Med., *30:* 772, 1932.
Light, R. V., Bishop, C. C., and Kendall, L. G.; J. Pharmacol. & Exper. Ther., *45:* 227, 1932.
Lindemann, E.:   Arch. Neurol. and Psychiat., *53:* 322, 1945.
Saul, L. J.:   Psychosom. Med., *8:* 204, 1946.
Sperling, M.:   Psychoanalytic Study of Ulcerative Colitis in Children, Psychoanal. Quart., *15:* 302, 1946.
Von Bergmann, G.:   Berl. Klin. Wchnschr., *55:* 524, 1918.
Weiss, E.:   Am. J. Digest. Dis. & Nutrition., *3:* 1, 1936.
Wolf, S. and Wolff, H. G.:   J.A.M.A., *120:* 670, 1942.

CHAPTER XIV

THE ENDOCRINE SYSTEM AND METABOLISM

Beach, F. A.:   Physiol. Reviews, *27:* 240, 1947.
Benedek, T., Psychosexual Function in Women, Encyclopedia of Psychology, Harriman, P. L., Philosophical Library, New York, p. 678, 1946.
Benedek, T., and Rubenstein, B. B.:   Psychosom. Med., *1:* 245 and 461, 1939.
Bennett, H. G., Jr., and TeLinde, R. W., J.A.M.A., *118:* 1341, 1942.
Heller, C. G., and Meyers, G. B.:   J.A.M.A., *126:* 472, 1944.
Kasanin, J., and Biskind, G. R.:   J.A.M.A., *121,* 1318, 1943.
Palmer, H. D., Hastings, D. W., and Sherman, S. H.:   Am. J. Psychiat., *97:* 1086, 1941.
Papanicolaou, G. N., and Shorr, Ephraim: Am. J. Obst. & Gynec., *31:* 806, 1936.
Pratt, J. P.:   Am. J. Obst. & Gynec., *31:* 782, 1936.
Rosenzweig, S., and Hoskins, R. G.:   Psychosom. Med., *3:* 87, 1941.
Schonfeld, W. A.:   J.A.M.A., *121:* 177, 1943.

Stoddard, F. J.: J.A.M.A., *129:* 508, 1945.
Tauber, E. S.: Psychosom. Med., *2:* 74, 1940.
Tauber, E. S., and Daniels, G. E.: Psychosom. Med., *3:* 72, 1941.

CHAPTER XV

THE ENDOCRINE SYSTEM AND METABOLISM (Continued)

Allan, F. N.: N. England J. Med., *231:* 414, 1944.
Benedek, T.: Psychoanalyt. Quart., *3:* 153, 1934.
Bram, I.: Am. J. Psychiat., *92:* 1077, 1936.
Conrad, A.: J. Nerv. & Ment. Dis., *79:* 505 and 656, 1934.
Deutsch, E.: Med. Klin., *19:* 678, 1923.
Hyman, H. T., and Kessel, L.: J.A.M.A., (*a*) *85:* 1017, 1925; (*b*) *88:* 1478, 1927; (*c*) *96:* 2014, 1931.
Lewis, N. D. C.: M. J. & Rec., *122:* 121, 1925.
Mittelman, B.: J. Nerv. & Ment. Dis., *77:* 465, 1933.
Moschcowitz, E.: Arch. Int. Med., *46:* 610, 1930.
Ruesch, J. Christiansen, C., Patterson, L. C., Dewees, S., and Jacobson, A.: Psychosom Med., *9:* 77, 1947.

CHAPTER XVI

THE ENDOCRINE SYSTEM AND METABOLISM (Concluded)

Bollmeier, L. N., and Meyer, A.: J. Arkansas Med. Soc., *41:* 121, Nov. 1944.
Bruch, H.: Am. J. Dis. Child., (*a*) *59:* 739, 1940; (*b*) *60:* 1082, 1940.
Bruch, H., and Hewlett, I.: Psychosom. Med., *9:* 205, 1947.
Bruch, H., and Touraine, G.: Psychosom. Med., *2:* 141, 1940.
Conn, J. W.: J.A.M.A., *115:* 1669, 1940.
Daniels, G. E.: Am. J. Psychiat., *93:* 711, 1936; Psychoan. Quart. *5:* 513, 1936.
Daniels, G. E.: Psychiatry, *7:* 121, 1944.
Dunbar, H. F.: J. Nerv. & Ment. Dis., *86:* 712, 1937.
Fischer, A. E., and Dolger, H.: Arch. Int. Med., *78:* 711, 1946.
Gull, W. W.: Tr. Clin. So . London., *7:* 22, 1874.
Haagensen, C. D., and Lloyd, Wyndham, E. B.: A Hundred Years of Medicine, Sheridan House, Inc., New York, 1943.
Houssay, B. A.: New England J. Med., *214:* 971, 1936.
Houssay, B. A., and Biasotti, A.: Endocrinology, *15:* 511, 1931.
Lorand, S.: Psychosom. Med., *5:* 282, 1943.
McCullough, E. P., and Tuffer, R.: Ann. Int. Med., *14:* 817, 1940.
Menninger, W. C.: (*a*) J. Nerv. & Ment. Dis., *81*: 1, 1935, (*b*) J. Ment. Sci., *81*: 332, 1935.
Meyer, A., Bollmeier, L. N., and Alexander, F.: Psychosom. Med., *7:* 335, 1945.
Mirsky, I. Arthur: (*a*) The Biology of Diabetes Mellitus in Man, Institute on Psychosomatics, University of Nebraska, February 11, 1948. (*b*) Emotional Factors in the Patient With Diabetes Mellitus, presented before Section on Nervous and Mental Diseases, Ohio State Medical Association, April 1, 1948, Cincinnati, Ohio.
Nicholson, W. M.: Am. J. Med. Sci., *211:* 443, 1946.
Richardson, H. B.: Obesity and Neurosis, Psychiat. Quart., *20:* 400, 1946.
Richardson, H. B.: Med. Clin. of North America, p. 1187, Sept., 1946.
Simmonds, M.: Deutsche med. Wchnschr., *40:* 322, 1914.
Waller, J. V., Kaufman, M. R., and Deutsch, F.: Psychosom. Med., *2:* 3, 1940.

CHAPTER XVII

THE GENITO-URINARY SYSTEM AND THE SEXUAL FUNCTION

Chadwick, M.: Psychological Effects of Menstruation. Nervous and Mental Disease Monographs, 1934.

Dunbar, F.: Emotions and Bodily Changes. 2nd ed. Columbia University Press, N. Y., 1938.

Frank, R. T.: Arch. Neurol. & Psychiat., *26:* 1053, 1931.

Furst, W.: J. Clin. Psychopath., *7:* 507, 1946.

Horney, K.: Am. J. Obst. & Gynec., *25:* 694, 1933.

Kinsey, A. C.: Jour. Clin. Endocrin., *1:* 424, 1941.

Menninger, K. A.: (*a*) Psychoanalyt. Quart., *3:* 173, 1934; (*b*) Psychoanalyt. Quart., *5:* 488, 1936; (*c*) Psychoanalyt. Rev., *28:* 117, 1941.

Montgomery, J.: The Diagnosis and Treatment of Dysmenorrhea. Post-Graduate Seminar, Phila. County Med. Soc., Phila., 1941.

Ruesch, J., et. al.: Chronic Disease and Psychological Invalidism, Psychosomatic Medicine Monograph, Paul B. Hoeber, Inc., New York, p. 126, 1946.

Whitacre, F. E. and Barrera, B.: J.A.M.A., *124:* 399, 1944.

Wittkower, E. and Wilson, A.T.M.: British M. J., *2:* 583, 1940.

CHAPTER XVIII

THE GENITO-URINARY SYSTEM AND THE SEXUAL FUNCTION (Concluded)

Farris, E. J.: Amer. J. Obst. & Gynec., *52:* 3, 1946.

Farris, E. J.: J. Urol., *58:* 85, 1947.

Menninger, K. A.: J. Urol., *34:* 166, 1935.

CHAPTER XIX

THE RESPIRATORY SYSTEM

Alexander, F.: Psychoan. Quart., *3:* 501, 1934.

Alexander, F., and Saul, L. J.: Psychosom. Med., *2:* 110, 1940.

Axelrad. R. K.: News Letter, Am. Assoc. Psychiatric Social Workers, *15:* 4, 1946.

Binger, C.: Ann. Int. Med., *11:* 195, 1937.

Christie, R. V.: Quart. J. Med., *4:* 427, 1935.

Coleman, J. V., Hurst, A., and Hornstein, R.: J.A.M.A., *135:* 699, 1947.

Engel, G. L., Ferris, E. B., and Logan, M.: Ann. Int. Med., *27:* 693, 1947.

Faulkner, W. B.: Northwest Med. J., *40:* 367, 1941.

Finesinger, J. E.: Am. J. Psychiat. (*a*) *100:* 159, 1943. (*b*) *100:* 659, 1944.

Hartz, J.: Psychosom. Med., *6:* 17, 1944.

Holmes, T., Goodell, H., Wolf, S. G., and Wolff, H. G.: The Nose, Charles C Thomas, Ref. 1, p. 590, Springfield, Ill., 1949.

Saul, L. J. et. al.: Internat. J. Psycho-Analysis, *19:* 451, 1938.

Spencer, E. C.: Jewish Social Service Quart., *19:* 307, 1943.

CHAPTER XX

THE RESPIRATORY SYSTEM (Concluded)

Alexander, F.: Psychosom. Med. Monograph IV, 1941.

Deutsch, F.: Internat. J. Psycho-Analysis, *20:* 1, 1939

Dunbar, H. F.: Psychoanalyt. Quart., *7:* 25, 1938.

French, T. M.: Am. J. Psychiat., *96:* 87, 1939.

French, T. M., and Alexander, F.: Psychosom. Med. Monograph IV, 1941.

Gillespie, R. D.: Brit. M. J., *1:* 1285, 1936.

Major, R. H.: Classic Description of Disease. P. 540. Chas. C Thomas, Springfield, Ill., 1932.

McDermott, N. T., and Cobb, S.: Psychosom. Med., *1:* 203, 1939.

Rapaport, B. Z., and Hecht, R.: Psychosom. Med. Monograph IV, 1941.

Rogerson, C. H., Hardcastle, D. H., and Duguid, K.: Guy's Hosp. Rep., *85:* 289, 1935.

Schatia, V.: Psychosom. Med., *3:* 157, 1941.

Strauss, E. B.: Guy's Hosp. Rep., *85:* 309, 1935.

CHAPTER XXI

THE CENTRAL NERVOUS SYSTEM

Alvarez, W. C.: Trained Nurse and Hosp. Rev., *104:* 495, 1940.

Editorial: J.A.M.A., *102:* 2188, 1934.

Engel, G. L., and Romano, J.: Arch. Neur. and Psychiat., *51:* 356, 1944.

Engel, G. L., Webb, J. P., Ferris, E. B., Romano, J., Ryder, H., and Blankenhorn, M. A.: War Medicine, *5:* 304, 1944.

Engel, G. L., Ferris, E. B., and Romano, J.: Am. J. Med. Sc., *209:* 650, 1945.

Friedman, A. P., Brenner, C., and Merritt, H. H.: J.A.M.A., *132:* 489, 1946.

Fromm-Reichmann, F.: Psychoanalyt. Rev., *24:* 26, 1937.

Gardner, J. W., Mountain, G. E., and Hines, E. A.: Am. J. M. Sc., *200:* 50, 1940.

Hunt, T. C.: Lancet, *2:* 279, 1933.

Kozol, H. L.: Arch. Neurol. and Psychiat., *56:* 245, 1946.

Lennox, W. G.: (*a*) Science and Seizures. P. 109. Harper & Bros., N. Y., 1941; (*b*) Letter: J.A.M.A., *117:* 1806, 1941.

Romano, J.: Bull. New England Med. Soc., *4:* 64, 1942.

Romano, J. and Engel, G. L.: M. Clin. North America, *28:* 629, 1944.

Romano, J. and Engel, G. L. Psychosom. Med., *7:* 3, 1945.

Ross, W. D., and McNaughton, F. L.: Canad. M. A. J., *53:* 12, 1945.

Ross, W. D., and McNaughton, F. L.: Psychosom. Med., *7:* 73, 1945.

Simons, D. J., and Wolff, H. G.: Psychosom. Med., *8:* 227, 1946.

Touraine, T. A., and Draper, G.: J. Nerv. & Ment. Dis., *80:* 1, 1934.

Weiss, E.: Bull. N. Y. Acad. Med., *23:* 604, 1947.

Wolff, H. G.: Arch. Neurol. and Psychiat., *37:* 895, 1937.

Wolff, H. G.: Lecture, Institute of Living, March 20, 1946.

Wolff, H. G.: Headache and Other Head Pain, Oxford Univ. Press, N. Y., 1948.

CHAPTER XXII

EAR AND EYE

Ear:

Furstenberg, A. C.: Ann. Otol., Rhin. & Laryng., *43:* 1035, 1934.

Simonton, K. M.: Proc. Staff Meet., Mayo Clin. *16:* 465, 1941.

Eye:

Culpin, M.: Recent Advances in the Psychoneuroses, J. A. Churchill, London, p 193, 1931.

Derby, G. S.: J.A.M.A., *95:* 913, 1930.

Freud, S.: Collected Papers. Vol. II, p. 110, Hogarth Press, London, 1924.

Halliday, J. L.: Psychosom. Med., *5:* 71, 1943.

Halliday, J. L.: Psychosocial Medicine, W. W. Norton and Co., New York, 1948.

Harrington, D. O.: J.A.M.A., *133:* 669, 1947.

Inman, W.: Lancet, *2:* 118, 1929.

Piers, Ten-Year Report, Inst. for Psychoanalysis, Chicago, p. 32, 1932-1942.

Rutherford, C. W.: J.A.M.A., *99:* 284, 1932.

Schoenberg, M.: Arch. Ophth., *23:* 76, 1940.

Wittkower, E. D., Rodger, T. F., et. al.: Brit. Med. J., *2:* 671, 1941.

Zeligs, M. A.: Psychosom. Med., *9:* 110, 1947.

CHAPTER XXIII

SKIN DISORDERS AND ALLERGIES

Abramson, H. A.: Psychosomatics and the Allergic Patient, Bruce Pub. Co., St. Paul, 1948.

Ackerman, N. W.: Psychosom. Med., *1:* 366, 1939.

French, T. M.: Psychosom. Med. Monograph IV, 1941.

Halliday, J. L.: Brit. J. M. Psychol., *19:* 367, 1943.

Harris, H. J.: Psychosom. Med., *6:* 336, 1944.

Klauder, J. V.: J. Nerv. & Ment. Dis., *84:* 249, 1936.

Menninger, K. A.: Man Against Himself. P. 359. Harcourt, Brace & Co., New York, 1938.

Miller, H. and Baruch, D. W.: Amer. Academy of Allergy, New York, Nov. 25, 1946.

Pearson, G. H. J.: Psychosom. Med., *2:* 22, 1940.

Rattner, H.: J.A.M.A., *99:* 1934, 1932.

Saul, L. J.: (*a*) Psychoanalyt. Quart., *7:* 336, 1938; (*b*) Psychosom. Med., *3:* 66, 1941.

Saul, L. J.: Psychosom. Med., *3:* 66, 1941.

Saul, L. J.: The Nervous Child, *5:* 332, 1946.

Stokes, J. H., and Beerman, H.: Psychosom. Med., *2:* 438, 1940.

Sulzberger, M. B.: Dermatologic Allergy. Chas. C Thomas, Springfield, Ill., 1940.

Sulzberger, M. B.: J.A.M.A., *136:* 156, 1948.

Wilson, G. W.: Psychosom. Med., *3:* 51, 1941.

Wittkower, E. D.: Bull. Menninger Clinic, *2:* 148, 1947.

CHAPTER XXIV

DENTISTRY, ARTHRITIS AND ORTHOPEDIC PROBLEMS

Binger, C.: Annals of Dentistry, *4:* 175, 1946.

Boland, E. W., and Corr, W. P.: J.A.M.A., *123:* 805, 1943.

Booth, G.: Psychosom. Med., *8:* 367, 1946.

Chamberlain, W. E.: Personal Communication, May, 1946.

Champion, W. M.: Medical Information for Social Workers. Wm. Wood & Co., Baltimore, 1938. Chapter by Harbin, M., p. 347.

Cobb, S., Bauer, W., and Whiting, I.: J.A.M.A., *113:* 668, 1939.

Dunbar, H. F.: Mind and Body, Psychosomatic Medicine, Random House, New York, p. 98, 1947.

Dunbar, H. F.: Ann. Int. Med., *14:* 839, 1940.

Editorial: J.A.M.A., *135:* 288, 1947.

Flind, J., and Barber, H. S.: Quart. J. Med., *14:* 57, 1945.

Gaston, S. R.: Personal Communication, October, 1947.

Gold, H.: Weekly Roster, Phila., Sept., 20, 1941. Quoted from New York State J. Med., *41:* 688, 1941.

Halliday, J. L.:   Ann. Int. Med., *15:* 666, 1941.

Halliday, J.:   Brit. Med. J., *1:* 213 and 264, 1937.

Hamlin, P. G.:   Mil. Surgeon, *92:* 295, 1943.

Irvine, J. H.:   Am. Soc. Research Psychosom.   Problems, Atlantic City, May 3, 1947.

Jelliffe, S. E.:   Tr. Am. Neurol.   Assoc., 1923, p. 419.

Johnson, A., Shapiro, L. B., and Alexander, F.:   Psychosom. Med., *9:* 1295, 1947.

Kapp, F. T., and Rosenbaum, M.:   Personal Communication, Sept., 1947.

Margolis, H. M.:   The Family, *25:* 331, 1945.

Menninger, K. A.:   Psychoan.   Quart., *3:* 173, 1934.

Meyer, A., in Strecker, E. A., and Ebaugh, F. G.:   Practical Clinical Psychiatry. 5th ed., p. 54.   The Blakiston Co., Phila., 1940.

Ryan, E. J.:   Psychobiologic Foundations in Dentistry, Charles C Thomas, Springfield, Ill., 1946.

Sandler, S. A.:   Psychosom. Med., *9:* 197, 1947.

Schless, B. G.:   The Family, *25:* 331, 1945.

Stimson, B. B.:   Psychosom. Med., *9:* 210, 1947.

Tarachow, S.:   N. Y. J. of Dentistry, *76:* 189, 1946.

Thomas, G. W.:   Am. J. Psychiat., *93:* 693, 1936.

Watkins, A. L., and Finesinger, J. E.:   J.A.M.A., *135:* 1050, 1947.

Weiss, E.:   Annals Int. Med., *26:* 890, 1947.

Zeno, L., and Crespo, E. P.:   Libreria Editorial El Ateneo, Argentina, 1945.

SELECTED REFERENCES

PSYCHOANALYSIS

The Basic Writings of Sigmund Freud. With an introduction by A. A. Brill. The Modern Library, Random House, Inc., N. Y., 1938. Contains Freud's writings on Psychopathology of Everyday Life; The Interpretation of Dreams; Three Contributions to the Theory of Sex; Wit and Its Relation to the Unconscious; Totem and Taboo; and the History of the Psychoanalytic Movement.

Fundamentals of Psychoanalysis, Franz Alexander, W. W. Norton & Co., 1948. The theories and applications of psychoanalysis dealing with the teachings of the author and his associates of the Institute of Psychoanalysis in Chicago.

Man Against Himself, Karl A. Menninger. Harcourt, Brace & Co., N. Y., 1938. A readable book which discusses many aspects of human behavior, particularly the workings of the aggresive impulses. There is an interesting section on psychological factors in organic disease.

Facts and Theories of Psychoanalysis, Ives Hendrick, 2nd. ed. Alfred A. Knopf, N. Y., 1939. One chapter concerns psychologic study of organic disease and another deals with the application of psychoanalysis to conditions other than medical. Clearly written.

Practial Aspects of Psychoanalysis, Lawrence S. Kubie. W. W. Norton & Co., N. Y., 1936. A short, well-written and easily understood account of psychoanalysis.

The Unconscious Mind and Medical Practice, Ernest Jones. British Medical Journal, *1*: 1354, 1938. An important paper by a leading authority in psychoanalysis.

Psychoanalysis and Medicine, Karin Stephen. The Macmillan Co., N. Y., 1935. The subtitle reads, *The Wish to Fall Ill,* and this succinctly describes the nature of its contents. It illustrates with case material some of the most important facts of psychopathology.

Psychoanalytic Therapy, Franz Alexander, Thomas M. French, and collaborators, Ronald Press, N. Y., 1947. A psychoanalytic contribution to brief psychotherapy from the directors and associates of the Chicago Institute of Psychoanalysis.

PSYCHOSOMATIC MEDICINE

The Journal of Psychosomatic Medicine. Established in 1939, published under the editorial supervision of the American Psychosomatic Society. A journal of experimental and clinical studies dealing with psychosomatic medicine, with Carl Binger as managing editor. Monograph supplements for experimental data resulting from longer studies have been published. Paul B. Hoeber, New York.

Emotions and Bodily Changes, Flanders Dunbar, 2nd. ed. Columbia University Press, N. Y., 1938. The first comprehensive survey of the literature of psychosomatic medicine. It is a standard work of reference for anyone interested in this field.

Studies in Psychosomatic Medicine, Franz Alexander and Thomas M. French, Ronald Press Company, N. Y., 1948. A collection of the most important papers written by the staff of the Chicago Institute for Psychoanalysis during the past sixteen years.

Sketches in Psychosomatic Medicine, Smith Ely Jelliffe. Nervous and Mental Disease Monograph, N. Y., 1939. A collection of interesting and important papers by a pioneer in psychosomatic medicine.

Psychotherapy in Medical Practice, Maurice Levine, The Macmillan Company, N. Y., 1942. A standard work of real help to the general physician.

Chronic Disease and Psychological Invalidism, Jurgen Ruesch, with collaborators, Psychosomatic Medicine Monograph number 9, Paul B. Hoeber, N. Y., 1947. A study of patients suffering from various chronic diseases with a careful inquiry into medical, psychiatric, social, economic, and cultural status.

Introduction to Psychosomatic Medicine, C. Albert Seguin, Emp. Grafica T. Scheuch, S. A., Lima, Peru, 1947. A South American contribution to the subject of psychosomatic medicine written by an earnest and capable student of the subject.

Teaching Psychotherapeutic Medicine, The Commonwealth Fund, N. Y., 1948. A transcript of the experimental course for general physicians sponsored by the Commonwealth Fund. Contains the principal teaching material of the course and much of the discussion.

PEDIATRICS

The Common Sense Book of Baby and Child Care, Benjamin Spock, Duell Sloan & Pearce, N. Y., 1947. One of the best books on this subject written by a skilled pediatrician trained in psychological medicine.

The Parents' Manual, Anna W. M. Wolf. Simon and Schuster, N. Y., 1941. A first-rate and readable manual on the emotional development of young children.

Some Special Problems of Children. A series of pamphlets for parents and teachers dealing with problems of aggression, destruction, bad language, thumb-sucking, enuresis, masturbation and fears. New York Committee on Mental Hygiene, 105 E. 22nd Street, New York 10, N. Y., 1947. Very useful for the pediatrician and general physician to give to parents.

Pediatrics and the Emotional Needs of the Child, The Commonwealth Fund, N. Y., 1948. Report of the Hershey conference of pediatricians, psychiatrists, and social workers, to further the practice and teaching of comprehensive pediatrics.

SOCIAL FACTOR

The Social Component in Medical Care; A Study of 100 Cases from the Presbyterian Hospital in N. Y., Janet Thornton, in collaboration with M. S. Knauth. Columbia University Press, N. Y., 1937. An intensive study of the social background of illness.

Psychosocial Medicine: A Study of the Sick Society, James L. Halliday, W. W. Norton & Co., New York, 1948. A novel presentation by a pioneer who has made many interesting and important contributions to psychosomatic medicine.

Patients Have Families, Henry B. Richardson, Commonwealth Fund, N. Y., 1945. A thoughtful consideration of health as affected by group and family relationships.

FOR THE PHYSICIAN AND LAYMAN

The Doctor's Job, Carl Binger, W. W. Norton & Co., N. Y., 1946. A well-written and interesting group of essays on many aspects of psychosocial medicine by a distinguished psychiatrist.

Mind and Body: Psychosomatic Medicine, Flanders Dunbar, Random House, N. Y., 1947. A popular presentation of the subject.

Emotional Problems of Living, O. Spurgeon English and Gerald H. J. Pearson, W. W Norton & Co., N. Y., 1945. A popular presentation of the emotional development and its aberrations.

Sexual Behavior in The Human Male, Alfred C. Kinsey, W. B. Saunders Co., Philadelphia, 1948. The first volume of a large scale study of human sexual behavior that throws new light on this fundamental aspect of living.

The Human Mind—An Outline of Psychiatry, Karl A. Menninger, 3rd Ed., Alfred A. Knopf, N. Y., 1947. A standard presentation of the subject for the intelligent layman.

Psychiatry in A Troubled World; Yesterday's War and Today's Challenge, William C. Menninger, The Macmillan Co., N. Y., 1948. A valuable work by the former army chief of psychiatry.

Emotional Maturity, Leon J. Saul, J. B. Lippincott & Co., Philadelphia, 1948. A well-written study of the concept of emotional maturity with extensive reference to wartime experience. Numerous, helpful case illustrations.

"What's the Score in a Case Like Mine?", War Department Pamphlet 20-35. A simple statement given to patients discharged from the service for psychoneurosis. Superintendent of Documents, Government Printing Office, Washington, D. C., 10 cents a copy. Useful in civil practice.

INDEX

"The Person in the Patent" P. 74